ENT

SECRETS

ENT SECRETS

FOURTH EDITION

MELISSA A. SCHOLES, MD
Assistant Professor
Department of Otolaryngology
University of Colorado
Aurora, CO

VIJAY R. RAMAKRISHNAN, MD
Assistant Professor
Department of Otolaryngology
Co-Director, CU Skull Base Program
University of Colorado
Aurora, CO

ELSEVIER

ELSEVIER

1600 John F. Kennedy Blvd.
Ste 1800
Philadelphia, PA 19103-2899

ENT SECRETS, FOURTH EDITION ISBN: 978-0-323-29856-8

Library of Congress Cataloging-in-Publication Data

ENT secrets / [edited by] Melissa A. Scholes, Vijay R. Ramakrishnan.—Fourth edition.
p. ; cm.—(Secrets series)
Includes bibliographical references and index.
ISBN 978-0-323-29856-8 (pbk. : alk. paper)
I. Scholes, Melissa A., editor. II. Ramakrishnan, Vijay R., editor. III. Series: Secrets series.
[DNLM: 1. Otorhinolaryngologic Diseases–Examination Questions. WV 18.2]
RF57
617.5′10076–dc23

2015009820

Senior Content Strategist: James Merritt
Content Development Specialist: Amy Meros
Publishing Services Manager: Hemamalini Rajendrababu
Senior Project Manager: Beula Christopher
Design Direction: Ryan Cook

Printed in United States

Last digit is the print number: 9 8 7 6 5 4 3 2 1

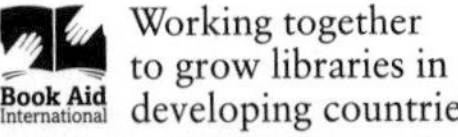

PREFACE

ENT Secrets has been a learning tool used by medical students, residents, and health care providers since the first edition, published in 1996 by Bruce Jafek and Anne Stark. Dr. Jafek went on to edit two subsequent editions with the goal of sharing knowledge and insight in the field of otolaryngology. Our newest edition aims to provide updates on that knowledge as well as introduce new concepts and technologies in the ever-changing field of otolaryngology. We were fortunate to be residents under Dr. Jafek, who loved teaching and training students of all types. We want to carry on that tradition with this latest edition of *ENT Secrets*. This has been possible with the support of the University of Colorado Otolaryngology Department faculty, alumni, and residents, and other contributors of this book. We sincerely thank them.

CONTRIBUTORS

Gregory C. Allen, MD, FACS, FAAP
Associate Professor
Departments of Otolaryngology—Head and Neck Surgery and Pediatrics
University of Colorado School of Medicine;
Department of Pediatric Otolaryngology
Children's Hospital Colorado
Aurora, CO

Jeremiah A. Alt, MD, PhD
Sinus and Skull Base Surgery Program
Division of Otolaryngology
University of Utah
Salt Lake City, UT

Marcelo B. Antunes, MD
Private Practice
Northwest Facial Aesthetic Center
Marietta, GA

Ronald Balkissoon, MD
Division of Pulmonology
National Jewish Health
Denver, CO

Renee Banakis Hartl, MD, AuD
Department of Otolaryngology
University of Colorado School of Medicine
Aurora, CO

Henry P. Barham, MD
Department of Otolaryngology—Head and Neck Surgery
University of Colorado
Aurora, CO

Kenneth T. Bellian, MD, MBA
Assistant Professor
Department of Otolaryngology—Head and Neck Surgery
University of Colorado;
Chief of Clinical Operations
Denver Health Medical Center
Denver, CO

Carly Bergey, MA, CCC-SLP
CCC-SLP- Rehabilitation
National Jewish Health
Denver, CO

Daniel W. Bowles, MD
Assistant Professor
Department of Medicine
University of Colorado School of Medicine
Aurora, CO

Allison Brower, AuD, MS
Department of Audiology
University of Colorado Hospital
Aurora, CO

Mariah Brown, MD
Assistant Professor
Department of Dermatology—Mohs Surgery
University of Colorado School of Medicine
Aurora, CO

Cristina Cabrera-Muffly, MD, FACS
Assistant Professor
Department of Otolaryngology
University of Colorado School of Medicine
Aurora, CO

Thomas L. Carroll, MD
Director
Voice Program
Brigham and Women's Hospital;
Division of Otolaryngology
Harvard Medical School
Boston, MA

Justin Casey, MD
Department of Otolaryngology—Head and Neck Surgery
University of Colorado Hospital
Aurora, CO

Stephen P. Cass, MD
Professor
Department of Otolaryngology
University of Colorado Denver School of Medicine
Aurora, CO

Jeffrey Chain, MD
Private Practice
Comprehensive ENT, Head and Neck Surgery
Denver, CO

Kenny H. Chan, MD
Department of Otolaryngology
University of Colorado School of Medicine;
Department of Pediatric Otolaryngology
Children's Hospital Colorado
Aurora, CO

Henry H. Chen, MD, MBA
Department of Otolaryngology
Facial Plastic and Reconstructive Surgery
Cedars-Sinai Medical Center
Los Angeles, CA

Tendy Chiang, MD
Department of Otolaryngology—Head and Neck Surgery
The Ohio State University College of Medicine;
Department of Pediatric Otolaryngology—Head and Neck Surgery
Nationwide Children's Hospital
Columbus, OH

Matthew S. Clary, MD
Department of Otolaryngology
University of Colorado School of Medicine
Aurora, CO

Stacy Claycomb, AuD
University of Colorado Hospital
Aurora, CO

Alexander Connelly, MD
University of Colorado School of Medicine
Aurora, CO

Mark S. Courey, MD
Department of Otolaryngology—Head and Neck Surgery
Division of Laryngology
University of California, San Francisco
San Francisco, CA

Brett W. Davies, MD, MS
Oculoplastic and Orbital Surgery
San Antonio Military Medical Center/Wilford Hall
San Antonio, TX

Allison M. Dobbie, MD
Department of Otolaryngology
University of Colorado School of Medicine;
Department of Pediatric Otolaryngology
Children's Hospital Colorado
Aurora, CO

Vikram D. Durairaj, MD, FACS
Oculoplastic and Orbital Surgery
Director
ASOPRS Fellowship
Texas Oculoplastic Consultants
Austin, TX

Marcia Eustaquio, MD
Assistant Professor
Department of Otolaryngology—Head and Neck Surgery
Denver Health Medical Center
University of Colorado Denver
Denver, CO

Vincent Eusterman, MD, DDS
Associate Professor
University of Colorado School of Medicine;
Director
Otolaryngology—Head and Neck Surgery
Denver Health Medical Center
Denver, CO

Geoffrey R. Ferril, MD
Resident Physician
Department of Otolaryngology—Head and Neck Surgery
Facial Plastic and Reconstructive Surgery
University of Colorado School of Medicine
Aurora, CO

Lindsay K. Finkas, MD
National Jewish Health;
Department of Allergy/Immunology
University of Colorado Denver
Denver, CO

Carol A. Foster, MD
Departments of Otolaryngology, Audiology, and Rehabilitative Medicine
University of Colorado Denver School of Medicine
Aurora, CO

Norman R. Friedman, MD
Department of Otolaryngology
University of Colorado School of Medicine;
Department of Pediatric Otolaryngology
Children's Hospital Colorado
Aurora, CO

Sandra Abbott Gabbard, PhD
Associate Professor
Department of Pediatrics
Department of Speech, Language, Hearing Sciences
University of Colorado;
President/CEO
Marion Downs Center
Denver, CO

Anne E. Getz, MD
Department of Otolaryngology—Head and Neck Surgery
University of Colorado
Denver, CO

Sarah A. Gitomer, MD
Baylor College of Medicine
Bobby R. Alford Department of Otolaryngology—Head and Neck Surgery
Houston, TX

John C. Goddard, MD
Associate
House Ear Clinic;
Clinical Instructor
University of Southern California
Los Angeles, CA

Julie A. Goddard, MD, FACS
Department of Otolaryngology—Head and Neck Surgery
University of California, Irvine
Orange, CA

Elizabeth A. Gould, BA
Department of Otolaryngology
University of Colorado
Aurora, CO

Leah J. Hauser, MD
Department of Otolaryngology—Head and Neck Surgery
University of Colorado
Aurora, CO

Herman Jenkins, MD
Department of Otolaryngology
University of Colorado School of Medicine
Aurora, CO

Kristina L. Johnston, MA, CCC-SLP
CCC-SLP-Rehabilitation
National Jewish Health
Denver, CO

Sana D. Karam, MD, PhD
Department of Radiation Oncology
University of Denver Colorado
Aurora, CO

Rohit K. Katial, MD, FAAAAI, FACP
Professor of Medicine
Program Director, Allergy/Immunology
Director
Weinberg Clinical Research Unit
Denver, CO

Peggy E. Kelley, MD
Department of Otolaryngology
University of Colorado School of Medicine;
Department of Pediatric Otolaryngology
Children's Hospital Colorado
Aurora, CO

Todd T. Kingdom, MD
Professor and Vice Chair
Department of Otolaryngology—Head and Neck Surgery
University of Colorado School of Medicine
Aurora, CO

Ted H. Leem, MD, MS
Department of Otolaryngology
University of Colorado School of Medicine
Aurora, CO

J. Eric Lupo, MD, MS
Clinical Fellow
House Ear Clinic
Los Angeles, CA

Jon Mallen-St. Clair, MD, PhD
Department of Otolaryngology—Head and Neck Surgery
University of California, Los Angeles
Los Angeles, CA

Scott Mann, MD
Assistant Professor
Department of Otolaryngology
University of Colorado Denver School of Medicine
Aurora, CO

Jameson K. Mattingly, MD
Department of Otolaryngology
University of Colorado School of Medicine;
Department of Pediatric Otolaryngology
Children's Hospital Colorado
Aurora, CO

Brook K. McConnell, MD
Department of Otolaryngology
University of Colorado School of Medicine;
Department of Pediatric Otolaryngology
Children's Hospital Colorado
Aurora, CO

Jessica D. McDermott, MD
Fellow
Division of Medical Oncology
University of Colorado School of Medicine
Aurora, CO

Benjamin Milam, MD
Resident Physician
Department of Otolaryngology—Head and Neck Surgery
University of Colorado
Aurora, CO

David M. Mirsky, MD
Pediatric Neuroradiologist
Children's Hospital Colorado;
Assistant Professor of Radiology
University of Colorado
Aurora, CO

Paul Montero, MD
Division of Gastrointestinal, Tumor, and Endocrine Surgery
University of Colorado Hospital
Aurora, CO

Pamela A. Mudd, MD
Assistant Professor
Pediatric Otolaryngology
Children's National Medical Center
Washington, DC

Vignesh Narayanan, MD
Division of Medical Oncology
University of Colorado School of Medicine
Denver, CO

Stephen S. Newton, MD
Assistant Professor of Otolaryngology
University of Colorado;
Pediatric Otolaryngologist
Children's Hospital of Colorado
Colorado Springs, CO

Sarah J. Novis, MD
Department of Otolaryngology—Head and Neck Surgery
University of Michigan
Ann Arbor, MI

Matthew Old, MD, FACS
Assistant Professor
Department of Otolaryngology—Head and Neck Surgery
The James Cancer Hospital and Solove Research Institute
Wexner Medical Center at The Ohio State University
Columbus, OH

Richard R. Orlandi, MD
Sinus and Skull Base Surgery Program
Division of Otolaryngology
University of Utah
Salt Lake City, UT

Anju K. Patel, MD
Otolaryngology Resident
Department of Otolaryngology—Head and Neck Surgery
Tufts Medical Center
Boston, MA

Erik Peltz, DO
Division of Trauma and Acute Care Surgery
University of Colorado Hospital
Aurora, CO

Daniel A. Pollyea, MD, MS
Division of Hematology
University of Colorado School of Medicine
Denver, CO

Kavitha K. Prabaker, MD
Instructor
Department of Internal Medicine
Division of Infectious Diseases
University of Colorado School of Medicine
Aurora, CO

Jeremy D. Prager, MD
Department of Otolaryngology
University of Colorado School of Medicine;
Department of Pediatric Otolaryngology
Children's Hospital Colorado
Aurora, CO

Craig Quattlebaum, MD
Resident Physician
University of Colorado
Aurora, CO

Jeevan B. Ramakrishnan, MD
Raleigh-Capitol Ear, Nose, and Throat, P.A.
Raleigh, NC

Brianne Barnett Roby, MD
Department of Pediatric ENT and Facial Plastic Surgery
Children's Hospitals and Clinics of Minnesota
St. Paul, MN;
Associate Professor
Department of Otolarynology
University of Minnesota
Minneapolis, MN

Victor I. Scapa, MD
Department of Otolaryngology—Head and Neck Surgery
Group Health Permanente
Seattle, WA

Ameer T. Shah, MD
Department of Otolaryngology—Head and Neck Surgery
Tufts Medical Center
Boston, MA

Kaylee Skidmore, MA, CCC-SLP
Speech Language Pathologist
Department of Rehabilitation
University of Colorado Hospital
Aurora, CO

Franki Lambert Smith, MD
Clinical Associate
Dermatology
Mayo Clinic Health System-Franciscan Healthcare
La Crosse, WI

Mofiyinfolu Sokoya, MD
Resident
Department of Otolaryngology—Head and Neck Surgery
Facial Plastic and Reconstructive Surgery
University of Colorado School of Medicine
Aurora, CO

John Song, MD
Associate Professor
Department of Otolaryngology
University of Colorado School of Medicine
Aurora, CO

Sven-Olrik Streubel, MD, MBA
Department of Otolaryngology
University of Colorado School of Medicine;
Department of Pediatric Otolaryngology
Children's Hospital Colorado
Aurora, CO

Jeffrey D. Suh, MD
Assistant Professor
Rhinology and Skull Base Surgery
Department of Head and Neck Surgery
David Geffen School of Medicine at UCLA
Los Angeles, CA

Masayoshi Takashima, MD
Director
Sinus Center at BCM;
Associate Professor
Bobby R. Alford Department of Otolaryngology—Head and Neck Surgery
Baylor College of Medicine
Houston, TX

Adam M. Terella, MD
Assistant Professor
Department of Otolaryngology—Head and Neck Surgery
Facial Plastic and Reconstructive Surgery
University of Colorado School of Medicine
Aurora, CO

Lisa Treviso-Jones, MS, CCC-SLP
Speech Language Pathologist
Department of Rehabilitation
University of Colorado Hospital
Aurora, CO

Kristin Uhler, PhD
University of Colorado Denver School of Medicine
Aurora, CO

Craig R. Villari, MD
Department of Otolaryngology—Head and Neck Surgery
Division of Laryngology
University of California, San Francisco
San Francisco, CA

Sean X. Wang, MD
Department of Otolaryngology—Head and Neck Surgery
Division of Laryngology
University of California, San Francisco
San Francisco, CA

Taylor M. Washburn, MD
Instructor
Division of Infectious Disease
University of Colorado Denver
Denver, CO

Timothy V. Waxweiler, MD
Department of Radiation Oncology
University of Denver Colorado
Aurora, CO

Edwin F. Williams, III, MD
Department of Otolaryngology
Albany Medical Center
Albany, NY;
Department of Facial Plastic and Reconstructive Surgery
Williams Center Plastic Surgery Specialists
Latham, NY

Todd M. Wine, MD
Children's Hospital of Colorado
University of Colorado Anschutz Medical Campus
Aurora, CO

Andrew A. Winkler, MD
Associate Professor
Department of Otolaryngology;
Director
Division of Facial Plastic and Reconstructive Surgery
University of Colorado Denver School of Medicine
Aurora, CO

Justin M. Wudel, MD
Renew Facial Plastic Surgery
Edina, MN

William C. Yao, MD
Assistant Professor
Department of Otorhinolaryngology—Head and Neck Surgery
University of Texas Medical School at Houston
Houston, TX

Patricia J. Yoon, MD
Department of Otolaryngology—Head and Neck Surgery
University of Colorado School of Medicine;
Department of Pediatric Otolaryngology
Children's Hospital Colorado
Aurora, CO

CONTENTS

VI Facial Plastic Surgery, Reconstruction and Trauma

VII Laryngology and Swallowing Disorders

TOP 100 EXAMINATION PEARLS

1. CT scan is best for looking at temporal bone fractures and lesions; MRI (of the internal auditory canal with contrast) is the best test for evaluation of acoustic neuromas.
2. The best imaging to evaluate thyroid nodules is ultrasound.
3. Malignant otitis externa usually occurs in an immunocompromised person with a disease such as diabetes. The most common pathogen is *Pseudomonas aeruginosa.*
4. Ludwig's angina is an odontogenic infection of the submental and submandibular spaces, causing progressive swelling of the floor of the mouth and upper airway obstruction.
5. The diagnosis of invasive fungal sinusitis relies on histopathologic findings of fungal invasion into submucosal tissues and vessels with associated necrosis.
6. Infections of the parapharyngeal, prevertebral, and retropharyngeal space can extend into the "danger space," allowing unrestricted spread of infection into the mediastinum.
7. The classic presentation of peritonsillar abscess includes trismus, uvular deviation, muffled voice, and soft palatal edema
8. Elevated risk factors for OSA:
   a. Age greater than 65 years
   b. Body mass index (BMI) greater than 30kg/m^2
   c. Postmenopausal female
   d. African American or Asian race
   e. Male gender
   f. Neck circumference greater than 17″ in men and 16″ in women
9. Mucor species demonstrate nonseptate, wide-angled branching hyphae on histology in contrast to *Aspergillus* species, which display septate hyphae with 45-degree branching angles.
10. Tension-type headache is the most common type of headache/facial pain.
11. First-line treatment of persistent idiopathic facial pain is tricyclic antidepressants.
12. Fungiform, foliate, circumvallate, and filiform are the four type of papillae on the tongue. Filiform papillae do not actually contain taste buds.
13. The second branchial cleft is the most common branchial cleft to develop an anomaly.
14. Depth of invasion is the most important prognostic factor in melanoma.
15. At least one cricoarytenoid joint must be preserved in conservation laryngeal surgery.
16. Hypopharyngeal cancer is notable for frequent submucosal spread and carries a worse prognosis than cancer of the larynx.
17. The most common benign salivary gland tumor is pleomorphic adenoma. The most common malignant salivary gland tumor is mucoepidermoid carcinoma.
18. Papillary carcinoma is the most common malignancy of the thyroid. Follicular adenomas are the most common neoplasms of the thyroid.
19. Factors such as tumor site, stage, thickness, presence of perineural and angiolymphatic invasion, and tumor differentiation can all increase the risk of regional lymphatic involvement.

20. Carotid body tumors are the most common head and neck paragangliomas, and present as a pulsatile neck mass that has characteristic CT, MRI, or angiography findings of splaying of the external and internal carotids (Lyre's sign).
21. A teenage male with unilateral nasal obstruction, epistaxis, and a bluish mass filling the nasal cavity is the typical presentation of a juvenile nasopharyngeal angiofibroma.
22. The classic radiographic findings for JNA are expansion of the PPF on axial view (Holman-Miller sign), widening of the sphenopalatine and vidian foramina, and bony destruction of the pterygoid process.
23. Adenocarcinoma of the paranasal sinuses is associated with exposure to wood and leather dust. Squamous cell carcinoma of the paranasal sinuses is associated with exposure to chromium, nickel, mustard gas, and aflatoxin.
24. Ohngren's line is an imaginary line drawn from the medial canthus to the angle of the mandible. Maxillary sinus tumors that are located above this line on presentation are associated with a poorer prognosis.
25. CN III, IV, V1, V2, VI, internal carotid artery, and venous channels are present in the cavernous sinus. CN VI is the most medial nerve in the cavernous sinus, and the most commonly injured.
26. CSF production is approximately 20 ml/hr.
27. Viruses are usually responsible for the symptoms in acute rhinosinusitis, not bacteria.
28. Know the Chandler classification for orbital infection: I, preseptal cellulitis; II, orbital cellulitis; III, subperiosteal abscess; IV, orbital abscess; V, cavernous sinus thrombosis.
29. The major nasal tip support mechanisms include the attachments between the septum, lower lateral cartilages, and upper lateral cartilages. The minor tip support mechanisms include the interdomal ligament, the dorsal septum, the membranous septum, the sesamoid complex, the skin and subcutaneous tissue of the nasal tip, and the maxillary spine.
30. How is the nose anomalous in a patient with unilateral cleft lip/palate?
    The ipsilateral lower lateral cartilage is displaced inferiorly, posteriorly, and laterally. The nasal tip, caudal septum, and columella are displaced toward the noncleft side. The bony septum is deviated toward the cleft side.
31. Septal perforation and saddle nose deformity are the most common complications of an untreated septal hematoma.
32. Toxic shock syndrome is a rare complication of *S. aureus* infection characterized by high fever, rash, hypotension, vomiting, diarrhea, and multiorgan failure. Treatment consists of removal of the nasal packing, IV antibiotics, and supportive/resuscitative care.
33. Know the Keros classification of olfactory fossa depth (Class I: 1 to 3 mm, Class II: 4 to 7 mm, Class III: 8 mm and greater)
34. The lateral lamella of cribriform is the most common site of iatrogenic CSF leak during functional endoscopic sinus surgery (FESS).
35. Spontaneous CSF leaks are likely associated with idiopathic intracranial hypertension.
36. Thyroid eye disease results from autoimmune inflammation of muscle and fat, where the TSH receptor is the autoantigen.
37. The cochlea is tonotopic, meaning specific areas of the cochlea are stimulated by specific tone frequencies. The physical properties of the cochlear basilar membrane (thick, stiff, narrow base and thin, flexible, wide apex) are responsible for its tonotopic properties.
38. The severity of cochlear deformities depends significantly on the gestational age at growth arrest or disruption.

39. Top causes of CHL
    1. Cerumen impaction
    2. Otitis media with effusion (most common cause in children)
    3. Tympanic membrane perforation
    4. Otosclerosis
40. Top causes of SNHL
    1. Presbycusis
    2. Noise exposure
    3. Hereditary
41. Most common ototoxic medications
    1. Aminoglycosides
    2. Cisplatin
    3. Loop diuretics
    4. Salicylates
42. The most common radiographic finding in pediatric SNHL is enlarged vestibular aqueduct.
43. Pure-tone average is the average air conduction hearing threshold at the frequencies associated with speech (500, 1000, and 2000 Hz).
44. Masking is the simultaneous presentation of sound to the nontest ear (to "mask" it) while actually testing the other ear with the stimulus.
45. Peripheral nystagmus becomes faster and more apparent when the patient gazes in the direction of the fast phase: A right-beating nystagmus worsens on right gaze, for example. This is called Alexander's Law.
46. A conventional hearing aid consists of four main components: microphone, amplifier, receiver, and battery.
47. Acoustic feedback occurs when amplified sound leaks out of the receiver back into the microphone.
48. The most common bacterial pathogens contributing to acute otitis media are *Streptococcus pneumoniae* (35% to 40%), *Haemophilus influenza* (30% to 35%), and *Moraxella catarrhalis* (15% to 25%).
49. Amoxicillin remains the first-line therapy for acute otitis media as approximately 80% of bacterial isolates remain susceptible.
50. For a diagnosis of otitis media, a middle ear effusion must be present and confirmed by pneumatic otoscopy or tympanometry.
51. A canal wall down mastoidectomy is indicated when there is a semicircular canal fistula or posterior canal wall damage due to cholesteatoma, a sclerotic mastoid prevents adequate visualization with a wall up mastoidectomy, or the patient is unable to follow up or undergo additional surgeries for proper monitoring of recurrent cholesteatoma.
52. The most common presentation of otosclerosis is progressive conductive hearing loss, although it can rarely present with sensorineural hearing loss, and many patients will have a positive family history.
53. Cholesteatomas are usually classified into congenital, primary acquired, and secondary acquired types.
54. Passive upper eyelid closure can occur by relaxation of the levator palpebrae muscle (innervated by the oculomotor nerve), so upper eyelid motion is not always indicative of an intact facial nerve.
55. The labyrinthine segment of the facial nerve is the narrowest portion of the fallopian canal, making it the area most susceptible to entrapment neuropathy during nerve swelling.

56. Superior semicircular canal dehiscence can mimic other otologic diseases because it can present with conductive hearing loss similar to otosclerosis, ear fullness and autophony similar to a patulous Eustachian tube, and vertigo similar to Ménière's disease.
57. The Hitzelberger sign is numbness of the medial, posterior, or superior external auditory canal caused by an acoustic neuroma compressing CN VII.
58. Periorbital and mastoid ecchymoses following basal skull fractures are known as "raccoon eyes" and "Battle's sign," respectively.
59. CSF leak is common in temporal bone fractures and usually stops within 7 days.
60. The pediatric airway is significantly smaller than the adult airway; inflammation and narrowing of the airway can be far more clinically significant in an infant than a similar degree of edema in an adult.
61. Bilateral choanal atresia classically presents with respiratory distress and cyanosis at birth that is relieved with crying.
62. Laryngomalacia is the most common cause of stridor in the infant. Unilateral vocal cord paralysis in the pediatric population is most commonly iatrogenic in etiology and represents the second most common cause of stridor.
63. The most common cause of subglottic stenosis is iatrogenic scarring related to endotracheal intubation.
64. Infantile hemangiomas are the most common tumors of infancy. The majority are found within the head and neck.
65. A "beard" distribution of hemangioma in a stridulous child should raise suspicion for subglottic hemangioma.
66. GLUT-1 positivity distinguishes hemangiomas from vascular malformations.
67. Propranolol is the first-line treatment for infantile hemangioma.
68. A submucous cleft palate is associated with a higher incidence of postadenoidectomy VPI.
69. If mononucleosis is suspected, amoxicillin should be avoided because it may cause a salmon-colored rash.
70. Branchial cleft anomalies track deep to the structures of their own arch and superficial to the structures of the subsequent arch.
71. The differential for pediatic midline nasal mass includes glioma, dermoid, and encephalocele. Imaging should always be obtained prior to excision for diagnosis and to rule out intracranial extension.
72. Cleft lip and palate most commonly occur together (50%). Cleft palate alone occurs in 35%, and cleft lip alone in 15%. Left unilateral cleft lip and palate is the most common.
73. The most common indication for tonsillectomy is sleep disordered breathing, followed by recurrent tonsillitis.
74. The majority of facial mimetic muscles are "superficially situated" and receive facial nerve innervation from their deep surface.
75. Nasal projection refers to how far the tip projects from the face. Nasal rotation refers to movement of the tip along an arc from the external auditory canal.
76. The interval nasal valve is comprised of the upper lateral cartilage, nasal septum, and nasal floor. The Cottle maneuver helps to diagnose internal nasal valve collapse.

77. A "pollybeak" deformity is a complication of rhinoplasty whereby supratip fullness results in the appearance of a parrot's beak; this can be the result of loss of tip support or supratip scar tissue.

78. The layers of the eyelid from anterior to posterior are the skin, orbicularis oculi, orbital septum, preaponeurotic fat, levator aponeurosis, Müller's muscle, and conjunctiva.

79. The Baker-Gordon formula's (phenol 88%, croton oil, septisol, and distilled water) depth of penetration is more dependent on the croton oil than the concentration of phenol.

80. Phenol chemical peels are associated with cardiac toxicity, and should be applied to individual facial subunits in 15-minute intervals.

81. The most common complication from facelift surgery is hematoma. It occurs in up to 10% of cases and is more common in men.

82. The most commonly injured nerve in facelift surgery is the great auricular nerve. The most commonly injured motor nerve in facelift surgery is the marginal mandibular.

83. Botulinum toxin works at the presynaptic neuromuscular junction by preventing acetylcholine release, leading to temporary muscle paralysis.

84. Utilization of a full-thickness skin graft, when possible, will limit graft contraction, and usually result in an improved texture and color match.

85. An early clinical finding of optic nerve injury in the traumatized eye is loss of red color vision.

86. The most common facial bone fractured is the nasal bone.

87. The most common site of mandible fracture is at the angle.

88. The posterior cricoarytenoid muscle is the only abductor muscle of the true vocal folds.

89. The cricothyroid muscle is the only intrinsic laryngeal muscle not innervated by the recurrent laryngeal nerve; it is innervated by the superior laryngeal nerve. The interarytenoid muscle is the only intrinsic laryngeal muscle with bilateral innervation.

90. Recurrent respiratory papillomatosis (RRP) is primarily caused by HPV types 6 and 11.

91. The primary management for vocal fold nodules is voice therapy.

92. Laryngeal EMG is a tool to measure motor unit recruitment. When muscle is denervated, fibrillation potentials and positive waves are seen, whereas polyphasic motor units are seen when reinnervation occurs.

93. What is the management for an airway fire?
    1. Turn off the flow of O_2
    2. Douse fire with saline
    3. Remove damaged tube
    4. Reintubate as atraumatically as possible
    5. Administer IV steroids and antibiotics
    6. Bronchoscopy before leaving the OR to remove any charred tissue or other debris, and evaluate extent of airway injury
    7. Delayed extubation with repeat endoscopic airway examinations

94. Patients with hearing loss and an enlarged vestibular aqueduct or Mondini dysplasia on imaging should be tested for mutations in *SLC26A4,* which is associated with Pendred syndrome.

95. The key to a Sistrunk procedure is not just resecting the central portion of the hyoid bone, but resecting tongue musculature between the hyoid bone and foramen cecum in the tongue.

96. Antibiotics associated with increased risk of *C. difficile* colitis are clindamycin, fluoroquinolones, cephalosporins, and carbapenems. Macrolides, penicillins, and sulfonamides are less frequently associated.

97. Be able to define and differentiate radical, modified radical, and selective or functional neck dissections.
98. Sinus disease can spread via vascular channels into the intracranial cavity and orbit.
99. If a patient requires posterior nasal packing, the patient should be admitted to the hospital and placed on telemetry and continuous pulse oximetry.
100. Most scars improve in appearance without revision 1 to 3 years after the inciting event. Patients should be counseled to wait at least 6 to 12 months before undergoing a scar revision surgery, unless there are obvious scar characteristics that aren't expected to improve.

I

GENERAL

GENERAL ANATOMY AND EMBRYOLOGY WITH RADIOLOGY CORRELATES

CHAPTER 1

Cristina Cabrera-Muffly, MD, FACS

KEY POINTS

1. Eight branches of the external carotid artery:
   - Superior thyroid
   - Ascending pharyngeal
   - Lingual
   - Facial
   - Occipital
   - Posterior auricular
   - Maxillary
   - Superficial temporal
2. Layers of fascia in the neck:
   - Superficial cervical fascia
   - Superficial layer of deep cervical fascia
   - Middle layer of deep cervical fascia
   - Deep layer of deep cervical fascia
3. Characteristics of malignant lymph nodes on neck CT with contrast:
   - Size >1–1.5 cm
   - Round shape
   - Necrotic center
   - Ill-defined margins
4. Facial nerve landmarks:
   - Tragal pointer
   - Tympanomastoid suture line
   - Insertion of the posterior belly of digastric muscle onto the mastoid
5. Best imaging study by region:
   - Cerebellopontine angle—MRI with contrast
   - Neck and salivary glands—CT with contrast or MRI with contrast
   - Sinus—CT without contrast
   - Temporal bone—CT without contrast
   - Thyroid—Ultrasound

Pearls

1. CT scan is better for looking at temporal bone masses and lesions, but MRI (of the internal auditory canal with contrast) is the best test for evaluation of acoustic neuromas.
2. When you suspect a temporal bone fracture, the best test is a fine cut CT temporal bones without contrast.
3. On T1 MRI, if the nasal turbinates light up, that means the study has contrast.
4. MRI scans commonly over call sinus disease. The most appropriate study to determine chronic sinus disease is CT without contrast (Figure 1-1).
5. The best imaging to evaluate thyroid nodules is ultrasound.

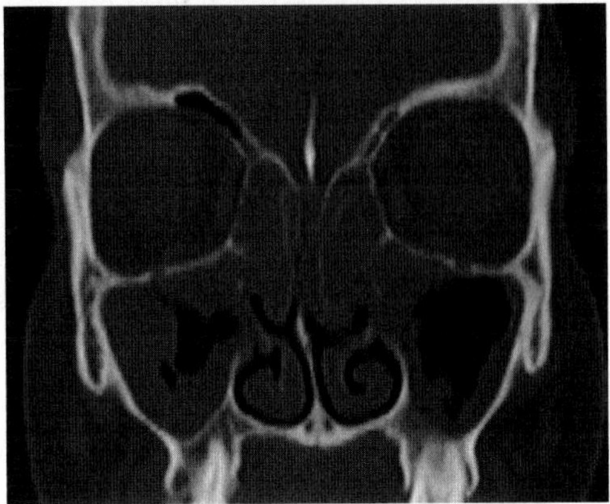

Figure 1-1. Chronic sinusitis with nasal polyposis on CT scan.

QUESTIONS

1. **When do the sinuses develop?**
   The maxillary sinus is the first to develop in utero. After birth, this sinus enlarges in two stages, once at age three and then again between ages 7 and 12. Neonates have three to four ethmoid cells at birth, which multiply to become ten to fifteen cells by the age of 12. The sphenoid sinus begins pneumatization at 3 years of age, while the frontal sinus is the last to develop at about age 5. The sphenoid and frontal sinuses do not reach adult size until the teenage years.

2. **What is the difference between agger nasi, Onodi, and Haller ethmoid cells?**
   The agger nasi cell is the most anterior of the ethmoid cells. It is found anterior and superior to the attachment of the middle turbinate to the lateral wall. The Onodi cell is an ethmoid cell that pneumatizes lateral or posterior to the anterior wall of the sphenoid. This cell can be adjacent to the optic nerve or carotid artery, so it is important to recognize this variation during sinus surgery. A Haller cell forms when the ethmoid pneumatizes into the medial and inferior orbital walls. If this cell is large, it can cause obstruction of the maxillary ostium.

3. **Name the branches of the internal carotid artery in the neck.**
   Trick question! The internal carotid artery does not branch in the neck.

4. **Name the eight branches of the external carotid artery in the neck.**
   From proximal to distal, the branches are: the superior thyroid, ascending pharyngeal, lingual, facial, occipital, posterior auricular, maxillary, and superficial temporal arteries.

5. **Name the four types of tongue papillae. Where are they located?**
   The four types are circumvallate, fungiform, foliate, and filiform papillae. The circumvallate are located at the junction of the anterior two thirds and posterior one third of the tongue in a V shape. Fungiform papillae are found at the tip and lateral edges of the anterior two thirds of the tongue. Foliate papillae are found at the posterolateral base of tongue. Filiform papillae are found all over the tongue, and do not participate in taste sensation.

6. **Describe the landmarks used to find the facial nerve during parotid surgery.**
   The typical landmarks used to find the facial nerve during parotid surgery are the tragal pointer, the tympanomastoid suture line, and the posterior digastric muscle. The tragal pointer refers to the tragus cartilage, which "points" to the location of the nerve one centimeter anterior, inferior, and deep to the cartilage. Another method of identification is to follow the tympanomastoid suture line inferiorly to its drop-off point. Six to eight millimeters medial to this point, the facial nerve can be found passing through the stylomastoid foramen. Finally, the nerve can be located just medial to the insertion of the posterior belly of the digastric on the mastoid.

7. **Name each of the major salivary glands and describe the types of saliva produced by each.**
There are three paired major salivary glands: the parotid, submandibular, and sublingual glands. Each gland has acinar cells that produce either serous or mucinous solution. The parotid glands produce mostly serous saliva. The sublingual glands produce mostly mucinous saliva, and the submandibular glands produce a mixture of the two.

8. **How do the salivary glands develop embryologically?**
The major salivary glands develop from the first pharyngeal pouch. The glands form during weeks 4 to 9 of gestation. The parotids form by an ectodermal outpouching into the surrounding mesenchyme. The submandibular and sublingual glands form from endoderm growing either into the submandibular triangle or the floor of the mouth (sublingual).

9. **Describe the embryology of the parathyroid glands.**
The superior parathyroid glands develop from the fourth dorsal branchial pouch, whereas the inferior parathyroid glands develop from the third dorsal branchial pouch. This apparent inversion occurs because the fourth branchial pouch does not migrate during development, but the third branchial pouch descends with the thymus to lie inferior to the fourth pouch. Ectopic parathyroid tissue is present in up to 20% of patients.

10. **Describe the fascial planes of the neck.**
The neck fascia has two main layers, the superficial and deep cervical fascia. The superficial cervical fascia envelops the platysma, muscles of facial expression, and SMAS. The deep cervical fascia splits into three parts, the superficial, middle, and deep layers. The superficial layer of the deep cervical fascia envelops the trapezius, sternocleidomastoid, and masseter muscles as well as the parotid and submandibular glands. The middle layer of the deep cervical fascia contains the strap muscles as well as the trachea, esophagus, thyroid, pharynx, and larynx. The deep layer of the deep cervical fascia envelops the cervical vertebrae and paraspinal muscles. All three layers of the deep cervical fascia come together to form the carotid sheath, enveloping the carotid artery, jugular vein, and vagus nerve (Figure 1-2).

11. **Describe the lymph node levels of the neck used for staging head and neck cancer.**
The neck is divided into six areas for the purposes of staging head and neck cancer. The location of the primary tumor determines the likelihood of spread to each particular area. Level I includes the

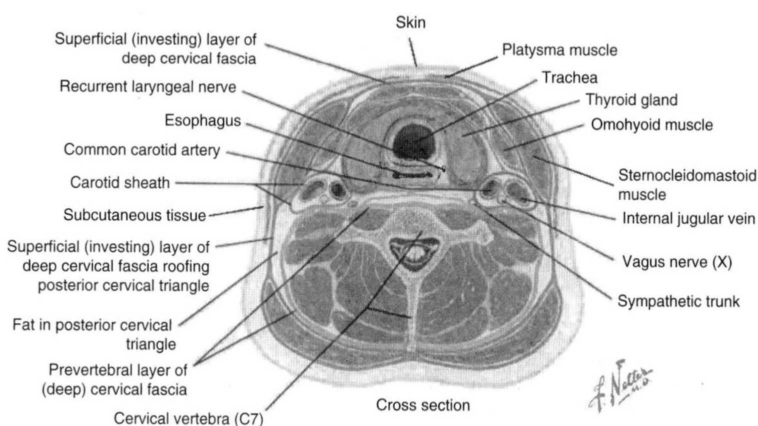

Figure 1-2. Fascial layers of the neck. *(From Goldstone: Netter's Surgical Anatomy and Approaches, 389–398 © 2014 by Saunders, an imprint of Elsevier Inc.)*

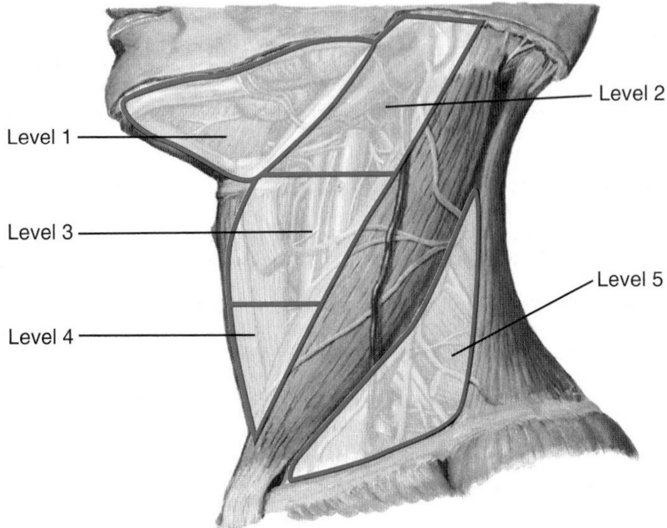

Figure 1-3. Lymph node levels of the neck, commonly used during head and neck cancer staging. *(From Goldstone: Netter's Surgical Anatomy and Approaches, 389–398, © 2014 by Saunders, an imprint of Elsevier Inc.)*

submandibular and submental triangles. Levels II through IV lie along the carotid sheath superiorly to inferiorly. The boundary between levels II and III is the hyoid bone. The boundary between levels III and IV is the cricoid cartilage. Level V encompasses the posterior triangle, while level VI is the central compartment (Figure 1-3).

12. **Describe the branchial arch derivatives as they relate to the ear.**
The first branchial arch contributes Meckel's cartilage, which includes the malleus head and neck, incus body and short process, and anterior malleal ligament. It also contributes the tensor tympani and the first three hillocks of His. The second branchial arch contributes Reichert's cartilage, which includes the manubrium of the malleus, the long process and lenticular process of the incus, and most of the stapes. It also contributes the last three hillocks of His. The first branchial pouch contributes the eustachian tube, mastoid air cells, and inner layer of the tympanic membrane. The first branchial cleft contributes the external auditory canal and outer layer of the tympanic membrane.

13. **Describe the branchial arch derivatives as they relate to the larynx.**
The third branchial arch contributes the stylopharyngeus muscle which elevates the larynx. The fourth branchial arch contributes thyroid and cuneiform cartilage, the superior laryngeal nerve, and cricothyroid muscle. The fifth and sixth branchial arches contribute the cricoid, arytenoid, and corniculate cartilages, recurrent laryngeal nerve, and all the intrinsic laryngeal muscles (except the cricothyroid).

14. **Name the 12 cranial nerves and their functions.**
I: Olfactory—olfaction
II: Optic—vision
III: Oculomotor—motor to all eye muscles except superior oblique and lateral rectus muscles; parasympathetic to ciliary muscle (accommodation) and sphincter pupillae muscle (pupil constriction)
IV: Trochlear—motor to superior oblique muscle
V: Trigeminal—sensation from the face; motor to muscles of mastication, tensor tympani, tensor veli palatine, mylohyoid, and anterior digastric muscles

VI: Abducens—motor to lateral rectus muscle
VII: Facial—motor to the muscles of facial expression, stapedial, external auricular, occipitofrontalis, stylohyoid, and posterior digastric muscles; parasympathetics to lacrimal gland (lacrimation), submandibular and sublingual glands (salivation); taste to anterior two thirds of the tongue; sensation from the concha, postauricular skin, wall of the EAC, and part of the tympanic membrane
VIII: Vestibulocochlear—balance and hearing
IX: Glossopharyngeal—taste; motor to stylopharyngeus muscle; sensation from the posterior one third of the tongue, tympanic membrane, and external auditory canal; visceral sensation from the carotid body; parasympathetics to parotid gland (salivation)
X: Vagus—motor to the pharyngeal muscles (except stylopharyngeal), levator veli palatini, uvulae, palatopharyngeus, palatoglossus, salpingopharyngeus, cricothyroid and pharyngeal constrictors (via superior laryngeal nerve), and all intrinsic muscles of the larynx (via the recurrent laryngeal nerve) except cricothyroid; parasympathetic innervation to and sensation from the thoracic and abdominal viscera; sensation from the laryngeal mucosa, postauricular skin, external auditory canal, tympanic membrane, and pharynx
XI: Spinal accessory—motor to the sternocleidomastoid and trapezius muscles
XII: Hypoglossal—motor to the tongue except palatoglossus muscle

15. What muscle is the only vocal fold abductor?
Posterior cricoarytenoid is the only ABductor of the larynx.

16. Name the layers of the vocal fold, from superficial to deep.
1. Squamous epithelium
2. Lamina propria (three layers: superficial, intermediate, and deep)
3. Thyroarytenoid muscle and vocalis muscle (vocal fold body)

17. Which layers of the vocal fold form the cover? Which form the ligament?
The cover is formed by the epithelium and superficial lamina propria. The intermediate and deep lamina propria form the vocal ligament.

18. What is the best type of imaging for the temporal bone?
CT scan without contrast is best for evaluation of the cortical bone and soft tissue lesions due to its ability to show bony detail.

19. What is the best type of imaging to evaluate the cerebellopontine angle?
MRI, with its superior ability to show soft tissue contrast, is best for evaluating tumors and lesions of the cerebellopontine angle. MRI of the internal auditory canals is usually done with contrast.

20. What is the best type of imaging to evaluate the thyroid?
The best type of initial imaging for evaluation of the thyroid is ultrasound.

21. If you suspect a peritonsillar abscess is present, do you need to obtain imaging?
No imaging is needed to diagnose a peritonsillar abscess, since this is usually a clinical diagnosis. If an abscess is suspected in the retropharyngeal or parapharyngeal space, imaging can be helpful for establishing a diagnosis.

22. How does a PET (positron emission tomography) scan work?
A radioactive tracer called fludeoxyglucose (very similar to glucose) is given via IV injection. The patient then waits one hour to allow for absorption of the tracer. The areas of the body that are most metabolically active (take up the most glucose), are detected by the scanner. A computer then turns this data into a three-dimensional image. PET scans are often used to determine whether cancer metastasis is present. Since cancer cells are usually more metabolically active than normal tissue, these areas will "light up" on the scan.

23. What changes to the appearance of a lymph node make it suspicious for malignancy on a CT scan with contrast?
Lymph nodes that are greater than one centimeter (1.5 centimeters in the jugulodigastric area), have a necrotic center, have ill-defined margins, or are round (instead of the usual oval shape) are suspicious for malignancy. Lymph nodes with these characteristics should undergo either needle or excisional biopsy depending on the rest of the clinical history (Figure 1-4).

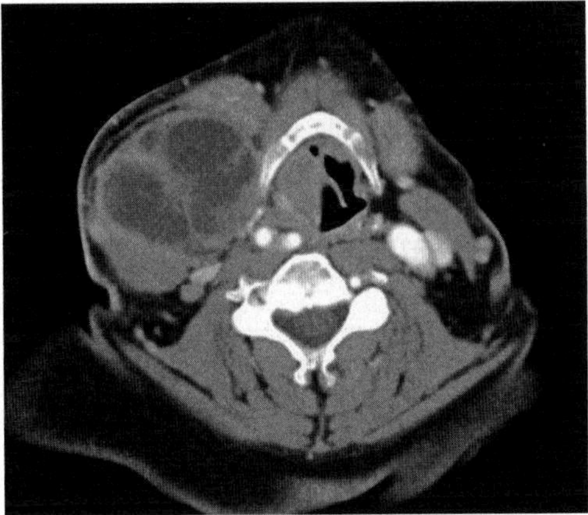

Figure 1-4. Malignant lymph node on CT scan—note large size, necrotic center, and round shape. *(Courtesy of Ted Leem, M.D., Department of Otolaryngology, University of Colorado.)*

Bibliography

Ahmad A, Branstetter BF: CT versus MR: still a tough decision, *Otolaryngol Clin North Am* 41(1):1–22, 2008.

Bailey BJ, Calhoun KH, Healy GB, et al: *Head and Neck Surgery—Otolaryngology*, ed 3, Philadelphia, 2001, Lippincott Williams & Wilkins.

Deschler DG, Day T, editors: *TNM Staging of Head and Neck Cancer and Neck Dissection Classification*, ed 3, Alexandria, Virginia, 2008, American Academy of Otolaryngology—Head and Neck Surgery Foundation.

Grevellec A, Tucker AS: The pharyngeal pouches and clefts: development, evolution, structure, and derivatives, *Semin Cell Dev Biol* 21(3):325–332, 2010.

Myers EN: *Operative Otolaryngology*, Philadelphia, 2008, Saunders Elsevier.

Netter FH: *Atlas of Human Anatomy*, East Hanover, NJ, 1997, Novartis.

Pasha R: *Otolaryngology Head and Neck Surgery: Clinical Reference Guide*, San Diego, 2006, Plural Publishing.

CHAPTER 2

ENT EMERGENCIES

Henry P. Barham, MD and Kenneth T. Bellian, MD, MBA

KEY POINTS

1. Airway management is the otolaryngologist's main role in emergencies.
2. Epiglottitis is an emergency because of the high potential for airway obstruction.
3. Angioedema involves the reticular dermis, subcutaneous, and submucosal layers of nondependent areas.
4. Malignant otitis externa most commonly affects immunocompromised or elderly patients.
5. The mylohyoid muscle is crossed as a boundary in Ludwig's angina.

Pearls

1. In patients with recurrent angioedema, hereditary angioedema must be considered in addition to medicines such as ACE inhibitors. For hereditary angioedema you should request C1 esterase inhibitor levels and complement evaluation (C4).
2. Malignant otitis externa usually occurs in an immunocompromised person with a disease such as diabetes. The most common pathogen is *Pseudomonas aeruginosa.*
3. Ludwig's angina is an infection that is odontogenic in nature. It arises in the submental and submandibular area and causes swelling of the floor of the mouth and subsequent displacement of the tongue posteriorly. This upper airway obstruction can proceed rapidly, making intubation difficult or impossible.
4. The definitive diagnosis of invasive fungal sinusitis requires histopathologic analysis, which confirms invasion of the fungal elements into the submucosal tissues including vessels. There is necrosis as well. Clinically this tissue lacks sensation.
5. A cricothyroidotomy is converted to a formal tracheotomy within 24 hours to minimize the risk of subglottic stenosis.

QUESTIONS

1. **What are the ABCDEs of any medical emergency?**

   A = **A**irway
   B = **B**reathing
   C = **C**irculation
   D = **D**isability/**D**rugs (what the patient is taking or what should be given)
   E = **E**xposure/**E**nvironmental control

2. **What is acute epiglottitis and why is it an emergency?**

   Epiglottitis is inflammation of the epiglottis, typically due to an infectious etiology resulting in rapid airway obstruction. Mortality rates can reach 20%, making urgent diagnosis and treatment essential. The incidence has rapidly declined since the introduction of *Haemophilus influenzae* type b vaccination. Commonly a childhood disease in the past, it is more common now in adults. The most common bacteria identified include *H. influenzae*, beta-hemolytic *Streptococcus*, *Staphylococcus aureus*, and *Streptococcus pneumoniae.* Current belief is that George Washington died from acute bacterial epiglottitis.

3. **How does the presentation of epiglottitis differ in adults and children?**

   Children often present with dyspnea, drooling, stridor, or fever. Adults often complain of severe sore throat, odynophagia, and hoarseness. Historically, patients presented acutely but now more patients are presenting in a subacute fashion. The "tripod sign" is classically seen on presentation.

4. **How should epiglottitis be diagnosed and treated?**
The classic radiographic finding is referred to as the "thumb print sign" described as swelling of the epiglottis on lateral soft tissue neck x-ray. In children, direct visualization via laryngoscopy in the operating room is recommended. Indirect laryngoscopy (fiber-optic nasopharyngeal laryngoscopy) can be considered in adults if the patient is stable enough to tolerate the procedure. Once the diagnosis is made, treatment should consist of airway management and prompt antibiotic administration. Patients with respiratory distress should be intubated. Patients who are deemed medically stable from a respiratory standpoint may be observed closely (ICU) with medical management including antibiotics with activity against *H. influenza* (second- or third-generation cephalosporin), humidified air, racemic epinephrine, and intravenous steroids. It is important to remember that patients who are being observed should always have equipment for intubation and cricothyroidotomy available at the bedside.

5. **Describe angioedema.**
Angioedema is the abrupt onset of nonpitting, nonpruritic edema involving the reticular dermis, subcutaneous, and sub-mucosal layers of nondependent areas. This can affect the lips, soft palate, larynx, and pharynx causing airway obstruction. The duration typically ranges from 24 to 96 hours. Approximately 25% of the U.S. population will have an episode of urticaria and/or angioedema during their lifetime. Acute angioedema is arbitrarily defined as symptom duration of less than 6 weeks.

6. **What causes angioedema?**
The most common causes of acute angioedema include medications, foods, infections, insect venom, contact allergens (latex), and radiology contrast material. The evaluation of chronic angioedema and/or urticaria can be challenging. In the majority of cases, no etiology is ever found.

7. **What is involved in the workup of angioedema?**
In addition to a good history and physical examination, fiber-optic laryngoscopy may be used to determine the degree of laryngeal edema. Patients with angioedema who complain of dyspnea, hoarseness, voice changes, odynophagia, or have stridor on physical exam are likely to have laryngeal involvement. All patients with laryngeal edema require admission to the ICU.

8. **What is the treatment of angioedema?**
For patients with both angioedema and urticaria, treatment may consist of epinephrine, antihistamines, and corticosteroids. For the majority of these patients, H1 antihistamines are the cornerstone of therapy. Although effective, they can also cause profound sedation. As a result of this, second-generation H1 antihistamines (loratadine, cetirizine, desloratadine, and fexofenadine) have become the treatment of choice for angioedema. H2 blockers, such as ranitidine, are necessary as well to completely interrupt the histamine cascade. Corticosteroids are indicated for patients with anaphylaxis, laryngeal edema, and severe symptoms unresponsive to antihistamines. Isolated angioedema is often caused by medications, most commonly ACE inhibitors. Patients with recurrent episodes should be evaluated for hereditary angioedema, a deficiency in C1 esterase inhibitor, with laboratory assessment of C1 inhibitor protein and C4 complement factor levels. Danazol has been the mainstay treatment for prophylaxis, although newer drugs with better side effect profiles are in clinical trials. During the acute illness, fresh frozen plasma can be given to replace C1 inhibitor levels.

9. **Describe malignant otitis externa (MOE).**
MOE is a potentially life-threatening ENT infection that involves the external auditory canal, temporal bone, and surrounding structures. Typically, MOE has an aggressive course and is associated with a high mortality rate, ranging from 50% to 80%. MOE typically occurs in immunocompromised elderly patients. The most common comorbid condition associated with MOE is diabetes mellitus (Types 1 and 2).

10. **What are the common bacteria associated with MOE?**
Pseudomonas aeruginosa is the causative agent in the majority of cases of MOE. This organism is particularly virulent due to its mucoid coating that deters phagocytosis. In addition, some strains release a neurotoxin that is thought to contribute to a number of intracranial complications. Patients with malignancy and HIV are at risk for infection with less common organisms, including *Aspergillus, S. aureus, Proteus mirabilis, Klebsiella oxytoca,* and *Candida species.*

11. **What is the presentation of MOE?**
Patients with MOE present with severe, unrelenting ear pain, temporal headaches, and purulent otorrhea. The hallmark physical examination finding is the presence of granulation tissue in the inferior portion of the external auditory canal, at the bone-cartilage junction. As the infection progresses, patients develop cranial nerve abnormalities, most commonly associated with the seventh cranial nerve. Once cranial nerve abnormalities develop, prognosis is poor. Mortality for patients with MOE and cranial nerve abnormalities approaches 100%.

12. **How is the diagnosis of MOE made?**
The diagnosis of MOE is confirmed with imaging studies including computed tomography (CT), magnetic resonance imaging (MRI), technetium bone scanning, and gallium citrate scintigraphy. CT of the temporal bone is considered by many to be the initial imaging modality of choice to evaluate for bone destruction. It is important to recognize that anywhere from 30% to 50% of bone must be destroyed before findings are evident on CT. For patients with a normal CT scan and high suspicion for MOE, either a bone scan or gallium scintigraphy has a high sensitivity for bone erosion.

13. **Describe the treatment of MOE.**
Treatment of MOE centers on antimicrobial therapy. Antipseudomonal antibiotics are the drugs of choice and must be initiated early. Fluoroquinolones and aminoglycosides are considered by many to be the antibiotic of choice with cure rates close to 90%. In addition to systemic antibiotics, patients should receive good aural toilet with debridement of granulation tissue. Recent studies have suggested an adjuvant role for hyperbaric oxygen therapy for MOE.

14. **What is acute invasive sinusitis and why is it considered an emergency?**
Acute invasive fungal sinusitis (AIFS) is a major cause of morbidity and mortality in the immunocompromised patient population. It is characterized as an aggressive and often fatal angioinvasive infection of the nose, paranasal sinuses, and neighboring structures. It has been increasingly diagnosed in immunocompromised patients with hematologic malignancies, immunosuppression, and poorly controlled diabetes mellitus.

15. **What are the typical causes of AIFS?**
The causative fungal organisms that typically function as saprophytes in the environment can become pathogenic in humans under certain circumstances. The typical species responsible for sinonasal invasive infections are *Aspergillus* and zygomycetes (*Rhizopus, Mucor, Rhizomucor*).

16. **How do you diagnose AIFS?**
The diagnostic gold standard is histopathologic evaluation and culture of nasal biopsies. Nasal endoscopy typically will demonstrate areas of mucosal ischemia or frank necrosis that lack sensation. Radiologic studies will typically show nonspecific findings of sinus mucosal thickening, soft tissue reaction, and possibly bony destruction. Histopathologic confirmation of the diagnosis requires the presence of invasive fungal elements within submucosal tissues and vessels.

17. **What is the survival associated with AIFS?**
Though both medical and surgical treatments have improved, mortality rates have remained high, and vary from 20% to 80% in the literature. Negative prognostic factors include the presence of hematologic malignancy, advanced age, and intracranial or orbital involvement. Survival success is determined by early diagnosis, prompt initiation of culture-directed antifungal therapy, surgical debridement, and reversal of the underlying medical disease.

18. **Describe Ludwig's angina.**
Named after Karl Friedrich Willhelm von Ludwig, it is characterized as a rapidly progressive cellulitis of the soft tissues of the neck and floor of the mouth. With progressive swelling of the soft tissues and elevation and posterior displacement of the tongue, airway obstruction is the most emergent concern. Prior to the development of antibiotics, mortality for Ludwig's angina exceeded 50%. With antibiotic therapy and improved imaging modalities and surgical techniques, mortality currently averages <10%.

19. **What causes Ludwig's angina?**
The majority of cases of Ludwig's angina are of odontogenic origin. The submandibular space is the primary site of infection. This space is subdivided by the mylohyoid muscle into the sublingual space superiorly and the submaxillary space inferiorly. Once infection develops, it can spread contiguously

to the sublingual space and can also spread to involve the pharyngomaxillary and retropharyngeal spaces, encircling the airway. Polymicrobial infection occurs in over 50% of cases. The most commonly cultured organisms include *Staphylococcus*, *Streptococcus*, and *Bacteroides* species.

20. **How do you diagnose Ludwig's angina?**
The majority of patients report dental pain or a history of recent dental procedures, and neck swelling. Less common complaints include neck pain, dysphonia, dysphagia, and dysarthria. Less than one third of adults will present in respiratory distress with dyspnea, tachypnea, or stridor. On physical examination, over 95% of patients have bilateral submandibular swelling and an elevated or protruding tongue.

21. **What is the management of Ludwig's angina?**
Any patient presenting in respiratory distress may require immediate intubation, either by routine orotracheal intubation or fiber-optic nasotracheal intubation. In nonintubated patients with Ludwig's angina, airway equipment, including tracheostomy and cricothyroidotomy instruments, should be kept at the bedside.

Antibiotics should be initiated as soon as possible. Antibiotics should initially be broad-spectrum and cover gram-positive, gram-negative, and anaerobic organisms. Combinations of penicillin, clindamycin, and metronidazole are typically used. Corticosteroid administration can be used in some cases to avoid the need for airway management.

More than 50% of patients with Ludwig's angina develop a suppurative fluid collection that requires surgical drainage. Physical examination alone is insufficient in determining which patients require a surgical procedure. CT scan with intravenous contrast is recommended to detect patients who have developed suppurative complications.

22. **What is a tracheo-innominate (TI) fistula?**
TI fistula is a rare but life-threatening complication of tracheostomy, long-term mechanical ventilation, neck tumors, and tracheal surgery. In patients with a tracheostomy, the incidence of TI fistula is less than 1% but mortality approaches 80%. Patients with a TI fistula secondary to tracheostomy typically present between the first and second week following the procedure. Risk factors for TI fistula include tracheal infection, steroid use, and an anomalous innominate artery. The most common site for fistula formation is at the level of the endotracheal cuff. A large percentage of patients will report a brief episode of bright red blood from the tracheal stoma, referred to as a "sentinel bleed".

23. **What is the treatment of a TI fistula?**
Definitive treatment of a TI fistula requires ligation of the innominate artery, often via a sternotomy. Because the most common site for hemorrhage is at the level of the endotracheal cuff, the first maneuver is to overinflate the cuff of the tracheostomy tube to help tamponade the bleeding. If there is still hemorrhage, the cuff should be placed distal to the site of bleeding to protect the airway. A final maneuver is simply to place a finger in the airway and compress the innominate artery against the posterior sternum. Patients with a sentinel bleed require urgent thoracic surgery consultation for bronchoscopy and ligation of the innominate artery.

24. **Describe nonsurgical management of the airway.**
Chin lift: The mandible is lifted to bring the chin anteriorly.
Jaw thrust: Pressure is applied bilaterally behind the angle of the mandible to displace it anteriorly. This is favored in patients with suspected cervical spine injury.
Oropharyngeal airway: Tube is inserted using a tongue blade into the oropharynx.
Nasopharyngeal airway: Well tolerated in conscious patients. Bypasses base of tongue.
Orotracheal intubation: This is the most common type of definitive airway management. Cervical spine immobilization must be maintained in suspected injuries.
Nasotracheal intubation: Useful with a known cervical spine injury. It is contraindicated in patients with extensive midface trauma.

25. **Describe emergent surgical management of the airway.**
Needle cricothyroidotomy: A large-bore intravenous catheter (12- to 14-gauge) is inserted into the cricothyroid membrane. High-flow oxygen or jet insufflation is used to ventilate the patient. The patient can be adequately ventilated for approximately 30 to 45 minutes until more definitive airway can be obtained (tracheotomy or intubation).

Surgical cricothyroidotomy: A horizontal incision is made through the skin and cricothyroid membrane. This incision is then dilated using a hemostat and an endotracheal or tracheostomy tube is inserted. A cricothyroidotomy should be converted to a tracheotomy within 24 hours to prevent possible subglottic stenosis. This procedure is not recommended in children under the age of 12 years.

Bibliography

Amorosa L, Modugno GC, Pirodda A: Malignant external otitis: review and personal experience, *Acta Otolaryngol Suppl* 521:3–16, 1996.

Bansal A, Miskoff J, Lis RJ: Otolaryngologic critical care, *Crit Care Clin* 19:55–72, 2003.

Berrouschot J, Oeken J, Steiniger L, et al: Perioperative complications of percutaneous dilational tracheostomy, *Laryngoscope* 107(Pt 1):1538–1544, 1997.

Carey MJ: Epiglottitis in adults, *Am J Emerg Med* 14:421–424, 1996.

Dibbern DA Jr, Dreskin SC: Urticaria and angioedema: an overview, *Immunol Allergy Clin North Am* 24:141–162, 2004.

Gillespie MB, Huchton DM, O'Malley BW: Role of middle turbinate biopsy in the diagnosis of fulminant invasive fungal rhinosinusitis, *Laryngoscope* 110:1832–1836, 2000.

Marple BF: Ludwig angina: a review of current airway management, *Arch Otolaryngol Head Neck Surg* 125:596–599, 1999.

Quinn FB Jr: Ludwig angina, *Arch Otolaryngol Head Neck Surg* 125:599, 1999.

Turner JH, Soudry E, Jayakar VN, et al: Survival outcomes in acute invasive fungal sinusitis: a systematic review and quantitative synthesis of published evidence, *Laryngoscope* 123(5):1112–1118, 2013.

CHAPTER 3

DEEP NECK INFECTIONS

Tendy Chiang, MD and Kavitha K. Prabaker, MD

KEY POINTS

1. Initial evaluation of deep neck space infections (DNSI) should be directed toward identifying the acuity and medical stability of the patient; hemodynamic and airway instability may require emergent intervention.
2. Trismus, dysphonia, "hot potato" voice, stridor, and stertor are signs of airway compromise and may require urgent evaluation with flexible fiber-optic laryngoscopy. Tachypnea and oxygen desaturations are late manifestations of airway obstruction and should not be relied on to determine clinical stability.
3. Management with intravenous antibiotics is indicated in stable, antibiotic naïve patients without any clinical or radiographic features of abscess formation.
4. Infections of the parapharyngeal, prevertebral, and retropharyngeal space can extend into the "danger space," allowing for unrestricted spread of infection into the mediastinum.

Pearls

1. Deep neck space infections most commonly originate from odontogenic sources in adults whereas tonsillitis and pharyngitis are the most common etiologies in children.
2. There has been a dramatic increase in the incidence of MRSA since the early 2000s, particularly community-acquired MRSA among children, and it is now a common organism seen in DNSI.
3. The classic presentation of peritonsillar abscess includes trismus, uvular deviation, muffled voice, and soft palatal edema.

QUESTIONS

1. **What are deep neck space infections?**
   Deep neck space infections (DNSI) encompass a wide spectrum of infectious disorders of the neck. DNSI are typically classified by the fascial space the infection occupies.

2. **What risk factors are associated with the development of DNSI?**
   Risk factors of DNSI include low level of education, living greater than 1 hour from a tertiary care center, presence of tonsils, *Streptococcus* infections, substance abuse, and poor dental hygiene.

3. **Describe how the neck is organized in terms of fascial planes.**
   The neck is compartmentalized in two main divisions of fascia: the superficial cervical fascia and the deep cervical fascia.

   The superficial cervical fascia includes subcutaneous tissue and envelops the muscles of facial expression. It is continuous with the superficial musculoaponeurotic system (SMAS) and extends inferiorly to involve the platysma.

   The deep cervical fascia is divided into superficial, middle, and deep layers.
   - The **superficial layer** invests parotid and submandibular glands, muscles of mastication, trapezius, sternocleidomastoid, and forms the stylomandibular ligament.
   - The **middle layer** is composed of two divisions: the *visceral division* invests the larynx, pharynx, trachea, esophagus, thyroid, and parathyroid; the *muscular division* invests the strap muscles.
   - The **deep layer** is composed of two divisions as well: the *prevertebral division* envelops the paraspinal muscles and vertebrae; the *alar division* lies atop the prevertebral layer and covers

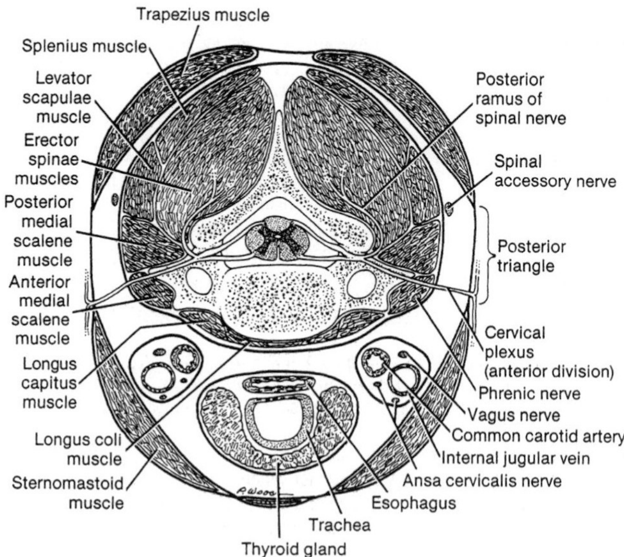

Figure 3-1. Structures contained by deep cervical fascia: transverse section at the level of CN VII. *(From Graney DO: Anatomy. In Cummings CW, et al [eds]: Otolaryngology—Head and Neck Surgery, 3 ed, St. Louis, 1998, Mosby.)*

the sympathetic trunk. The carotid sheath represents the confluence of the deep layers of the deep cervical fascia (Figure 3-1).

4. **Identify the deep neck spaces as well as anatomic sites that contribute to the infections within these spaces.**
Deep neck spaces can either be suprahyoid, infrahyoid, or span the entire length of the neck. It is important to understand the boundaries of the deep neck spaces because infections often follow these boundaries (or lack thereof) as they spread. DNSI typically are the result of suppuration of lymph nodes from infection at a primary anatomic site.
   a. Suprahyoid:
      i. Peritonsillar: tonsil
      ii. Parapharyngeal: tonsil, pharynx
      iii. Submandibular: odontogenic, gingiva, submandibular gland
      iv. Sublingual: odontogenic, gingiva, sublingual gland
   b. Infrahyoid: visceral
   c. Span entire length of neck
      i. Retropharyngeal: nasal cavity, paranasal sinuses, nasopharynx, vertebral bodies
      ii. Prevertebral: hematogenous spread from vertebrae and intervertebral discs
      iii. "Danger" space: parapharyngeal, retropharyngeal space infections
      iv. Carotid sheath: parapharyngeal, retropharyngeal space infections

5. **What conditions can present in a similar fashion to DNSI?**
Congenital anomalies can either masquerade as a DNSI or become more clinically apparent when they become infected. Thyroglossal duct cysts, lymphatic malformations, and branchial cleft cysts can rapidly increase in size and present with signs and symptoms identical to DNSI. Prior history of a mass or fullness that waxes and wanes suggests the presence of an underlying congenital lesion.
    Neoplastic processes can present with rapid neck swelling and features consistent with an infectious process as well. Fevers, night sweats, and weight loss can be presenting signs of lymphoma. New neck masses in adults are more likely to be malignant when compared to pediatric patients.

6. **What is the "danger space"?**
The danger space is bound by the alar fascia anteriorly and the prevertebral fascia posteriorly. It extends from the skull base to the thoracic cavity, providing an unrestricted path for spread of infection into the mediastinum, causing mediastinitis. Infections of the parapharyngeal, retropharyngeal, and prevertebral space can easily extend to this space.

7. **What is the most common major complication of DNSI?**
Mediastinitis is the most common major complication of DNSI. It typically presents with tachycardia, dyspnea, and pleuritic chest pain. Chest x-ray can demonstrate mediastinal widening. Further evaluation with contrast chest CT is necessary to identify fluid collections that require drainage. Broad-spectrum intravenous antibiotics, early consultation with the thoracic surgery service, and close surveillance in the intensive care unit are recommended.

8. **How are prevertebral space infections different from infections of other deep neck spaces?**
Prevertebral space infections are generally the result of hematogenous seeding or contiguous spread of infection from discitis or vertebral osteomyelitis. Gram-positive bacteria, especially *Staphylococcus aureus*, are the most common pathogens in these infections; anaerobes are uncommon.

9. **What are the most common etiologies of DNSI?**
The etiology of DNSI varies with age. Bacterial pharyngitis and tonsillitis with resultant suppuration of parapharyngeal, retropharyngeal, and jugulodigastric lymph nodes are the most common etiologies in children. Odontogenic infections are the most common etiology in adults; bacteria within dental plaque erode tooth enamel to form periapical abscesses that may penetrate the mandible or maxilla to enter the deep spaces of the neck. Other etiologies include cellulitis, trauma, foreign body, intravenous drug use, or congenital lesions such as thyroglossal duct cysts or branchial cleft anomalies.

10. **What are the most common pathogens causing deep neck space infections?**
Because most of these infections are odontogenic in origin, pathogens are typically part of normal oral flora. These infections are usually polymicrobial, involving a large proportion of anaerobic bacteria, especially as the infections spread into deeper neck spaces. Common bacteria include: *Streptococcus* species, *Peptostreptococcus*, *Actinomyces*, *Fusobacterium*, and *Prevotella*. *Staphylococcus aureus* (including MRSA), *Pseudomonas aeruginosa*, and other gram-negative rods are more common among immunocompromised hosts, diabetics, and postoperative infections.

11. **What is the role of methicillin-resistant *Staphylococcus aureus* (MRSA) in deep neck space infections in the United States?**
Streptococcal species, particularly *group A streptococcus*, remain the most common pathogen responsible for nonpurulent skin and soft tissue infections, such as cellulitis and erysipelas. Purulent skin and soft tissue infections involving the head and neck (abscesses, furuncles, carbuncles, wound infections), on the other hand, are most commonly caused by *S. aureus*. There has been a dramatic increase in the incidence of MRSA since the early 2000s, particularly community-acquired MRSA among children. Up to 70% of pediatric neck abscesses are due to MRSA in some communities. Patients less than 16 months of age with lateral neck abscesses are 10 times more likely to have a *S. aureus* infection than non-*S. aureus*.

12. **What signs and symptoms are common in DNSI?**
The most common symptoms are neck pain, fever, dysphagia, neck swelling, and odynophagia. Referred pain resulting in otalgia and odynophagia is also common.

13. **What are the key physical exam findings in the evaluation of a patient with DNSI?**
A complete head and neck exam is essential in all patients with DNSI. Initial interview should devote attention to hoarseness, dyspnea, stridor, stertor, muffling or "hot potato" voice. Dysphonia should be evaluated with flexible fiber-optic laryngoscopy for possible airway compromise if the patient is stable.

Inspection and palpation of the head and neck should begin away from the primary site of infection, reserving that portion of the exam for last. Evaluation of the involved area should focus on the size of the area, presence of induration, swelling or fluctuance, and any color change or cellulitic change of the overlying skin. Any cellulitic change should be marked along its periphery to permit accurate surveillance. Presence of crepitus suggests infection with gas-producing organisms.

Cranial neuropathies can suggest retrograde spread of infection along the valveless venous system of the midface from soft tissue, nasal cavity, or the paranasal sinus infections.

14. What is trismus and why is it significant?

Trismus refers to the reduced ability to open the mouth. In the setting of DNSI, it is a sign of inflammation of the parapharyngeal, masseteric, pterygoid, and/or temporal spaces. While seen commonly in odontogenic infections, trismus is also seen with peritonsillar, parapharyngeal, and floor of mouth infections. Severe trismus can lead to difficulty managing secretions and cause airway compromise, presenting challenges for airway intervention should it be needed.

15. How should suspected deep space neck infections be worked up?

Typical diagnostic workup of DNSI includes complete blood count with differential and radiographic evaluations. Atypical presentations (painless, slow growing, association with weight loss and night sweats) should raise suspicion for malignancy. Atypical infectious etiologies should be evaluated with placement of a PPD with chest x-ray, HIV testing, and titers for *Bartonella henselae.*

Anterior-posterior and lateral neck plain films are useful in evaluation of the retropharyngeal space (Figure 3-2). Ultrasound and computed tomography are the most common radiographic modalities employed when evaluating DNSI. Ultrasound is effective in differentiating cellulitic change from a fluid collection and can also be used for guidance to localize an abscess cavity. Computed tomography with contrast can demonstrate an abscess in the form of a hypodense focus centrally with peripheral rim enhancement.

16. How can submandibular space infections be distinguished from sublingual space infections?

Submandibular space infections involve the area inferior to the mylohyoid muscle. They are usually the result of apical abscesses of the second or third molars. Sublingual infections, which involve the

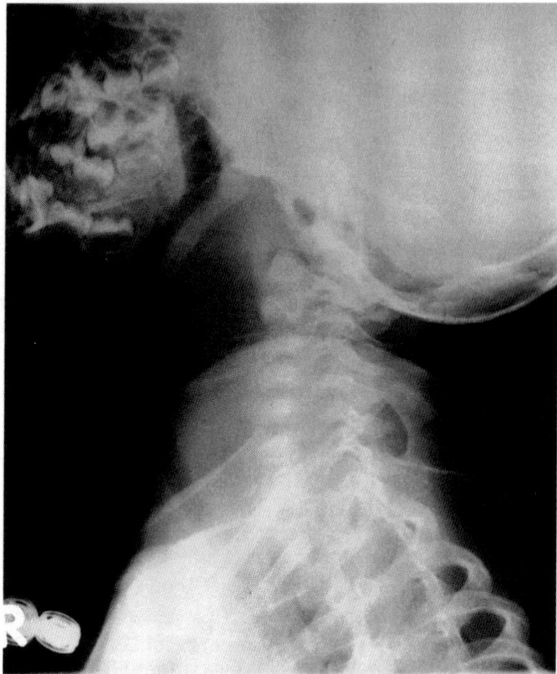

Figure 3-2. Lateral neck plain film of a pediatric patient with a retropharyngeal abscess showing significant prevertebral thickening.

space superior to the mylohyoid muscle, on the other hand, are usually the result of infections of the mandibular incisors.

17. **Which DNSI pose the greatest risk to the contents of the carotid sheath?**
The parapharyngeal and retropharyngeal spaces are adjacent to the carotid sheath. Infections of the carotid sheath may lead to complications such as Horner's syndrome (ptosis, miosis, anhydrosis from involvement of the cervical sympathetic chain), cranial nerve palsies, carotid artery rupture, and septic phlebitis of the jugular vein. This can present with neck fullness, a pulsatile neck mass with ecchymosis, and bright red bleeding from the nose, mouth, or external auditory canal.

18. **What are the classic signs of peritonsillar abscess?**
Peritonsillar abscess is a clinical diagnosis and does not typically require additional diagnostic and radiographic testing. Patients typically present with trismus, muffled voice, uvular deviation, and fullness of the soft palate.

Management of peritonsillar abscess involves surgical incision and drainage. This procedure is generally tolerated with local anesthesia alone in the clinic or emergency department in cooperative patients, typically the adolescent and adult population. Pediatric patients typically require general anesthesia for management.

Isolated peritonsillar abscess requires completion of a course of oral antibiotics following drainage. Tonsillectomy is indicated in the setting of recurrent peritonsillar abscess.

19. **What are the indications for surgical intervention for DNSI?**
The indications for surgical intervention depend on the medical stability of the patient. Patients who are antibiotic naïve, do not have any airway compromise, and do not have any radiographic features of abscess formation can be managed initially with systemic antibiotic therapy. Any signs of airway compromise, lack of marked improvement after 24 to 72 hours of intravenous antibiotic therapy, or clinical or radiographic signs of abscess formation should undergo incision and drainage.

The goal of incision and drainage should including collection of culture specimens, blunt dissection into the abscess cavity, and disruptions of loculations within the abscess cavity to promote drainage. Packing is placed and removed gradually during the postoperative period to prevent reaccumulation of fluid.

20. **What is Lemierre's syndrome?**
Lemierre's syndrome is septic thrombophlebitis of the internal jugular vein, which is usually the result of hematogenous extension through tonsillar veins. Typical symptoms of pharyngitis lead to fever, lethargy, neck pain, and swelling. Septic emboli can seed in the lungs, resulting in nodular infiltrates on chest x-ray. Contrast CT of the neck demonstrates occlusion of the internal jugular vein. *Fusobacterium necrophorum* is the pathogen isolated in over 90% of cultures. Metronidazole is the treatment of choice.

21. **What is the hallmark of *Actinomyces israelii* infections involving the head and neck?**
Infections caused by this bacteria frequently cross fascial planes, forming sinus tracts that drain grainy material commonly referred to as "sulfur granules." Actinomyces is a gram-positive, branching, facultative anaerobe. Fifty percent of cases involve the head and neck. Infections typically present as a nontender, hard, slowly progressive mass in the perimandibular area ("lumpy jaw"). Treatment is with a long-term course of penicillin or amoxicillin.

22. **What is Ludwig's angina and what is its major complication?**
Ludwig's angina is a rapidly spreading infection of the submandibular and sublingual spaces, typically odontogenic in origin. Infection superior to the mylohyoid muscle places the patient at risk for rapid swelling of the floor of mouth and tongue, resulting in airway obstruction. Patients typically present with trismus, fever, drooling, dysphonia, and dysphagia. On exam, tense swelling of the floor of the mouth and tongue protrusion are present, which can deteriorate quickly into respiratory distress. Intubation can rapidly become difficult if not impossible. Emergent tracheostomy may be indicated in addition to antibiotics and surgical drainage.

23. **What empiric antibiotic regimens are appropriate for DNSI?**
Empiric antibiotics should be administered parenterally and have activity against *Streptococcus* species and oral anaerobes. Appropriate cultures should be obtained if possible prior to initiation of any antimicrobial therapy. Penicillin G plus metronidazole or ampicillin-sulbactam are good choices.

For patients who are allergic to penicillin, clindamycin, moxifloxacin, levofloxacin plus metronidazole, or ciprofloxacin plus metronidazole may be used.

A complete course of antimicrobial therapy is typically 10 to 14 days. Marked clinical improvement should be observed prior to conversion from intravenous to oral therapy.

24. **What is the most common cause of chronic unilateral regional lymphadenopathy in children?**
Cat-scratch disease (CSD) presents as lymphadenopathy from infection by *Bartonella henselae*, typically several weeks after inoculation. A history of cat exposure is present in most patients. Lymphadenopathy typically resolves within 2 months but can last up to a year. Early treatment (within the first 30 days) with azithromycin for 5 days demonstrated significant decrease in lymph node volume while delayed treatment (after 30 days) demonstrated no change in rate of resolution. Surgical treatment is reserved for persistent discomfort, suppuration, and diagnostic purposes.

25. **Describe the typical presentation of cervical lymphadenitis caused by atypical mycobacterial infection.**
Atypical mycobacterial infections typically present with firm, painless lymphadenopathy that typically does not respond to antibiotic therapy. The infectious process becomes more superficial in time, resulting in violaceous change of the overlying skin, resulting in drainage and scarring. Natural resolution occurs over a period of months to years. Medical management consists of long-term antibiotic therapy accompanied with surgical excision to prevent skin breakdown and unfavorable scarring.

26. **What is the most common manifestation of tuberculosis of the head and neck?**
Scrofula is tuberculous lymphadenitis of the cervical region. It typically presents as a unilateral, painless, firm mass without fevers or other systemic symptoms. Diagnosis is via biopsy with culture. Treatment includes complete excision of the lymph node, in addition to antimycobacterial therapy.

27. **Discuss the risk factors and typical presentation of necrotizing fasciitis.**
Necrotizing fasciitis is a rapidly progressive DNSI of the fascial planes that typically occurs in immunosuppressed patients (diabetes, chronic illness, patients undergoing chemotherapy, malnutrition) and presents with pain disproportionate with physical exam. Gas-forming bacteria can produce crepitus and gas bubbles may be seen on imaging within the soft tissues. Progression of disease is rapid; early medical management with broad-spectrum IV antibiotics coupled with aggressive surgical debridement of infected tissue is required.

Bibliography

Barber BR, Dziegielewski PT, Biron VL, et al: Factors associated with severe deep neck space infections: targeting multiple fronts, *J Otolaryngol Head Neck Surg* 43:35, 2014.

Daramola OO, Flanagan CE, Maisel RH, et al: Diagnosis and treatment of deep neck space abscesses, *J Otolaryngol Head Neck Surg* 141:123–130, 2009.

Duggal P, Naseri I, Sobol SE: The increased risk of community-acquired methicillin-resistant *Staphylococcus aureus* neck abscesses in young children, *Laryngoscop* 121:51–55, 2011.

Fraser L, Moore P, Kubba H: Atypical mycobacterial infection of the head and neck in children: a 5-year retrospective review, *Otolaryngol Head Neck Surg* 138:311–314, 2008.

Hull MW, Chow AW: An approach to oral infections and their management, *Curr Infect Dis Rep* 7:17, 2005.

Mandell GL, Bennett JE, Dolin R, editors: *Mandell, Douglas, and Bennett's Principles and Practice of Infectious Diseases*, ed 7, Philadelphia, 2010, Churchill Livingstone Elsevier, pp 855–870.

Marioni G, Rinaldi R, Staffieri C, et al: Deep neck infection with dental origin: analysis of 85 consecutive cases (2000–2006), *Acta Otolaryngol* 128(2):201–206, 2008.

Massei F, Gori L, Macchia P, et al: The expanded spectrum of bartonellosis in children, *Infect Dis Clin North Am* 19: 691–711, 2005.

Munson PD, Boyce TG, Salomao DR, et al: Cat-scratch disease of the head and neck in a pediatric population: surgical indications and outcomes, *Otolaryngol Head Neck Surg* 139:358–363, 2008.

Reynolds SC, Chow AW: Severe soft tissue infections of the head and neck: a primer for critical care physicians, *Lung* 187:271, 2009.

Smego RA Jr, Foglia G: Actinomycosis, *CID* 26(6):1255–1261, 1998.

Velargo PA, Burke EL, Kluka EA: Pediatric neck abscesses caused by methicillin-resistant *Staphylococcus aureus*: a retrospective study of incidence and susceptibilities over time, *Ear Nose Throat J* 89(9):459–461, 2010.

CHAPTER 4

ANTIMICROBIALS AND PHARMACOTHERAPY

Taylor M. Washburn, MD

KEY POINTS

1. Knowledge of antibiotic methods of action and microbial resistance mechanisms and patterns can facilitate appropriate drug selection.
2. The most directed antimicrobial therapy is preferred, and may require a sample to be obtained for culture and sensitivity testing.
3. Factors to consider when choosing an antibiotic:
   - Antibiotic must have activity against the organism(s)
   - Consider local resistance patterns
   - Location of the infection and antibiotic penetration
   - Mechanism of action (bacteriocidal versus bacteriostatic)
   - Host factors: age, drug allergy, renal or liver dysfunction, pregnancy, immune status, other medications that may cause drug–drug interactions
4. Can cephalosporins be used if there is a history of penicillin allergy?
   - Yes, cephalosporins can be used. If penicillin skin testing is available, this should be done to verify the presence of penicillin allergy. If penicillin skin testing is not available, then the nature of the allergy should be considered. If the allergy was serious (anaphylaxis), then penicillins should be avoided.
5. Antibiotics with excellent oral absorption
   - Fluoroquinolones
   - Clindamycin
   - TMP-SMX
   - Doxycycline
   - Linezolid
6. Antibiotics with activity against *Pseudomonas aeruginosa*
   - Antipseudomonal penicillins: piperacillin-tazobactam, ticarcillin-clavulanate
   - Cephalosporins with pseudomonal activity: ceftazidime, cefepime
   - Fluoroquinolones: levofloxacin, ciprofloxacin
   - Carbapenems (all but ertapenem)
   - Aztreonam
   - Aminoglycosides
   - Colistin/polymyxin B
7. Antibiotics with activity against methicillin-resistant *Staphylococcus aureus*
   - Vancomycin
   - Daptomycin
   - Linezolid
   - TMP-SMX
   - Clindamycin
   - Tetracyclines

Pearls

1. Ertapenem is the least broad of the carbapenems due to its lack of activity against *Enterococcus* sp. and *P. aeruginosa*.
2. Clindamycin has efficacy against oral cavity anaerobes, and is an ideal antibiotic for odontogenic infection.
3. Antibiotics associated with increased risk of *C. difficile* colitis are clindamycin, fluoroquinolones, cephalosporins, and carbapenems. Macrolides, penicillins, and sulfonamides are less frequently associated.
4. The tetracyclines should not be used in children or pregnant women due to the effect on developing teeth and bones.
5. Liposomal amphotericin B is more commonly used than conventional amphotericin B because the liposomal form of the drug has less nephrotoxicity.

QUESTIONS

1. Describe the key factors that influence antibiotic choice.

- An antimicrobial active against the organism causing the infection should be used. If this is not known, then the typical organisms known to cause the infection should be considered and treatment directed toward these organisms.
- The anticipated resistance pattern of the organism must be considered. If the organism has been cultured, resistance testing should be done. If susceptibility testing is not possible, local resistance patterns should be taken into consideration when choosing antibiotics.
- The location of the infection, and delivery and penetration of the antibiotic must be considered.
- The mechanism of action of the antibiotic is important. If the patient does not have an intact immune system, a bacteriocidal antibiotic should be chosen over a bacteriostatic one if possible.
- Host factors such as age, history of drug allergy, renal or liver dysfunction, pregnancy, drug–drug interactions due to other medications the patient is taking, and the immune status must be taken into consideration. Drug dosage adjustment is required for many antibiotics in the setting of renal or hepatic dysfunction.

2. What facts must the clinician consider when deciding between oral and intravenous antibiotic therapy?

Severity of infection: Oral antibiotics are typically used in mild infections whereas intravenous (IV) antibiotics are chosen for moderate to severe infections. Intravenous antibiotics should be given to patients who are in shock, because oral absorption can be erratic.

Degree of systemic absorption: If an oral antibiotic is given, the absorption of the antibiotic must be considered. For example, some antibiotics such as aminoglycosides are not given orally due to poor absorption. On the other hand, some antibiotics have excellent oral bioavailability and can be used nearly interchangeably with IV antibiotics. Examples of antibiotics with excellent oral bioavailability include fluoroquinolones, clindamycin and linezolid.

3. What are some advantages of topical antibiotics?

Optimal delivery to the site, ability to deliver higher concentration, ability to overcome resistance mechanisms, minimized systemic side effects

4. Describe the mechanism of action and spectrum of activity of the penicillin class of antibiotics.

Penicillins are β-lactam antibiotics and are bactericidal. They kill bacteria by inhibiting cell wall synthesis (Table 4-1).

5. Explain the spectrum of activity of the different classes of cephalosporin antibiotics.

First generation cephalosporins (intravenous cefazolin, oral cephalexin) primarily have activity against gram-positive cocci, such as *Staphylococcus* sp. and *Streptococcus* sp.

Second generation cephalosporins (cefuroxime) have increased activity against gram-negative respiratory pathogens, including *Haemophilus influenza* and *Moraxella catarrhalis*. However, the second generation cephalosporins have limited activity against many *Enterobacteriaceae*. Cefuroxime is active against penicillin-sensitive strains of *Streptococcus pneumoniae*.

Table 4-1. Clinically Relevant Penicillin Classes and Spectrum of Activity

Classes of Penicillins and Spectrum of Activity				
NATURAL PENICILLINS	**ANTISTAPHYLOCOCCAL PENICILLINS**	**AMINOPENICILLINS**	**CARBOXYPENICILLINS**	**ACYL UREIDO-PENICILLINS**
Penicillin G and V	Oxacillin, nafcillin, dicloxacillin	Ampicillin, amoxicillin	Ticarcillin-clavulanate	Piperacillin-tazobactam
GPC, GNC, and some GNR. Also spirochetes and actinomyces	Methicillin sensitive staphylococci, penicillin suspectible stains of *Streptococci*, anaerobic GPC	Essentially the same as natural penicillins, including *Haemophilus influenza*	Increased gram-negative coverage including *Pseudomonas aeruginosa*	Excellent gram-positive and gram-negative coverage, including *Pseudomonas aeruginosa*
Susceptible to all β-lactamases	Not active against gram-negative organisms	Susceptible to β-lactamases	Less active against penicillin-resistant *Streptoccoccus* sp.	Enhanced activity against some β-lactamases

GPC, gram-positive cocci; GNC, gram-negative cocci; GNR, gram-negative rods.

Third generation cephalosporins (intravenous ceftriaxone and ceftazidime, oral cefixime and cefditorin) demonstrate increased activity against gram-negative organisms. Some of the drugs in this class, such as ceftriaxone, also have activity against penicillin-resistant *S. pneumoniae.*

Fourth generation cephalosporins (cefepime is the only drug in this class available in the United States) have the broadest activity against gram-negative organisms, including *P. aeruginosa.*

Fifth generation or methicillin-resistant *Staphylococcus aureus* (MRSA) active cephalosporins (only approved agent in this class is ceftaroline) have excellent activity against MRSA and other gram-positive organisms including *S. pneumoniae.* The gram-negative activity of this drug is similar to ceftriaxone. Currently, ceftaroline is FDA approved only for treatment of pneumonia and skin and soft tissue infections, but likely will be approved for other indications in the future.

6. Like the penicillin class of antibiotics, the cephalosporin antibiotic class possesses a β-lactam ring. Can the cephalosporins be safely used in patients who report a history of penicillin allergy?

Penicillin skin testing is recommended if available. Many patients who report a history of penicillin allergy (assumed to be an allergy to any antibiotic in the penicillin class) in fact have negative penicillin skin tests. If the penicillin skin test is negative, then there is no increased risk for cross-reactivity to cephalosporins. However, if penicillin skin testing is positive, then the patient is at increased risk for cephalosporin reaction and antibiotics should be administered via graded challenge, rapid desensitization or should be avoided all together.

Penicillin skin testing is frequently not available. Of patients with a history of penicillin allergy, only 10% have positive penicillin skin tests and studies have shown that 3.4% of patients with a positive skin test to penicillin have allergy to cephalosporins. Therefore, the risk is low, but risk is still present. In this case, the nature of the penicillin allergy should be considered. If the reaction is severe (anaphylaxis), options are to avoid cephalosporins or to administer antibiotics via a graded challenge.

7. In addition to the penicillin and cephalosporin class of antibiotics, the carbapenems are also β-lactam antibiotics. What is their range of antimicrobial activity?

There are four carbapenems available for use in the United States—ertapenem, imipenem, doripenem, and meropenem. All have a very broad range of antimicrobial activity, including

Table 4-2. Antimicrobial Activity of the Fluoroquinolones

Common coverage	Gram-negative bacilli, including *Enterobacteriaceae* and respiratory pathogens such as *Haemophilus influenza* Gram-positive respiratory pathogens such as *Neisseria* sp. and *Moraxella catarrhalis.* Atypical respiratory pathogens that can cause pneumonia, such as *Legionella pneumophilia, Mycoplasma pneumoniae,* and *Chlamydophilia pneumonia*
Ciprofloxacin	Broadest gram-negative activity, including *Pseudomonas aeruginosa.* Limited activity against *Streptococcus* sp. (not typically used for head and neck infections)
Levofloxacin, moxifloxacin, gatifloxacin	Best activity against *Streptococcus sp.* Levofloxacin also has activity against *Pseudomonas aeruginosa.*

gram-positive organisms, gram-negative organisms (including drug-resistant gram-negatives) and anaerobic organisms. Ertapenem is the least broad of the carbapenems due to its lack of activity against *Enterococcus* sp. and *P. aeruginosa.*

8. **There are differences in antimicrobial coverage between the various agents of the fluoroquinolone class of antibiotics. Describe the mechanism of action of the fluoroquinolones and the differences in coverage between the drugs in this class.**
   Fluoroquinolones are bactericidal antibiotics that work by inhibiting bacterial DNA synthesis (Table 4-2).

9. **The macrolides are used frequently for infections of the head and neck. How do they work and what is their antimicrobial activity?**
   There are three members of the macrolide class of antibiotics—erythromycin, azithromycin, and clarithromycin. They are bacteriostatic antibiotics which inhibit RNA protein synthesis. Erythromycin has fairly broad antimicrobial activity, with activity against gram-positive and gram-negative organisms. Azithromycin and clarithromycin are the newest agents in the class and were developed with an even broader range of antimicrobial activity. Azithromycin and clarithromycin are more easily absorbed than erythromycin with fewer gastrointestinal side effects.

10. **Describe the spectrum of activity of clindamycin.**
    Clindamycin has good activity against gram-positive organisms, including *Staphylococcus aureus* (including MRSA) and *Streptococcus sp.* including *S. pyogenes*, *S. pneumonia*, and members of the viridans streptococcus group. The special quality of clindamycin is the anaerobic coverage it provides. The adage is to use clindamycin for "anaerobic infections above the diaphragm" because clindamycin has activity against the anaerobes found in the oral cavity including *Peptostreptococcus sp.* and *Veillonella sp.*

11. **Describe the signs and symptoms of *Clostridium difficile* colitis.**
    Patients with *Clostridium difficile* colitis typically complain of diffuse watery diarrhea, up to several times daily. Leukocytosis is a very common manifestation and can present prior to development of symptoms of diarrhea. Fever, bloody diarrhea, and abdominal pain can be present in severe disease. Prior antibiotic use is the primary risk factor for development of disease. The antibiotics associated with increased risk are clindamycin, fluoroquinolones, cephalosporins, and carbapenems. Macrolides, penicillins, and sulfonamides are less frequently associated.

12. **Trimethaprim-sulfamethoxazole (TMP-SMX) is a bactericidal antibiotic that works by inhibiting bacterial production of folic acid. Describe the antimicrobial spectrum of action of the drug and its major side effects.**
    TMP-SMZ is a fairly broad spectrum antibiotic, with activity against a wide range of aerobic gram-positive and gram-negative bacteria. Examples include *Staphylococcus aureus* (both methicillin

sensitive and methicillin resistant), *S. pneumoniae*, *M. catarrhalis*, and *H. influenza* and enteric aerobic gram-negative bacilli.

The most common side effects of TMP-SMX are gastrointestinal upset and dermatologic reactions such as rash. More severe dermatologic reactions can occur including Stevens-Johnson syndrome and toxic epidermal necrolysis. Nephrotoxicity can also occur.

13. **Describe the mechanism of action of the tetracyclines and their spectrum of activity.**
Tetracyclines (doxycycline, minocycline, tetracycline) are bacteriostatic antibiotics which work by inhibiting bacterial protein synthesis. Tetracyclines are active against a wide range of gram-positive and gram-negative organisms, including respiratory pathogens such as *S. pneumonia, H. influenza*, and *Mycoplasma pneumoniae*. Tigecycline, a new IV tetracycline, also has activity against drug-resistant gram-negative organisms. The tetracyclines should not be used in children or pregnant women due to the effect on developing teeth and bones.

14. **Name the antibiotics with activity against MRSA.**
The most commonly used IV agent is vancomycin, which is an inhibitor of bacterial cell wall synthesis. Other intravenous agents with MRSA activity include daptomycin, linezolid, and ceftaroline.
There are also a number of oral agents with activity against MRSA. These include TMP-SMX, clindamycin, tetracyclines, and oral linezolid. The fluoroquinolones do have activity against *Staphylococcus aureus* including MRSA, but should not be used as monotherapy for Staphylococcal infections as resistance can rapidly develop on therapy.

15. **Fungal infections of the head and neck are uncommon, but can be devastating. What are the classes of antifungal medications and what infections do they treat?**
The azoles are the most commonly used antifungal medications. Examples of medications in this class include fluconazole, itraconazole, posaconazole, and voriconazole. Fluconazole is commonly used for infections due to *Candida* sp., whereas voriconazole is first line therapy for aspergillosis.
Micafungin, caspofungin, and anidulafungin are all echinocandins. These are used for invasive candidiasis due to certain species of *Candida*, including *Candida krusei* and *Candida glabrata*.
The polyene amphotericin B is typically reserved for serious fungal infections, including invasive rhinosinusitis due to mucormycosis. The different formulations of the medication are conventional amphotericin B and liposomal amphotericin B. The liposomal form of the drug has less nephrotoxicity, so it is more commonly used.

Table 4-3. Overview of Characteristics of Antibiotics Used in Head and Neck Infections

CLASS	ACTIVITY	MECHANISM OF ACTION
Penicillins	Bactericidal	Inhibit cell wall synthesis
Cephalosporins	Bactericidal	Interfere with cell wall synthesis
Carbapenems	Bactericidal	Inhibit cell wall synthesis
Fluoroquinolones	Bactericidal	Inhibit DNA gyrase
Macrolides	Bacteriostatic	Inhibit protein synthesis
Clindamycin	Bacteriostatic	Inhibit protein synthesis
Trimethoprim/sulfamethoxazole	Bacteriostatic	Folate antagonist/inhibit folate synthesis
Vancomycin	Bactericidal	Inhibit cell wall synthesis and RNA synthesis
Tetracyclines	Bacteriostatic	Inhibit protein synthesis
Aminoglycosides	Bactericidal	Inhibit protein synthesis

16. **Herpes simplex virus (HSV) is a frequent cause of orolabial infections. What are the oral antiviral medications used for this infection?**
    Acyclovir is commonly used for orolabial HSV infections. Other oral antiviral medications used for HSV are valacyclovir and famciclovir.

BIBLIOGRAPHY

Andes DR, Craig WA: Cephalosporins. In *Mandell, Douglas, and Bennett's Principles and Practice of Infectious Diseases* (vol 1), ed 7, Philadelphia, 2009, Churchill Livingstone, pp 323–339.
Chang C, Mahmood MM, Teuber SS, et al: Overview of penicillin allergy, *Cinic Rev Allerg Immunol* 43:84–97, 2012.
Jorgenson MR, DePestel DD, Carver PL: Ceftaroline fosamil: a novel broad-spectrum cephalosporin with activity against methicillin-resistant *Staphylococcus aureus*, *Ann Pharmacother* 45(11):1384–1398, 2011.
Kachrimanidou M, Malisiovas N: Clostridium difficile infection: a comprehensive review, *Crit Rev Microbiol* 37(3): 178–187, 2011.
Nathwani D, Wood MJ: Penicillins: A current review of their clinical pharmacology and therapeutic use, *Drugs* 45(6): 866–894, 1993.
Roberts MC: Tetracycline therapy: update, *Clin Infect Dis* 36(4):462–467, 2003.
Wolfson JS, Hooper DC: Fluoroquinolone antimicrobial agents, *Clin Microbiol Rev* 2(4):378–424, 1989.
Zhanel GG, Dueck M, Hoban DJ, et al: Review of macrolides and ketolides: focus on respiratory tract infections, *Drugs* 61(4):443–498, 2001.
Zhanel GG, Wiebe R, Dilay L, et al: Comparative review of the carbapenems, *Drugs* 67(7):1027–1052, 2007.
Zinner SH, Mayer KH: Sulfonamides and trimethoprim. In *Mandell, Douglas, and Bennett's Principles and Practice of Infectious Diseases*, ed 7, Philadelphia, 2009, Churchill Livingstone, pp 475–486.

CHAPTER 5

SNORING AND OBSTRUCTIVE SLEEP APNEA

Masayoshi Takashima, MD and Sarah A. Gitomer, MD

KEY POINTS

1. History and physical exam can help differentiate between snoring and sleep apnea. A thorough history and physical, input from a bed partner, and the Epworth Sleepiness Scale can help determine which patients need further diagnostic workup, such as polysomnography.
2. OSA is a major problem in the United States with serious health complications. Although noninvasive treatments such as CPAP are readily available, compliance with these is highly variable. For this reason, surgery may be an excellent option for many patients with OSA.
3. Identification of the site of airway obstruction should be performed prior to any attempted OSA surgery. Drug induced sleep endoscopy may help define the site of obstruction. There are a wide variety of surgical techniques used in the treatment of OSA. Surgery should be tailored for each patient based on anatomic variations, severity of sleep apnea, and patient preference.

Pearls

1. Elevated risk factors for OSA
   a. Age greater than 65 years
   b. Body mass index (BMI) greater than 30 kg/m^2
   c. Postmenopausal female
   d. African American or Asian race
   e. Male gender
   f. Neck circumference greater than 17 inches in men and 16 inches in women
2. Although the severity of OSA is frequently associated with obesity, a thin patient may also have severe OSA.
3. OSA patients most likely to respond best to surgical therapy are those with “kissing” or 4+ tonsils.
4. Tracheotomy remains the gold standard in the treatment of OSA. It bypasses the upper airway entirely and is effective in almost all patients, including those with severe disease.
5. Patients with craniofacial anomalies frequently require correction of their skeletal deformity prior to soft tissue surgery for treatment of their OSA.

QUESTIONS

1. **What is the difference between snoring and obstructive sleep apnea (OSA)? What about sleep disordered breathing (SDB)? Upper airway resistance syndrome (UARS)?**

   Snoring is simply noisy breathing during sleep that occurs due to the vibration of lax tissue in the upper airway. SDB is characterized by snoring along with symptoms suggestive of OSA, including daytime somnolence and snoring. Sleep disordered breathing exists along a continuum of severity. UARS presents with symptoms of OSA without meeting the criteria of OSA as determined by the apnea hypopnea index (AHI) and/or respiratory disturbance index (RDI). OSA, the most severe form of SDB, affects quality of life and is potentially life threatening. OSA is defined by AHI or RDI greater than 5 during sleep as revealed by polysomnography. OSA is caused by upper airway tissue collapse resulting in airway obstruction.

2. **How common is snoring? What about sleep apnea?**
Snoring is very common across the population. Based on self-report and questionnaires, 40% of middle-aged men and 28% of middle-aged women snore. This increases to as high as 84% and 73%, respectively, in the seventh decade of life. It is estimated that as many as 3% to 7% of men and 2% to 5% of women have OSA. It has been shown that the prevalence is even higher in obese, senior, postmenopausal, and minority populations. The risk of OSA is higher when a person has a close relative (parent, child, sibling) with OSA.

3. **What causes snoring? OSA?**
Snoring is caused by variations in airflow across dynamic portions of the upper airway, which results in vibrations of the soft tissues. Most commonly, it occurs in the area of the uvula, soft palate, tonsillar pillars, and/or pharyngeal walls. Occasionally, it may also occur at the base of tongue. OSA occurs secondary to collapse at the anatomic levels mentioned above but also may occur due to obstruction by the lingual tonsils or epiglottis. Obesity often contributes to snoring and apnea because of increased weight of the neck tissues, increased fat in the parapharyngeal space that narrows the pharynx, redundancy in the soft palate, and fullness in the tongue base.

4. **What is obstructive sleep apnea (OSA)?**
OSA refers to a collection of conditions and syndromes that have periods of *apnea*, a temporary cessation of breathing (defined as intermittent cessation of airflow during sleep that lasts 10 seconds or longer), as key occurrences. It was initially described in the early 1800s. One of the first accounts was written by Charles Dickens in 1837 and entitled *The Posthumous Papers of the Pickwick Club*. Subsequently, William Osler coined the term “pickwickian” in 1918 to describe the obese, hypersomnolent patient. The pathogenesis and pathophysiology of OSA have been studied extensively. During sleep, the upper airway becomes occluded, resulting in an episode of obstructive apnea. As a result, the patient experiences a brief arousal from sleep. With the return of breathing, the patient typically returns to sleep quickly. This sequence is repeated over and over.

5. **What are the subclassifications of sleep apnea?**
Over the years, various sleep apnea syndromes have been described and classified into three main types: *central, obstructive,* and *mixed.* Central sleep apnea refers to apnea with origins in the central nervous system. Obstructive sleep apnea refers to apnea due primarily to collapse of the upper airway during sleep. Mixed apnea refers to apnea with both central and obstructive characteristics. Of the three main types of apneas, OSA is the most common and has received the most scientific interest and study.

6. **What are common symptoms of obstructive sleep apnea?**
Snoring, restless sleep, witnessed episodes of choking or gasping for air while sleeping, excessive daytime somnolence, morning headaches, nocturia, changes in mood (depression, irritability, anxiety, aggression), poor concentration, memory loss, night sweats, bruxism.

7. **What medical comorbidities can predispose to sleep apnea?**
   - **Hypothyroidism:** There appears to be a link between hypothyroidism and OSA beyond increased BMI alone. It is thought that mucoprotein and hyaluronic acid deposition in the upper airway may be related to increased airway compression. Treating underlying hypothyroidism often improves sleep apnea independent from weight change or pulmonary function.
   - **Acromegaly:** Tongue enlargement and skeletal changes including increased head size can also impact the airway and predispose patients to OSA.
   - **Obesity:** Obesity is very common in the OSA population. Although being overweight is not necessary for OSA, truncal obesity predisposes patients to sleep apnea. In patients with a small airway diameter at baseline, even a modest weight gain can cause OSA.
   - **Gastro-esophageal reflux disease (GERD):** GERD is commonly present alongside OSA. Changing intrathoracic pressures and obesity predispose to reflux and the inflammation caused by untreated GERD has been shown to worsen sleep apnea.
   - **Polycystic ovarian syndrome:** Hormone dysregulation in PCOS can lead to increased frequency of apneic episodes in women with anatomic predisposition for pharyngeal collapse. Hormonal changes associated with postmenopausal women have also been shown to cause higher incidences of OSA.

8. **What medical complications can arise if OSA is untreated?**
Systemic hypertension, myocardial infarction, vascular accidents, congestive heart failure, cor pulmonale, atherosclerosis, atrial fibrillation, ventricular arrhythmias, pulmonary hypertension, glaucoma, decreased seizure threshold, diminished libido, death

9. **What are the medical consequences of OSA in children?**
   - ADHD
   - Growth delay
   - Nocturnal enuresis

10. **An in-office clinical exam of the snoring and OSA patient should include what?**
A complete head and neck examination should be performed. The nose should be examined for signs of obstruction due to a deviated septum, hypertrophic turbinates or allergic rhinitis. Frequently, improving nasal congestion will decrease the intensity and frequency of snoring. Examination of the oral cavity may reveal potential obstruction due to large tonsils, redundant soft palate and uvula, redundant lateral pharyngeal walls, and/or a full base of the tongue. Patients may also have a high arched hard palate, retrognathia, and micrognathia. The Friedman tongue position classification system can be used together with BMI and tonsil size to predict patients' response to uvulopalatopharyngoplasty (UPPP) and a tonsillectomy (Figure 5-1). The system grades the view of the uvula and tonsillar pillars while the patient opens his or her mouth with the tongue in a neutral position. Higher grades are associated with better response to UPPP. Müller's maneuver may be helpful in confirming the diagnosis and the site of obstruction (Figure 5-2).

11. **What is Müller's maneuver?**
Müller's maneuver is performed as part of an extensive physical examination and involves passing a flexible fiber-optic scope from the nose into the hypopharynx to obtain a view of the entire hypopharynx and larynx. The examiner then pinches the nostrils closed, and the patient closes his or her lips while attempting to inhale. If the hypopharynx and/or larynx collapse, then the test result is positive. A positive test helps delineate the location of antomic obstruction which occurs with OSA.

12. **How is OSA diagnosed?**
The gold standard for diagnosing OSA is an in-lab monitored polysomnography. The history and physical, along with supplementary studies such as the Epworth Sleepiness Scale (ESS), help identify patients who would benefit from a sleep study to diagnose sleep apnea. Sleep studies measure brain activity, leg muscle movements, cardiac rhythm, eye movements, oxygen saturation, respiratory effort, and air movement at the nose and mouth. Polysomnography can differentiate between snoring without OSA, pure OSA, and central sleep apnea and can characterize the severity of the apnea. This test requires the patient to spend a night in a formal sleep laboratory. Portable monitoring devices for home sleep studies, which are not as comprehensive as in-lab studies, have recently been approved by the Center for Medicare and Medicaid Services (CMS) as appropriate for the diagnosis of OSA.

13. **What defines obstructive sleep apnea on polysomnography in adults? What is the difference between AHI and RDI?**
The diagnostic criteria for OSA is an apnea-hypopnea index (AHI) greater than 5 or a respiratory disturbance index (RDI) greater than 5. AHI is defined as the number of obstructive apneic or hypopneic episodes a patient has per hour. On polysomnography, obstructive apnea is defined as cessation of airflow due to anatomic airway obstruction for 10 seconds and hypopnea is defined as reduction in ventilation by at least 30% of baseline for 10 seconds associated with at least a 4% oxygen desaturation. RDI is similar to AHI but also includes respiratory effort related arousals (RERAs). RERAs do not fulfill the criteria of an apnea or hypopnea but still result in an arousal from sleep. AHI or RDI between 5 and 15 is considered mild OSA, 16 to 30 is moderate OSA, and any number greater than 30 is considered severe OSA.

14. **Are sleep studies always used in children?**
Formal sleep studies are not done as often in children as in adults. Some physicians use 24-hour pulse oximetry or sleep sonography, which is recording of nocturnal breathing sounds. Usually a history and physical (usually large tonsils and adenoids) consistent with OSA are enough to make a surgical decision for a child. Other causes of sleep disturbed breathing include nasopharyngeal

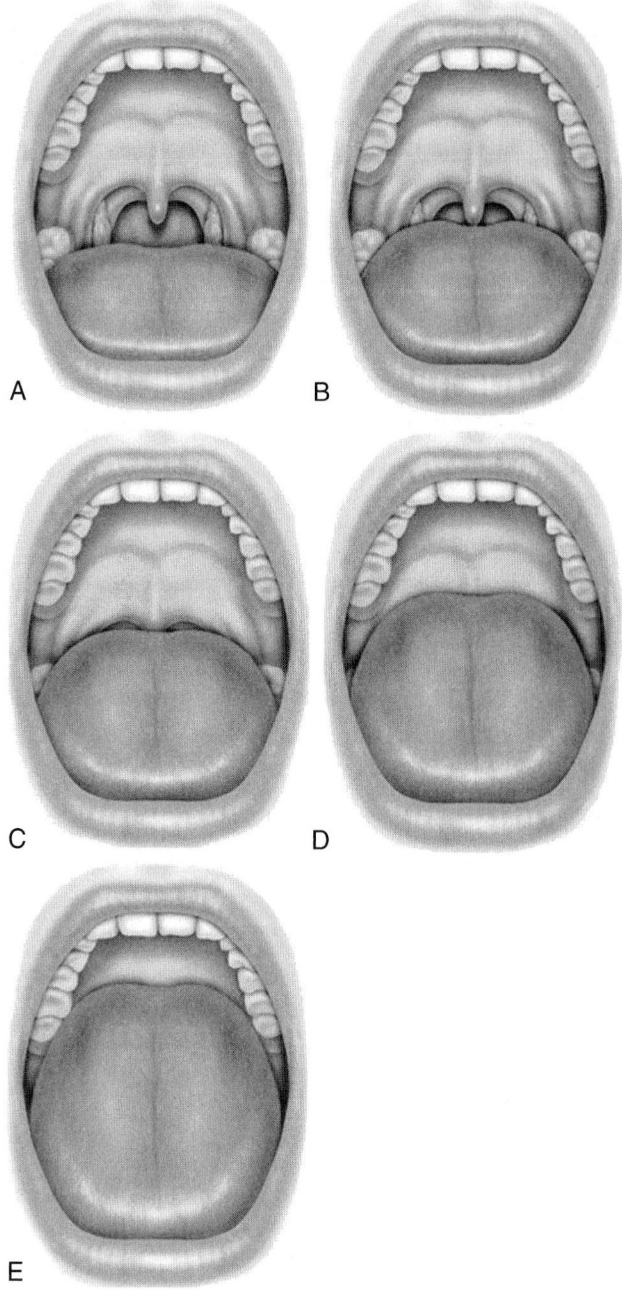

Figure 5-1. Friedman tongue position. **A)** I: visualization of the entire uvula and tonsils/pillars. **B)** IIa: visualization of most of the uvula, but tonsils/pillars are absent. **C)** IIb: visualization of the entire soft palate to the base of the uvula. **D)** III: visualization of some of the soft palate, but structures distal to this are not seen. **E)** IV: visualization of the hard palate only. *(Reprint permission obtained from Dr. Michael Friedman.)*

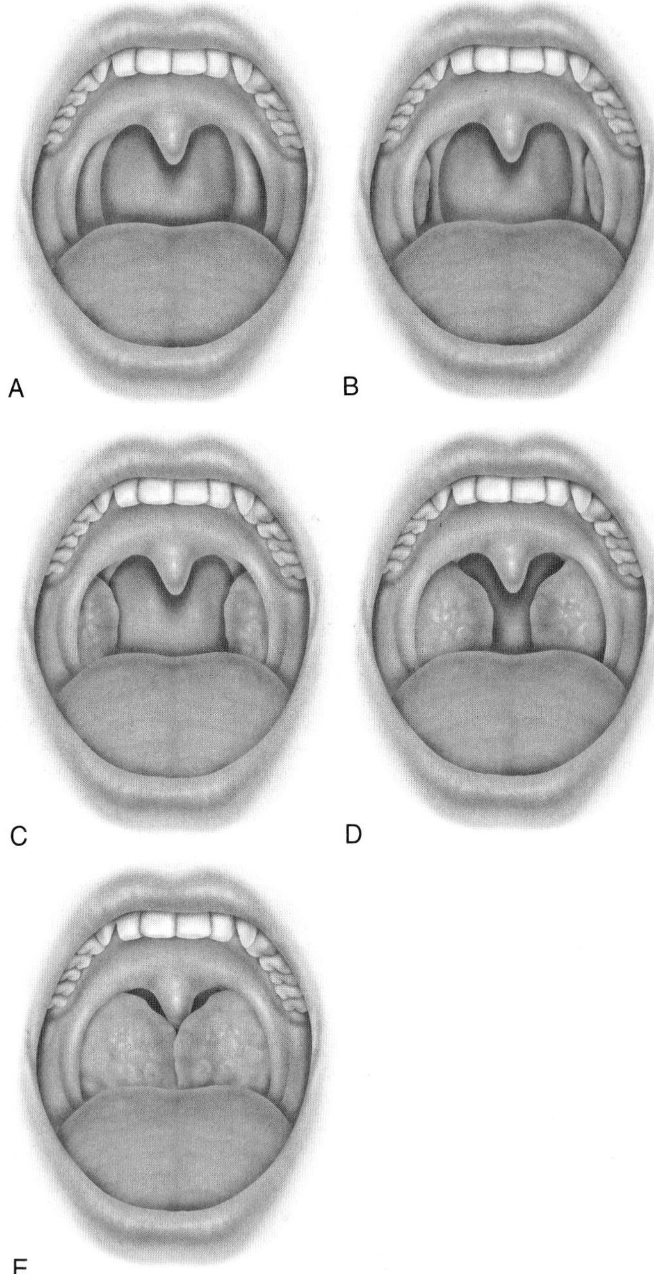

Figure 5-2. **A)** Tonsil grade 0, post surgical; **B)** Tonsil grade 1; **C)** Tonsil grade 2; **D)** Tonsil grade 3; **E)** Tonsil grade 4. *(Reprint permission obtained from Dr. Michael Friedman.)*

cysts, encephaloceles, choanal atresia, a deviated nasal septum, and craniofacial or orthodontic malformations. When in doubt, a formal sleep study is still indicated.

15. **Describe the classic sleep pattern seen in OSA.**
Typically, OSA patients exhibit a quick onset of sleep and multiple arousals. The patient maintains relatively more stage I and II sleep and less stage III, IV, and rapid eye movement (REM) sleep. This lack of deep sleep results in the symptoms of sleep deprivation.

16. **During which stage of sleep do most obstructive events occur?**
Most obstructive events occur during the deeper stages of sleep, including stages III and IV and REM sleep. It is during these stages that muscles are most relaxed, and thus upper airway collapse is most likely. OSA patients are therefore being deprived of deep sleep. This explains the restless sleep patterns and daytime somnolence. In fact, the hallmark of successful treatment of OSA is REM rebound, or a significant increase in REM sleep (clinical increase in dreaming) due to correction of previous sleep deprivation.

17. **Should everyone who snores undergo a sleep study?**
When snoring is accompanied by symptoms of OSA, such as hypersomnolence, morning headache, and restless sleep, a thorough examination and sleep study are indicated. When snoring is socially disruptive but not accompanied by symptoms of sleep apnea, the picture is not so clear. Unfortunately, even "apneas" witnessed by bed partners may not be predictive of OSA. The only reasonably accurate method of detecting OSA remains the formal sleep study. Therefore, current recommendations suggest obtaining a sleep study prior to any surgery for sleep apnea or snoring.

18. **What are some treatments for snoring?**
Weight loss, tonsillectomy, and improving nasal breathing are the most common treatments for snoring because they decrease vibrations of the soft palate. Stiffening of the soft palate can also be accomplished with a variety of techniques. The standard technique, UPPP, can be completed with cold steel, Bovie, or coblation. Another, in-office procedure under local anesthesia is laser-assisted uvulopalatoplasty (LAUP), which causes soft palate scarring by a laser burn and is accomplished in multiple stages. A newer advancement in palate surgery is submucosal radiofrequency ablation which can also be a staged palatal scarring/stiffening in-office procedure. Snoreplasty involves sclerosants injected into the palate to cause scarring and shrinkage, which will also result in palatal stiffening. Placement of soft palate pillar woven polyester implants may also be performed to treat snoring.

19. **What are conservative, nonsurgical management options for treating OSA?**
    - Reducing or eliminating alcohol or sedatives as they may cause excess relaxation of tissues which may exacerbate soft tissue collapse.
    - Treatment of underlying medical conditions: antireflux medications, thyroid replacement, hormone replacement therapy.
    - Weight loss has been shown to result in improvement in OSA severity.
    - Continuous positive airway pressure (CPAP) involves the administration of air through the nose or mouth by an external device at a fixed pressure. The pressure of the airflow stents the airway open, particularly during the inspiratory phase when negative pressure would otherwise cause the pharyngeal walls to collapse. Bi-level positive airway pressure (BiPAP) is similar to CPAP, but these devices are capable of generating a second, lower level of pressure during expiration that improves patient comfort.
    - There are also multiple types of dental appliances that can be used to treat mild sleep disordered breathing and snoring. These devices target mandibular advancement or tongue positioning.
    - Changing the position that patients sleep in is another conservative technique that can improve mild symptoms as many people have worse OSA when supine.

20. **What minimally invasive procedures are available for treating sleep apnea?**
    - **Pillar procedure:** Under local anesthetic, one midline and two lateral woven polyester implants are implanted into the muscle of the soft palate.
    - **Tongue base suspension:** A titanium screw attached to a suture is inserted into the inner table of the mandibular symphysis. The suture is then passed through the base of the tongue to suspend the tongue base, effectively preventing collapse of the base of tongue.

- **Radiofrequency ablation (RFA) of the palate and tongue base** to increase tissue stiffness can be performed in the office. It may require multiple sessions to achieve adequate soft tissue reduction.
- **RFA of the inferior turbinates** can be performed in the office to improve nasal airflow and decrease nasal resistance. By improving airflow through the nose and decreasing upper airway resistance, the patient may also become more tolerant to the use of a CPAP because the pressure requirements of the machine also decrease.

21. Why would you recommend surgery over CPAP alone?

CPAP can be uncomfortable, and it is recognized that there is a low compliance rate over time. Some patients are unable to tolerate CPAP even after desensitization. This may be due to claustrophobia, inability to sleep supine, or the inadvertent removal of the CPAP while sleeping. Patients with a high nasal bridge also suffer from frequent air leaks associated with an inadequate mask seal. Nasal surgery to decrease airway resistance can make wearing nasal CPAP more tolerable by decreasing the required pressures. Younger patients typically have a lower compliance rate in using CPAP than older adults, especially if they are dating or live in a college dormitory. Patients who frequently travel overseas to countries with undeveloped electrical utility may also be better surgical candidates. Children with OSA have a high cure rate with a tonsillectomy and adenoidectomy alone.

22. If surgery is indicated, how do you select the operation to be performed?

Surgery is effective in treating snoring and less effective in treating sleep apnea. The challenge confronting the surgeon is to know what part of the upper airway is causing the obstruction to airflow. There are multiple possible sites, and conventional sleep testing does not usually identify the area the surgeon should modify. If the surgeon treats the wrong part of the airway, or if there are multiple sites of obstruction, it is less likely that sleep apnea will improve to a degree at which no other treatment is needed. Given the several sites where airway obstruction may exist, a diagnostic drug induced sleep endoscopy to identify the site of obstruction while the patient is asleep may be helpful. There are several types of operations currently used to treat sleep apnea. The most common is UPPP. The success rate of this operation is about 50%. Some surgeons have achieved very high success rates using multiple, staged operations.

- **Nose:** Nasal obstruction can be treated by septoplasty, turbinate reduction, and sinus surgery, if appropriate.
- **Adenoids:** Adenoidectomy in children is often done. It is 80% to 90% effective, often in conjunction with tonsillectomy, for improving nasal airway, snoring, and apnea in children. This operation is rarely necessary in adults.
- **Tonsils:** Tonsillectomy for tonsillar hypertrophy. In adults with OSA, tonsillectomy is often done as part of a UPPP.
- **Palate:** Palate reduction can be achieved by snoreplasty (sclerosants injected into the palate to cause scarring and shrinkage), laser-assisted uvulopalatoplasty (LAUP), submucosal radiofrequency device, electrocautery (termed "Bovie-assisted uvulopalatoplasty" or BAUP), or UPPP (or "U-triple-P").
- **Tongue base:** Transoral robotic surgery, coblation or radiofrequency tongue base reduction, lag screw and suture suspension of the tongue and hyoid, advancement genioplasty combined with a hyoid suspension, distraction osteogenesis, partial midline glossectomy, and maxillomandibular advancement are used to reduce obstruction at the tongue base.
- Most authorities recommend a repeat polysomnogram 3 months after surgery.

23. What is a drug induced sleep endoscopy (DISE)?

It is hard to predict which patients are likely to have a successful surgical outcome. Part of the reason is the difficulty associated with accurately identifying the site(s) of obstruction. Sleep endoscopy, a relatively new technique, helps define this better. Patients are examined in a drug induced sleep-resembling relaxed state. A flexible fiber-optic scope is passed through the nose to evaluate the upper airway to reveal the site of obstruction. This enables the surgeon to adequately address those sites while preserving areas that are not involved. The data on the validity of this procedure are scant yet promising, but this procedure may not be widely available in all areas.

24. What is UPPP? What are the complications associated with it?

Uvulopalatopharyngoplasty or "U triple-P" is the most commonly performed surgical procedure for OSA. It has the best outcomes for patients with retropharyngeal collapse that have mild to moderate sleep apnea. Under general anesthesia, the tonsils are removed along with a portion of the anterior and posterior pillars, and part of the soft palate. The remaining tonsillar pillars are sutured together and the uvula is shortened. The operation decreases the amount of soft tissue collapse in the oropharynx, and as such, it is most successful for patients with isolated palatal collapse. The efficacy of UPPP alone in improving AHI over time ranges from 40% to 70%, depending on the patient selection. Bleeding is by far the most common postoperative complication, occasionally requiring another visit to the operating room for control. Transient velopharyngeal insufficiency with nasal regurgitation occurs in 5% to 10% of patients but is rarely permanent. Nasopharyngeal stenosis is a very rare but devastating complication in which the nasopharynx scars down completely. Patients may also complain of dry mouth, tightness in the throat, increased gag reflex, and/or change in taste; however, these symptoms are usually transient.

25. **What are some new directions for OSA surgery?**
Pharmacologic treatments for obesity have recently been FDA approved as a prescription weight loss medication, and outcomes with bariatric surgery are being explored. Transoral robotic surgery (TORS) is becoming more popular for base of tongue reduction for OSA. The benefits of using the robot include improved visualization and instrument access. However, this surgical approach is limited to centers that have a robotic system, and remains expensive compared to more standard procedures. There are only preliminary data currently available about this technique, and outcomes data comparing this to more standard techniques are lacking. Hypoglossal nerve stimulators are a newer technique aimed at increasing the tone of the tongue during inspiration and, though limited, early data show promise.

CONTROVERSIES

1. Questions exists as to the usefulness of the Müller's maneuver as this is a test performed while the patient is awake with good tone as opposed to when asleep with less muscle tone.
2. There currently exist two different but accepted definitions of hypopnea.
   a. Recommended:
      i. Ventilation drop by ≥30% of pre-event baseline.
      ii. The duration of the ≥30% drop in signal excursion is ≥10 seconds.
      iii. There is a ≥3% oxygen desaturation from pre-event baseline and/or the event is associated with an arousal.
   b. Alternate version:
      i. Ventilation drops by ≥30% of pre-event baseline.
      ii. The duration of the ≥30% drop in signal excursion is ≥10 seconds.
      iii. There is a ≥4% oxygen desaturation from pre-event baseline.

Bibliography

Clinical indicators: palatopharyngoplasty for obstructive sleep apnea. American Academy of Otolaryngolgy–Head and Neck Surgery. Aug 7, 2014. Apr 11, 2015. http://www.entnet.org/sites/default/files/UPPP-CI%20Updated%208-7-14.pdf.

Friedman M, Ibrahim H, Bass L: Clinical staging for sleep-disordered breathing, *Otolaryngol Head Neck Surg* 127:13–21, 2002.

Hohenhorst W, Ravesloot MJL, Kezirian EJ, et al: Drug-induced sleep endoscopy in adults with sleep-disordered breathing: technique and the VOTE classification system, *Oper Tech Otolaryngol Head Neck Surg* 23(1):11–18, 2012.

Katsantonis GP: Uvulopalatopharyngoplasty for obstructive sleep apnea and snoring, *Oper Tech Otolaryngol Head Neck Surg* 2(2):100–103, 1991.

Punjabi NM: The epidemiology of adult obstructive sleep apnea, *Proc Am Thorac Soc* 5(2):136–143, 2008.

Strollo PJ Jr, Soose RJ, Maurer JT, et al: Upper-airway stimulation for obstructive sleep apnea, *N Engl J Med* 370(2):139–149, 2014.

Terris DJ: Multilevel pharyngeal surgery for obstructive sleep apnea: indications and techniques, *Oper Tech Otolaryngol Head Neck Surg* 11:12–20, 2000.

Walker RP: Chapter 46: Snoring and Obstructive Sleep Apnea. In Bailey BJ, Johnson JT, Newlands SD, editors: *Head & neck surgery–otolaryngology*, ed 4, Philadelphia, 2006, Lippincott Williams & Wilkins, pp 645–665.

Weaver EM, Maynard C, Yueh B: Survival of veterans with sleep apnea: continuous positive airway pressure vs. surgery, *Otolaryngol Head Neck Surg* 130:659–665, 2004.

Young T, Palta M, Dempsey J, et al: The occurrence of sleep-disordered breathing among middle-aged adults, *N Engl J Med* 328:1230–1235, 1993.

CHAPTER 6

GRANULOMATOUS AND AUTOIMMUNE DISEASES OF THE HEAD AND NECK

Victor I. Scapa, MD

KEY POINTS

1. Many systemic autoimmune and granulomatous diseases may initially present with sinonasal symptoms. Refractory or severe disease should raise suspicion for possible granulomatous disease.
2. A detailed history, careful exam, and high index of suspicion may allow the otolaryngologist an opportunity to diagnosis a systemic inflammatory process earlier in the disease course, thus allowing the patient to receive more timely treatment.
3. Careful histopathologic review as well as laboratory evaluation may further assist in establishing a diagnosis.
4. Appropriate medical treatment is critical for systemic autoimmune or granulomatous disease. Surgical intervention is usually reserved for select cases/indications.

Pearls

1. Sarcoidosis demonstrates noncaseating granulomas on histology and may be associated with hilar lymphadenopathy and an elevated serum angiotensin-converting enzyme (ACE) level.
2. Granulomatosis with polyangiitis (GPA) involves the formation of necrotizing granulomas and is associated with cytoplasmic-staining anti-neutrophil cytoplasmic antibody (c-ANCA) positivity. Up to 16% of patients may develop subglottic stenosis.
3. Churg-Strauss syndrome (CSS) is a systemic vasculitic disorder featuring eosinophilia, asthma, and sinonasal disease. Eosinophilic myocarditis and coronary artery vasculitis are the leading causes of death for patients.
4. Bacterial granulomatous diseases of the nose and sinuses may include rhinoscleroma, tuberculosis, leprosy, syphilis, and actinomycosis.
5. *Mucor* species demonstrate nonseptate, wide-angled branching hyphae on histology in contrast to *Aspergillus* species, which display septate hyphae with 45-degree branching angles.

QUESTIONS

1. What is sarcoidosis?
   Sarcoidosis is a systemic inflammatory disease leading to noncaseating granuloma formation. Although pulmonary manifestations are most common, multiple organs may be affected including the liver, skin, heart, and eyes. A small percentage of patients may experience central nervous system involvement, a condition known as neurosarcoidosis. Head and neck disease occurs in 10% to 15% of patients. Symptoms may include nasal crusting, hyposmia, postnasal drip, epistaxis, sinus infections, nasal obstruction, parotid gland enlargement, xerostomia, and uveitis. Sarcoidosis may also affect the supraglottic larynx causing cough, hoarseness, and dyspnea. The cause of sarcoidosis is not well understood. Etiologic factors may include genetic predisposition, infectious agents, or occupational exposure. This disease more commonly affects African American populations

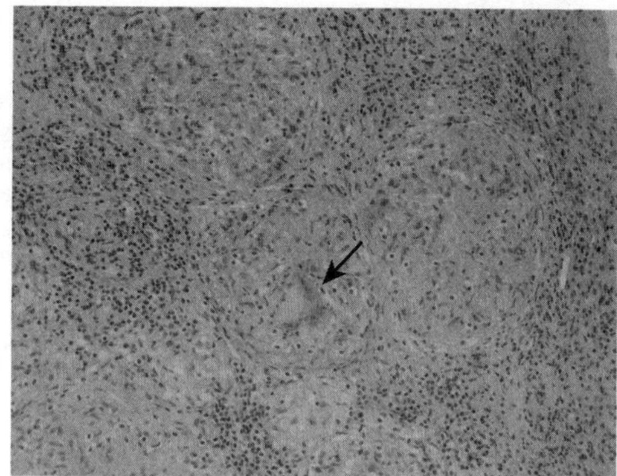

Figure 6-1. Sinonasal sarcoidosis. Biopsy demonstrating noncaseating granuloma formation. The arrow highlights a multinucleated giant cell. Hematoxylin and eosin stain, original magnification ×10.

with most diagnoses occurring between the ages of 20 and 40. The clinical course may range from spontaneous resolution to severe, long-standing disease.

2. What physical findings and laboratory results may be suggestive of sarcoidosis?
Physical examination may reveal inflamed sinonasal mucosa and polypoid changes. More advanced sinonasal disease may present with septal perforation, saddle-nose deformity, or submucosal pearly nodules. Diagnosis of sarcoidosis requires excluding other potential causes of granulomatous inflammation, including infectious causes. Tissue biopsy demonstrates noncaseating granuloma formation with multinucleated giant cell formation (Figure 6-1). Serum angiotensin-converting enzyme (ACE) may be elevated, as well as serum or urine calcium levels (due to increased activation of vitamin D within granulomas). Hilar lymphadenopathy is a common finding on chest radiographs.

3. How is sarcoidosis treated?
Sinonasal sarcoidosis is usually treated with nasal irrigations, topical nasal steroids, and potentially intralesional steroid injections. Endoscopic sinus surgery may be considered for medically refractive disease in select patients with chronic sinusitis and sarcoidosis. Severe sarcoidosis may require treatment with systemic steroids or other immune-modulating drugs such as methotrexate, azathioprine, or cyclophosphamide.

4. What is Heerfordt syndrome?
Heerfordt syndrome is a rare form of sarcoidosis presenting with parotid gland enlargement, uveitis, facial nerve palsy, and fever.

5. Describe granulomatosis with polyangiitis.
Granulomatosis with polyangiitis (GPA) is a systemic vasculitic disease and was previously known as Wegener granulomatosis. While the cause of GPA is not well understood, the disease is believed to be autoimmune mediated. Many patients will present with sinonasal complaints including congestion, pain, epistaxis, crusting, and foul-smelling discharge. Examination reveals inflamed, erythematous mucosa with possible crusting. Septal perforation is a common finding and saddle-nose deformity may occur in more severe cases. Other head and neck manifestations of GPA can include gingival hyperplasia, hearing loss (conductive or sensorineural), nasolacrimal duct obstruction, and conjunctivitis. Up to 16% of patients may develop subglottic stenosis. Childhood onset of GPA increases the likelihood of subglottic stenosis. Pulmonary involvement and progressive glomerulonephritis may cause significant morbidity.

6. How is GPA diagnosed and treated?
Histologic examination of suspicious lesions reveals necrotizing granulomas, inflammatory cells, and multinucleated giant cells. Small and medium-sized blood vessels undergo vasculitic changes. Laboratory evaluation demonstrates elevated C-reactive protein (CRP) and erythrocyte sedimentation rate (ESR). A positive cytoplasmic-staining anti-neutrophil cytoplasmic antibody (c-ANCA) is associated with GPA. Greater than 90% of patients diagnosed with GPA are white, with male and female patients being equally affected. Medical treatment involves corticosteroids and other immune-modulating drugs such as cyclophosphamide, azathioprine, or methotrexate. Surgical

treatment of subglottic stenosis or tracheostomy may be necessary for patients with airway compromise.

7. **Which sinonasal granulomatous disease is associated with eosinophilia?**
Churg-Strauss syndrome (CSS) is a systemic vasculitic disorder featuring eosinophilia, asthma, and sinonasal disease. Early stages of the disease present with asthma and sinonasal symptoms, including crusting, rhinorrhea, nasal obstruction, and nasal polyp formation. Later stages of the disease are marked by hypereosinophilia and vasculitis. Symptoms associated with advanced disease may include weight loss, fever, malaise, night sweats, and gastrointestinal involvement. Eosinophilic myocarditis or coronary artery vasculitis are the leading causes of death for patients with CSS. Tissue biopsy reveals necrotizing vasculitis affecting small to medium-sized vessels as well as eosinophilic granulomas. Laboratory evaluation may demonstrate elevated CRP, ESR, and eosinophilia. Perinuclear anti-neutrophil cytoplasmic antibody (p-ANCA) testing may be positive as well. Sinonasal disease is usually treated with nasal irrigations and topical nasal steroids. Endoscopic sinus surgery and nasal polypectomy may be necessary to provide symptomatic relief. Treatment of CSS typically includes systemic corticosteroids and potentially other immune-modulating drugs.

8. **Which autoimmune disorder prominently features xerostomia, xerophthalmia, and xerorhinia?**
Sjögren syndrome is a chronic autoimmune disease that targets exocrine glands leading to decreased salivary and lacrimal function. Frequent presenting symptoms may include parotid enlargement, xerostomia, xerophthalmia, and xerorhinia. Patients affected by Sjögren syndrome are more commonly female than male and have a higher incidence of non-Hodgkin lymphoma compared to the general population. Laboratory testing for anti-SS-A/Ro and anti-SS-B/La antibodies may be positive. Minor salivary gland biopsy is performed at times to establish a diagnosis. Histologic confirmation of Sjögren syndrome requires at least one aggregate of >50 lymphocytes in a 4-mm^2 region of salivary gland tissue. Treatment of head and neck symptoms is symptomatic and may include the use of humidifiers, artificial saliva products, sialogogues, and nasal saline irrigations. Systemic pilocarpine and cevimeline can be used to treat xerostomia but are associated with many adverse effects. Sialoendoscopy is a potential treatment option for patients with recurrent parotitis associated with Sjögren syndrome.

9. **How might systemic lupus erythematosus affect the head and neck?**
Systemic lupus erythematosus (SLE) is a chronic autoimmune disease that may affect multiple organ systems. Head and neck presenting symptoms may include oral ulcerations and a malar rash. Nasal mucosal involvement is possible with some reports of nasal septal perforation as well. Glottic bamboo nodules have been identified in patients with SLE, as well as other autoimmune diseases such as rheumatoid arthritis and Sjögren syndrome. The majority of affected patients are female and the clinical course is variable, ranging from mild cases to severe, fatal disease. Immune complex deposition is a prominent feature of SLE.

10. **Which autoimmune disease may present with episodic auricular and nasal swelling?**
Relapsing polychondritis is a rare autoimmune disorder directed at the cartilaginous tissues of the ears, nose, and airway. Symptoms are typically episodic in nature. Auricular chondritis is the most common manifestation of this disease, causing lobule-sparing erythema and swelling of the auricles. Nasal chondritis is also relatively common, leading to recurrent episodes of nasal pain and erythema. Long-standing disease may lead to saddle-nose deformity and nasal collapse. Severe airway involvement may require tracheal stent placement or tracheostomy. Medical treatment involves the use of systemic corticosteroids and potentially other immune-modulating drugs.

11. **What is Behçet syndrome?**
Behçet is an autoimmune small-vessel vasculitic disease characterized by recurrent oral aphthous ulcers, genital ulcers, and uveitis. More advanced disease may affect the central nervous system, gastrointestinal tract, kidneys, or extremity joints. Coronary artery thrombosis as well as pulmonary artery aneurysms may also occur. Sporadic cases of nasal mucosal involvement are reported. Nonspecific inflammatory markers are usually elevated during laboratory evaluation of active disease. Clinical criteria for diagnosis include recurrent oral aphthous ulcers along with two of the following: genital ulcers, skin lesions, ocular lesions, or a positive pathergy test (papule formation in

response to a needle prick). Medical treatment may involve corticosteroids or other immune-modulating drugs.

12. **List bacterial pathogens that may cause granulomatous infections.**
Klebsiella rhinoscleromatis (rhinoscleroma), *Mycobacterium tuberculosis* (tuberculosis), *Mycobacterium leprae* (leprosy), *Treponema pallidum* (syphilis), *Actinomyces* species (actinomycosis), and *Bartonella henselae* (cat-scratch disease).

13. **Describe rhinoscleroma.**
Rhinoscleroma is a chronic granulomatous disease involving the nose and potentially other sites within the upper respiratory tract. The disease is caused by a gram-negative, encapsulated bacillus, *Klebsiella rhinoscleromatis.* Some studies suggest the disease may also involve an inherited genetic predisposition leading to the chronic inflammation. Endemic regions include East Africa, Central and South America, Central Europe, and the Indian subcontinent. The disease is subdivided into three stages: *catarrhal, granulomatous,* and *sclerotic* stages. The catarrhal stage is remarkable for purulent, foul-smelling nasal discharge. Friable, granulomatous masses occur in the second stage. Epistaxis and nasal deformity due to destruction of nasal cartilages may occur. The final stage involves fibrosis of tissues and further deformity. Histologic findings include granuloma formation and *Mikulicz cells*, large histiocytes with intracellular bacilli. Treatment involves long-term antibiotic therapy.

14. **Which head and neck structures may be affected by the acid-fast bacillus *Mycobacterium tuberculosis*?**
Extrapulmonary tuberculosis may affect several different head and neck structures, including the cervical lymph nodes, larynx, middle ear, and nasal cavity. Findings may include cervical lymphadenopathy, laryngeal granulation tissue, refractory otorrhea, or nodular hypertrophy of the nasal mucosa. Histologic examination of affected tissues demonstrates caseating and noncaseating granuloma formation. Positive staining for acid-fast bacilli and culture results are used to confirm diagnosis. Treatment typically involves a prolonged regimen of antituberculosis antibiotics.

15. **What disease does *Mycobacterium leprae* cause?**
Leprosy is a chronic infection caused by the acid-fast bacillus *Mycobacterium leprae.* Most cases involve the nasal mucosa with an early finding of nodular thickening. As the disease progresses, granulomas enlarge and patients may suffer from nasal obstruction and nasal deformity. Diagnosis may be confirmed with tissue biopsy and positive staining for acid-fast bacilli. Treatment involves prolonged regimens of antileprosy drugs, such as dapsone or rifampin.

16. **Which granulomatous disease is caused by a sexually transmitted spirochete?**
Syphilis is a sexually transmitted granulomatous infection caused by the spirochete *Treponema pallidum.* Multiple phases of infection are described: primary, secondary, latent, and tertiary. Primary syphilis involves a painless chancre at the initial site of inoculation. Secondary syphilis occurs weeks later and most frequently involves the skin, mucosal membranes, and lymph nodes. Patients are without active symptoms during the latent phase. Tertiary disease may involve formation of disfiguring gummata. If the nasal septum is involved, patients may develop nasal obstruction, septal perforation, or nasal collapse. Syphilis may also cause sensorineural hearing loss as well as laryngeal disease. Serologic testing for *T. pallidum* or dark-field microscopy may be used to confirm the diagnosis. Penicillin remains the first-line treatment choice for syphilis.

17. **Describe infection caused by the genus *Actinomyces*.**
Multiple species from the genus *Actinomyces* can cause granulomatous infections of the head and neck. The gram-positive, mainly anaerobic bacteria are part of the normal oral flora. Actinomycosis may then develop after dental work, mandible trauma, or due to poor oral hygiene and periodontal disease. Infection may lead to mass formation and abscess. Histologic examination reveals gram-positive branching, filamentous bacteria and sulfur granules. Medical treatment of choice consists of prolonged penicillin therapy. Surgical debridement may be necessary in select cases.

18. **List granulomatous fungal diseases that may occur in the head and neck.**
Multiple fungal granulomatous diseases may occur in the head and neck, including blastomycosis, histoplasmosis, coccidiomycosis, mucormycosis, and aspergillosis. Many of these fungal species may cause severe, life-threatening disease in immunocompromised hosts. In these cases, aggressive use of antifungal medication is indicated.

- **Blastomycosis:** *Blastomyces dermatitidis* infection is endemic in eastern North America. The fungus is present in soil and most commonly affects the lung and skin. Sinonasal involvement is relatively rare. Laryngeal disease may present with progressive hoarseness or aphonia. Fungal staining of sputum or tissues demonstrates spherical, broad-based budding yeast.
- **Histoplasmosis:** *Histoplasma capsulatum* infection is endemic in the central region of the United States, particularly the Ohio River valley. The fungus is present in soil contaminated by bird or bat droppings and infection initially causes nonspecific respiratory symptoms. Head and neck manifestations may result from disseminated disease. Mucosal lesions of the upper aerodigestive tract may resemble carcinoma. Methenamine silver staining reveals macrophages with intracellular oval and round fungi.
- **Coccidiomycosis:** This fungal disease is caused by *Coccidioides immitis* and is sometimes referred to as San Joaquin Valley fever. Endemic regions include parts of the southwest United States, particularly California and Arizona. Pulmonary disease may occur as well as cutaneous disease or disseminated disease. Head and neck involvement has been reported. Methenamine silver staining of sputum or tissues demonstrates spherules filled with small endospores.
- **Mucormycosis:** This fungal disease may be caused by species from the *Mucor*, *Absidia*, or *Rhizopus* genera. These species may cause severe, life-threatening disease in immunocompromised hosts. Poorly controlled diabetic patients are also at risk. Infection frequently involves the nose, paranasal sinuses, orbit, or brain. Anterior rhinoscopy or nasal endoscopy may demonstrate black, necrotic tissues. Invasive nonseptate, wide-angled branching hyphae are visible on tissue biopsy. Prognosis may still be poor despite attempts to reverse the immunocompromised state, aggressive medical treatment, and surgical debridement of affected tissues.
- **Aspergillosis:** This fungal disease may be caused by species from the *Aspergillus* genus. These species may cause noninvasive disease (i.e., sinus fungus balls) or severe, life-threatening disease in immunocompromised hosts. Tissue biopsy demonstrates septate hyphae with 45-degree branching angles.

19. Which infectious disease may present with a friable, strawberry-like polypoid mass?

Rhinosporidiosis is a granulomatous disease caused by *Rhinosporidium seeberi* infection and often presents with a friable, strawberry-like polypoid mass. This disease may affect mucosal membranes including the nose, nasopharynx, oropharynx, larynx, or conjunctiva. Historically classified as a fungus, *R. seeberi* is now believed to be an aquatic protozoan. Although cases have been reported worldwide, most occur in patients living in the Indian subcontinent. Presenting symptoms may including nasal obstruction, epistaxis, rhinorrhea, or foreign body sensation. Histologic evaluation typically shows thick-walled sporangium-like structures, infiltration of immune cells, multinucleated giant cells, and scattered granulomas. Treatment typically includes surgical excision with cauterization at the site of attachment. Medical treatment with antimicrobials (i.e., dapsone) may not be effective and recurrent disease is common.

20. Which parasitic granulomatous disease is transmitted by the bite of a female sandfly?

Multiple protozoan species of the genus *Leishmania* may cause parasitic infection and granulomatous disease known as leishmaniasis. Most disease is transmitted by the bite of an infected female sandfly; human to human transmission is atypical. Cases are concentrated in tropical and subtropical countries. Manifestations include cutaneous disease, mucocutaneous involvement, and disseminated visceral leishmaniasis. Cutanenous findings may include red papules, skin plaques or nodules, or ulcerative lesions. Mucocutaneous disease may affect the nasal septum leading to possible nasal septal perforation or nasal collapse. Diagnosis may be made clinically in endemic regions. Biopsy and culture may help confirm cases of leishmaniasis. Histologic findings include mononuclear inflammatory cells and visualization of Leishman-Donovan bodies, small encapsulated protozoa with peripheral nuclei and a rod-shaped kinetoplast (Figure 6-2). Medical treatment is used to control the disease. Regimens typically include antimonials, amphotericin B, or miltefosine.

21. What is idiopathic midline destructive disease?

Idiopathic midline destructive disease (IMDD) describes a spectrum of neoplastic and nonneoplastic diseases that may present with similar sinonasal complaints as well as nasal or midface collapse.

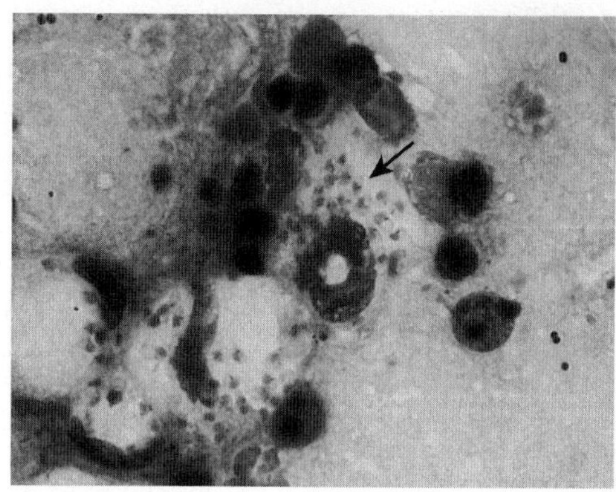

Figure 6-2. Mucocutaneous leishmaniasis/Leishman-Donovan bodies. Biopsy demonstrating small encapsulated protozoa *(arrow)* with peripheral nuclei and a rod-shaped kinetoplast. Giesma stain, oil immersion, original magnification ×100.

Infectious and other nonneoplastic granulomatous conditions that may present in this fashion are previously described throughout this chapter. Sinonasal lymphoma represents the most common neoplastic disease presenting within the IMDD spectrum. Lethal midline granuloma is a historical term that describes this rare and aggressive non-Hodgkin lymphoma variant. This particular sinonasal lymphoma variant is now more accurately referred to as an extranodal natural killer (NK)/T-cell lymphoma.

22. Can intranasal drug abuse lead to granuloma formation?
    Yes, chronic intranasal cocaine or narcotic abuse may lead to granulomatous inflammation as well as local tissue destruction and nasal collapse.

Bibliography

Cantarini L, Vitale A, Brizi MG, et al: Diagnosis and classification of relapsing polychondritis, *J Autoimmun* 48:53–59, 2014.

Ferguson BJ: Mucormycosis of the nose and paranasal sinuses, *Otolaryngol Clin North Am* 33:349–365, 2000.

Fuchs HA, Tanner SB: Granulomatous disorders of the nose and paranasal sinuses, *Curr Opin Otolaryngol Head Neck Surg* 17:23–27, 2009.

Gerber ME, Rosdeutscher JD, Seiden AM, et al: Histoplasmosis: the otolaryngologist's perspective, *Larngoscope* 105: 919–923, 1995.

Justice JM, Soylar AY, Davis KM, et al: Progressive left nasal obstruction and intermittent epistaxis, *JAMA Otolaryngol Head Neck Surg* 139:955–956, 2013.

Kleidermacher P, Vito KJ, Strome M: Otolaryngologic manifestations of acquired syphilis, *Otolarngol Head Neck Surg* 119:399–402, 1998.

Kohanski MA, Reh DD: Granulomatous diseases and chronic sinusitis, *Am J Rhinol Allergy* 27:S39–S41, 2013.

Malinvaud D, Mukundan S, Crevier-Buchman L, et al: Glottic bamboo nodules from systemic lupus erythematosus, *Ann Otol Rhinol Laryngol* 122:496–499, 2013.

Mukara BK, Munyarugamba P, Dazert S, et al: Rhinoscleroma: a case series and review of the literature, *Eur Arch Otorhinolaryngol* 271:1851–1856, 2014.

Nadler C, Enk CD, Leon GT, et al: Diagnosis and management of oral leishmaniasis—case series and literature review, *J Oral Maxillofac Surg* 72:927–934, 2014.

Rucci J, Eisinger G, Miranda-Gomez G, et al: Blastomycosis of the head and neck, *Am J Otolaryngol* 35:390–395, 2014.

Shahram F, Zarandy MM, Ibrahim A, et al: Nasal mucosal involvement in Behçet disease: a study of its incidence and characteristics in 400 patients, *Ear Nose Throat J* 89:30–33, 2010.

Taylor SC, Clayburgh DR, Rosembaum JT, et al: Progression and management of Wegener granulomatosis in the head and neck, *Laryngoscope* 122:1695–1700, 2012.

Turner MD: Salivary gland disease in Sjögren's syndrome: sialoadenitis to lymphoma, *Oral Maxillofac Surg Clin North Am* 26:75–81, 2014.

CHAPTER 7

FACIAL PAIN AND HEADACHE

Benjamin Milam, MD and Vijay R. Ramakrishnan, MD

KEY POINTS

1. Headaches can be classified as primary, secondary, or both. Primary headaches occur in the absence of another disorder known to cause headaches (e.g., tension-type or migraine headache). Secondary headaches occur in the presence of another disorder that is known to cause headaches (e.g., headache attributed to rhinosinusitis).
2. The great majority of patients with "sinus headaches" will meet ICHD (International Classification of Headache Disorders) criteria for migraine disorder.
3. *Cortical spreading depression* is the leading theory for the etiology of migraine disorder. It is a slowly propagated wave of depolarization followed by suppression of brain activity and results in the release of neuropeptide transmitters such as substance P, calcitonin gene-related peptide, and neurokinin A.
4. Patients with temporomandibular disorder can be divided into three groups: myofascial disorder, disc displacement, and arthritis/arthrosis/arthralgia.

Pearls

1. Postherpetic neuralgia occurs in about 25% of patients previously diagnosed with herpes zoster.
2. Tension-type headache is the most common type of headache/facial pain.
3. First-line treatment of persistent idiopathic facial pain is tricyclic antidepressents.
4. Triptans are the first-line medical abortive therapy for migraine disorder.
5. Substance P is a neuropeptide that has been associated with the sensation of pain during a migraine and is released from trigeminocervical axons promoting plasma protein extravasation.

QUESTIONS

1. **What is the difference between primary and secondary headache?**
A headache is labeled a primary headache if it occurs in the absence of a disorder that is known to cause headaches. A secondary headache is a new headache that occurs in close temporal relation to another disorder that is known to cause headache. Headaches can also be categorized as having both primary and secondary components, such as a primary headache that becomes chronic or at least two-fold worsened by another headache-causing disorder.

2. **What is the differential diagnosis for facial pain?**
   - Primary Headache:
     - Tension-type headache
     - Migraine headache
     - Trigeminal autonomic cephalalgias
   - Secondary Headache:
     - Trigeminal neuralgia
     - Persistent idiopathic facial pain
     - Temporomandibular disorder
     - Headache attributed to acute and/or chronic rhinosinusitis
     - Trauma or injury to the head and/or neck
     - Cranial or cervical vascular disorder
     - Neoplasm

- Substance abuse and/or withdrawal
- Intracranial infection
- Somatization disorder
- Headache attributed to disorder of eyes (acute glaucoma, refractive error, heterophoria, heterotropia)
- Psychotic disorder

3. **What is the prevalence of headache?**
Worldwide headache prevalence for the adult population is 46% for headache in general, 42% for tension-type headache, 11% for migraine, and 3% for chronic daily headache. Based on years lived with disability, headaches are one of the 10 most disabling conditions, and one of the five most disabling for women.

4. **How do you diagnose and treat tension-type headache?**
Tension-type headaches are diagnosed by history: episodic headache, typically bilateral, pressing or tightening in quality, of mild to moderate intensity, and lasting minutes to days. The pain does not worsen with routine physical activity and is not associated with nausea. Photophobia or phonophobia may be present. Treatment consists of aspirin, acetaminophen, or NSAIDs for occasional mild tension-type headache while more severe headaches usually require a prescription analgesic. Amitriptyline is the most effective prophylactic pharmaceutical for tension-type headaches.

5. **What is the adult diagnostic criteria for migraine headache without aura?**
For a headache to meet ICHD-III (3rd edition of the International Classification of Headache Disorders) criteria as a migraine without aura, a person must suffer at least five headaches that include the following characteristics: (1) must last between 4-72 hours; (2) have at least two of the following: unilateral location, pulsating quality, moderate/severe pain intensity, or aggravation by physical activity; (3) must have either nausea and/or vomiting or photophobia/phonophobia; (4) must not meet other criteria.

6. **Why do migraine headaches occur?**
Cortical spreading depression (CSD) is the currently accepted etiology for migraine with aura. CSD is a transient neuronal and glial cell excitation followed by long-lasting depression, slowly propagating across the cerebral cortex and gray matter. During CSD, there are significant changes in the levels of extracellular ions and neurotransmitters (such as glutamate, acetylcholine, and substance P), leading to activation of dural nociceptors and central trigeminovascular neurons in the superficial and deep laminae of the trigeminocervical complex contributing to the clinical manifestation of migraines.

7. **What is the first-line medical option for abortive therapy for migraine headache?**
Triptans are the main first-line medical option for abortive therapy for migraines. They are synthetic serotonin analogs that activate the 5-HT_{1B} and 5-HT_{1D} serotonin receptors, constricting cranial blood vessels and inhibiting release of proinflammatory neuropeptides.

8. **Is "sinus headache" recognized as a type of headache?**
The ICHD-III lists "sinus headache" as a type of secondary headache. Specifically, sinus headache has been divided into headache attributed to acute or chronic rhinosinusitis.

9. **Is imaging necessary to diagnose someone with a sinus headache?**
While imaging can help contribute to diagnosing someone with a sinus headache, it is not mandatory. ICHD-III states that headache attributed to rhinosinusitis must demonstrate clinical, endoscopic, and/or imaging evidence of current or past infection or inflammation. In addition, evidence of headache causation is established by at least two of the following: (1) headache with a temporal relation to rhinosinusitis, (2) headache correlates with rhinosinusitis symptoms, (3) headache is exacerbated by pressure over the sinuses, (4) headache localizes to side of rhinosinusitis.

10. **What percentage of patients presenting with complaints of sinus headache will meet IHS for migraine headache syndrome?**
Many patients that have a chief complaint of sinus headache actually fulfill IHS criteria for migraine. One large study screened patients with a history of sinus headache and found that 88% actually fulfilled IHS criteria for migraine-type headache.

11. **Describe the diagnostic criteria and initial management of trigeminal neuralgia.**
Trigeminal neuralgia is characterized by paroxysmal attacks of severe facial pain. Diagnosis is based on five characteristics: (1) paroxysmal, (2) provoked by light touch, (3) confined to the trigeminal distribution, (4) unilateral, (5) normal clinical sensory exam. First-line pharmacotherapy is carbamazepine.

12. **What is the most common division of trigeminal nerve to be affected by post-herpetic trigeminal neuropathy?**
The first division of the trigeminal nerve is most commonly affected in post-herpetic trigeminal neuropathy. However, the second and third divisions can also be involved. Post-herpetic trigeminal neuropathy is unilateral head and/or facial pain persisting or recurring for at least 3 months in the distribution of one or more branches of the trigeminal nerve, with variable sensory changes, caused by herpes zoster. Typically, the pain is burning and may be pruritic. Patients can also have sensory abnormalities and allodynia in the affected territory. Pale or light purple scars may be present as sequelae of the herpetic eruption. Postherpetic neuralgia occurs in about 10% of patients with herpes zoster ophthalmicus. Treatment is difficult and often ineffective. Tricyclic antidepressants, gabapentin, pregabalin, opioids, and lidocaine patches are medical options with inconsistent efficacy. Denervation procedures have been used in the past, but little evidence has supported their use and these have largely been abandoned.

13. **What is persistent idiopathic facial pain?**
Persistent idiopathic facial pain, formerly referred to as atypical facial pain, is a type of secondary headache. It is a type of facial and/or oral pain that occurs in the absence of clinical neurologic deficit and dental etiology. It can have many types of presentations but must recur daily for more than 2 hours per day over greater than 3 months. Treatment includes tricyclic antidepressants and/or other medications used to treat neuropathic pain, such as gabapentin.

14. **Describe contact point headaches.**
Contact point headaches are assumed to be associated with an intranasal contact point, where two structures within the nasal cavity meet (most commonly a large septal spur). The contact point can be identified on clinical exam with endoscopy or radiologically. It is believed that stimulation from the mucosal contact point can result in referred pain of the face due to the cross innervation of the trigeminal nerve. Therefore, there should be a correlation between the headache and contact point regarding time, symptoms, and location. ICHD-III recognizes contact point headaches as a category of secondary headaches that are attributed to a disorder of the nasal mucosa, turbinates, or septum.

15. **Is there evidence that patients with headache and contact points may benefit from surgical intervention?**
Level 4 evidence suggests a potential benefit from surgery in these patients. However, interestingly, the majority of people who have mucosal contact points have no associated facial pain. There is also debate whether the improvement in facial pain following removal of contact points in some patients may be due to cognitive dissonance and/or neuroplasticity. A trial of topical anesthesia to the contact point region can be used as a diagnostic test prior to considering surgical intervention.

16. **What are the three groups of temporomandibular disorders?**
    1. Muscle disorders with myofascial pain
    2. Disc displacement with or without reduction
    3. Arthralgia, arthritis, arthrosis

17. **What is the prevalence of temporomandibular disorders?**
In a meta-analysis of TMD patients, 45.3% patients had Group I disorders (myofascial), 41.1% had Group II disorders (disc displacement), and 30.1% had group III disorders (arthralgia, arthritis, arthrosis). Some patients may have more than one type. Group I and Group II disorders are more common in the general population, each with a prevalence of approximately 10%.

18. **Describe the criteria for diagnosis of TMJ pain disorders.**
    - Criteria for temporomandibular pain:
        - Pain should relate directly to jaw movements and mastication.
        - Tenderness to palpation of the muscles of mastication and/or over the temporomandibular joint.
        - Confirmation of presence and location of pain source with relief from anesthetic blocking.

- Criteria for temporomandibular dysfunction:
  - Interference with mandibular movement
  - Restriction of mandibular movement
  - Sudden change of occlusal relationship of teeth

First-line treatment for TMJ disorders typically involves conservative management with analgesics, anti-inflammatory agents, application of local heat, and bite appliances. If these fail, in severe cases, surgical management may be considered.

19. What is the CSF pressure level used as a cut-off for diagnosing idiopathic intracranial hypertension (IIH)?

25 cm H_2O is the common pressure limit used as diagnostic criteria for IIH. However, children can have normal opening pressures of up to 28 cm H_2O. This is measured by lumbar puncture performed in the lateral decubitus position, without sedative medications or other medications that have the potential to alter intracranial pressure.

CONTROVERSIES

1. What causes the neurologic symptoms of migraine headache?

The exact causative mechanism of the symptoms of migraine headache is still controversial. Recent literature has supported that the cortical spreading depression that initiates migraines leads to release of proinflammatory mediators, such as substance P, calcitonin gene-related peptide, and neurokinin A. These inflammatory pathways provide a persistent stimulus that sensitizes trigeminal nerve endings. The parenchymal inflammatory response and trigeminal stimulation leads to pain.

2. Is there a role for empiric triptan therapy in patients with a diagnosis of sinus headache?

Studies have shown that a high percentage of patients with a self- or physician diagnosis of sinus headache may have a migraine-type headache. It has been proposed that empiric migraine therapy (triptans) may be employed in patients with sinus headache, with one study demonstrating improvement in 82% of patients that had a self- or physician diagnosis of sinus headache.

3. Is there a role for interventional therapies in patients with facial pain and headache?

The role of interventional procedures is still being defined, such as the use of neural blockade in the anterior ethmoid and sphenopalatine region with a steroid and local anesthesia mixture. Radiofrequency ablation of the pterygopalatine ganglion has also been anecdotally described, but the efficacy of these treatment options and their possible complications is still poorly understood.

BIBLIOGRAPHY

Daroff RB, Bradley WG: *Bradley's Neurology in Clinical Practice*, Philadelphia, 2012, Elsevier/Saunders.

Flint PW, Cummings CW: *Cummings Otolaryngology: Head & Neck Surgery*, Philadelpha, 2010, Mosby Elsevier.

Harrison L, Jones NS: Intranasal contact points as a cause of facial pain or headache: a systematic review, *Clin Otolaryngol* 38(1):8–22, 2013.

Headache Classification Committee of the International Headache Society (IHS): The International Classification of Headache Disorders, 3rd edition (beta version), *Cephalalgia* 33(9):629–808, 2013.

Kari E, Delgaudio JM: Treatment of sinus headache as migraine: the diagnostic utility of triptans, *Laryngoscope* 118(12):2235–2239, 2008.

Manfredini D, Guarda-Nardini L, Winocur E, et al: Research diagnostic criteria for temporomandibular disorders: a systematic review of axis I epidemiologic findings, *Oral Surg Oral Med Oral Pathol Oral Radiol Endod* 112(4):453–462, 2011.

Mokbel KM, Abd Elfattah AM, Kamal el-S: Nasal mucosal contact points with facial pain and/or headache: lidocaine can predict the result of localized endoscopic resection, *European Arch Oto-rhino-laryngol* 267(10):1569, 2010.

Rodman R, Dutton J: Endoscopic neural blockade for rhinogenic headache and facial pain: 2011 update, *Int Forum Allergy Rhinol* 2(4):325–330, 2012.

Schreiber CP, Hutchinson S, Webster CJ, et al: Prevalence of migraine in patients with a history of self-reported or physician-diagnosed "sinus" headache, *Arch Intern Med* 164(16):1769–1772, 2004.

Stovner L, Hagen K, Jensen R, et al: The global burden of headache: a documentation of headache prevalence and disability worldwide, *Cephalalgia* 27:193–210, 2007.

Tfelt-Hansen P, De Vries P, Saxena PR: Triptans in migraine: a comparative review of pharmacology, pharmacokinetics and efficacy, *Drugs* 60(6):1259–1287, 2000.

Wang M: Cortical spreading depression and calcitonin gene-related peptide: A brief review of current progress, *Neuropeptides* 47(6):463–466, 2013.

CHAPTER 8

TASTE AND SMELL

Elizabeth A. Gould, BA and Vijay R. Ramakrishnan, MD

KEY POINTS

1. Chemosensation (the perception of chemicals) relies on three sensory systems: taste, olfaction, and somatosensory.
2. Chemosensory dysfunction can severely detract from quality of life, ranging from safety issues such as detection of a gas leak, to higher functions such as emotion and memory.
3. Flavor results from the combination of taste, smell, and somatosensory-mediated sensations of temperature, texture, and pungency.

Pearls

1. There are 5 described tastes: salty, sour, sweet, bitter, and umami.
2. Fungiform, foliate, circumvallate, and filiform are the four type of papillae on the tongue. Filiform papillae do not actually contain taste buds.
3. Anosmia is the absence of olfactory function. Hyposmia describes reduced olfactory function. Dysosmia means changes in odor quality, including parosmia (altered perception of an odor) and phantosmia (perception of an odor when that odor is not present).
4. Common causes of olfactory dysfunction include upper respiratory infection, head trauma, sinonasal disease, medication, and chemical exposure.

QUESTIONS

1. **What is the purpose of the chemosensory system?**
   Chemosensation is the perception of chemicals. We detect chemicals through three different sensory systems: taste, olfaction, and somatosensory. Taste refers to the sensation arising from taste receptors and is used to evaluate the nutritious content of food and avoid ingestion of toxic substances. Smell is the detection of volatile odorants though olfactory and somatosensory systems. Olfaction is the perception of odorants through activation of odorant receptors, and is mediated by cranial nerve (CN) I. Smell is important for social interactions and memory. Trigeminal somatosensory fibers of CN V detect thermal, mechanical, and chemical stimuli in the head and neck, and initiate protective respiratory reflexes from noxious chemicals.

2. **What are the consequences of taste or smell dysfunction?**
   Chemosensation is an integral aspect of how we interact with the environment and guides our behavior. Loss of these senses can lead to hazardous situations, such as food poisoning and the inability to detect fire or gas. The disruption of appetitive cues can lead to weight changes and nutritional deficiencies. People without taste often lose the desire to eat and may require medical intervention to restore their appetite.

3. **What is the impact of taste or smell dysfunction on quality of life?**
   There is a well-established relationship between olfaction, emotion, and memory, in which odorants can strongly evoke emotions related to the previous experiences associated with that odor. Odor-associated memories are long-lasting and salient. The loss of chemosensation impairs the ability to feel motivated and engage in pleasurable activities, and is correlated with lower perception of quality of life, changes in mood, and depression.

Social chemical cues play a role in determining our social behavior. It has been shown that odorants are reported to influence mate selection and cause females to synchronize their menstrual cycle, indicating a biological importance for olfactory cues. Smell dysfunction can lead to impaired social interactions and social isolation.

4. **What is the relationship between taste, smell, and flavor?**
The flavor of our food is the combination of taste, smell, and the somatosensory-mediated sensations of temperature, texture, and pungency. Thus, patients presenting with taste complaints may often really suffer from olfactory dysfunction.

5. **Describe the trigeminal (CN V) contribution to smell.**
The trigeminal system mediates the perception of touch, pressure, temperature, and nociception (pain or irritation), and displays a limited spectrum of sensations compared to olfaction. The ophthalmic and maxillary branches of the trigeminal nerve innervate the nasal cavity. Most odorants can activate the trigeminal system, and individuals with impaired olfaction (CN I) may still be able to detect odors (often strong irritating odors such as gasoline or ammonia) through trigeminal sensations.

6. **What are the five basic tastes?**
Taste is limited to a spectrum of five tastes: salty, sour, sweet, bitter, and umami. Umami is the detection of L-amino acids and is also described as savory. Sweet is indicative of energy-rich foods. The detection of salt allows us to control proper dietary electrolytic balance. Sour and bitter are used to warn against noxious/poisonous compounds.

7. **Where are taste receptors located?**
Taste receptors are located on taste receptor cells. *Taste buds* are bundles of taste receptor cells. Taste receptors are also found on specialized chemosensory cells, ciliated cells, and smooth muscle cells in the airway and are thought to mediate the perception of irritants. Taste-sensing of food also occurs within the gastrointestinal tract as taste receptors are expressed by enteroendocrine cells.

8. **Where are taste buds located?**
Taste buds are located on a large portion of the tongue dorsum within small protrusions of epithelium called *papillae.* Taste buds are also found on the soft palate, larynx, pharynx, and epiglottis, and these taste buds are innervated by the vagus nerve (CN X).

9. **Describe the four types of papillae.**
The anterior two-thirds of the tongue contains *fungiform* papillae. Fungiform papillae contain 1 to 15 taste buds each and are innervated by the chorda tympani branch of the facial nerve (CN VII). There are approximately 750 fungiform papillae.
The posterior aspects of the tongue contain *circumvallate* and *foliate* papillae and are innervated by the glossopharyngeal nerve (CN IX). Humans have 8 to 12 circumvallate papillae arranged in a V-shape on the dorsal tongue and a few foliate papillae on the lateral sides, each housing dozens of taste buds.
Filiform papillae are distributed throughout the tongue dorsum. They contribute to the mechanical distribution of chemicals on the tongue, and do not contain taste buds.

10. **Describe the central processing of taste.**
Taste receptor cells transmit taste information to neural fibers within the taste bud, which project from neurons located in the sensory ganglia of cranial nerves VII, IX, and X. The cranial nerves enter the central nervous system at the brainstem and converge to form the solitary tract. Afferent information enters the thalamus and proceeds to the gustatory cortex.

11. **Where is olfactory epithelium found?**
The olfactory epithelium is located in the superior and posterior aspect of the nasal cavity, including the nasal septum and superior and middle turbinates. The precise location of the olfactory epithelium varies between individuals.

12. **Describe the cellular composition of the olfactory epithelium.**
The olfactory epithelium is a pseudostratified columnar epithelial tissue comprised of several cell types. *Bipolar sensory neurons* extend an apical dendrite to the epithelial surface from which cilia extend to detect odors. The basal pole extends into an axon, which crosses the cribriform plate and enters the olfactory bulb. The axons of the sensory neurons are ensheathed by *olfactory ensheathing*

cells, which have received clinical interest for their ability to support axon growth. *Basal cells* produce new olfactory sensory neurons as the old neurons die or are damaged. Supporting or *sustentacular* cells regulate and maintain the mucus layer into which odorants dissolve. Flask-shaped *microvillar* cells have no known role, but can respond to odorants and may play a role in reception.

13. **Where are olfactory receptors located?**
We are able to distinguish over 1,000 odorants through a large multigene family of receptors that detect specific chemical structures within odorant molecules. Olfactory receptors are located on the cilia of bipolar sensory neurons within the olfactory epithelium. Each sensory neuron expresses only one type of receptor.

14. **Describe the central processing of olfactory stimuli.**
Odorant molecules that enter the nasal cavity and diffuse through the mucus layer bind to specific odorant receptors depending on their chemical structure. Odor-evoked responses are conducted through the sensory neuron axons, which converge with axons expressing the same receptor type into circular structures called *glomeruli* in the olfactory bulb. Information about the odorant is encoded by the pattern of sensory neurons and the glomeruli they activate forming a chemotopic map. Second-order neurons (mitral and tufted cells) transmit the response through the olfactory tract to regions in the frontal lobe and dorsomedial temporal lobe. There is a structural overlap of olfactory-responsive regions and those related to emotion, memory, and motivation. These regions include the amygdala, entorhinal cortex, orbital cortex, striatum, hypothalamus, and hippocampus. The structural overlap is thought to contribute to the salience of olfactory memories and emotional responses.

15. **What are the terms used to describe olfactory dysfunction?**
Anosmia is the absence of olfactory function. *Hyposmia* describes reduced olfactory function. *Dysosmias* are changes in odor quality, including *parosmia* (altered perception of an odor) and *phantosmia* (perception of an odor when that odor is not present).

16. **What are the terms used to describe taste dysfunction?**
Ageusia is the absence of the ability to taste. *Hypogeusia* describes reduced taste perception. *Dysgeusias* are changes in taste quality, including *parageusia* (altered perception of tastant) and *phantogeusia* (taste detection in the absence of stimulus).

17. **How are sensory dysfunctions classified?**
Disruption of the transmission of sensory information can occur at multiple levels from the peripheral elements to areas within the central nervous system.
    - Transport or *conductive losses* refer to conditions that interfere with access to receptor cells. Transport losses in taste can result from infections, oral inflammation, and dry mouth (xerostomia). Transport losses in olfaction can result from mucosal inflammation, structural obstructions, and alterations in nasal mucus.
    - *Sensory losses* refer to conditions that disrupt receptor cell function, including the loss of receptor cells due to injury. Olfactory neuron disruption can occur from head injury, sinonasal disease, respiratory tract infections, and chemical exposure. Taste receptor cell loss may be caused by medications, radiation therapy, infection, and endocrine disorders.
    - *Neural losses* refer to disruptions in the transmission of information upstream of receptor cells. For olfaction this includes injury to the olfactory bulb and cortex. Neural losses in taste can occur following damage to the chorda tympani, facial, vagus, and glossopharyngeal nerves as well as with brain injury.

18. **What are the major causes of taste disorders?**
Respiratory infections, head trauma, radiation therapy, medication side effects, chemical exposure, endocrine disorders, and poor oral hygiene. Isolated taste dysfunction is very rare, with a prevalence of 0.001% of the population.

19. **What are the major causes of olfactory disorders?**
Olfactory dysfunction occurs in 1% to 2% of the population. The prevalence of olfactory dysfunction increases with age with estimates of 24% to 40% in individuals over 50 years of age. Causes include upper respiratory infection, head trauma, sinonasal disease, medication, and chemical exposure.

20. **What are key questions to ask during evaluation of the patient with a taste or smell problem?**
Inquire about any prior history of dysfunction, including any upper respiratory infections, nasal obstruction, sinonasal disease, head trauma, or prior ear surgery. Ask if the onset was gradual of sudden, or if it fluctuates. Determine whether the loss is complete or partial, and if there are any distortions/hallucinations in taste or olfaction. Inquire about cognition, medication use, appetite, and changes in weight.

21. **What should you look for on physical examination of a patient with a taste or smell problem?**
Nasal examination should assess for septal deviation, turbinate enlargement, allergic appearance of mucosa, or presence of nasal polyps or purulence. Mucus character and signs of epithelial irritation or inflammation should be assessed in the nasal cavity and oral cavity. Ear examination should assess the middle ear space to rule out disease affecting the chorda tympani.

22. **How do you proceed with the workup for taste and/or smell dysfunction?**
Formal testing may include threshold and odorant identification tests for olfactory loss. MRI may be indicated to rule out central processes, and can demonstrate presence of sinus inflammation.

23. **How do you assess olfactory function?**
Patients often do not accurately report deficits in olfaction; therefore, it can be important to obtain a more objective measurement of olfactory function. Several standardized tests of olfactory function have been developed. The two most frequently used are the Smell Identification Test (SIT), an odor identification "scratch and sniff" test, and Sniffin Sticks, an odor identification, discrimination, and threshold assessment using odor-dispensing pens. Odor identification and discrimination tasks are generally thought to assess peripheral and central processing, while threshold testing reflects mainly peripheral processing. Direct measures of odor-evoked responses are not often used, but the ability of sensory neurons to respond can be measured using electroolfactograms (EOGs) and cortical responses can be assessed using electroencephalograms (EEGs) or imaging.

24. **Will steroid administration help sense of smell?**
Steroid administration is frequently used to reduce inflammation and clear obstruction of the olfactory cleft. Rapid improvement of olfactory function is often observed, however, this is usually transient and permanent restoration of normal function is unlikely. Systemic administration is more effective then topical application, but extended administration of systemic steroids puts the patient at risk of side effects.

25. **Will surgery help sense of smell?**
If the deficit is due to obstruction of the olfactory cleft, then restoring airflow with surgery will aid in recovery of olfactory function. Sinus surgery to decrease infection and/or inflammation often provides some degree of benefit, particularly in patients with nasal polyps. While improvement of olfactory function is possible, it is frequently transient and incomplete.

Bibliography

Chandrashekar J, Hoon MA, Ryba NJP, et al: The receptors and cells for mammalian taste, *Nature* 444:288–294, 2006.

Doty R: The Olfactory System and Its Disorders, *Semin Neurol* 29:74–81, 2009.

Gottfried JA: Central mechanisms of odour object perception, *Nat Rev Neurosci* 11:628–641, 2010.

Holbrook EH, Wu E, Curry WT, et al: Immunohistochemical characterization of human olfactory tissue, *Laryngoscope* 121:16871701, 2011.

Hummel T, Livermore A: Intranasal chemosensory function of the trigeminal nerve and aspects of its relation to olfaction, *Int Arch Occup Environ Health* 75:305–313, 2002.

Keller A, Malaspina D: Hidden consequences of olfactory dysfunction: a patient report series, *BMC Ear* 13(1):8, 2013.

Kinnamon SC: Taste receptor signalling—from tongues to lungs, *Acta Physiol* 204:158–168, 2011.

Leopold DA, Hummel T, Schwob JE, et al: Anterior distribution of human olfactory epithelium, *Laryngoscope* 110: 417–421, 2000.

London B, Nabet B, Fisher AR, et al: Predictors of prognosis in patients with olfactory disturbance, *Ann Neurol* 63: 159–166, 2008.

Pribitkin E, Rosenthal MD, Cowart BJ: Prevalence and causes of severe taste loss in a chemosensory clinic population, *Ann Otol Rhinol Laryngol* 112:971–978, 2003.

II

HEAD AND NECK

HEAD AND NECK ANATOMY AND EMBRYOLOGY WITH RADIOLOGY CORRELATES

CHAPTER 9

Ted H. Leem, MD, MS, Benjamin Milam, MD and Mofiyinfolu Sokoya, MD

KEY POINTS

1. The six branchial arches form the skeletal and muscular derivatives of the head and neck while the six pharyngeal pouches form the endothelium and glands of the head and neck. Each is associated with a nerve and artery.
2. Aberrant embryological development can cause branchial cleft anomalies. These can subsequently become infected and require surgical removal. Anomalies of the first, second, third, and fourth branchial clefts can occur. The most common anomaly is from the second branchial cleft. Branchial cleft anomalies can have associated sinus tracts, which pass deep to their associated aortic arch derivatives.
3. Cervical lymphadenectomy (neck dissection) is based on lymphatic drainage patterns to regional lymph nodes delineated by sublevels of the neck.
4. The upper aerodigestive tract is divided into the nasal cavity, oral cavity, nasopharynx, oropharynx, hypopharynx, and larynx.
5. Deep neck space infections can travel through the neck and into other parts of the body via the retropharyngeal space, danger space, and prevertebral space.

Pearls

1. The second branchial cleft is the most common branchial cleft to develop an anomaly.
2. The soft palate divides the nasopharynx from the oropharynx and the hyoid bone separates the oropharynx from the hypopharynx.
3. Retropharyngeal space contains lateral and medial lymph nodes. The most common cancer to metastasize to these lymph nodes is nasopharyngeal cancer.
4. The retropharyngeal space extends from the skull base to the mediastinum, the danger space extends from the skull base to the diaphragm, and the prevertebral space extends from the clivus to the coccyx.
5. The pterygopalatine fossa is a deep space in the face that contains the maxillary artery, maxillary branch of the trigeminal nerve, and the pterygopalatine ganglion.

QUESTIONS

1. What are the skeletal derivatives of the six branchial arches?

Table 9-1.

BRANCHIAL ARCH	SKELETAL DERIVATIVES
1st	Body and ramus of the mandible, the sphenomandibular ligament, anterior malleolar ligament, malleus (except for the manubrium), and the incus (except for its long process)
2nd	Stylohyoid ligament, styloid process, the manubrium of the malleus, the long process of the incus, the stapes superstructure, and the body of the hyoid and the lesser cornu of the hyoid bone
3rd	Body and greater cornu of the hyoid bone
4th, 5th, 6th	Thyroid, cricoid, arytenoid, corniculate, and cuneiform laryngeal cartilages

2. What are the muscular derivatives of the six branchial arches?

Table 9-2.

BRANCHIAL ARCH	MUSCLE DERIVATIVES
1st	Muscles of mastication: the temporalis, masseter, and medial and lateral pterygoid muscles as well as the tensor tympani, tensor veli palatini, anterior belly of the digastric, and mylohyoid muscles
2nd	Muscles of facial expression: the posterior belly of the digastric, the stylohyoid, and the stapedius
3rd	Stylopharyngeus muscle
4th, 5th, 6th	Pharyngeal muscles (superior, middle, and inferior constrictor muscles), striated muscle of the upper half of the esophagus, as well as all of the extrinsic and intrinsic muscles of the larynx

3. What do the six pharyngeal pouches form?
The pharyngeal pouches are composed of endoderm and therefore will form glandular structures.

Table 9-3.

PHARYNGEAL POUCH	POUCH DERIVATIVES
1st	Epithelial lining of the middle ear and the tympanic membrane
2nd	Epithelial lining of the palatine tonsil
3rd	Superior: inferior parathyroid glands; inferior: thymus
4th	Superior parathyroid glands
5th and 6th	Parafollicular (C) cells

4. What cranial nerve innervates the derivatives of each branchial arch?

Table 9-4.

BRANCHIAL ARCH	CRANIAL NERVES
1st	Trigeminal nerve
2nd	Facial nerve
3rd	Glossopharyngeal nerve
4th, 5th, 6th	Vagus nerve

5. Where are the potential tracts of the branchial cleft sinuses?
The tracts for the associated sinuses typically have a pattern of passing deep to the associated aortic arch derivatives. First branchial cleft anomalies are duplications of the membranous part of the external auditory canal. They are typically divided into two types. Type I is of ectodermal origin and is a duplication anomaly of the external auditory canal. This cyst may be located antero-inferior to the lobule. Type II is of ectodermal and mesodermal origin and duplicates the cartilage as well. Type II first branchial cleft sinuses typically present below the angle of the mandible and pass through the parotid gland in close proximity to the facial nerve either inferior to the external auditory canal or into the canal at the bony cartilaginous junction.

Second branchial cleft anomalies typically present below the angle of the mandible and at the anterior border of the sternocleidomastoid muscle. The potential tract for this sinus passes deep to the external carotid artery, stylohyoid, and digastric muscle and superficial to the internal carotid artery opening in the tonsillar fossa.

Third branchial cleft anomalies typically present anterior to the sternocleidomastoid muscle and lower in the neck than either first or second branchial cleft anomalies. The potential tract for this sinus passes deep to the glossopharyngeal nerve and the internal carotid artery and superficial to the vagus nerve opening in the pharynx at the thyrohyoid membrane or piriform sinus.

Fourth branchial cleft anomalies are predominantly left-sided, presenting as thyroid masses or paratracheal masses inferiorly in the lateral neck. The potential tract of this sinus passes deep to the superior laryngeal nerve and superficial to the recurrent laryngeal nerve opening into the hypopharynx. If these tracts are present, it is important to attempt surgical excision of them along with the cyst.

6. **What is the most common branchial cleft anomaly?**
Second branchial cleft anomalies are the most common, representing approximately 95% of all anomalies. First branchial cleft anomalies are the second most common. Third and fourth branchial cleft anomalies are rare.

7. **What are the boundaries and subsites of the oral cavity?**
   - Anterior: Vermillion border of the lip
   - Superior: Hard-soft palate junction
   - Lateral: Tonsillar pillars
   - Posterior/inferior: Circumvallate papillae of the tongue
   - Subsites: Lip, oral tongue (anterior two thirds), buccal mucosa, floor of mouth, hard palate, upper and lower gingiva (alveolar ridges), and retromolar trigone

8. **What are the boundaries of the nasopharynx?**
   - Anterior: Posterior nasal cavity
   - Superior: Sphenoid sinus
   - Posterior: First and second vertebrae
   - Inferior: Soft palate
   - Lateral: Eustachian tube, torus tubarius, and the fossa of Rosenmuller (most common site of origin for nasopharyngeal carcinoma)

9. **What are the boundaries and subsites of the oropharynx?**
   - Anterior: Oral cavity
   - Superior: Soft palate
   - Posterior: Posterior pharyngeal wall
   - Inferior: Hyoid
   - Subsites: Base of tongue (posterior third), palatine tonsil/lateral pharyngeal wall, soft palate, and posterior pharyngeal wall

10. **Where is HPV-associated squamous cell carcinoma (SCCA) most commonly located?**
The oropharynx, specifically the tonsils and base of tongue, is the most common location for HPV SCCA.

11. **What are the boundaries and subsites of the hypopharynx?**
   - Anterior: Larynx
   - Superior: Hyoid bone and pharyngoepiglottic folds
   - Posterior: Retropharyngeal space
   - Inferior: Esophageal introitus at the cricopharyngeus muscle
   - Subsites: The piriform sinuses, the postcricoid region, and the posterior pharyngeal wall

12. **Describe the subsites of the hypopharynx.**
The piriform sinuses are an inverted pyramid with the base at the level of the pharyngoepiglottic fold and the apex extending to just below the cricoid cartilage. The second subsite, the postcricoid region, is the anterior wall of the hypopharynx. It extends from the just inferior to the posterior

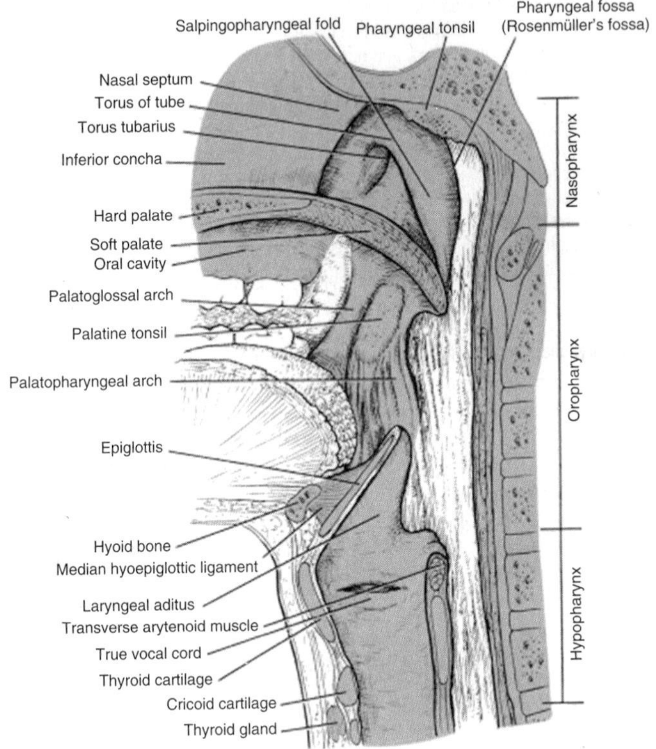

Figure 9-1. Anatomic subsites and structures of the upper aerodigestive tract.

aspect of the arytenoid cartilages to the esophageal introitus. The third region of the hypopharynx, the posterior pharyngeal wall, extends from the hyoid bones to the superior aspect of the cricopharyngeus muscle.

13. **Describe the different layers of the deep cervical fascia.**
    Deep fascia is divided into three layers: the external, middle, and internal layers. The external layer is underneath the platysma layer and invests the superficial neck structures. The middle layer encloses the visceral structures including the trachea and esophagus. The most internal layer surrounds the deep muscles of the neck and cervical vertebrae.

14. **Where are the retropharyngeal space, danger space, and prevertebral space?**
    - Retropharyngeal Space Boundaries
      - Superior: Skull base
      - Inferior: Mediastinum at the tracheal bifurcation
      - Anterior: Buccopharyngeal fascia that lines the posterior pharynx and esophagus
      - Posterior: Alar fascia over the danger space
      - Lateral: Carotid sheath
    - Danger Space Boundaries
      - Superior: Skull base
      - Inferior: Diaphragm
      - Anterior: Alar fascia and retropharyngeal space
      - Posterior: Prevertebral fascia and prevertebral space
      - Lateral: Transverse process of the vertebrae

- Prevertebral Space Boundaries
  - Superior: Clivus of the skull base
  - Inferior: Coccyx
  - Anterior: Prevertebral fascia and danger space
  - Posterior: Vertebral bodies
  - Lateral: Transverse process of the vertebrae

15. **Describe the lymphatics of the retropharyngeal space.**
There are two groups of retropharyngeal lymph nodes, lateral and medial. The lateral retropharyngeal lymph nodes (RPLNs) are also known as the Rouvière nodes and are subdivided into the lateral nasopharyngeal and lateral oropharyngeal lymph nodes.

The number of lateral RPLNs ranges from 1 to 3 and they are normally 2 to 5 mm in size. The medial RPLNs are inferior to the lateral nodes and are subclassified into upper and lower lymph nodes. Retropharyngeal lymph nodes typically become smaller in adults and medial retropharyngeal lymph nodes are rarely present in adults

Nasopharyngeal cancer is the most common primary tumor that metastasizes to the retropharyngeal lymph nodes.

16. **Describe the cervical triangles of the neck.**
The sternocleidomastoid muscles divide each side of the neck into two major triangles, anterior and posterior. The anterior triangle of the neck is further divided by the strap muscles into the superior and inferior carotid triangles. The posterior triangle is formed by the sternocleidomastoid anteriorly, the clavicle inferiorly, and the anterior border of the trapezius posteriorly. The omohyoid divides the posterior triangle into a small inferior subclavian triangle and a larger posterior occipital triangle.

17. **Describe the contents of the posterior cervical triangle.**
The cutaneous branches of the cervical plexus, the spinal accessory nerve, and the suprascapular and transverse cervical vessels can all be found in the posterior cervical triangle.

18. **What are the boundaries of the lymphatic levels of the neck (Figure 9-2)?**
- Level Ia (Submental Triangle)
  - Anterior: Mandible
  - Lateral: Anterior belly of the digastric
  - Posterior: Hyoid
  - Superior: Mylohyoid

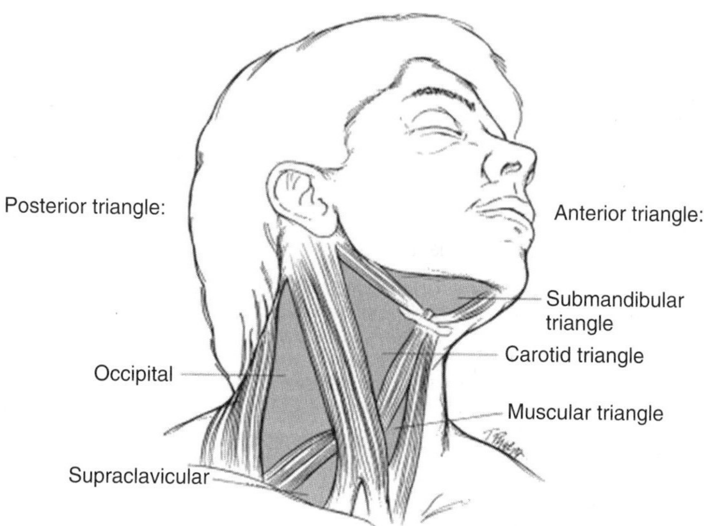

Figure 9-2. Boundaries of the lymphatic levels of the neck.

- Level Ib (Submandibular Triangle)
  - Superior: Mandible
  - Posterior/Inferior: Posterior belly of the digastric
  - Anterior/Inferior: Anterior belly of the digastric
- Level II (Upper Jugular Region)
  - Superior: Skull base
  - Inferior: Hyoid bone
  - Lateral: Posterior border of the sternocleidomastoid muscle
  - Medial: Lateral border of the sternohyoid and stylohyoid muscles
    - IIa: Region anterior to the spinal accessory nerve
    - IIb: Region postero-superior to the nerve
- Level III (Middle Jugular Region)
  - Superior: Hyoid bone
  - Inferior: Junction of the omohyoid and internal jugular vein
  - Lateral: Posterior border of the sternocleidomastoid muscle
  - Medial: Lateral border of the sternohyoid muscle
- Level IV (Lower Jugular Region)
  - Superior: Omohyoid
  - Inferior: Clavicle
  - Lateral: Posterior border of the sternocleidomastoid muscle
  - Medial: Lateral border of the sternohyoid muscle
- Level V (The Posterior Triangle)
  - Medial: Posterior border of the sternocleidomastoid muscle
  - Lateral: Anterior border of the trapezius muscle
  - Inferior: Clavicle
    - Va: Region superior to the inferior border of the cricoid cartilage
    - Vb: Region inferior to the inferior border of the cricoid cartilage
- Level VI (The Anterior Compartment)
  - Superior: Hyoid
  - Inferior: Suprasternal notch
  - Lateral: Medial border of the carotid sheaths

19. Name the cranial nerves and skull base foramina where they exit.
- Cranial Nerve 1: Olfactory Nerve—Cribriform plate of the ethmoid bone
- Cranial Nerve II: Optic Nerve—Optic canal
- Cranial Nerve III: Oculomotor Nerve—Superior orbital fissure
- Cranial Nerve IV: Trochlear Nerve—Superior orbital fissure
- Cranial Nerve V: Trigeminal Nerve
  - V1: Ophthalmic Nerve—Superior orbital fissure
  - V2: Maxillary Nerve—Foramen rotundum
  - V3: Mandibular Nerve—Foramen ovale
- Cranial Nerve VI: Abducens Nerve—Superior orbital fissure
- Cranial Nerve VII: Facial Nerve—Enters at internal acoustic meatus
  - Motor Root—Exits through stylomastoid foramen
  - Nervus Intermedius:
    - Chorda Tympani—Exits through petrotympanic fissure
    - Greater Superficial Petrosal Nerve—Exits through the pterygoid canal
- Cranial Nerve VIII: Vestibulocochlear Nerve—Internal acoustic meatus
- Cranial Nerve IX: Glossopharyngeal Nerve—Jugular foramen
- Cranial Nerve X: Vagus Nerve—Jugular foramen
- Cranial Nerve XI: Accessory Nerve—Jugular foramen
- Cranial Nerve XII: Hypoglossal Nerve—Hypoglossal canal

20. Describe the pterygopalatine fossa (Figure 9-3).
- Boundaries of the Pterygopalatine Fossa
  - Anterior: Maxilla
  - Superior: Medial half of the inferior orbital fissure
  - Posterior: Pterygoid plates of the sphenoid bone
  - Inferior: Upper end of the palatine canal

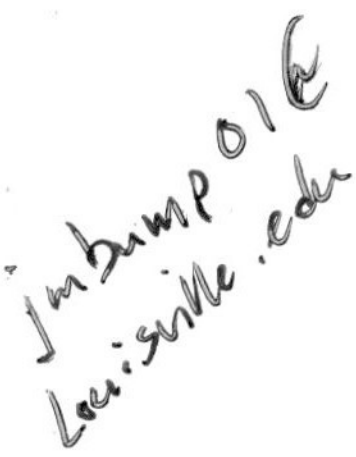

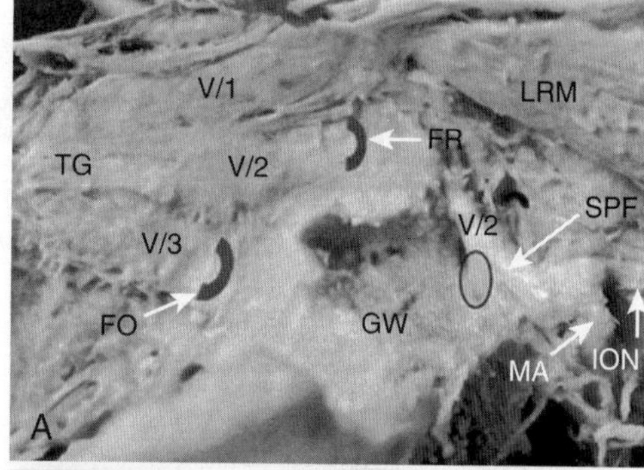

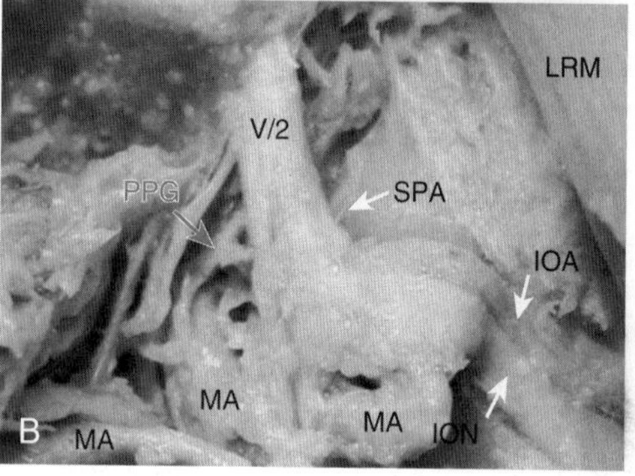

Figure 9-3. Boundaries of the pterygopalatine fossa. **A,** lateral view; **B,** superior view. V1, ophthalmic division of trigeminal nerve; V2, maxillary division of trigeminal nerve; V3, maxillary division of trigeminal nerve; TG, trigeminal ganglion; FR, foramen rotundum; FO, foramen ovale; SPF, sphenopalatine foramen; GW, greater wing of sphenoid; LRM, lateral rectus muscle; MA, maxillary artery; ION, infraorbital nerve; IOA, infraorbital artery; PPG, pterygopalatine ganglion.

  - Lateral: Pterygomaxillary fissure
  - Medial: Sphenopalatine foramen and perpendicular plate of the palatine bone
- Communications of the Pterygopalatine Fossa
  - Anterior: Maxillary sinus (no direct communication)
  - Superior: Orbital cavity through the inferior orbital fissure
  - Posterior: Middle cranial fossa through foramen rotundum and the pterygoid canal
  - Inferior: Oral cavity through the palatine canal
  - Lateral: Infratemporal fossa through the pterygomaxillary fissure
  - Medial: Nasal cavity through the sphenopalatine foramen
- Contents of the Pterygopalatine Fossa
  - Fat
  - Maxillary artery
  - Maxillary division of the trigeminal nerve
  - Pterygopalatine ganglion: Parasympathetic ganglion where post-parasympathetic nerves innervate the lacrimal gland and nasal mucosa.

21. What are the branches of the external carotid artery in approximate order from proximal to distal?
    - Superior thyroid artery
    - Ascending pharyngeal artery
    - Lingual artery
    - Facial artery
    - Occipital artery
    - Posterior auricular artery
    - Maxillary artery *(terminal branch)*
    - Superficial temporal artery *(terminal branch)*

BIBLIOGRAPHY

Bailey BJ, Johnson JT, Newlands SD: *Head and Neck Surgery—Otolaryngology*, Philadelphia, 2006, Lippincott Williams & Wilkins.

Cummings CW, Flint PW: *Cummings Otolaryngology: Head & Neck Surgery*, Philadelphia, 2010, Mosby Elsevier.

Coskun HH, Ferlito A, Medina JE, et al: Retropharyngeal lymph node metastases in head and neck malignancies, *Head Neck* 33(10):1520–1529, 2011.

Kreimer AR, Clifford GM, Boyle P, et al: Human papillomavirus types in head and neck squamous cell carcinomas worldwide: a systematic review, *Cancer Epidemiol Biomarkers Prev* 14(2):467–475, 2005.

Lalwani AK: *Current Diagnosis & Treatment in Otolaryngology: Head & Neck Surgery*, New York, 2008, McGraw-Hill Medical.

TUMOR BIOLOGY

Jessica D. McDermott, MD and Daniel W. Bowles, MD

CHAPTER 10

KEY POINTS

1. Cancer development requires an accumulation of genetic and cellular alterations.
2. The most common risk factors associated with head and neck squamous cell cancer in the United States are tobacco use, alcohol use, and the HPV virus (type 16).
3. HPV-positive and HPV-negative HNSCC have different drivers of carcinogenesis.
4. There are recurring DNA translocations in a number of different salivary gland cancers.
5. There are often driver mutations or translocations in differentiated thyroid cancers, including BRAF (papillary thyroid cancer), RET (medullary and papillary thyroid cancers), and PPAR-gamma-1 (follicular thyroid cancer).
6. Dysregulation of cell cycle progression and angiogenesis are hallmarks of tumorigenesis.
7. Targeted therapies, such as the use of EGFR-inhibitors, are being explored in the development of novel agents for cancer treatment.

QUESTIONS

1. **What is the multi-hit theory of carcinogenesis?**
   This theory postulates that cells must acquire multiple mutations or aberrations in order to develop into cancer. Different types of tumors may result from different cellular changes.

2. **What biological processes are thought to contribute to cancer development, growth, and persistence?**
   1. Aberrant cell signaling controlling mitosis and cell differentiation
   2. Decreased apoptosis, or programmed cell death
   3. Angiogenesis, or the growth of new blood vessels

3. **What are some molecular techniques used to analyze causes of head and neck cancer development?**
   1. Immunohistochemistry (IHC): Stains for proteins in tumor specimens.
   2. Fluorescent in situ hybridization (FISH): Uses fluorescent probes to analyze for DNA translocations.
   3. Next generation sequencing: Several methods that allow a wide number of genes to be analyzed for mutations simultaneously.

4. **What are oncogenes, proto-oncogenes, and tumor suppressor genes?**
   An oncogene is a gene that confers the potential to cause cancer, and a proto-oncogene is a normal gene that can contribute to cancer formation when mutated. A tumor suppressor gene is one that protects a cell from transitioning to cancer. Mutations in tumor suppressor genes that cause loss of function may allow the cell to progress to cancer, especially when combined with overexpression of oncogenes and mutations in proto-oncogenes.

Squamous Cell Carcinomas of the Head and Neck

5. **What are the most common risk factors for head and neck squamous cell cancer (HNSCC) worldwide?**
   1. Tobacco use
   2. Alcohol consumption
   3. Human papillomavirus (HPV) infection, especially in oropharyngeal cancer
   4. Betel nut chewing

6. **What is the concept of field cancerization?**
Field cancerization refers to epithelium changes adjacent to an invasive cancer showing precancerous alterations such as dysplasia or carcinoma in situ. This is more common in smoking-related cancers, implying that such risk factors may be more broadly impacting the tissues.

7. **Which "high-risk" HPV virus type is most commonly implicated in HNSCC?**
HPV type 16

8. **How does HPV cause HNSCC?**
HPV is a DNA virus that will insert genes into host DNA which then act as oncogenes.
    1. E6 protein: An oncoprotein that inactivates p53, a host tumor suppressor protein that blocks apoptosis
    2. E7 protein: An oncoprotein that inactivates the retinoblastoma (Rb) tumor suppressor protein and promotes host DNA synthesis and cell cycle progression

9. **How is HPV tested for in patients with HNSCC?**
    1. HPV in-situ hybridization: This looks for HPV DNA in cancer cells.
    2. P16 protein over expression by immunohistochemistry: P16 is downstream of Rb and, when Rb is destroyed by HPV oncoproteins, P16 protein levels increase.

10. **What key molecular pathways appear to be important in HNSCC for pathogenesis and potential treatment targets?**
    1. p53, a tumor suppressor altered in most HPV-negative HNSCC
    2. Epidermal growth factor receptor (EGFR)
    3. Phosphoinositide 3-kinase (PI3K)
    4. NOTCH-1
    5. Cyclin D1

11. **How do p53 mutations cause oncogenesis in HNSCC?**
    1. Wild-type p53 is a tumor suppressor protein that plays a role in apoptosis and cell cycle regulation. Mutations of the TP53 gene allow increased cell survival and growth in an unregulated fashion.
    2. Mutations are present is most HPV-positive HNSCC but only a minority of HPV-negative tumors

12. **What is the role of EGFR in HNSCC?**
    1. EGFR is a member of a family of tyrosine kinases that is overactivated in HNSCC. This results in increased activation of downstream pathways including Ras/Raf/MAPK, PI3K-Akt, and transcription pathways promoting angiogenesis, proliferation, metastasis, and invasion.
    2. EGFR is upregulated in up to 90% of HNSCC.
    3. It may have different levels of importance in HPV-positive and HPV-negative tumors.

13. **Which molecular pathway has the only FDA-approved targeted drug for treatment of HNSCC?**
EGFR is the only molecular pathway that has a FDA-approved targeted drug to treat HNSCC. The targeted therapy is cetuximab, an IgG1-human monoclonal antibody against the extracellular domain of EGFR.

14. **What is the role of the PI3K pathway in HNSCC?**
    1. The PI3Ks are a family of enzymes that play a role in cellular regulatory mechanisms. In HNSCC their signaling is increased, activating mTOR proteins resulting in increased cell growth, survival, proliferation, and migration.
    2. Mutations of the PI3KCA gene have been found in 6% to 20% of HNSCC.
    3. PIK3CA mutations appear to be more common in HPV-positive cancers.

15. **How does the NOTCH pathway play a role in HNSCC?**
    1. The NOTCH family of receptors are thought to play a tumor suppressor role in squamous cell cancers. Patients with a NOTCH-1 inactivation mutation have a dysregulated pathway thought to promote cancer cell survival.
    2. NOTCH is mutated in 12% to 15% of HNSCC.

Salivary Gland Cancers

16. What receptors are overexpressed in salivary gland tumors and may be exploited as potential biological targets for treatment?

1. c-kit is a proto-oncogene that can stimulate growth and differentiation. It is mainly increased in adenoid cystic carcinoma (78% to 92%) and some mucoepidermoids (0% to 40%). Clinical trial with c-kit inhibitors have been disappointing to date.
2. EGFR is increased in adenoid cystic carcinoma (36% to 85%), mucoepidermoid (53% to 100%), adenocarcinoma (60%), salivary duct cancers (9% to 40%), and others.
3. HER-2/neu receptor is involved in cell growth and differentiation. It is increased mostly in salivary duct cancers (44% to 83%), but can also be found in adenocarcinomas (14% to 21%), mucoepidermoids (0% to 38%), and adenoid cystic carcinoma (2% to 36%).
4. Androgen receptor is increased in salivary duct cancers (43% to 100%) and adenocarcinomas (21%).

17. What recurring translocations occur commonly in salivary gland cancers?

1. t(11;19) producing a fusion protein CRTC1-MAML2 is seen in mucoepidermoid carcinomas (found in about 30%).
2. t(6;9) MYB-NFIB translocations are seen in adenoid cystic carcinomas. It is estimated that 80% to 90% of adenoid cystic carcinomas have MYB activation by gene fusion.
3. t(12;15) ETV-NTRK3 translocations are seen in mammary analogue secretory carcinomas (found in >90%).

Thyroid Cancers

18. What are the different histologic types of thyroid cancer and what cells do they arise from?

1. Papillary: well differentiated tumor of the thyroid epithelium
2. Follicular: well differentiated tumor of the thyroid epithelium
3. Medullary: neuroendocrine tumor of the parafollicular or C cells of the thyroid gland
4. Anaplastic: undifferentiated tumors of the thyroid follicular epithelium
5. Hürthle cell: follicular epithelium

19. What genetic mutations are commonly found in papillary thyroid cancer (PTC)?

1. RET/PTC: RET codes for a glial cell line–derived neurotrophic factor receptor that has tyrosine kinase activity.
   a. Patients can have somatic or germline mutations (MEN-2 syndromes).
   b. Mutations occur in about 40% of PTC.
2. NTRK1: A nerve growth factor with tyrosine kinase activity
3. BRAF: Activates the RAF/MEK/MAPK signaling pathway promoting tumorigenesis, invasion, metastasis, and recurrence. Mutations occur in 40% to 60% of PTC.

20. What genetic mutations are commonly found in follicular thyroid cancers (FTC)?

1. Translocation t(2;3)[q13:p25]: Resulting in a fusion protein of PAX8 (a thyroid transcription factor) and PPAR-gamma-1 (a transcription factor that stimulates cell differentiation and inhibits cell growth). Estimated to be in about 40% of FTC.
2. HRAS/KRAS/NRAS: Proto-oncogenes that affect the MAPK and PI3K-AKT pathways promoting tumorigenesis, invasion, and metastasis (30% to 45% of FTC).
3. PTEN: The mutation or deletion inactivates the gene which activates the PI3K pathway promoting tumorigenesis and invasiveness (10% to 15% of FTC)

21. What genetic mutations are commonly found in anaplastic thyroid cancer (ATC)?

1. BRAF: V600E activating mutation (25% of ATC)
2. TP53: An inactivating mutation that promotes tumor progression. Seen in 70% to 80% of ATCs
3. PIK3CA: An activating mutation affecting the PI3K-AKT pathway promoting tumorigenesis and invasiveness (15% to 25% of ATC)
4. RAS: Activating mutation affecting the MAPK and PI3K-AKT pathways (20% to 30% of ATC)

22. What is the major gene mutated in medullary thyroid cancer (MTC)?

1. RET: A proto-oncogene that has gain-of-function mutations in medullary thyroid cancer resulting in tumor pathogenesis

a. Sporadic MTC: Somatic mutations seen in 20% to 80%, often associated with worse prognosis
b. Familial MTC: >95% have RET mutations. Seen in patients with MEN2A, MEN2B, and familial MTC.

Bibliography

Agrawal N, Frederick MJ, Pickering CR, et al: Exome sequencing of head and neck squamous cell carcinoma reveals inactivating mutations in NOTCH1, *Science* 333:1154, 2011.

Guzzo M, Locati LD, Prott FJ, et al: Major and minor salivary gland tumors, *Crit Rev Oncol Hematol* 74(2):134–148, 2010.

Kroll TG, Sarraf P, Chen CJ, et al: PAX8-PPARgamma1 fusion oncogene in human thyroid cancer, *Science* 289(5483): 1357, 2000.

Psyrri A, Seiwert TY, Jimeno A: Molecular pathways in head and neck cancer: EGFR, PI3K, and more, *Am Soc Clin Oncol Educ Book* 33:246–255, 2013.

Rampias T, Sasaki C, Psyrri A: Molecular mechanisms of HPV induced carcinogenesis in head and neck, *Oral Oncol* S1368-8375(13)00642-8, 2013.

Sankaranarayanan R, Masueyer E, Swaminathan R, et al: Head and neck cancer: a global perspective on epidemiology and prognosis, *Anticancer Res* 18(6B):4779–4786, 1998.

Stenman G: Fusion oncogenes in salivary gland tumors: molecular and clinical consequences, *Head Neck Pathol* 7(Suppl 1):S12–S19, 2013.

Stransky N, Egloff AM, Tward AD, et al: The mutational landscape of head and neck squamous cell carcinoma, *Science* 333:1157, 2011.

Xing M: Molecular pathogenesis and mechanisms of thyroid cancer, *Nat Rev Cancer* 13(3):184–199, 2013.

CHAPTER 11

SKIN CANCER

Franki Lambert Smith, MD and Mariah Brown, MD

KEY POINTS

1. Skin cancer incidence
   - Normal population: BCC > SCC > melanoma > Merkel cell carcinoma
   - Transplant population: SCC > BCC > melanoma > Merkel cell carcinoma
2. Patients at higher risk for nonmelanoma skin cancer
   - Fair skinned with light eyes
   - Previous history of significant sun exposure and blistering sunburns
   - Family history of skin cancer
   - Previous skin cancer
   - History of chemical exposure
   - Genetic syndromes
   - Immunosuppression
   - Male
   - Older age
3. Important prognostic factors for melanoma
   - Breslow depth
   - Ulceration
   - Mitotic figures
   - Presence of nodal or distant metastases

Pearls

1. What is the most important prognostic factor in melanoma? Breslow depth
2. What is the most common type of skin cancer in transplant patients? Squamous cell carcinoma

QUESTIONS

1. **What are the common cutaneous malignancies?**
Cutaneous malignancies are classified into melanoma and nonmelanoma skin cancers. Nonmelanoma skin cancers include basal cell carcinoma and squamous cell carcinoma, which account for the majority of all skin cancers. Melanoma skin cancers account for only 5% of cutaneous malignancies, but result in 90% of the mortality from skin cancer in patients less than 50 years old. Rare nonmelanoma skin cancers include Merkel cell carcinoma, dermatofibrosarcoma protuberans, sebaceous carcinoma, and cutaneous T-cell lymphoma. Overall there are more skin cancers in the United States population than all other malignancies combined, and it is estimated that 20% of the population will develop a skin cancer during their lifetime.

2. **What is a basal cell carcinoma?**
Basal cell carcinoma (BCC) is a cutaneous neoplasm that arises from the basal layer of the epidermis. It is the most common skin cancer in humans, representing 75% of all nonmelanoma skin cancers with estimates of up to 1.5 million BCCs being diagnosed in the United States each year. There are many different classifications of BCC based on the tumor's histologic appearance under the microscope, including *superficial, nodular, micronodular, desmoplastic, pigmented,* and *basosquamous* BCCs. The classic appearance of a BCC is a skin-colored to pink, pearly papule or plaque with a rolled border and possibly central ulceration (Figures 11-1A and 11-1B). Superficial BCCs present as thin, pink, scaly papules or plaques and are most common on the trunk in younger patients (Figure 11-1C). Desmoplastic BCCs, also known as morpheaform, infiltrating or

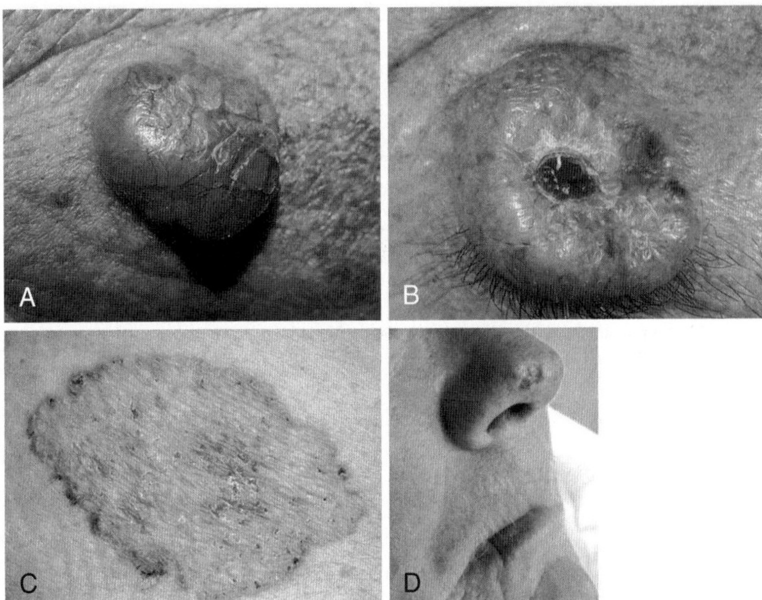

Figure 11-1. Variants of basal cell carcinoma (BCC). **A)** Nodular BCC with classic pearly appearance and dilated blood vessels. **B)** Ulcerated nodular BCC. **C)** Superficial BCC demonstrating pink plaque with scale. **D)** Desmoplastic BCC with scarred appearance. *(From Fitzsimons Army Medical Center.)*

sclerosing BCCs, may have a more subtle clinical appearance, presenting as a flat, slightly atrophic lesions, similar to a scar (Figure 11-1D). Desmoplastic and basosquamous BCCs have a more aggressive clinical course and a higher risk of recurrence. Risk factors for BCC include fair skin, ultraviolet exposure, immunosuppression, ionizing radiation, exposure to chemicals such as arsenic, and rare genetic syndromes. Although BCCs can be locally aggressive, they almost never metastasize.

3. What is squamous cell carcinoma?
Squamous cell carcinoma (SCC) is the second most common cutaneous malignancy and arises from the keratinocytes within the epidermis. SCC represents up to 25% of all skin cancers, but can have a more aggressive clinical course than BCC. SCC-in-situ, also known as Bowen's disease, is confined to the epidermis and presents as a thin, pink, scaly papule or plaque (Figure 11-2A). Invasive SCC presents as a pink, crusted papule or nodule on sun-damaged skin (Figure 11-2B). Common locations are sun-exposed areas such as the face, forearms and dorsal hands. SCCs associated with human papillomavirus (HPV) can occur on the hands, feet, and genitals. SCCs can also occur in areas of chronic inflammation such as a stasis ulcer or burn site (Marjolin's ulcer). Risk factors for SCCs include fair skin, ultraviolet exposure, immunosuppression, smoking, HPV, ionizing radiation, exposure to chemicals such as arsenic, certain medications, and rare genetic syndromes. The risk of metastatic SCC is less than 5% in sun-exposed skin but can be significantly higher for high-risk tumors. Metastases are most commonly found in regional lymph nodes but can also be distant. The role of sentinel lymph node biopsy in high-risk SCC is debated.

4. What makes a squamous cell carcinoma high risk?
SCCs are considered high risk based on several factors including location, etiology, histologic features, and host immune status. High risk factors include the following:
- **Location**: ear, lip, and genitalia
- **Etiology**: association with HPV, chronic inflammation, radiation, chemical exposures

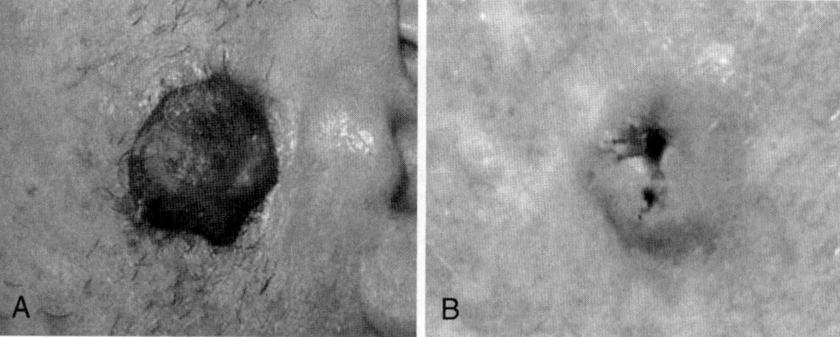

Figure 11-2. Squamous cell carcinoma (SCC). **A)** Large SCC composed of fungating hyperkeratotic plaque. **B)** Pink hyperkeratotic papule with central ulceration.

- **Histology**: poor differentiation, >2 cm size, >4 mm depth of invasion, perineural invasion, recurrence
- **Host immune status**: immunosuppression, genetic DNA repair defects such as xeroderma pigmentosum

5. **What are the most common cutaneous malignancies in the transplant population?**
   Transplant patients are more likely to develop numerous, aggressive nonmelanoma skin cancers and should be counseled on the importance of sun protective measures, regular skin exams, and self skin checks. While BCCs are the most common cutaneous malignancy in the general population, SCCs are by far the most common cutaneous malignancy in transplant patients. Transplant patients are 100 times more likely to develop SCCs than the general population and 10 times more likely to develop BCCs. Reported increased incidence of melanoma varies from 0 to 17 times higher for transplant patients. Merkel cell carcinoma is also seen more commonly in transplant patients. Rates of skin cancer development and skin cancer mortality increase with the length of immunosuppression, level of immunosuppression, and in patients with a baseline high risk for skin cancer. Mortality from skin cancer may approach 27% in cardiac transplant patients.

6. **What is Merkel cell carcinoma?**
   Merkel cell carcinoma (MCC) is a rare cutaneous neoplasm that is more common in older, immunosuppressed individuals. It presents as a rapidly enlarging pink or violaceous nodule on the head and neck or other sun-exposed areas. MCC was felt to have a neuroendocrine origin for many years, however in 2008 it was discovered that a polyomavirus was present in the majority of MCCs and the tumor is now considered to be infectious in origin, similar to HPV-induced malignancies. MCCs rapidly grow and up to 30% are metastatic at presentation. Treatment consists of surgical excision, often with sentinel lymph node biopsy and lymph node dissection if necessary, followed by adjuvant radiation therapy to the surgical site and nodal basin. Even with therapy, outcomes are poor with 5-year mortality at 30%.

7. **What is a keratoacanthoma and how is it treated?**
   Keratoacanthoma (KA) is a controversial entity that presents as an enlarging skin-colored or red nodule often with a central crater that may be filled with keratinous debris (Figure 11-3). KAs usually develop over a few weeks and then are often reported to spontaneously resolve over months, leaving a scar. KAs are generally solitary but can be multiple in certain genetic syndromes. Given the difficulty in distinguishing a KA from a well-differentiated SCC both clinically and histologically, these tumors are best considered a variant of well-differentiated SCC and treated as such.

8. **What is an actinic keratosis and how is it treated?**
   An actinic keratosis (AK) is a precancerous lesion that presents as a skin-colored to pink, rough papule on sun-exposed skin (Figure 11-4). Often, AKs are more easily felt than seen and patients

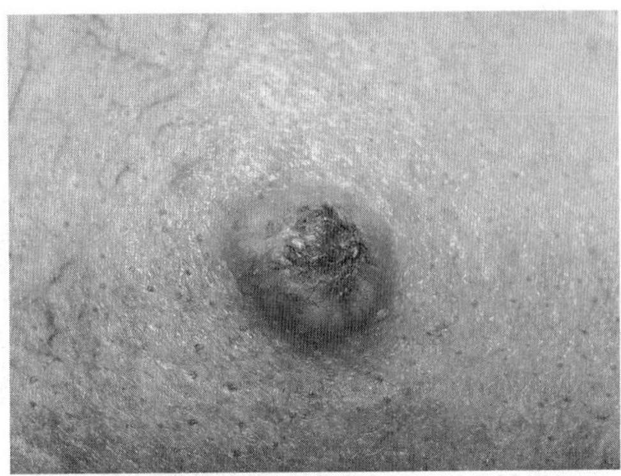

Figure 11-3. Keratoacanthaoma. Dome-shaped nodule with central crater. *(From Fitzpatrick JE, Aeling JL. Dermatology Secrets in Color, 2 ed, Philadelphia, 2000, Hanley & Belfus.)*

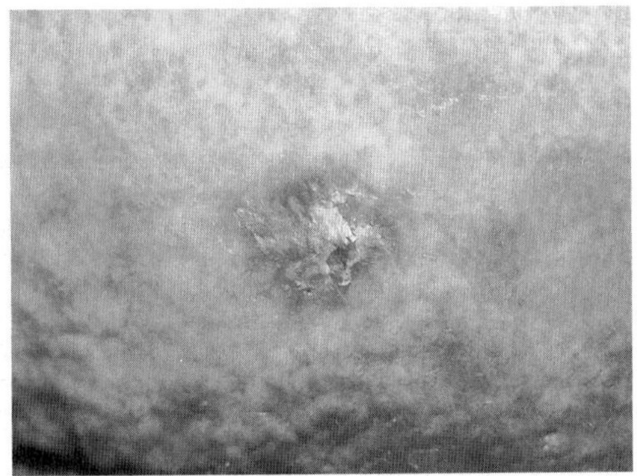

Figure 11-4. Actinic keratosis. Scaly pink papule on sun-exposed skin. *(From Fitzpatrick JE, Aeling JL. Dermatology Secrets in Color, 2 ed, Philadelphia, 2000, Hanley & Belfus.)*

describe them as areas that develop a crust that later falls off and reforms. If left untreated, AKs can develop into invasive SCC at a rate of 1/10 to 1/1000 per year, which presents a significant risk in patients with a large burden of these lesions. As a result, it is recommended that AKs be treated in most cases rather than observed. AKs can be treated individually with destructive mechanisms such as liquid nitrogen cryotherapy. Larger numbers of actinic keratoses can be field treated with multiple modalities, including topical chemotherapy (5-fluorouracil), topical immunomodulators (imiquimod), photodynamic therapy (δ-aminolevulinic acid exposed to 415 nm blue light), chemical peels or laser therapy. AKs are not treated surgically, being nonmalignant, ill-defined, and often diffusely present across sun-damaged skin. The risk factors for AKs are similar to those for SCC.

9. **What is actinic cheilitis?**
Actinic cheilitis describes the precancerous sun-damage changes that typically occur on the lower lip of older adults. It is the mucosal equivalent of an actinic keratosis, but because of its location has a higher risk of transformation to SCC. Actinic cheilitis can present as discrete, rough papules or encompass the entire lower lip with scaling of the lip and blurring of the vermillion border. Actinic cheilitis can be treated similar to AKs with cryotherapy, topical agents, or photodynamic therapy. However, once squamous cell carcinoma has formed within large areas of actinic cheilitis, removal

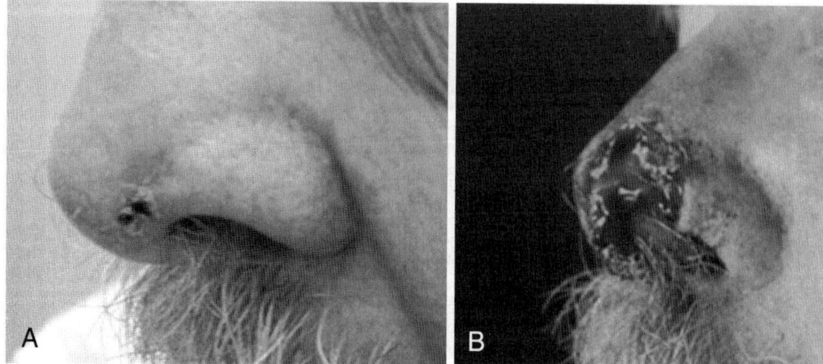

Figure 11-5. Before and after Mohs. **A)** Pre-Mohs. Desmoplastic BCC on the nasal tip. It is difficult to determine extent and depth of tumor. **B)** Post-Mohs. Large defect involving cartilage and nasal mucosa after four stages of Mohs surgery. This was reconstructed using a free cartilage graft and paramedian forehead flap.

of the entire affected area with vermillionectomy and mucosal advancement flap or CO_2 laser ablation may be indicated.

10. **What is Mohs micrographic surgery?**
Mohs micrographic surgery (MMS) is a technique for treating skin cancer developed by Dr. Frederic Mohs in 1938. The modern technique of MMS is a single-day procedure performed under local anesthesia designed to provide high cure rates and conserve normal, uninvolved skin. During MMS, a lesion is removed in a specific beveled disc shape and the resected tissue is mapped out with ink to provide accurate orientation. This tissue is then processed into frozen sections and stained, using a method of horizontal *en face* sections that allows for visualization of 100% of the peripheral and deep margins (standard tissue processing examines <1% of the surgical margin). The tissue is examined under the microscope by the Mohs surgeon and the areas of tumor are precisely mapped out. If needed, the patient then has additional tissue removed only in the areas that were positive for tumor. Each excision and visualization of tissue is referred to as a stage. As many stages as necessary are taken to ensure that the entire tumor is completely removed (Figure 11-5), at which time surgical reconstruction may be performed. Because all margins are examined during MMS, it offers high cure rates—approximately 99% for primary BCCs and SCCs—along with tissue conservation. Cure rates are lower for recurrent tumors and high-risk tumors.

11. **What tumors can be treated with Mohs surgery?**
MMS is predominantly used to treat BCC and SCC, as these comprise 95% of all skin cancers. However, more rare cutaneous tumors can also be treated with MMS (see Table 11-1). Certain types of cutaneous tumors may be treated with MMS using immunohistochemistry tissue stains to help better visualize the tumor cells. Many Mohs surgeons use immunohistochemistry stains such as MART-1 and/or Mel-5 to treat melanoma-in-situ (particularly the lentigo maligna variant) with MMS. Special stains have been used in MMS for extramammary Paget's disease (cytokeratin 7) and SCC (AE1-AE3—high molecular weight keratin stain).

12. **What are the indications for Mohs micrographic surgery?**
MMS is reserved for skin cancers in anatomic locations where tissue conservation is key or for high-risk tumors, due to the cost and time-consuming nature of the procedure. MMS is usually considered appropriate for skin cancers of the face, neck, scalp, hands, feet, and genitalia. Skin cancers in other anatomic locations may be candidates for MMS if they are recurrent, large, have an aggressive histologic subtype of SCC or BCC, present in an immunocompromised host or are a less common skin cancer (see Table 11-1). Appropriate use criteria have been determined to stratify which tumors are appropriate for MMS and these algorithms can be found at http://www.aad.org/education/appropriate-use-criteria/mohs-surgery-auc or by downloading the Mohs AUC mobile app.

Table 11-1. Rare Nonmelanoma Skin Cancers Appropriate for Mohs Surgery
Adenocystic carcinoma
Apocrine/eccrine carcinoma
Atypical fibroxanthoma
Dermatofibrosarcoma protuberans
Extramammary Paget's disease
Leiomyosarcoma
Undifferentiated pleomorphic sarcoma
Merkel cell carcinoma
Microcystic adnexal carcinoma
Mucinous carcinoma
Sebaceous carcinoma

13. **What are other treatments for nonmelanoma skin cancer besides Mohs surgery?**
Other treatment options for nonmelanoma skin cancer include excision, electrodesiccation and curettage, cryosurgery, topical therapies or radiation therapy. Excision can be performed for BCCs and SCCs, anticipating margins of 4 to 5 mm from clinically visible tumor, and clear margins should be confirmed with histologic examination. Electrodesiccation and curettage is a destructive technique that allows for localized treatment of low-risk skin cancers without the need for sutures or histologic examination. However, the technique can result in suboptimal scars and lower cure rates than excision or MMS. Cryosurgery or topical treatments, including 5-fluorouracil, imiquimod, and photodynamic therapy, are best limited to treatment of superficial variants of SCC and BCC. Radiation can be used to treat skin cancers, but is often reserved for inoperable tumors, patients who cannot tolerate surgery, or adjuvant therapy after complete surgical removal.

14. **What is vismodegib?**
Vismodegib is an oral small molecule chemotherapy that targets a mutation present in the majority of sporadic BCCs and in basal cell nevus syndrome. These BCCs have a mutation in the *PTCH* gene that leads to constitutive activation of the receptor "Smoothened," which in turn leads to gene replication and BCC formation. Vismodegib inhibits this hedgehog signaling pathway and can lead to the resolution of existing BCCs and prevention of new BCCs. However, there is often tumor recurrence or rebound after discontinuing the drug. The medication is currently approved for locally advanced BCC or metastatic BCC. Vismodegib has several side effects including nonscarring alopecia, dysgeusia, and muscle cramps and is teratogenic.

15. **What is melanoma?**
Melanoma is a malignancy that arises from aberrant growth of melanocytes, the pigment-containing cells that exist in the basal cell layer of the epidermis and also within moles (Nevi). Melanoma is most frequently seen in fair-skinned individuals with histories of intense, intermittent ultraviolet exposure. It is the most common cancer in female patients 25 to 29 years old. Approximately 75% of melanomas arise de novo and the remainder arise from existing nevi. The four main types of melanoma are *superficial spreading* melanoma (70%), *nodular* melanoma (15% to 30%), *lentigo maligna* melanoma (up to 15%), and *acral lentiginous* (5% to 10%). Less common variations of melanoma are *desmoplastic* melanoma and *amelanotic* melanoma.

16. **What is the clinical appearance of melanoma?**
Melanomas are usually heavily pigmented, with color variations of brown, black, and blue, but may also include red or pink areas as well as lighter areas that represent tumor regression (Figure 11-6). Melanomas are often asymmetric with irregular borders and variegated color. Common symptoms are pain, itching or bleeding. Amelanotic (nonpigmented) melanomas are much more difficult to diagnose clinically and often present as a pink, rapidly enlarging nodule that may ulcerate and bleed.

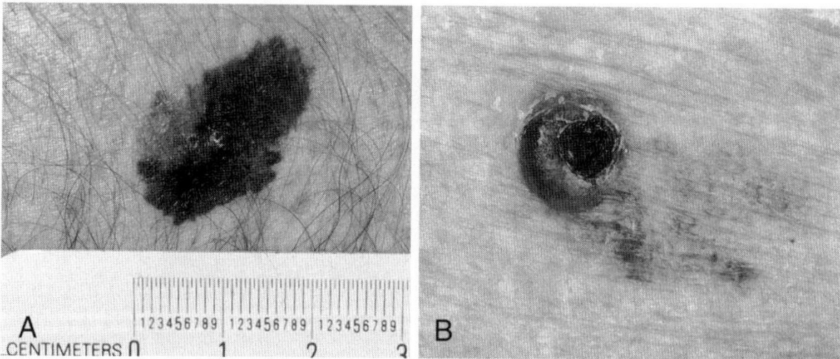

Figure 11-6. Melanoma. **A)** Superficial spreading melanoma with asymmetry, irregular borders, and color variegation. **B)** Superficial spreading and nodular melanoma with ulceration. *(From Fitzpatrick JE, Aeling JL. Dermatology Secrets in Color, 2 ed, Philadelphia, 2000, Hanley & Belfus.)*

17. What are the ABCDEs of melanoma?

Table 11-2. ABCDEs of Melanoma

A	Asymmetry: Melanomas are not uniform in size, shape or color.
B	Border: Melanomas often have borders that are not smooth or clearly demarcated.
C	Color: Melanomas may contain varying shades of pigment and also colors such as red, white, and blue.
D	Diameter: Most melanomas are >6 mm (the diameter of a pencil eraser); however suspicious lesions <6 mm should still be biopsied.
E	Evolution: Patients with melanoma often note changes in shape, size, color or symptomatology. Any new pigmented lesion in a patient >35 years old should be evaluated.

18. What are lentigo maligna and lentigo maligna melanoma?

Lentigo maligna is defined as a variant of in situ melanoma with a characteristic histologic and clinical appearance. Lentigo maligna presents clinically as a slow-growing, irregularly hyperpigmented patch on sun-exposed skin (Figure 11-7). Lentigo maligna melanoma (LMM) represents lentigo maligna with areas of tumor invasion into the dermis, and is the third most common type of melanoma (up to 15%). Lentigo maligna and lentigo maligna melanoma are most commonly seen in elderly patients on sun-exposed areas.

19. What are risk factors for melanoma?

Risk factors for melanoma consist of genetic, skin type, and environmental factors. Most commonly, genetic susceptibility is related to an inherited phenotype of fair skin. Patients with multiple benign moles (>50) also have an increased risk of melanoma development, and the development of moles is linked with childhood sun exposure. Melanoma risk is increased in individuals with a first degree relative with a melanoma. True genetic predisposition (i.e., familial melanoma) is much more rare and is most commonly associated with defects in *CDKN2A*, the gene that encodes the proteins p16 and p14. Patients with multiple atypical moles and a family history of melanoma, described as dysplastic nevus syndrome, have an elevated risk of melanoma. Patients with large congenital nevi (>20 cm) also have an elevated risk of developing melanoma. Sun exposure is the most important environmental risk factor and it has been shown that people living at latitudes closer to the equator (i.e., Florida, Australia) have a much higher incidence of melanoma. Times of intense, intermittent sun exposure is associated with the development of superficial spreading and nodular melanoma, while a high cumulative sun exposure is associated with the development of lentigo maligna melanoma.

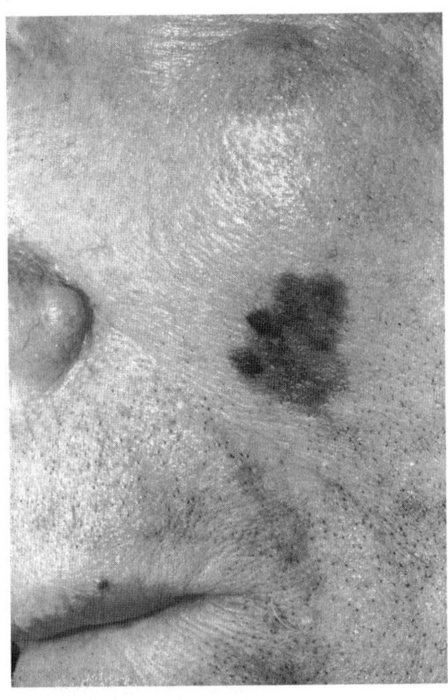

Figure 11-7. Lentigo maligna. Irregular pigmented patch on sun-exposed skin. *(From Fitzpatrick JE, Aeling JL. Dermatology Secrets in Color, 2 ed, Philadelphia, 2000, Hanley & Belfus.)*

20. What is Breslow depth?
Breslow depth is a measurement in millimeters of the tumor depth from the granular layer of the epidermis to the base of the melanoma. It is the most important prognostic indicator for melanomas. Clark's level, a measurement of melanoma depth based on skin anatomy, is no longer used for melanoma staging, but may still be reported by some pathologists.

21. How is melanoma staged?
Melanoma is staged by the TNM staging system from the American Joint Commission on Cancer (AJCC). This staging system was first published in 2000 and was modified in 2009 to include data on mitotic rate and micrometastases (Table 11-3).
- Micrometastases are diagnosed after sentinel or elective lymphadenectomy.
- Macrometastases are defined as clinically detectable nodal metastases confirmed by therapeutic lymphadenectomy or when nodal metastasis exhibits gross extracapsular extension.
- In-transit metastases are >2 cm from the primary tumor but not beyond the regional lymph nodes, while satellite lesions are within 2 cm of the primary (Table 11-4).

22. What is a sentinel lymph node biopsy and how is it performed?
Sentinel lymph node biopsy (SLNB) is performed to determine whether or not cancer has spread from the skin to the regional draining lymphatics. Sentinel lymph node status is an important prognostic indicator used in the staging of melanoma. A radioactive tracer and/or a blue dye is injected into the melanoma site and then the lymph node (or sometimes multiple lymph nodes) that most strongly picks up these markers is removed and examined for the presence of melanoma cells. Normally, wide local excision of the melanoma is done at the time of SLNB to prevent disruption of lymphatics, which could alter the normal drainage pattern. If the SLNB is positive, a completion lymph node dissection is recommended. SLNB is a prognostic tool rather than a treatment modality, as studies have not shown a clear survival benefit for patients who undergo the procedure.

23. When is a sentinel lymph node biopsy recommended for melanoma patients?
SLNB is recommended for patients with a melanoma with Breslow depth greater than 1.0 mm. For patients with melanomas between 0.75 mm and 0.99 mm, especially those with ulceration or

Table 11-3. Melanoma TNM Classification

T CLASSIFICATION	THICKNESS	ULCERATION STATUS/ MITOSES	5-YEAR % SURVIVAL
Tis	NA	NA	
T1	≤1.0 mm	a: Without ulceration and mitosis <1/mm^2 b: With ulceration or mitoses ≥1/mm^2	97 90
T2	1.01–2.0 mm	a: Without ulceration b: With ulceration	90 78
T3	2.01–4.0 mm	a: Without ulceration b: With ulceration	78 65
T4	>4.0 mm	a: Without ulceration b: With ulceration	65 45
N CLASSIFICATION	**NUMBER OF METASTATIC NODES**	**NODAL METASTATIC MASS**	
N0	0	NA	
N1	1 node	a: Micrometastasis b: Macrometastasis	
N2	2–3 nodes	a: Micrometastasis b: Macrometastasis c: In-transit met(s)/satellite(s) without metastatic node(s)	
N3	4 or more metastatic nodes, matted nodes, or in-transit met(s)/ satellite(s) with metastatic node(s)		
M CLASSIFICATION	**SITE**	**SERUM LACTATE DEHYDROGENASE (LDH)**	
M0	No distant metastases	NA	
M1a	Distant skin, subcutaneous or nodal metastases	Normal	
M1b	Lung metastases	Normal	
M1c	All other visceral metastases Any distant metastasis	Normal Elevated	

Data from the American Joint Committee on Cancer website https://cancerstaging.org/Pages/default.aspx.

mitotic figures (pT1b), it is generally recommended to discuss with them the pros and cons of SLNB and offer treatment. SLNB is not indicated for patients who present with evidence of metastatic disease at the time of diagnosis.

24. **What is the treatment for thin melanoma?**
The treatment for localized, primary melanoma is surgical excision. Surgical margins for melanoma are based on Breslow depth (Table 11-5). There is some debate whether or not >2 cm margins should be taken on thicker melanomas (>2 mm Breslow depth).

25. **What is the treatment for metastatic melanoma?**
Once melanoma has spread to the lymph nodes or other distant sites, mortality sharply increases and treatment options are more limited. Metastatic melanoma is not very responsive to radiation or traditional chemotherapy. Recently, melanoma treatment has been advanced by the development of targeted molecular therapies such as vemurafenib. This chemotherapy agent targets a mutation in

Table 11-4. Stage Groupings for Cutaneous Melanoma

	5-YEAR % SURVIVAL	*Clinic Staging*			*Pathologic Staging*		
		T	**N**	**M**	**T**	**N**	**M**
0		Tis	N0	Mo	Tis	N0	M0
IA	97	T1a	N0	M0	T1a	N0	M0
IB	93	T1b T2a	N0	M0	T1b T2a	N0	M0
IIA	82 79	T2b T3a	N0	M0	T2b T3a	N0	M0
IIB	68 71	T3b T4a	N0	M0	T3b T4a	N0	M0
IIC	53	T4b	N0	M0	T4b	N0	M0
III		Any T	N1 N2 N3	M0			
IIIA	78				T1-4a T1-4a	N1a N2a	M0 M0
IIIB	59				T1-4b T1-4b T1-4a T1-4a T1-4a	N1a N2a N1b N2b N2c	
IIIC	40				T1-4b T1-4b T1-4b Any T	N1b N2b N2c N3	M0
IV	9–27	Any T	Any N	Any M1	Any T	Any N	Any M1

Data from the American Joint Committee on Cancer website https://cancerstaging.org/Pages/default.aspx.

Table 11-5. Excisional Margins for Melanoma

MELANOMA BRESLOW DEPTH	MARGIN IN CM
Melanoma-in-situ (excluding lentigo maligna which may need larger margins)	0.5
≤1 mm	1
1.01–2.0 mm	1–2
>2 mm	2

the BRAF pathway present in 40% to 60% of melanomas. Initial studies cite a 64% relative reduction in the risk of death and a 74% relative reduction in disease progression. However, further mutations in the melanoma lead to eventual inefficacy of the medication and disease progression. Combining BRAF inhibitors with MEK inhibitors such as trametinib further increases progression-free survival in advanced melanoma. The side effects of vemurafenib include arthralgias, rashes, photosensitivity, and the development of squamous cell carcinoma. Another important new medication for metastatic melanoma patients is ipilimumab. This medication is a monoclonal antibody against CTLA-4 that activates T-cells to attack tumor cells. The main side effects of ipilimumab are autoimmune in nature, including colitis, hypophysitis, hepatitis, and iridocyclitis.

26. **What is the association between ultraviolet light and skin cancer?**
Ultraviolet radiation (UVR) emitted from the sun consists of ultraviolet C (UVC), ultraviolet B (UVB), and ultraviolet A (UVA). UVC is almost completely blocked by the Earth's atmosphere and UVB is

somewhat blocked by the atmosphere; 95% of UVR that reaches the Earth's surface is UVA and the remainder is UVB. Exposure to ultraviolet radiation has repeatedly been shown to increase the risk of nonmelanoma and melanoma skin cancer by inducing DNA mutations and causing immunosuppression within the skin, which decreases DNA repair. It was previously thought that UVB is responsible for the majority of skin cancers; however, now UVA is thought to play a larger role. Tanning beds, which predominantly emit UVA light, have been associated with an increased risk of BCC, SCC, and melanoma. UVC is profoundly carcinogenic, but does not contribute to skin cancer formation because it is blocked from reaching the ground by the Earth's atmosphere (Table 11-6).

27. **What are important methods of photoprotection?**
Photoprotection should be recommended for all patients, especially those at high risk for skin cancer or with a history of skin cancer. Photoprotection is multifactorial and includes avoidance of sun during peak hours of UV radiation (10 am to 2 pm), protective clothing, wide brimmed hats, and sunscreen for exposed areas. Photoprotection is measured in UV protection factor (UPF) for clothing and hats and sun protection factor (SPF) for sunscreens. Sunscreens are composed of organic and inorganic compounds that absorb and scatter UV light. Sunscreens should be "broad spectrum," meaning they block both UVB and UVA for optimal photoprotection. It is important to note that protocols to determine sunscreen SPF include application of 2 mg/cm^2 of sunscreen, but the majority of people apply a much smaller density of sunscreen. As a result, frequent reapplications (every 2 to 4 hours) and use of high SPF products is recommended.

CONTROVERSIES

28. **How are squamous cell carcinoma tumors staged?**
Squamous cell carcinoma is traditionally staged using the AJCC staging system, which was most recently revised in 2010 (Table 11-7). Recently an alternative staging system was proposed in 2013 to better stratify SCCs, specifically T2 tumors. The alternative staging system has divided T2 into T2a and T2b because of significantly higher risk of nodal metastasis in T2b tumors. The alternative system also does not include a T4 stage.

Table 11-6. Ultraviolet Spectrum

ULTRAVIOLET RADIATION TYPE	WAVELENGTH IN NM
UVC	270–290
UVB	290–315
UVA	315–400

Table 11-7. American Joint Committee on Cancer Squamous Cell Carcinoma Tumor Staging System

Tx	Primary tumor cannot be assessed
T0	No evidence of primary tumor
Tis	Carcinoma in situ
T1	Tumor ≤2 cm with <2 high-risk features*
T2	Tumor >2 cm OR Tumor with >2 high-risk features
T3	Tumor with invasion of maxilla, mandible, orbit, or temporal bone
T4	Tumor with invasion of skeleton (axial or appendicular) or perineural invasion of skull base.

*AJCC High-risk factors: Breslow thickness >2 mm, Clark's level ≥4, site on ear or lip, poorly differentiated.
(From Farasat S, Yu SS, Neel VA, et al. A new American Joint Committee on Cancer staging system for cutaneous squamous cell carcinoma: creation and rationale for inclusion of tumor (T) characteristics, J Am Acad Dermatol 64(6):1051–1059, 2011.)

29. **When should sentinel lymph node biopsies be used for squamous cell carcinoma?**
There have been no randomized clinical trials establishing when SLNBs are appropriate in SCC. A recent meta-analysis reviewed case reports and cases series using both the AJCC and the alternative staging system (see above) to determine which SCCs had a high risk of sentinel lymph node positivity. The results showed that patients who fell into the T2b alternative staging system had a 29% risk of positive SLNB and patients with T3 cancers had a 50% risk of positive SLNB. More studies are needed to make definitive recommendations on SLNB in squamous cell carcinoma.

30. **Should Mohs surgery be performed on melanoma-in-situ?**
Because Mohs surgery employs frozen sections while viewing tissue, some argue that the freezing artifact makes it very difficult to correctly identify melanocytes on standard hematoxylin and eosin processed slides. Some Mohs surgeons believe that melanoma-in-situ is best treated with the slow (modified) Mohs technique. With this technique, the tissue is embedded in paraffin and sectioned en face for permanent sections. If needed, special stains can be performed with melanocytic markers such as MART-1 or SOX-10. The disadvantage of this protocol is a longer wait time for the patient (as only one stage can be performed each day) and the tissue leaving the surgeon's hands for pathologic processing, increasing the risk for error in embedding or mapping. Many Mohs surgeons instead advocate performing Mohs surgery on melanoma-in-situ using special immunohistochemistry stains, usually MART-1, on frozen tissue within their own laboratories. The advantages of this technique are shorter wait time for the patients and increased control in the hands of the surgeon for mapping purposes.

Bibliography

Amber K, McLeod MP, Nouri K: The Merkel cell polyomavirus and its involvement in Merkel cell carcinoma, *Dermatol Surg* 39(2):232–238, 2013.

Balch CM, Gershenwald JE, Soong SJ, et al: Final version of 2009 AJCC melanoma staging and classification, *J Clin Oncol* 27:6199–6206, 2009.

Bolognia J, Jorizzo JL, Rapini RP: *Dermatology*, St. Louis, MO, 2008, Mosby/Elsevier. Print.

Chapman PB, Hauschild A, Robert C: Improved survival with vemurafenib in melanoma with BRAF V600E mutation, *N Eng J Med* 364:2507–2516, 2011.

Costantino D, Lowe L, Brown DL: Basosquamous carcinoma-an under-recognized, high-risk cutaneous neoplasm: case study and review of the literature, *J Plast Reconstr Aesthet Surg* 59(4):424–428, 2006.

Jambusaria-Pahlajani A, Kanetsky PA, Kria PS, et al: Evaluation of AJCC tumor staging for cutaneous squamous cell carcinoma and a proposed alternative tumor staging system, *JAMA Dermatol* 149(4):402–410, 2013.

Mudigonda T, Levender MM, O'Neill JL, et al: Incidence, risk factors, and preventative management of skin cancers in organ transplant recipients: a review of single- and multicenter retrospective studies from 2006 to 2010, *Dermatol Surg* 39:345–364, 2013.

Rigel DS, Friedman RJ, Kopf AW: Lifetime risk for development of skin cancer in the U.S. population: current risk is now 1 in 5, *J Am Acad Dermatol* 35:1012–1013, 1996.

Schmitt AR, Brewer JD, Bordeaux JS, et al: Staging for cutaneous squamous cell carcinoma as a predictor of sentinel lymph node biopsy results: meta-analysis of American Joint Committee on Cancer criteria and a proposed alternative system, *JAMA Dermatol* 150(1):19–24, 2014.

Sladden MJ, Balch C, Barzilai DA, et al: Surgical excision margins for primary cutaneous melanoma, *Cochrane Database Syst Rev* (4):CD004835, 2009.

CHAPTER 12

DISEASES OF THE ORAL CAVITY AND OROPHARYNX

Julie A. Goddard, MD, FACS

KEY POINTS

1. Despite their proximity, oral cavity and oropharyngeal cancers often behave differently and thus are treated differently.
2. Premalignant lesions of the oral cavity warrant evaluation and follow-up. There are no specific premalignant lesions of the oropharynx.
3. Depth of invasion is utilized in treatment decisions for oral cancer, and cervical lymph node metastasis is a key driver of prognosis.
4. Human papilloma virus (HPV) has changed the evaluation and management of oropharyngeal cancer.

Pearls

1. Oral cavity cancer most commonly spreads to lymph nodes in Levels I, II, and III. Oropharyngeal cancer most commonly spreads to lymph nodes in Levels II, III, IV.
2. Staging of oral cavity and oropharyngeal tumors can generally be remembered by size criteria: T1 = 0 to 2 cm, T2 = 2 to 4 cm, T3 = > 4 cm, T4 = extension to adjacent structures.
3. Oral cavity cancer is primarily treated with surgery, whereas oropharyngeal cancer is commonly treated with radiation.

QUESTIONS

1. **Describe the anatomy of the oral cavity and name the eight subsites within it.**
   The oral cavity extends from the vermilion border of the lip (mucocutaneous junction) to the circumvallate papillae of the tongue inferorly and the junction of the hard and soft palate superiorly. The eight subsites are:
   1. Lips
   2. Buccal mucosa
   3. Lower (mandibular) alveolar ridge/gingiva
   4. Upper (maxillary) alveolar ridge/gingiva
   5. Retromolar trigone
   6. Hard palate
   7. Floor of mouth
   8. Oral tongue (anterior two thirds)
2. **What is the most common type of malignancy within the oral cavity?**
   Squamous cell carcinoma. As in all head and neck sites, squamous cell carcinoma (SCC) is by far the most common type of tumor seen. More than 90% of oral cavity cancers are SCC. Other malignant tumors include minor salivary gland malignancies, Kaposi's sarcoma, other sarcomas, melanoma, and rarely lymphoma.
3. **Where in the oral cavity are minor salivary gland malignancies most commonly seen? What is the most common type?**
   Within the oral cavity, minor salivary gland malignancies most commonly occur on the hard palate. Adenoid cystic carcinoma is the most common tumor of the minor salivary glands in the oral cavity.

4. What are the most common subsites for oral cavity squamous cell carcinoma?

1. **Lips:** Incidence varies by geographic location, but overall 15% to 30% of oral cavity cancers occur on the lips. The lower lip is much more common than the upper lip (>90% arise in lower lip). Though still considered oral cavity SCC by the American Joint Committee on Cancer (AJCC), lip cancer can be considered separately because the vermilion of the lip is exposed to external environmental factors (such as UV radiation from the sun) and sometimes behaves more like cutaneous SCC.
2. **Oral tongue:** 20% to 30% of oral cavity cancers. Lateral tongue is more common than dorsal tongue.

5. Discuss three premalignant clinical lesions or conditions of the oral cavity.

1. **Leukoplakia:** White keratotic plaque or patch that cannot be rubbed off. Often seen due to chronic trauma or irritation of oral mucosa. Most are benign, but malignant potential/transformation rate is very difficult to predict. Baseline biopsy and follow-up or excision is recommended depending on pathologic findings.
2. **Erythroplakia:** Red mucosal plaque not arising from an obvious mechanical or inflammatory cause. This lesion has a much higher malignant potential than leukoplakia (estimated to be 7 times more malignant potential), and can be seen in conjunction with leukoplakia. More aggressive therapy is recommended than that for leukoplakia, including complete excision with adequate margins.
3. **Oral lichen planus:** Lacy white lines primarily noted on buccal mucosa (but changes can be seen throughout the oral cavity). Exact cause is unknown but thought to be immune mediated (lymphocytic infiltration of epithelial layers seen). Associated with pain and burning and clinical course waxes and wanes. Treated with topical steroids, systemic steroids, and sometimes other immunosuppressants. Lifetime malignant transformation risk is 5% to 10%.

Note: The above are *clinical*, rather than *pathologic*, descriptions of premalignant conditions. *Dysplasia*, which can be seen in any of these lesions, is the pathologic description of premalignant change describing degrees of cellular change. Dysplasia can be described as mild, moderate, and severe. Severe dysplasia and carcinoma in situ are often utilized interchangeably by pathologists.

6. Are oral cavity SCCs commonly caused by human papilloma virus (HPV)?

No. Whereas *oropharynx* SCC is very commonly driven by the HPV virus (some reports >80%), only a small percentage (<3%) of oral cavity cancers are truly HPV driven.

7. Where in the neck do regional metastases of oral cavity SCC most commonly appear and how is this clinically significant?

Regional nodal disease from oral cavity SCC most commonly presents in the upper cervical lymph nodes: level I (submental and submandibular), level II, and level III (upper and middle jugular nodes). This relatively predictable nodal drainage of oral cavity subsites has led to the use of what is termed the supraomohyoid neck dissection (includes levels I, II, and III) for elective nodal dissection in oral cavity cancers. The finding of microscopic nodal disease in levels III and IV without level I and II disease in greater than 15% of *oral tongue* cancer patients has led to some recommending inclusion of level IV in elective neck dissections for oral tongue cancer.

8. How is cancer of the oral cavity staged?

SCC of the oral cavity is staged according to the tumor, node, metastasis (TNM) sytem by the American Joint Committee for Cancer (AJCC), currently in its seventh iteration. Within the oral cavity, size of the tumor is the major factor determining T-stage.

- Tx: No information available on primary tumor
- T0: No evidence of primary tumor
- Tis: Carcinoma in situ
- T1: Tumor <2 cm
- T2: Tumor size 2 to 4 cm
- T3: Tumor size >4 cm
- T4a: Moderately advanced local disease.
  - Lip: Tumor invades through cortical bone, inferior alveolar nerve, floor of mouth, or skin of face
  - Oral cavity: Tumor invades adjacent structures only (e.g., through cortical bone [mandible or maxilla], into deep [extrinsic] muscle of tongue [genioglossus, hyoglossus, palatoglossus,

styloglossus], maxillary sinus, skin of face) Note: superficial erosion alone of bone/tooth socket by gingival primary is not sufficient to classify a tumor as T4.
- T4b: Very advanced local disease. Tumor invades masticator space, pterygoid plates, or skull base, and/or encases internal carotid artery

Nodal staging is the same for most head and neck squamous cell cancers.
- Nx: Regional lymph nodes cannot be assessed
- N0: No regional lymph node metastasis
- N1: Metastasis in a single ipsilateral lymph node, 3 cm or less in greatest dimension
- N2a: Metastasis in single ipsilateral lymph node more than 3 cm but not more than 6 cm
- N2b: Metastasis in multiple ipsilateral lymph nodes, none more than 6 cm in greatest dimension
- N2c: Metastasis in bilateral or contralateral lymph nodes, none more than 6 cm in greatest dimension
- N3: Metastasis in a lymph node more than 6 cm in greatest dimension

9. How is depth of invasion utilized in treatment of early oral tongue cancers?

Depth of tumor invasion is correlated with risk of nodal metastasis (and also correlates with prognosis and risk of recurrence). Depth of invasion refers to the depth below the surface epithelium into which the tumor extends. Depth of invasion and tumor thickness are not technically synonymous, as exophytic tumors can be very thick but have shallow depth of invasion into underlying structures. In oral tongue cancer, depth of invasion has been studied as a deciding factor regarding elective treatment of a clinically node-negative neck. Multiple trials have supported tumor depth of invasion of 4 mm as the cutoff point regarding elective treatment of the neck. Tumors with depth of invasion of 4 mm or greater are associated with greater than 20% incidence of microscopic nodal metastasis and thus elective neck treatment is indicated.

10. What does the initial workup for patients with oral cavity or oropharynx cancer typically include?

Complete history and physical examination, imaging (most commonly CT neck with contrast; MRI with gadolinium can be useful, especially if dental artifact on CT scan obscures view of tumor), dental evaluation, tissue biopsy, chest radiograph. Chest radiograph is still considered acceptable evaluation for distant metastasis or second primary malignancy, though CT chest and PET/CT are being utilized more recently. However, use of PET/CT as the primary staging imaging modality for all head and neck cancer patients is controversial and is the subject of ongoing debate. Generally, most patients will have laboratory evaluation including liver function tests (though abnormal liver function tests leading to the finding of liver metastases at initial presentation is a rare scenario).

11. What is the recommended treatment for oral cavity cancer?

Primary surgery is accepted as first-line therapy for all oral cavity sites. Surgical excision of all involved structures including a margin of normal tissue is performed. The generally accepted pathologically negative margin is 5 mm, but due to tissue shrinkage, clinical margins measured and excised by the surgeon intraoperatively are 1 to 1.5 cm.

12. What factors are indications to consider giving postoperative adjuvant therapy after resection of oral cavity SCC to minimize risk of locoregional recurrence?

Tumor Factors

1. Locally advanced T3 or T4 lesions
2. High-grade histology
3. Presence of perineural invasion or lymphovascular invasion on pathology
4. Infiltrating rather than pushing borders of tumor
5. Positive or close (<5 mm on pathologic specimen) margins of surgical resection
6. Surgeon concern regarding adequacy of resection regardless of histologic surgical margins

Nodal Factors

7. N stage higher than N1
8. Surgical contamination (excisional or incisional nodal biopsy prior to definitive surgery)
9. Presence of extracapsular extension

Note: Positive margins and presence of extracapsular extension are even higher risk features for recurrence and are used as indications to give chemotherapy with radiation postoperatively.

13. **What are the subsites within the oropharynx?**
The oropharynx is bounded by the junction of the hard and soft palate and circumvallate papillae anteriorly, superior surface of the soft palate superiorly, and pharyngoepiglottic fold inferiorly. Subsites include:
    1. Tonsils
    2. Base of tongue and vallecula
    3. Soft palate
    4. Tonsillar pillars (palatoglossus and palatopharyngeus muscles)
    5. Pharyngeal walls

14. **What is the primary lymphatic drainage of the oropharynx?**
Lymphatic drainage is primarily to the jugular lymphatics in level II, III, and IV. Nodal metastases are most commonly seen in level II. Isolated nodal metastasis to levels I and V is rare from oropharynx tumors. Subsites within the oropharynx known specifically to have rich bilateral lymphatic drainage are the base of tongue and soft palate (as well as posterior pharyngeal well, which is generally a much less common primary site for SCC). Oropharyngeal structures also drain to retropharyngeal and parapharyngeal lymph nodes.

15. **Which more commonly presents as an isolated neck mass, oral cavity or oropharyngeal SCC?**
Oropharyngeal cancer may commonly present as an isolated neck mass without other symptoms whereas oral cancer more commonly presents with oral cavity symptoms such as pain, bleeding, ulcer/visible lesion, change in speech, ear pain.

16. **List common symptoms of oropharynx cancer.**
Oropharyngeal cancer commonly presents with throat pain or fullness, dysphagia, odynophagia, referred ear pain, neck mass, change in voice (muffled voice), foul breath or foul taste, expectorating bloody secretions. With more advanced disease, patients may have trismus, difficulty with tongue mobility due to deep infiltration, or airway obstruction.

17. **How do oral and pharyngeal neoplasms refer pain to the ipsilateral ear?**
Otalgia is referred from the pharynx by way of the pharyngeal cranial nerves IX and X, which also supply sensory innervation to the ear. The tongue and floor of mouth are supplied by the lingual branch of V3. V3 also provides sensation to the external auditory canal, tympanic membrane, and temporomandibular joint through the auriculotemporal nerve. In some patients, the sensation of otalgia is much more prominent than oral or throat pain.

18. **Why should one be wary of the diagnosis of "branchial cleft cyst" in a 55-year-old former smoker?**
Oropharynx subsites very commonly present with cystic nodal metastases. Since the most common cervical location of these is level II of the neck, these metastases are located in the presenting location of a second branchial cleft cyst. These cystic metastases can have a thin wall and be full of clear/serous appearing fluid just like the branchial cleft cyst. We often cannot rely on fine needle aspiration (FNA) for diagnosis because the fluid obtained from either type of neck mass may look similar under the microscope—degenerated squamous cells and debris can be seen in the fluid of both a malignant metastasis or a branchial cleft cyst. Though it is possible for older persons to have their congenital branchial anomaly present later in life, this is an uncommon scenario and one must think of a cystic neck mass in an adult as cancer until proven otherwise.

19. **The incidence of many head and neck malignancies in the United States has been declining slowly in the recent past (likely due to decreased rates of smoking); however, the rate of oropharynx cancer is increasing significantly. To what factor is this attributed?**
Human papilloma virus (HPV)-associated oropharynx cancer is increasing dramatically in the United States and some European countries. Since the late 1990s and early 2000s, HPV has risen to the forefront of discussion in oropharynx SCC. Primary sites most associated with HPV are the tonsil and the base of tongue. Overall prognosis associated with HPV-positive SCC is significantly better than that of HPV-negative SCC, and research is ongoing to determine causes of this difference.

20. **Which subtype of HPV is considered to be highest risk for association with oropharyngeal malignancy?**
HPV 16 is by far the most common subtype of HPV associated with oropharynx SCC. Types 18, 31, and 33 are also considered high-risk subtypes, but are actually not that commonly seen in oropharyngeal cancer. Overexpression of the p16 protein can be evaluated by immunohistochemistry on pathologic specimens and is commonly utilized as a surrogate marker for HPV-positive tumors.

21. **How does HPV cause oropharyngeal cancer?**
Viral proteins E6 and E7 cause inactivation/degradation of p53 tumor suppressor gene allowing malignant cells to proceed through normal cell cycle check points and continue to replicate.

22. **How do oropharyngeal cancer patients diagnosed today differ from those seen 30 years ago?**
We are more commonly seeing oropharyngeal cancer in younger (40s to 50s) patients with little to no smoking history. Specifically, incidence is expanding in the white male population (though female incidence is expanding as well). These are classic HPV-associated oropharyngeal cancer patients. HPV-associated tumors present with early cervical nodal metastases, but these patients are noted to have overall better prognosis than their HPV-negative counterparts, suggesting a need to include HPV status in staging information and perhaps revise the future staging schema.

23. **How does primary treatment of oropharynx SCC differ from oral cavity SCC?**
Whereas recommendation for primary treatment of oral cavity cancer is surgical excision, oropharyngeal cancer is very commonly treated primarily with radiation with or without chemotherapy. Based initially on studies from the 1990s and 2000s regarding "organ preservation" therapy for laryngeal cancer that showed similar oncologic outcomes between nonsurgical therapy and laryngectomy for laryngeal cancer, further evidence has amassed for nonsurgical treatment of oropharyngeal cancer providing similar oncologic outcomes to surgery with postoperative radiation and significantly less morbidity. Thus, radiation-based therapy became standard of care for treatment of most oropharyngeal SCC over the last 30 years. With improved technology to allow for less invasive access to the oropharynx (TLM and TORS; see below), surgical therapy for oropharyngeal cancer is being revisited and is the subject of much ongoing research.

24. **Describe two techniques for a minimally invasive approach to the oropharynx.**
With the following techniques, surgeons can have access to the oropharynx for resection of tumors via the transoral route.
    1. Transoral Laser CO_2 Microsurgery (TLM): Initially described in the 1970s, this is a technique utilized initially for laryngeal surgery and subsequently applied to tumors of the oropharynx and hypopharynx. It utilizes laryngoscopes of various types to provide access to the pharynx and a microscope for magnified view of the tumor. A CO_2 laser is used as a cutting and coagulating instrument. This technique is traditionally limited by line of sight—the structures being visualized are in a straight line with the laryngoscope used and the CO_2 laser travels in a straight line from the microscope (though use of a CO_2 laser fiber has allowed for some angled use of the CO_2 laser).
    2. Transoral Robotic Surgery (TORS): In this technique, described in 2005, a surgeon seated at a distant console utilizes robotic arms inserted into the mouth to perform the dissection. Zero-degree or 30-degree angled, high-definition binocular endoscopy is utilized for enhanced visualization, and the robotic arms can be fitted with various grasping, cautery, or cutting instruments (including the laser fiber). This technique has become much more widely utilized than TLM for access to the oropharynx.

25. **How does presence of cervical nodal metastasis affect overall prognosis for oral cavity and oropharynx cancer?**
Cervical nodal metastasis is associated with worse prognosis, with survival rates diminished by up to 50% compared with patients lacking cervical nodal disease.

BIBLIOGRAPHY

Bernier J, Domenge C, Ozsahin M, et al: Postoperative irradiation with or without concomitant chemotherapy for locally advanced head and neck cancer, *N Engl J Med* 350:1045, 2004.

Byers RM, Weber RS, Andrews T, et al: Frequency and therapeutic implications of "skip metastases" in the neck from squamous cell carcinoma of the oral tongue, *Head Neck* 19:14, 1997.

Chaturvedi AK, Engels EA, Pfeiffer RM, et al: Human papillomavirus and rising oropharyngeal cancer incidence in the United States, *J Clin Oncol* 29:4294, 2011.

Cooper JS, Pajak TF, Forastiere AA, et al: Postoperative concurrent radiotherapy and chemotherapy for high-risk squamous-cell carcinoma of the head and neck, *N Engl J Med* 350:1937, 2004.

Edge S, Byrd DR, Compton CC, et al: *AJCC Cancer Staging Manual*, ed 7, New York, 2010, Springer.

Holsinger FC, Sweeney AD, Jantharapattana K, et al: The emergence of endoscopic head and neck surgery, *Curr Oncol Rep* 12:216, 2010.

Huang SH, Hwang D, Lockwood G, et al: Predictive value of tumor thickness for cervical lymph node involvement in squamous cell carcinoma of the oral cavity: a meta-analysis of reported studies, *Cancer* 115:1489, 2009.

Liang XH, Lewis J, Foote R, et al: Prevalence and significance of human papillomavirus in oral tongue cancer: the Mayo Clinic experience, *J Oral Maxillofac Surg* 66:1875, 2008.

Machado J, Reiss PP, Zhang T, et al: Low prevalence of human papillomavirus in oral cavity carcinomas, *Head Neck Oncol* 12:2, 2011.

Monroe MM, Gross ND: Management of the clinical node-negative neck in early-stage oral cavity squamous cell carcinoma, *Otolaryngol Clin N Am* 45:1181, 2012.

Myers EM, Suen JY, Myers JN, et al: *Cancer of the Head and Neck*, ed 4, Philadelphia, 2003, Saunders.

Shah JP, Patel SG, Singh B: *Jatin Shah's Head and Neck Surgery and Oncology*, ed 4, Philadelphia, 2012, Elsevier Mosby.

Zafereo ME: Evaluation and staging of squamous cell carcinoma of the oral cavity and oropharynx—limitations despite technological breakthroughs, *Otolaryngol Clin N Am* 46:599, 2013.

CHAPTER 13

CANCER OF THE HYPOPHARYNX, LARYNX, AND ESOPHAGUS

Marcia Eustaquio, MD and Craig Quattlebaum, MD

KEY POINTS

1. The most commonly affected subsite for laryngeal cancer is the glottis.
2. Smokers are approximately 20 times more likely than nonsmokers to develop laryngeal cancer. Smoking and alcohol intake are synergistic risk factors for the development of laryngeal cancer.
3. Conservation surgery or radiation are treatment options for voice preservation in early laryngeal cancer.
4. The supraglottis has bilateral lymphatic drainage.
5. Hypopharyngeal cancers have a poor prognosis and are usually discovered at a later stage than laryngeal cancers.

Pearls

1. Smoking through treatment for laryngeal cancer increases the chance for treatment failure and recurrence.
2. Both surgery and radiation therapy have similarly good outcomes for early glottic SCC.
3. An immobile vocal cord always warrants a workup for an etiology and is important in the staging of laryngeal and hypopharyngeal squamous cell carcinoma.
4. At least one cricoarytenoid joint must be preserved in conservation laryngeal surgery.
5. Hypopharyngeal cancer is notable for frequent submucosal spread and carries a worse prognosis than cancer of the larynx.

QUESTIONS

1. Describe the general anatomic divisions of the larynx.
   Vertically, the larynx is subdivided into three regions: the supraglottis, the glottis, and the subglottis. The division of these three subsites reflects embryologic development and natural barriers to cancer spread. The supraglottis can be thought of as a three-dimensional box containing a suprahyoid and infrahyoid epiglottis, the aryepiglottic folds, arytenoids, ventricles, and false vocal folds. It extends from the superior surface of the epiglottis and the superior edge of the aryepiglottic folds to a horizontal plane passing through the lateral margin of the ventricle and the superior surface of the true vocal folds. The supraglottis has bilateral lymphatic drainage to the upper and middle jugular lymph nodes. The glottis begins at the superior surface of the true vocal fold and extends inferiorly 1 cm. Laterally it is bordered by the thyroid cartilage with the lateral ventricle coming to the superior most extent. It contains the anterior and posterior commissures. The vocal folds themselves have sparse lymphatics, therefore deep invasion is needed for unilateral lymphatic spread. The subglottis begins at the inferior border of the glottis (1 cm below the supraglottis) and proceeds to the inferior border of the cricoid cartilage.

2. Regarding the divisions of the larynx, where does laryngeal cancer commonly occur?
   Laryngeal cancer most commonly arises in the glottis (60%), followed by supraglottis (35%), and subglottis (2%); another 3% are transglottic and involve multiple subsites. An overwhelming 95% of

glottic cancers arise from the true vocal cords. Because of natural barriers to spread and early presenting symptoms, laryngeal cancer is often confined to the larynx at time of diagnosis (60% of cases).

3. **How common is laryngeal cancer?**
Laryngeal cancer is the second most common malignancy of the head and neck (after oral cavity/ oropharynx). Currently, in the United States, there are over 12,000 new cases of laryngeal cancer annually. One third of these patients will die from their disease. The number of new cases is declining by roughly 2% to 3% per year due to decreased smoking. Laryngeal cancer is 3.8 times more common in men than women, though the gender disparity has narrowed in recent years due to the increased proportion of female smokers.

4. **What are the risk factors for laryngeal cancer?**
Tobacco and alcohol are the primary risk factors for laryngeal cancer. The risk is thought to be directly proportional to the duration and intensity of exposure. Smoking and alcohol are synergistic in increasing cancer risk rather than merely additive. Risk does decrease slowly after cessation but does not return to baseline for at least 20 years. Patients who continue to smoke through their treatment are at a higher risk of recurrence and development of a second primary. There is conflicting data as to whether laryngopharyngeal reflux could be a risk factor, though a causal relationship has yet to be established.

5. **What types of cancers are found in the larynx?**
Squamous cell carcinoma (SCC) is the most common type of malignancy found in the larynx, accounting for more than 95% of all tumors. Variations of SCC include verrucous carcinoma (2% to 4%) and spindle cell carcinoma. Verrucous carcinoma carries an improved prognosis while spindle cell variants are more aggressive. Both subtypes are typically treated with surgical excision.

Less common nonepithelial tumors include adenoid cystic carcinoma, mucoepidermoid carcinoma, sarcoma (e.g., fibrosarcoma, chondrosarcoma, liposarcoma), neuroendocrine tumor (e.g., paragangliomas, carcinoid), contiguous lesions (i.e., thyroid), and metastatic lesions.

6. **How might a patient with laryngeal cancer present?**
Hoarseness, dysphagia, odynophagia, referred otalgia, globus sensation, weight loss, and neck mass can all be presenting symptoms. Glottic cancers tend to present early with hoarseness, whereas airway obstruction and hemoptysis are later findings. Supraglottic cancers often present with dysphagia and odynophagia. Otalgia can occur due to pharyngeal extension. Hoarseness occurs secondary to transglottic extension or arytenoid involvement. Airway obstruction can be gradual with bulky disease, or may be acute in onset from a ball-valve type of obstruction. Supraglottic tumors are usually discovered later and have a poorer prognosis as these symptoms arise with progression beyond the supraglottis. Subglottic carcinomas present with signs and symptoms of early airway obstruction such as biphasic stridor.

7. **Discuss the workup of laryngeal cancer.**
History and physical exam should address symptoms such as dyspnea, stridor, dysphagia, odynophagia, otalgia, weight loss, and hoarseness. Special attention should be paid to risk factors for carcinoma, primarily smoking, alcohol, and history of cancer. It is important to determine overall health and functional status as this will play a key role in determining treatment. A complete head and neck exam should be performed with careful visualization and palpation of oral cavity, oropharynx, and neck. Laryngoscopy should be performed with any lesions characterized by location, size, endophytic or exophytic nature, vocal cord mobility, and patency of the airway.

In cases other than a T1 glottic primary, additional imaging should be ordered to evaluate extent of disease and metastatic potential. A computed tomography CT scan of the neck with contrast is the most utilized modality. MRI can also be useful and is more sensitive in differentiating soft tissue and cartilage involvement. PET scan may be helpful in advanced stages for metastatic workup. Operative endoscopy should be pursued with direct visualization, palpation, and tissue sampling. In select cases debulking and/or airway stabilization will also be warranted.

8. **What is the significance of a paralyzed vocal fold?**
A fixed or paralyzed vocal fold is one that appears immobile on exam, and can be associated with hoarseness or aspiration. A cord can be rendered immobile in several ways, including mass effect of the tumor, cricoarytenoid joint involvement, or recurrent laryngeal nerve involvement. Vocal cord

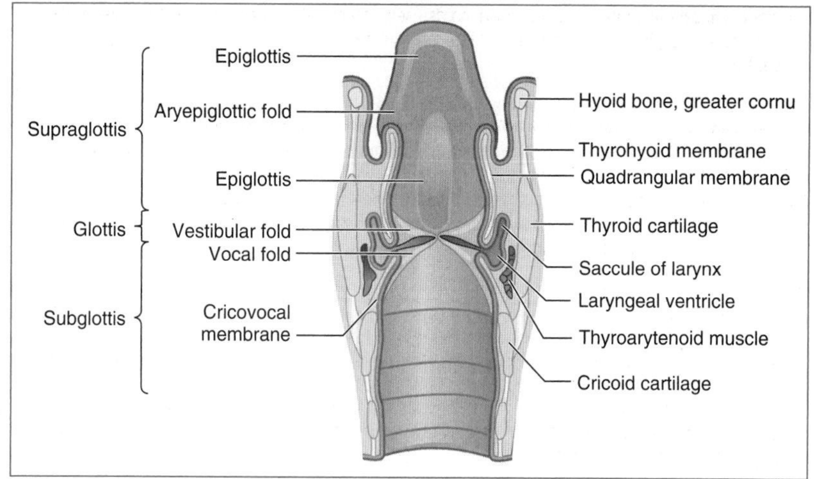

Figure 13-1. Coronal view of the internal larynx with quadrangular membrane and conus elasticus (cricovocal membrane). *(From Bogart Bl and Ort V. Elsevier's Integrated Anatomy and Embryology, 1 ed, Philadelphia, 2007, Elsevier.)*

immobility upstages laryngeal and hypopharyngeal cancers to T3. This is in contrast to a partially immobile or paretic vocal fold. A vocal fold with decreased mobility is characterized as at least a T2 cancer.

9. **What membranous structures help prevent the spread of cancer outside of the larynx?**
There are two fibroelastic membranes that help prevent cancer spread from the larynx. The *conus elasticus* helps support the vocal folds and extends from the cricoid cartilage to the vocal ligaments. It is the lower part of the elastic membrane of the larynx. The *quadrangular membrane* supports the supraglottis and begins superiorly at the lateral margin of the epiglottis and proceeds inferiorly to the false cords. This is the upper part of the elastic membrane of the larynx. This quadrangular membrane and the conus elasticus are separated by the laryngeal ventricle and form the medial boundary of the paraglottic space (Figure 13-1).

10. **Discuss the routes of local spread and nodal metastasis of SCC of the different laryngeal regions.**
Laryngeal cancer may spread by direct extension or through the lymphatics. Local extension may occur through the paraglottic space, which is a fibrofatty-filled space bounded medially by the conus elasticus and quadrangular membrane, laterally by the thyrohyoid membrane and thyroid cartilage lamina, and posteriorly by the medial mucosa of the piriform sinus. Entry of a mass into this space, commonly from the laryngeal ventricle, allows for transglottic extension. Paraglottic space involvement upstages any laryngeal carcinoma to T3. The pre-epiglottic space is a fibrofatty-filled space bounded superiorly by the hyoepiglottic ligament, anteriorly by the thyrohyoid membrane and thyroid cartilage, and posteriorly by the epiglottis and thyroepiglottic membrane. It is continuous laterally with the paraglottic space. Glottic cancer can invade from the anterior commisure along Broyle's ligament into the thyroid cartilage and via lacunae of the epiglottis into the pre-epiglottic space.
Regional lymphatic spread also occurs. The lymphatics of the supraglottis follow the superior laryngeal arteries draining to the upper and middle jugular lymph nodes in levels 2 and 3. Bilateral lymphatics allow cancer to spread to the ipsilateral or contralateral lymph nodes. The incidence of nodal metastasis varies from 0% to 57% depending on the primary tumor stage. The glottis is without notable lymphatic drainage; regional nodal spread for glottic cancer is below 10%. Subglottic carcinoma extends to and through the cricothyroid membrane to involve the lateral paratracheal and cervical lymphatics as well as the medial prelaryngeal (Delphian) node. There is also rich lymphatic drainage from the postcricoid area.

Table 13-1. Tumor Staging

Supraglottis	T1	Limited to one subsite, with normal vocal cord mobility
	T2	Invades mucosa of more than one adjacent subsite of the supraglottis or glottis or a region outside the supraglottis, without fixation of larynx
	T3	Limited to the larynx with vocal cord fixation and/or invasion of the postcricoid area, pre-epiglottic tissues, paraglottic space, and/or erosion of the inner laminae of the thyroid cartilage
	T4a	Invades through the thyroid cartilage and/or tissues beyond the larynx
	T4b	Invades the prevertebral space, encases the carotid artery, or invades the mediastinal structures
Glottis	T1a	Limited to one vocal cord
	T1b	Involves both vocal cords
	T2	Extends to the supraglottis and/or subglottis, and/or with impaired cord mobility
	T3	Limited to the larynx with vocal cord fixation or involvement of the inner layer of cartilage
	T4a	Invades through the thyroid cartilage and/or tissues beyond the larynx
	T4b	Invades the prevertebral space, encases the carotid artery, or invades the mediastinal structures
Subglottis	T1	Limited to the subglottis
	T2	Extends to the vocal cord(s) with normal/impaired mobility
	T3	Limited to the larynx with vocal cord fixation
	T4a	Invades the cricoid or thyroid cartilage and/or tissues beyond the larynx
	T4b	Invades the prevertebral space, encases the carotid artery, or invades the mediastinal structures

11. **How is a primary tumor in laryngeal carcinoma staged?**
Cancers of the larynx are described using the TNM classification system of the American Joint Committee on Cancer (AJCC). Cancers are staged based on their site of origin in the supraglottis, glottis, or subglottis. Regional nodal involvement and distant metastasis are staged similary to other sites in the head and neck (Table 13-1).

12. **How is laryngeal cancer treated?**
The patient's functional status, location of the cancer, and its stage are critical in determining the appropriate modality. Early cancers, defined typically as Stage 1 and Stage 2 lesions, are usually addressed with single-modality therapy. Radiation therapy and surgical excision have been shown to be statistically equivalent in terms of disease-free and overall survival. Advanced laryngeal cancers Stages 3 and 4 should be addressed by multimodality therapy. For high-volume tumors this may mean conservation surgery in select cases or total laryngectomy with postoperative radiation plus or minus chemotherapy. High-level evidence favors combined chemotherapy and radiation over radiation alone as a primary treatment modality for advanced stage cancers.

13. **What are the surgical options for early laryngeal cancer?**
Many early laryngeal cancers may be treated via conservation surgery with excellent local control rates. Traditional surgical resection has included open approaches, but transoral robotic and transoral laser techniques are now more commonly utilized. T1 and T2 lesions are usually amenable to surgery but other factors such as whether the tumor is exophytic or endophytic and the precise location of the tumor are important. Exophytic tumors located on the central portion of the cord or on the epiglottis are more easily excised than endophytic tumors located near the arytenoid or anterior commissure, for instance. Contraindications to conservation laryngeal surgery include: more than 5 mm of subglottic extension, extension into the postcricoid space, involvement of the base of tongue or piriform sinus, cartilage invasion, bilateral vocal cord fixation or bilateral arytenoid involvement. Glottic T1a tumors are treated with cordectomy while larger T1 or T2 lesions may be amenable to vertical partial laryngectomy through an open or transoral approach. Supraglottic T1 and T2 lesions may be treated with supraglottic (horizontal) laryngectomy or supracricoid partial laryngectomy through an open or transoral approach.

14. What is the difference between horizontal hemilaryngectomy and vertical partial laryngectomy?

In both instances the resection must be oncologically sound with preservation of at least one cricoarytenoid unit (the cricoid cartilage, one arytenoid cartilage, associated musculature, and superior and recurrent laryngeal nerves). Horizontal hemilaryngectomy, or supraglottic laryngectomy, is indicated for early T1, T2, or select T3 supraglottic tumors that do not involve the true vocal fold or associated cartilages. The open procedure removes the bilateral supraglottis but spares the true vocal folds and arytenoids. Voice and swallowing outcomes are typically good. If the tumor involves one vocal fold or cricoarytenoid joint a supracricoid laryngectomy may be performed. This leaves one cricoarytenoid joint intact and removes a portion of the thyroid cartilage. Vertical partial laryngectomy, or hemilaryngectomy, is indicated for T1, T2, and select T3 glottic lesions (not involving commissure or associated cartilages). This procedure removes the ipsilateral vocal fold, false cord, ventricle, and overlying thyroid cartilage. Post-operatively, patients have a functional glottic voice.

15. What are the subsites of the hypopharynx and important oncologic considerations?

1. The *piriform sinus* is the inferior extent of the hypopharynx. It is typically subdivided into anterior, lateral, posterior, and apical walls. The medial limits of the piriform sinus are the larynx, aryepiglottic folds, arytenoids, and cricoid. The piriform sinus is the most common site for hypopharyngeal cancer (65% to 75%). Cancer may extend from here into the subglottis, thyroid cartilage, postcricoid region, or cricoarytenoid joint. Three of every four patients presenting with hypopharyngeal cancer within the piriform sinus have regional metastasis, resulting in a poorer prognosis.
2. The *postcricoid space* spans from the posterior aspect of the arytenoids to the esophageal introitis, anterior to the posterior pharyngeal wall. Cancer here can directly invade the cricoid and can also involve the recurrent laryngeal nerve by spreading laterally into the tracheo-esophageal groove.
3. The *posterior pharyngeal wall* extends from the level of the hyoid bone to the cricopharyngeus muscle which marks the transition to cervical esophagus. Extension posteriorly through the potential retropharyngeal space can lead to involvement of the prevertebral tissues.

16. After total laryngectomy, what voice options are available for the patient?

Immediately after surgery all patients should be supplied with a writing board or picture board to assist in communication while in the hospital. For long-term rehabilitation the most commonly used methods of speech are the electrolarynx, esophageal speech, and a tracheoesophogeal prosthesis. The electrolarynx is the most common method of postlaryngectomy speech. This inexpensive device is easier to master than other voicing techniques. It uses patient-induced upper aerodigestive tract vibrations to create a mechanical voice. Drawbacks include the need for an independent power supply, difficultly being understood by others (particulary on the phone), and the need for additional equipment. Esophageal speech is another option with good voice quality for some, but is harder to learn. With this method, patients use vibration of the pharyngoesophageal mucosa along with oral air trapping to produce speech. It requires much patience and practice, but no extra equipment is required. Finally, placement of a tracheoesophageal prosthesis is another common method of voice management. This method allows expired air from the tracheal stoma to enter the esophagus via a surgically created tracheoesophageal fistula. This method allows a stronger more natural voice. Creation of the tracheoesophageal puncture requires a procedure that may be complicated by breakdown of the surrounding tissue or a fistulous tract. This is sometimes done at the time of laryngectomy or as an additional procedure after completion of treatment and healing. Success may be hampered by pharyngeal constrictor spasm and increased risk of aspiration. Proficient use of the tracheoesophageal prosthesis requires practice and training with speech therapy, and the prosthesis itself requires dexterity, can be costly, and must be replaced and cleaned on a regular basis.

17. What is the prognosis for laryngeal and hypopharyngeal cancers? Has this improved over the last few years?

Survival of patients with laryngeal cancer has not improved over the past several decades. Only early stage glottic cancer carries a good prognosis. Hypopharyngeal cancer survival has increased slightly over the same time period. Unfortunately, most hypopharyngeal and laryngeal tumors present late and thus have poor survival rates. See Table 13-2.

Table 13-2. Survival Data from the American Cancer Society

	STAGE	5-YEAR SURVIVAL RATE
Supraglottis	I	59%
	II	59%
	III	53%
	IV	34%
Subglottis	I	65%
	II	56%
	III	47%
	IV	32%
Glottis	I	90%
	II	74%
	III	56%
	IV	44%
Hypopharynx	I	53%
	II	39%
	III	36%
	IV	24%

(Data from American Joint Committee on Cancer: Larynx. In AJCC Cancer Staging Manual, 7 ed, New York, 2010, Springer, p. 41–49.)

18. **What are risk factors for esophageal cancer?**
The predominant risk factors for squamous cell carcinoma of the esophagus are smoking and alcohol consumption. Additional risk factors are poor socioeconomic status, low intake of fresh fruits and vegetables, copious consumption of hot tea, and hookah smoking. An increased risk of adenocarcinoma has also been shown in smokers but alcohol has not been implicated as an independent risk factor. The primary risk factor for adenocarcinoma is thought to be dysplasia (Barrett's esophagus) as a result of GERD (gastro-esophageal reflux disease). It has been postulated that the increasing rate of obesity is responsible for the rising rates of esophageal adenocarcinoma by increasing the severity of GERD as an independent risk factor.

19. **What is the most common type of esophageal cancer in the different parts of the esophogus?**
Esophageal cancer is a relatively uncommon cancer that carries a poor prognosis. Worldwide, squamous cell carcinoma is the most common form of esophageal cancer and this was historically true in the United States. Over the last forty years the epidemiology has shifted in the United States with adenocarcinoma accounting for over 70% of all new cases. The esophagus can be divided into a proximal, middle, and distal third. Adenocarcinoma is found most commonly in the distal third while SCC can be found along the entire length of the esophagus with predilection for the upper two thirds.

CONTROVERSIES

20. **Discuss the treatment options for early glottic cancers.**
Both radiation therapy and conservation surgery offer excellent and equal cure rates. The decision therefore often falls to the preferences of the patient. Benefits of surgery include a one-time treatment, histopathologic confirmation of free tumor margins, and sparing of radiation therapy for future treatment if needed. Radiation therapy offers a nonsurgical alternative and generally a better voice outcome when compared to open procedures or tumors involving the full thickness of the cord. Drawbacks to radiation include length of treatment, expense, and a decreased chance of laryngeal preservation with recurrence. A key point to remember is that the T1-T2 definition of

"early glottic cancers" encompasses a broad range of tumors. Each case should be evaluated, preferrably by a multidisciplinary panel, with regard to ease of surgical resection and radiation therapy and the risks and benefits of each.

21. **How should the N0 neck be addressed in laryngeal cancer?**
Treatment options for the N0 neck include observation, elective neck dissection, or radiation therapy. Before deciding on a treatment plan the location of the primary cancer and any previous treatments must be considered. For glottic tumors that have not extended into the supraglottis, elective treatment of the neck is not necessary because there is poor lymphatic drainage from the glottis. For more advanced glottic tumors with supraglottic extension or for primary tumors of the supraglottis staged T2 or greater there is debate on whether or not to electively treat the neck. There are no randomized controlled trials, and the literature relies heavily on retrospective reviews. Many of these do not show a benefit with treatment; however, some of the larger series support elective treatment of the neck based on improved locoregional control. In the case of recurrent laryngeal cancer after radiation treatment, if there has never been clinical evidence of neck disease, there is not strong evidence to support elective treatment of the neck. Elective neck dissection in such cases may also lead to an increased rate of postoperative complications.

Bibliography

American Cancer Society statistics on laryngeal and hypopharyngeal cancer, 2014. Accessed February 9, 2014, at https://www.cancer.org/cancer/laryngealandhypopharyngealcancer/detailedguide.

Armstrong WB, Vokes DE, Maisel RH: Malignant tumors of the larynx. In Flint P, et al, editors: *Cummings Otolaryngology: Head and Neck Surgery*, ed 5, Philadelphia, 2010, Mosby, p 1482.

Flint PW: Minimally invasive techniques for management of early glottic cancer, *Otolaryngol Clin North Am* 35:1055–1066, 2002.

Forastiere A, Koch W, Trotti A, et al: Head and neck cancer, *N Engl J Med* 345:1890–1900, 2001.

Gilbert J, Forastiere AA: Organ preservation trials for laryngeal cancer, *Otolaryngol Clin North Am* 35:1035–1054, 2002.

Goudakos JK, Markou K, Nikolaou A, et al: Management of the clinically negative neck (N0) of supraglottic laryngeal carcinoma: a systematic review, *EJSO* 35:223–229, 2008.

Redaelli de Zinis LO, Nicolai P, Tomenzoli D, et al: The distribution of lymph node metastases in supraglottic squamous cell carcinoma: Therapeutic implications, *Head Neck* 24:913–920, 2002.

Talamini R, Bosetti C, La Vecchia C, et al: Combined effect of tobacco and alcohol on laryngeal cancer risk: a case-control study, *Cancer Causes Control* 13:957–964, 2002.

Tufano RP: Organ preservation surgery for laryngeal cancer, *Otolaryngol Clin North Am* 35:1067–1080, 2002.

Zhang Y: Epidemiology of esophageal cancer, *World J Gastroenterol* 19(34):5598–5608, 2013.

CHAPTER 14

DISEASES OF THE SALIVARY GLANDS

Mofiyinfolu Sokoya, MD and Ted H. Leem, MD MS

KEY POINTS

1. Know multiple ways for identifying the facial nerve in parotid surgery. These can be used in combination to triangulate the likely location of the facial nerve.
2. Not all parotid masses are primary parotid neoplasms. Metastatic disease to the parotid gland should be included in the differential diagnosis of a parotid neoplasm.
3. Parotid surgery should be performed in the absence of neuromuscular blockade to help identify stimulation of the facial nerve during its dissection.

Pearls

1. Mumps is still possible in vaccinated children.
2. Salivary gland masses should be evaluated by FNA biopsy and imaging. This provides information relating to the nature of the disease.
3. The most common benign salivary gland tumor is pleomorphic adenoma.
4. The most common malignant salivary gland tumor is mucoepidermoid carcinoma.
5. HIV workup is important in a patient that presents with a cystic parotid mass.

QUESTIONS

1. **Describe the anatomy, including surrounding structures and involved neurovascular innervation, of the parotid gland.**
   - The parotid gland (Figure 14-1) is located in the lateral face, bordered by the masseter anteriorly and medially, the zygomatic arch superiorly, the tragal cartilage and the sternocleidomastoid muscle (SCM) posteriorly, and the ramus of the mandible and SCM inferiorly.
   - The external carotid artery lies medial to the parotid and gives off the maxillary artery and the superficial temporal artery, which course through the gland. Venous drainage uses the maxillary and superficial temporal veins that form the retromandibular vein, which joins the external jugular vein via the posterior facial vein.
   - Stensen's duct courses superficial to the masseter muscle and enters into the oral mucosa adjacent to the second upper molar.
   - After it exits from the stylomastoid foramen, the facial nerve **branches** to form the the postauricular and posterior belly of the diagastric before entering the parotid gland posteriorly.
   - Parasympathetic secretomotor innervation is provided through the glossopharyngeal nerve.

2. **Describe the relevant anatomy of the submandibular gland.**
   The submandibular gland is found inferior and deep to the mandible, in the submandibular triangle. This triangle is defined by the anterior and posterior bellies of the digastric muscle, and the mandibular body. Wharton's duct courses deep to the lingual nerve and enters the oral cavity at the anterior floor of the mouth. Parasympathetic secretomotor innervation is provided through the chorda tympani nerve.

3. **Describe the anatomy of the sublingual gland.**
   The sublingual gland is located adjacent to the lingual frenulum and superficial to the mylohyoid muscle. The parasympathetic innervation is provided by the chorda tympani nerve. The sublingual gland drains into the oral cavity through the ducts of Rivinus.

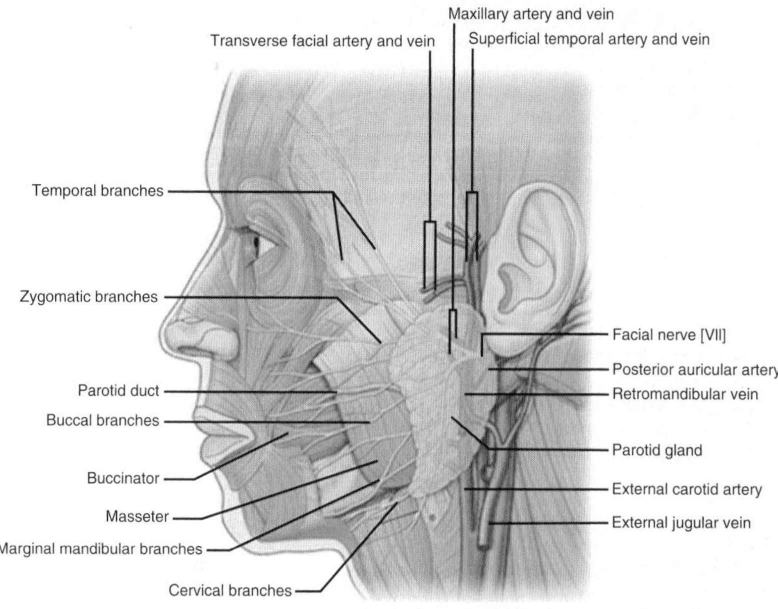

Figure 14-1. Anatomy of the parotid gland and surrounding structures. *(From Drake R, Vogl AW, Mitchell AWM: Gray's Anatomy for Students. Philadelphia, PA, 2009, Elsevier.)*

4. **What is the most commonly implicated bacteria in acute suppurative sialadenitis? How is it treated?**
   Staphylococcus aureus is the most common bacteria causing sialadenitis. Treatment consists of antibiotics with β-lactamase resistance such as amoxicillin-clavulanate, hydration, warm compresses, and sialagogues (such as lemon wedges).

5. **What are some available treatment options for sialolithiasis?**
   1. Conservative management with sialagogues, warm compresses, antibiotics, and hydration
   2. Open sialolithotomy
   3. Sialendoscopy with use of wire baskets, balloons, and grasping forceps
   4. Lithotripsy (laser, shockwave—not FDA approved in the U.S.)
   5. Excision of salivary gland

6. **What is the most common viral infection of the parotid?**
   Mumps is still the most common cause of viral parotitis. Peak age is 4 to 6 years of age and bilateral involvement is common. It is associated with orchitis, encephalitis, and sensorineural hearing loss. Most, but not all, mumps infections have been eliminated with vaccination.

7. **What is the most common parotid abnormality associated with HIV?**
   Diffuse lymphoepithelial cystic disease. HIV should be ruled out in any patient with cystic parotid disease.

8. **Describe common granulomatous diseases of the salivary glands and some pertinent features.**
   1. Tuberculosis: Diagnosed by PPD, FNA, culture showing acid-fast bacilli, and chest x-ray
   2. Atypical mycobacteria: Workup includes chest x-ray, PPD, and tissue culture
   3. Actinomycosis: Gram-positive actinomyces with pathognomonic sulfur granules. Treatment includes penicillin G, erythromycin, clindamycin

4. Cat-scratch disease: Caused by *Bartonella henselae*. Treated with azithromycin
5. Toxoplasmosis: Caused by *Toxoplasma gondii*. Treated with pyrimethamine and sulfadiazine plus folinic acid
6. Sarcoidosis: Noncaseating granulomas are the hallmark of this disease. Usually responds to steroids

9. What is the diagnostic test of choice for Sjogren syndrome?

Minor salivary gland biopsy of 3 to 5 glands is submitted from a lower lip biopsy, looking for lymphocytic infiltration. A positive test requires more than 1 focus per 4 mm^2, where each focus contains at least 50 lymphocytes.

10. List benign tumors of the salivary glands. Which is most common? Which can present bilaterally?

- Pleomorphic adenoma
- Basal cell carcinoma
- Sebaceous lymphadenoma
- Oncocytoma
- Myoepithelioma
- Inverted ductal papilloma
- Monomorphic adenoma
- Clear cell adenoma
- Warthin's tumor
- Oncocytic papillary cystadenoma
- Sialadenoma papilliferum
- Hemangioma

The most common benign tumor of salivary glands is pleomorphic adenoma.
Warthin's tumor presents bilaterally in up to 10% of cases (Table 14-1).

Table 14-1. Relative Incidence of Benign Salivary Gland Tumors

Distribution of 2807 Salivary Neoplasms		
HISTOLOGY	**NUMBER OF PATIENTS**	**PERCENT**
Pleomorphic adenoma	1274	45.4
Warthin's tumor	183	6.5
Benign cyst	29	1.0
Lymphoepithelial lesion	17	0.6
Oncocytoma	20	0.7
Monomorphic adenoma	6	0.2
Mucoepidermoid carcinoma	439	15.7
Adenoid cystic carcinoma	281	10.0
Adenocarcinoma	225	8.0
Malignant mixed tumor	161	5.7
Acinic cell carcinoma	84	3.0
Epidermoid carcinoma	53	1.9
Other (anaplastic)	35	1.3
Total	2807	100

(In Flint PW, et al: *Cummings Otolaryngology: Head & Neck Surgery*. Elsevier-Mosby, 2010. From Spiro RH: Salivary neoplasms: overview of a 35-year experience with 2,807 patients. *Head Neck Surg* 8:177–184, 1986.)

11. Warthin's tumor is an eponym for what? What are some of the epidemiologic features?
Warthin's tumor is an eponym for papillary cystadenoma lymphomatosum. It is more often found in women in the sixth or seventh decade of life. It is also related to cigarette smoke exposure even though it is benign.

12. List malignant tumors of the salivary glands. Which is most common? Which can present bilaterally?

- Mucoepidermoid carcinoma
- Adenoid cystic carcinoma
- Acinic cell carcinoma
- Basal cell carcinoma
- Epithelial-myoepithelial tumor
- Hyalinizing clear cell carcinoma
- Squamous cell carcinoma
- Undifferentiated carcinoma
- Malignant mixed tumor
- Salivary duct carcinoma
- Adenocarcinoma
- Carcinoma ex pleomorphic adenoma
- Polymorphous low-grade adenocarcinoma
- Metastases

The most common malignancy of the parotid gland is mucoepidermoid carcinoma. Acinic cell carcinoma presents bilaterally in 3% to 5% of cases (Table 14-2).

13. Describe the initial workup of a salivary gland mass.
Fine needle aspiration biopsy and imaging (contrasted CT or MRI) are frequently ordered during the workup. The combination can help differentiate benign from malignant processes and often provide a diagnosis.

14. Describe the staging of salivary gland tumors.
TX: Primary tumor cannot be assessed.
T0: No evidence of primary tumor.

Table 14-2. Relative Incidence of Malignant Salivary Gland Tumors

Relative Incidence of Malignant Salivary Gland Neoplasms

HISTOLOGIC TYPE	NUMBER	PERCENT
Mucoepidermoid	439	34
Adenoid cystic carcinoma	281	22
Adenocarcinoma NOS	225	18
Malignant mixed tumors	161	13
Acinic cell carcinoma	84	7
Squamous cell carcinoma	53	4
Other (anaplastic etc.)	35	3
Total	1278	

(In Flint PW, et al: *Cummings Otolaryngology: Head & Neck Surgery*. Elsevier-Mosby, 2010. From Spiro RH: Salivary neoplasms: overview of a 35-year experience with 2,807 patients. *Head Neck Surg* 8:177–184, 1986.)

T1: Tumor ≤2 cm in greatest dimension without extraparenchymal extension.
T2: Tumor >2 cm but ≤4 cm in greatest dimension without extraparenchymal extension.
T3: Tumor >4 cm and/or tumor having extraparenchymal extension.
T4a: Moderately advanced disease. Tumor invades skin, mandible, ear canal, and/or facial nerve.
T4b: Very advanced disease. Tumor invades skull base and/or pterygoid plates and/or encases carotid artery.
NX: Regional lymph nodes cannot be assessed.
N0: No regional lymph node metastasis.
N1: Metastasis in a single ipsilateral lymph node, ≤3 cm in greatest dimension.
N2: Metastasis in a single ipsilateral lymph node, >3 cm but ≤6 cm in greatest dimension.

N2a: Metastasis in a single ipsilateral lymph node, >3 cm but ≤6 cm in greatest dimension.
N2b: Metastases in multiple ipsilateral lymph nodes, ≤6 cm in greatest dimension.
N2c: Metastases in bilateral or contralateral lymph nodes, ≤6 cm in greatest dimension.

N3: Metastasis in a lymph node, >6 cm in greatest dimension.

15. **Describe the histology of mucoepidermoid carcinoma. How does this affect prognosis?**
Mucoepidermoid carcinoma is highlighted by the presence of mucinous and epidermoid cells. The amount of mucinous cells and the level of epidermoid differentiation determines the tumor grade. Low-grade tumors have a greater amount of mucinous cells compared to well-differentiated epidermoid cells. High-grade tumors have a dearth of mucinous cells with a preponderance of poorly differentiated epidermoid cells.

16. **Describe the histology of adenoid cystic carcinoma. How does this affect prognosis?**
Adenoid cystic carcinoma is divided into three histologic subtypes:
- The tubular pattern is characterized by tumor cells arranged in nests surrounded by variable amounts of eosinophilic, often hyalinized stroma. It has the best prognosis.
- The cribriform subtype occurs most frequently. It is composed of islands of basaloid cells surrounding variably sized cyst-like spaces forming a "swiss cheese" pattern. It has an intermediate prognosis (Figure 14-2).
- The solid pattern contains aggregates of basaloid cells without tubular or cystic formation. It has the worst prognosis.

17. **What is the Hayes-Martin maneuver in submandibular gland removal?**
The facial vessels run deep to the marginal mandibular nerve. Ligation of the vessels and subsequent superior retraction lift the nerve out of the surgical field and protect it from iatrogenic injury.

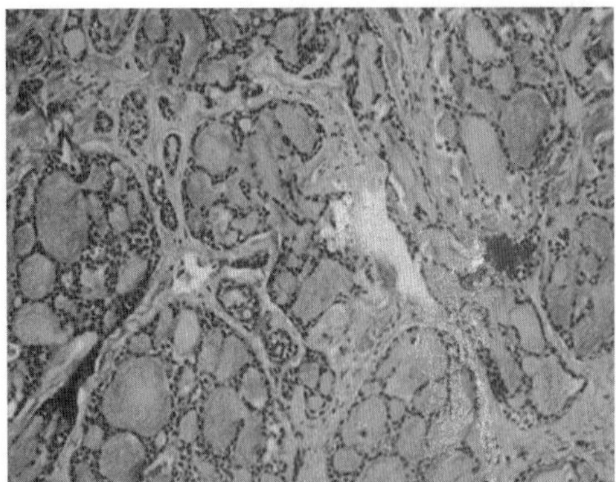

Figure 14-2. Cribriform (grade II) Adenoid cystic carcinoma with basaloid cells arranged around multiple rounded collections of central basophilic material giving a "Swiss-cheese" appearance (200×). *(From Flint PW, Haughey BH, Lund VJ, et al, editors: Cummings Otolaryngology: Head & Neck Surgery, ed 5, Philadelphia, 2010, Mosby.)*

18. **During a parotidectomy, what are some ways the facial nerve can be identified?**
    - 1 cm deep and inferior to the tragal pointer
    - 6 to 8 mm anterior and inferior to the tympanomastoid suture line
    - Superior to the cephalic portion of the posterior belly of the digastric muscle
    - Superficial/lateral to the styloid process
    - Retrograde dissection after finding the marginal mandibular branch as it passes over the facial artery and vein at the anterior border of the masseter muscle
    - Retrograde dissection after finding the zygomatic branch as it courses over the zygomatic arch two thirds of the way from the tragus to the lateral canthus of the eye
    - Mastoidectomy with anterograde nerve dissection

19. **List the indications for postoperative radiotherapy of a parotid neoplasm.**
    - High-grade tumors
    - Gross or microscopic residual disease
    - Lymph node metastasis
    - Extraparotid extension
    - Tumors involving the facial nerve
    - Some deep lobe cancers
    - Recurrent disease

20. **What is Frey's syndrome? How is it treated?**
    Frey's syndrome is defined by gustatory sweating of the skin overlying the surgical site of a parotidectomy. This is caused by postoperative growth of the interrupted preganglionic parasympathetic nerve branches of the parotid into the superficial sweat glands. It is best avoided, but treatments do exist. These include: botox injection, topical antiperspirants, surgery to place an intervening layer of tissue or allograft between the skin and parotid bed, and Jacobson's neurectomy (surgical interruption of the Jacobson's nerve, which carries preganglionic parasympathetic nerves to the parotid).

CONTROVERSIES

21. **What is the utility of facial nerve monitoring during a parotidectomy?**
    The use of facial nerve monitoring during a parotidectomy is a matter of surgeon preference. The monitor can be useful in confirming an anatomically identified nerve. It should never be relied on as the only means of identification. There are no data proving whether or not its use decreases rates of facial nerve injury.

22. **What is the role of elective neck dissection in treating a salivary gland malignancy?**
    Elective neck dissection is generally reserved for high-grade tumors as the risk of microscopic metastasis to the neck is greater than 20 percent. Radiation therapy may be used, but surgical treatment of the neck allows for accurate staging. Recent evidence indicates that the risk of lymph node metastases may be higher than previously reported, even in low-grade tumors, and may support the need for neck dissections.

BIBLIOGRAPHY

Cummings CW, Flint PW: *Cummings Otolaryngology Head & Neck Surgery*, ed 5, Philadelphia, 2010, Elsevier-Mosby.

Drake R, Vogl AW, Mitchell AWM: *Gray's Anatomy for Students*, Philadelphia, PA, 2009, Elsevier.

Jaso J, Malhotra R: Adenoid cystic carcinoma, *Arch Pathol Lab Med* 135(4):511–515, 2011.

Lee KJ: *Essential Otolaryngology: Head and Neck Surgery*, ed 8, San Francisco, CA, 2003, McGraw-Hill, pp 731–732.

Pather N, Osman M: Landmarks of the facial nerve: implications for parotidectomy, *Surg Radiologic Anat* 28(2):170–175, 2006.

Steger J, Tennyson H, Gal TJ, et al: Salivary gland tumors. In *ENT Secrets*, ed 2, Philadelphia, 2005, Elsevier-Mosby, pp 211–217.

CHAPTER 15

DISEASES OF THE THYROID AND PARATHYROID GLANDS

John Song, MD

KEY POINTS

1. Thyroid nodules found incidentally on PET scan warrant special attention as some studies suggest that as many as two thirds of these nodules are later diagnosed as malignancies.
2. Pathologic risk features for radioactive iodine (RAI) remnant ablation include:
   - Size of the primary tumor
   - Presence of lymphovascular invasion
   - Invasion of thyroid capsule
   - Number of involved lymph nodes

Pearls

1. Evaluation of palpable thyroid nodules should always include an ultrasound and FNA.
2. Exposure to ionizing radiation as a child and a strong family history of thyroid cancer are known risk factors for thyroid cancer.
3. Papillary carcinoma is the most common malignancy of the thyroid. Follicular adenomas are the most common neoplasms of the thyroid.
4. The presence of nodal metastasis in thyroid cancer should always be treated with a comprehensive neck dissection. Selective nodal biopsy or "berry-picking" is not recommended.
5. Molecular testing for common genetic mutations in thyroid cancer may be useful in diagnosing thyroid nodules with indeterminate cytopathology.

QUESTIONS: THYROID TUMOR

1. What is the incidence of a thyroid nodule?
   Clinically palpable nodules occur in 4% to 7% of the population, whereas the rate of incidental nodule found on ultrasound is higher (20% to 67% of patients) with more than half the thyroids containing more than one nodule. Nodules are more common in women (F : M ratio of 4 : 1). Thyroid cancer occurs in 5% to 10% of palpable nodules.
2. What is the workup of a thyroid nodule?
   - Comprehensive history and physical including a visualization of the vocal cords (laryngoscopy)
   - Laboratory studies including thyroid function assay and serum calcium
   - Ultrasound evaluation of nodule
3. What features indicate a higher risk of malignancy in the thyroid?
   - Age <30 years and >60 years
   - Male

- Positive family history
- Radiation exposure as child
- Elevated TSH/Hashimoto's thyroiditis
- Rapid growth
- Pain
- Compressive symptoms
- Hoarseness
- Cervical lymph nodes

4. **What ultrasound features are indications for a fine needle aspiration (FNA)?**
   - All nodules >1 cm, or smaller if other high-risk features are present (as below)
   - Microcalcification
   - Irregular margins
   - Solid rather than cystic nodule
   - Internal vascularity
   - Multiple nodules
   - Enlarged cervical lymph nodes on the same side of the neck

5. **What is the diagnostic accuracy of FNA cytology?**
   Accuracy 95%; false negative rate 2.3%; false positive 1.1%

6. **What are the FNA cytopathologic categories of thyroid nodules?**
   - Benign: 70%
   - Malignant: 5%
   - Suspicious: 10%
   - Indeterminate: 15%

   Of suspicious lesions, 10% to 20% will likely be follicular carcinomas on surgical pathology. With follicular lesions, I-123 scan may be helpful. If the lesion is "hot," it is unlikely to be malignant.

7. **What is the role of molecular testing for thyroid cancer?**
   Molecular testing allows for nodules in the "indeterminate" cytopathologic category (30% of all nodules) to be "ruled in" as cancer or "ruled out" as benign nodules. Proponents argue that this would save unnecessary surgeries and prevent two-surgery approaches (lobectomy followed by completion thyroidectomy).

8. **What molecular tests are currently available for thyroid cancer?**
   - Mutation panel testing: tests for mutations most commonly seen in thyroid cancer including BRAF, RAS, RET/PTC and PAX8/PPARY rearrangements. When positive, this test "rules in" a likely malignancy with a positive predictive value of 100%. However, 30% of thyroid cancers do not currently have a known mutation.
   - Gene expression testing: tests for 142 genes expressed differently between benign and malignant nodules. Test "rules out" nodules as benign and has a negative predictive value greater than 95%. The test is proprietary and expensive ($3,000).

9. **What is the recommended follow-up for a benign thyroid nodule?**
   Most authors recommend serial ultrasounds (every 6 to 12 mos) to look for changes in size or internal characteristics. Any significant changes may warrant a repeat FNA. Cysts that recur after multiple FNAs should be considered for surgical excision to establish a diagnosis. Suppression by exogenous thyroxine is NOT recommended.

10. **What is the differential diagnosis of thyroid cancers?**
    - Papillary carcinoma: 70% to 85%
    - Follicular carcinoma: 15% to 20%
    - Hurthle cell carcinoma: 3% to 5%
    - Medullary carcinoma: 3% to 10%
    - Anaplastic carcinoma: <2%
    - Insular or poorly differentiated carcinoma: rare
    - Other: lymphoma, squamous cell carcinoma, metastases

11. **What is the TNM staging for well-differentiated thyroid cancer?**

Table 15-1. TNM Staging for Well-Differentiated Thyroid Cancer

T1	The tumor is 2 centimeters (cm) or smaller and limited to the thyroid.
T1a	The tumor is 1 cm or smaller.
T1b	The tumor is bigger than 1 cm but less than 2 cm.
T2	The tumor is at least 2 cm, but it is not larger than 4 cm and is limited to the thyroid.
T3	The tumor is larger than 4 cm, but the tumor does not extend beyond the thyroid gland.
T4	The tumor is any size and has extended beyond the thyroid.
T4a	The tumor has spread beyond the thyroid to nearby soft tissues, the larynx, trachea, esophagus or recurrent laryngeal nerve.
T4b	The tumor has spread beyond the regions stated in T4a (above).
N0	There is no evidence of cancer in the regional lymph nodes.
N1	Cancer has spread to the lymph nodes.
N1a	Cancer has spread to the central compartment: pretracheal, paratracheal, and prelaryngeal nodes.
N1b	Cancer has spread beyond the central compartment, including unilateral, bilateral, contralateral or mediastinal nodes.
M0	Cancer without distant mets.
M1	Cancer with distant mets.
Mx	Distant mets not assessed.

12. **What is the staging for well-differentiated thyroid cancers?**

Table 15-2. Staging for Well-Differentiated Thyroid Cancer

Papillary or Follicular Thyroid Tumors <45 yrs. Old
Stage I: Any T, any N, M0
Stage II: Any T, any N, M1
Papillary or Follicular Thyroid Tumors >45 yrs. Old
Stage I: T1N0M0
Stage II: T2 or T3 N0M0
Stage III: T4 N0 M0 or any T any N M1
Stage IVA: T4a, any N M0 or T1-3 N1b M0
Stage IVB: T4b, any N M0
Stage IVC: Any T, any N M1

13. **What are the clinical prognostic indicators for thyroid cancer?**
   - **AMES:** Age; Metastasis; Extent, and Size of primary tumor
     - Low risk: age <40 (M) or <50 (F); tumor <4 cm and within thyroid gland
     - High risk: Age >41 (M) or >51 (F); extrathryoid invasion; size >5 cm
   - **MACIS:** Metastasis; Age; Completeness of resection; Invasion; Size of tumor
     - High risk: age >40; invasion of thyroid gland; incomplete tumor resection; size >4 cm

14. **What is the difference between total thyroidectomy (TT), near-total thyroidectomy (NT), and sub-total thyroidectomy?**
Total thyroidectomy is the complete removal of all visible thyroid tissue. In near-total thyroidectomy, the surgeon elects to leave a very small amount of thyroid tissue around the parathyroid glands or

recurrent laryngeal nerve to reduce morbidity. A sub-total thyroidectomy is ill-defined and results in large amounts of thyroid tissue left behind. A sub-total thyroidectomy is NOT an acceptable surgery for thyroid cancer.

15. **What is the treatment for Stage I and II papillary or follicular thyroid cancer?**
The treatment for well-differentiated thyroid cancer is a total thyroidectomy. Lobectomy alone results in a higher risk of local recurrence and death, except in some micro PTC <1 cm (see Question # 25). Total thyroidectomy also allows for radioactive iodine (RAI) I-131 thyroid ablation, which can improve the specificity of thyroglobulin assays and allows the detection of persistent disease by total body scanning.

16. **What is the treatment for Stage III papillary or follicular thyroid cancer?**
The current recommendation includes:
   - Total thyroidectomy plus removal of involved lymph nodes or other sites of extrathyroid disease
   - I-131 ablation following total thyroidectomy if the tumor demonstrates uptake
   - External-beam radiation therapy if I-131 uptake is minimal

17. **What is the treatment for Stage IV papillary or follicular thyroid cancer?**
   - Surgery: total thyroidectomy and neck dissection as indicated. Treatment of distant metastases is usually not curative but may produce good palliation. Metastases with uptake may be ablated by I-131. External-beam radiation is used for localized lesions that are unresponsive to RAI.
   - Resection of limited metastases, especially symptomatic metastases, should be considered when the tumor has no uptake of I-131. Removal of structures that will cause functional deficits (i.e., larynx, pharynx, trachea) should be thoroughly discussed with the patient.
   - Patients unresponsive to I-131 should be considered for chemotherapy such as inhibitors of vascular endothelial growth-factor (VEGF) receptors.

18. **What is the role of neck dissection in well-differentiated thyroid cancer?**
Papillary and medullary thyroid cancers have a high propensity to spread to regional lymph nodes whereas follicular carcinomas rarely do. A careful assessment of the central compartment (zone VI) and lateral neck (zones II-IV) should be done prior to surgery. Elective neck dissection beyond the central compartment is controversial. Some authors advocate routine central compartment dissection for PTC larger than 3 cm. Zone Ib (submandibular gland) is rarely involved by locoregional metastasis and can be preserved in thyroid cancer surgery.

19. **What is multiple endocrine neoplasia (MEN)?**
The term **multiple endocrine neoplasia** (**MEN**) encompasses several distinct syndromes featuring tumors of endocrine glands, each with its own characteristic pattern.
   - MEN type I: pancreas, pituitary, parathyroid adenomas
   - MEN type IIa: medullary carcinoma of thyroid, pheochromocytoma, parathyroid hyperplasia
   - MEN type IIb: MEN IIa and mucosal neuromas; no parathyroid involvement

20. **What is the staging for medullary thyroid cancer (MTC)?**

Table 15-3. Staging for Medullary Thyroid Cancer

Stage I:	T1 N0 M0
Stage II:	T2, T3 N0 M0
Stage III:	T1-3 N1a M0
Stage IVA:	T4a, any N M0 or T1-3, N1b M0
Stage IVB:	T4b, any N, M0
Stage IVC:	Any T, any N, M1

21. **What important characteristics are unique to medullary thyroid cancer?**
   - More aggressive than well-differentiated thyroid cancers (PTC and FTC)
   - Derive from parafollicular or C-cells and can secrete calcitonin and carcinoembryonic antigen (CEA) as well as prostaglandins, histaminases, and serotonin
   - High propensity for invasion into muscle and trachea as well as hematogenous spread to lungs and viscera (50% at presentation)
   - *RET* proto-oncogene mutation at codon 634 results in MEN IIa; codon 918 mutation results in MEN IIb.
   - MEN IIb type is the most aggressive. Familial medullary thyroid carcinoma (FMTC) has the best prognosis and MEN IIa has an intermediate prognosis
   - Sporadic unifocal lesions: 70%; familial/genetic: 30%

22. **What is the workup for medullary thyroid cancer?**
   Patients positive for RET mutation should be screened for MEN type II tumors: (i) pheochromocytoma: 24-hr urine catecholamine study and abdominal scan to rule out pheochromocytoma; (ii) parathyroid adenoma: serum calcium and PTH. Family members should have genetic screening for *RET* proto-oncogene and MEN type II tumors. Imaging should evaluate both locoregional and distant metastasis and include MRI, PET, sestamibi and indium-labeled somatostatin scans.

23. **What is the treatment for medullary thyroid cancer?**
   Total thyroidectomy and neck dissection (as needed) with resection of any additional structures involved is recommended. Children with MTC should have total thyroidectomy at age younger than 2 years old. Long-term follow-up with serial serum calcitonin and carcinoembryonic antigen (CEA) levels is recommended.

24. **What is anaplastic thyroid cancer?**
   - Extremely aggressive malignancy, usually occurs in older patients
   - 80% occur in pre-existing thyroid mass suggesting malignant de-differentiation within existing tumor
   - Presents as sudden growth in pre-existing mass associated with pain, hoarseness, dysphagia, and dyspnea

25. **What is the staging for anaplastic thyroid cancer?**
   - **Stage IV:** All anaplastic thyroid tumors are classified as stage IV, regardless of tumor size, location, or metastasis.
   - **IVA:** Anaplastic tumor that has spread to nearby structures, T4a
   - **IVB:** Tumor that has spread beyond nearby structures, T4b
   - **IVC:** There is evidence of metastasis (any N or M)

26. **What is the treatment for anaplastic thyroid cancer?**
   Almost all cases are advanced at time of presentation and median survival is less than 6 months. Doxorubicin, radiation, and palliative surgery (debulking and tracheostomy) can be considered for palliation and to improve QOL. Incidentally found anaplastic cancer and locally limited disease have somewhat better prognosis.

27. **How is RAI given?**
   RAI is given with thyroid hormone withdrawal or recombinant human TSH (rhTSH). Studies show that rhTSH maintains quality of life and reduces the radiation dose delivered to the body compared with thyroid hormone withdrawal.

28. **What is the treatment for recurrent thyroid cancer?**
   - 10% to 30% of patients develop recurrence and/or metastases.
   - 80% develop recurrence with disease in the neck alone; 20% develop recurrence with distant metastases (lungs).
   - 50% of the patients operated on for recurrent tumors can be rendered free of disease with a second operation.
   - Recurrences detected by I-131 scan and not clinically apparent can be treated with I-131 ablation with excellent prognosis.
   - Patients with iodine-refractory advanced thyroid cancer may respond to multi-tyrosine kinase inhibitor therapy.

QUESTIONS: PARATHYROID TUMOR

29. **What is the embryology of the parathyroid glands?**
The superior parathyroid glands develop from the fourth branchial pouch and the inferior parathyroid gland develops from the third pharyngeal pouch along with the thymus. Although most people have four parathyroid glands, 3% to 7% have five to seven glands, and 3% to 5% have fewer than four glands.

30. **What are the normal characteristics of parathyroid glands?**
The average parathyroid gland weighs 35 to 50 mgs and is 1 to 5 mm in diameter. Its primary blood supply is from the inferior thyroid artery, or more rarely from the posterior branch of the superior thyroid artery.

31. **What is primary hyperparathyroidism?**
Primary hyperparathyroidism is caused by the overproduction of PTH. Etiology is usually due to:
    - Solitary parathyroid adenoma (85%)
    - Multiple hyperplastic glands (10% to 15%)
    - Multiple adenomas (3% to 4%)
    - Parathyroid carcinoma (<1%)

    Primary hyperparathyroidism may be related to overexpression of PRAD1 oncogene or low-dose radiation exposure, but the true etiology is unknown.

32. **What are secondary and tertiary hyperparathyroidism?**
Secondary hyperparathyroidism is seen in patients with chronic renal failure causing elevated phosphate and decreased 1-alpha-hydroxylase in the kidney resulting in low vitamin D. It is associated with mild hypercalcemia but high PTH. Surgery is recommended for osteopenia and is usually a sub-total (three and one half glands) parathyroidectomy. Tertiary hyperparathyroidism is the result of long-term secondary hyperparathyroidism that results in autonomous parathyroid function, even when the underlying causes are corrected. Cinacalcet (calcimimetic agent) can be effective in treating patients with secondary hyperparathyroidism.

33. **What are the classic symptoms of hypercalcemia?**
"Moans, groans, stones, and psychic overtones": the most common symptoms include GI disturbance (nausea, constipation, peptic ulcer, pancreatitis), muscle weakness, renal stones, hypertension, cardiac arrhythmia, polydipsia, and neuropsychiatric symptoms including depression, fatigue, and memory loss. Renal stones and bone disorders such as osteitis fibrosa cystica are rare since the advent of routine parathyroid hormone (PTH) testing.

34. **What is the differential diagnosis for hypercalcemia?**

Table 15-4. Causes of Hypercalcemia
Metastatic cancer from lung, breast, prostate, breast primary
Multiple myeloma: leukemia, lymphoma
PTH-secreting tumors: small cell lung cancer, ovarian cancer, thymoma
Granulomatous diseases: sarcoidosis, tuberculosis, histoplasmosis, leprosy, Wegener
Drugs: thiazide diuretics, lithium, theophylline, hypervitaminosis A & D
Immobilization
Milk alkali syndrome
Benign familial hypocalciuric hypercalcemia
Adrenal insufficiency
Hyperphosphatasia
Paget's bone disease

35. **How is the diagnosis of primary hyperparathyroidism made?**
   - Increased serum total calcium and increased or very high PTH.
   - Serum phosphate is decreased or low-normal.
   - If PTH is elevated *but* serum calcium is normal or low normal, rule out vitamin D insufficiency or malabsorption.
   - If both calcium and phosphate levels are elevated, rule out hypervitaminosis D.

36. **What are available localization imaging studies for primary hyperparathyroidism?**
   - Noninvasive Localization
     - Technetium 99m sestamibi (Tc99m MIBI): Sestamibi localizes into the mitochondria of parathyroid cells. Late phase images at 2 hours allows for sestamibi to clear from the thyroid gland, but not the parathyroid. Single adenoma detection is high with sensitivity of 100% and specificity of 90%. Less useful for four-gland hyperplasia.
     - Tc 99m MIBI plus single photon emission CT (SPECT): Addition of SPECT gives a higher resolution three-dimensional image and some report superior detection of adenomas within the carotid sheath or mediastinum.
     - Tc 99m + thallium 201 subtraction: Thallium is taken up by the parathyroid and less by the thyroid gland. Subsequent subtraction image can detect enlarged parathyroid glands. Sensitivity rates are varied (30% to 90%), but more widely available than MIBI.
     - Ultrasound: Superior than other techniques for identifying intrathyroid parathyroid adenomas, quicker, and involves no radiation. Ectopic adenomas of retroesophageal, trachea and mediastinum are more difficult to localize with US. False positive rate is 15% to 20%.
     - MRI: Adenomas appear with high signal intensity on T-2 weighted images. May be useful in identifying ectopic adenomas and in patients requiring re-exploration after initial surgery.
   - Invasive Localization
     - Intraoperative gamma probe: Tc 99m MIBI is injected 2 hours prior to surgery and radioactive parathyroid glands are localized using handheld gamma probes.
     - Parathyroid angiography/arteriography.
     - Venous sampling of PTH: Angiographic sampling of selective veins preferred, but even large vein sampling (internal jugular vein) can help lateralize the gland and can be useful in re-exploration.
     - US guided parathyroid fine needle aspiration (FNA).

37. **What are the most common ectopic locations of parathyroid glands?**
   Ectopic parathyroid glands can be found in the superior mediastinum, thymic capsule, retro-esophagus, within the carotid sheath, and medial to the superior thyroid pole. The inferior parathyroid gland has more variability in its final location because it descends with the thymus gland. The superior parathyroid gland tends to be more closely associated with the lateral lobe of the thyroid.

38. **What is the most recent NIH recommendation for surgery in the asymptomatic primary hyperparathyroidism patient?**

Table 15-5. 2008 NIH Guidelines for Surgery in Asymptomatic Primary Hyperparathyroidism

Serum calcium (above upper limit or normal):	1.0 mg/dl
24-hour urine calcium:	no longer an indication
Renal function:	GFR < 60 ml/min
Bone density:	T score < 2.5 at any site; and/or previous fracture or fragility
Age:	<50 years old
Patient desires surgery or cannot be reliably followed	

39. **How is intraoperative PTH monitoring used in parathyroid surgery?**
PTH has a half-life of 3 to 5 minutes. In parathyroid surgery, the goal is to see a decrease in PTH level by more than 50% at 10 minutes after removal of a parathyroid adenoma or hyperplasia. Intraoperative PTH monitoring allows focused parathyroid surgery (i.e., one-gland surgery) and can prevent unnecessary bilateral four-gland exploration.

40. **How is autotransplantation of parathyroid tissue performed?**
Parathyroid tissue can either be autotransplanted at the time of surgery or cryopreserved for up to 18 months and transplanted at a later date. Transplantation occurs most commonly into the sternocleidomastoid (SCM) of the neck or into the brachioradialis of the arm. Transplanted parathyroid tissue usually functions within 3 months and has a success rate of 50%. One advantage of transplanting into the arm is the ability to remove parathyroid tissue under local anesthetic if it becomes hyperplastic.

41. **What are the surgical options for hyperparathyroidism?**
- Single gland disease plus positive MIBI scan: Directed unilateral exploration with intraoperative PTH monitoring to assess adequacy of resection
- MEN syndrome: Bilateral cervical exploration and four-gland identification
- Negative MIBI scan: Bilateral exploration with selective biopsy of suspicious glands and intraoperative PTH monitoring to assess adequacy of resection
- Secondary or tertiary hyperparathyroidism: 3½ gland resection or total parathyroidectomy with possible autotransplantation or cryopreservation of parathyroid tissue

42. **What strategies are used for parathyroid re-exploration?**
In re-exploration, the strategy is to dissect lateral to medial, from the SCM to retroesophageal tissue overlying the cervical spine. Inferiorly, the thymus is resected. Medially, the prevertebral space (retroesophageal, retropharyngeal) is explored. The thyroid lobe is mobilized and palpated for an intrathyroid parathyroid. The carotid sheath is opened from hyoid to the mediastinum. If unilateral exploration is negative, contralateral exploration is then performed. Mediastinal exploration should be performed only after imaging (i.e., MIBI and MRI) has been done.

CONTROVERSIES

43. **Does the presence of lymph node metastasis in well-differentiated thyroid cancers worsen the prognosis?**
This is unclear. Some studies demonstrate increased risk of local recurrence and lower disease-specific survival with nodal metastasis while other studies demonstrate survival difference only in patients older than 45 years old.

44. **What is the optimal surgery for micropapillary thyroid cancer (<1 cm)?**
According to the NCI, thyroid lobectomy alone may be sufficient treatment for small (<1 cm), low-risk, unifocal, intrathyroidal papillary carcinomas in the absence of prior head and neck irradiation or radiologically or clinically involved cervical nodal metastases. Lobectomy is associated with a lower incidence of complications, but approximately 5% to 10% of patients will have a recurrence in the contralateral thyroid. Completion thyroidectomy is often curative in these cases.

45. **What is the role of RAI in low-risk thyroid cancer patients?**
In low-risk patients (complete tumor resection; no nodal involvement; T1 or T2 stage I patients older than 45 years), there was no difference in overall survival and disease-specific survival between RAI and no RAI groups. Long-term complications of RAI include second malignancies, sialadenitis, and lacrimal and salivary gland dysfunction. Reducing the amount of radiation exposure by lowering the dosage of RAI and giving it in combination with rhTSH have been explored for low-risk thyroid cancer patients.

46. **Is molecular diagnostics for thyroid cancer cost-effective?**
This is unclear. Recent studies show that if unnecessary surgery and two-surgery approaches are eliminated by molecular testing, there is a cost savings even with the high cost of the tests. Additional value of molecular testing may be as a quality control for cytopathology and as a prognostic test for the aggressiveness of a thyroid cancer.

Bibliography

Bilimoria KY, Bentrem DJ, Ko CY, et al: Extent of surgery affects survival for papillary thyroid cancer, *Ann Surg* 246(3):375–381, discussion 381–384, 2007.

Bilezikian JP, Khan AA, Potts JT Jr: Guidelines for the management of asymptomatic primary hyperparathyroidism: summary statement from the third international workshop, *J Clin Endocrinol Metab* 94(2):335–339, 2009.

Carling T, Udelsman R: Thyroid tumors. In DeVita VT Jr, Lawrence TS, Rosenberg SA, editors: *Cancer: Principles and Practice of Oncology*, ed 9, Philadelphia, 2011, Lippincott Williams & Wilkins, pp 1457–1472.

Kebebew E, Clark OH: Medullary thyroid cancer, *Curr Treat Options Oncol* 1(4):359–367, 2000.

Mazzaferri EL: Thyroid cancer in thyroid nodules: finding a needle in the haystack, *Am J Med* 93:359–362, 1992.

Mazzaferri EL: Management of a solitary thyroid nodule, *N Engl J Med* 328:553–559, 1993.

Mazzaferri EL, Jhiang SM: Long-term impact of initial surgical and medical therapy on papillary and follicular thyroid cancer, *Am J Med* 97(5):418–428, 1994.

Schlumberger M, Catargi B, Borget I, et al: Strategies of radioiodine ablation in patients with low-risk thyroid cancer, *N Engl J Med* 366(18):1663–1673, 2012.

Shaha AR: Controversies in the management of thyroid nodule, *Laryngoscope* 110(2 Pt 1):183–193, 2000.

Thyroid. In Edge SB, Byrd DR, Compton CC, et al, editors: *AJCC Cancer Staging Manual*, ed 7, New York, 2010, Springer, pp 87–96.

Walsh RM, Watkinson JC, Franklyn J: The management of the solitary thyroid nodule: a review, *Clin Otolaryngol* 24:388–397, 1999.

NECK DISSECTION

John Song, MD

CHAPTER 16

KEY POINTS

1. Clinical or occult regional lymphatic involvement can be found in up to 50% of patients with SCC of the head and neck (SCCHN). The presence of cervical lymphadenopathy is the single most significant prognostic indicator in SCCHN.
2. Knowledge and identification of first echelon nodes for various primary head and neck tumor sites allows for selective neck dissection of nodes at greatest risk for metastatic disease.
3. The first muscle you see in Level I/II dissection is the anterior belly of the digastric muscle: it is NOT the mylohyoid muscle. The mylohyoid is always deep to the lymphatics of Level Ia and runs perpendicular and medial to the anterior belly of the digastric. Retracting the mylohyoid muscle medially helps identify the deeper structures of the submandibular fossa including the lingual nerve, the hypoglossal nerve, and submandibular ganglion and duct.
4. The digastric muscle is often referred to as the "resident's friend" because it is lateral to many of the most important structures of the neck including the IJV, carotid artery, and the hypoglossal nerve. Dissecting the digastric muscle in an anterior to posterior direction prevents injury to these structures.
5. The best way to prevent a chyle leak is to dissect laterally from the IJV as you dissect below the omohyoid muscle (i.e., Level IV). Careful ligation of the lymphatic vessels must be done to prevent further tearing these fragile structures. Increasing the intrathoracic pressure during surgery can help identify the source of the chyle leak.

Pearls

1. The floor of the posterior neck dissection is formed by the splenius capitis and levator scapulae muscles superiorly, and the scalene muscles (anterior, middle, posterior) inferiorly.
2. Factors such as tumor site, stage, thickness, presence of perineural and angiolymphatic invasion, and tumor differentiation can all increase the risk of regional lymphatic involvement.
3. Be able to define and differentiate radical, modified radical, and selective or functional neck dissections.

QUESTIONS

1. **According to the AJCC, what constitutes the Level I nodal group?**
   Level I includes both the submental (Ia) and the submandibular (Ib) lymph node basins. Anatomically, Ia includes the triangle formed by the anterior belly of the digastric muscle bilaterally and the hyoid bone. The mylohyoid muscle forms the floor of Level Ia. Level Ib is bound by the posterior belly of the digastric muscle and the mandible, and includes the perivascular lymph nodes around the facial artery and vein (Figure 16-1).

2. **What constitutes the Level II nodal group?**
   Level II includes the uppermost jugular nodes and is divided into Level IIa (nodes anterior to the spinal accessory nerve: cranial nerve XI) and Level IIb (nodes posterior to CN XI). Anatomically, this includes all nodes adjacent to the great vessels from the skull base to the carotid bifurcation, and from the sternohyoid muscle to the posterior border of the sternocleidomastoid muscle (SCM) (see Figure 16-1).

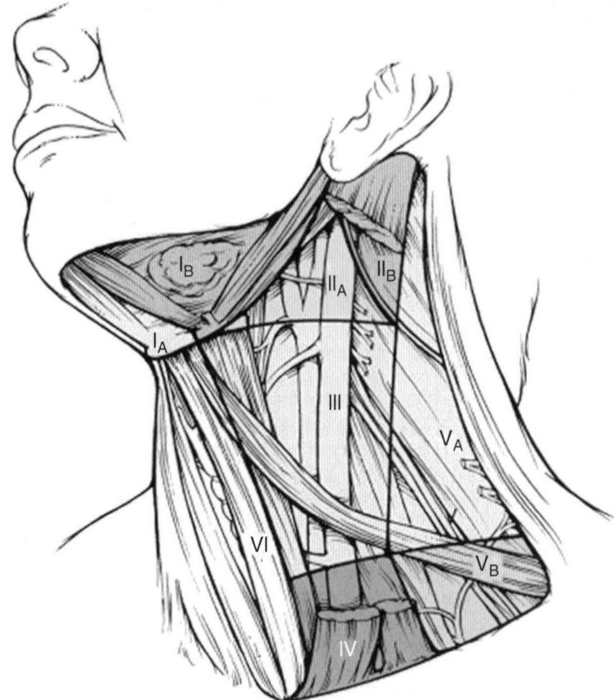

Figure 16-1. The six sublevels of the neck for describing the location of lymph nodes within Levels I, II, and V. *IA,* submental group; *IB,* submandibular group; *IIA,* upper jugular nodes along the carotid sheath including the subdigastric group; *IIB,* upper jugular nodes in the submuscular recess; *VA,* spinal accessory nodes; and *VB,* the supraclavicular and transverse cervical nodes. *(Redrawn from art provided courtesy of Douglas Denys, MD. From Cummings Otolaryngology: Head & Neck Surgery, 5 ed, Philadelphia, 2010, Mosby Elsevier, p. 1705.)*

3. **What constitutes the Level III nodal group?**
   Level III includes the mid-jugular nodes extending from the carotid bifurcation to the omohyoid muscle, and from the sternohyoid muscle to the posterior border of the SCM (see Figure 16-1).

4. **What constitutes the Level IV nodal group?**
   Level IV includes the inferior-most jugular nodes extending from the omohyoid muscle to the clavicle, and from the sternohyoid muscle to the posterior border of the SCM (see Figure 16-1).

5. **What constitutes the Level V nodal group?**
   Level V includes the posterior triangle bounded by the posterior border of the SCM, the anterior edge of the trapezius muscle, and the clavicle inferiorly. It includes Level Va (spinal accessory nodes) and Vb (supraclavicular and transverse cervical nodes) (see Figure 16-1).

6. **What constitutes the Level VI nodal group?**
   Level VI includes the central compartment nodes extending from the hyoid bone to the suprasternal notch, and laterally by the carotid arteries. These include the pretracheal, paratracheal, and Delphian (precricoid) nodes. Perithyroidal nodes and nodes occurring along the recurrent laryngeal nerves are also in Level VI (see Figure 16-1).

7. **Which primary sites are most likely to metastasize to these nodal groups?**
   Level Ia: Anterior oral tongue, floor of mouth, lower alveolar ridge and gingiva, lower lip
   Level Ib: Oral cavity (including tongue, lateral floor of mouth, buccal mucosa), anterior nasal cavity, maxillary sinus, submandibular gland

Level II: This nodal basin drains most of the primary SCCHN sites including the oral cavity, nasal cavity, nasopharynx, oropharynx, hypopharynx, larynx, parotid gland
Level III: Oral cavity, oropharynx, nasopharynx, hypopharynx, larynx
Level IV: Hypopharynx, thyroid, larynx, cervical esophagus
Level V: Cutaneous malignancies of posterior scalp and neck, nasopharynx, oropharynx
Level VI: Thyroid, larynx (glottic and subglottic), cervical esophagus, apex of piriform sinus (see Figure 16-1)

8. **What is the AJCC staging for nodal disease for head and neck tumors (excluding nasopharynx and thyroid)?**

Table 16-1. AJCC Staging for Nodal Disease for Head and Neck Tumors

NX	Regional lymph nodes cannot be assessed.
N0	There is no regional node metastasis.
N1	Metastasis in a single ipsilateral lymph node, 3 cm or less in greatest dimension.
N2	Metastasis in a single ipsilateral lymph node, more than 3 cm but not more than 6 cm in greatest dimension; or metastasis in multiple ipsilateral lymph nodes, none more than 6 cm in greatest dimension; or metastasis in bilateral or contralateral lymph nodes, none greater than 6 cm in greatest dimension.
N2a	Metastasis in a single ipsilateral lymph node, more than 3 cm but not more than 6 cm in greatest dimension.
N2b	Metastasis in multiple ipsilateral lymph nodes, none more than 6 cm in greatest dimension.
N2c	Metastasis in bilateral or contralateral lymph nodes, none more than 6 cm in greatest dimension.
N3	Metastasis is in a lymph node more than 6 cm in greatest dimension.

U, L: A designation of "U" or "L" may be given in addition to indicate the level of metastasis above the lower border of the cricoid cartilage (U) or below the lower border of the cricoid cartilage (L).
(From http://www.springer.com/gb/book/9780387884400)

9. **What is the AJCC nodal staging for nasopharyngeal tumors?**

Table 16-2. AJCC Nodal Staging for Nasopharyngeal Tumors

N0	No regional lymph node metastasis.
N1	Unilateral metastasis in lymph node(s) is 6 cm or less in greatest dimension, above the supraclavicular fossa.
N2	Bilateral metastasis in lymph nodes is 6 cm or less in greatest dimension, above the supraclavicular fossa.
N3	Metastasis in lymph node(s) is greater than 6 cm and/or to the supraclavicular fossa.
N3a	Tumor is greater than 6 cm in dimension.
N3b	Tumor extends to the supraclavicular fossa.

(From http://www.cancer.gov/cancertopics/pdq/treatment/nasopharyngeal/HealthProfessional/page3)

10. **What is the AJCC nodal staging for thyroid tumors?**

Table 16-3. AJCC Nodal Staging for Thyroid Tumors

NX	Regional lymph nodes cannot be assessed.
N0	No regional lymph node metastasis.
N1	There is regional lymph node metastasis.
N1a	There is metastasis to Level VI (pretracheal, paratracheal, and prelaryngeal/Delphian lymph nodes).
N1b	There is metastasis to unilateral, bilateral, or contralateral cervical or superior mediastinal lymph nodes.

(From http://www.cancer.gov/cancertopics/pdq/treatment/thyroid/HealthProfessional/page3)

11. **What is a radical neck dissection (RND)?**
This neck dissection, first popularized by George Crile in the early twentieth century and later by Hayes Martin in the 1950s, espoused the concept of radical en bloc resection of cervical lymph nodes for cancers of the head and neck. RND included removal of lymph node Levels I through V, along with the SCM, IJV, and spinal accessory nerve (CN XI). Morbidities resulting from RND include shoulder dysfunction due to sacrifice of CN XI (winged scapula, inability to raise the arm above 90 degrees, shoulder pain), and limited bilateral surgery due to IJV sacrifice.

12. **What are the indications for an RND?**
RND is indicated for patients whose cervical node metastasis has extended beyond the capsule of the lymph node to invade the SCM, the spinal accessory nerve, or IJV.

13. **What is a modified radical neck dissection (MRND)?**
In an MRND, lymph node Levels I through V are removed, but one or more of the nonlymphatic structures (spinal accessory nerve, SCM, or IJV) are spared. This significantly reduces the morbidity associated with a RND.

14. **What are the indications for a MRND?**
Unless there is fixation or infiltration of the nonlymphatic structures by tumor, the SCM, IJV, and spinal accessory nerve are preserved. Given that hypoglossal and lingual nerves are routinely preserved in neck dissection, sacrificing an uninvolved spinal accessory nerve in an en bloc resection of the neck cannot be justified. In bilateral neck dissections, removal of both internal jugular veins can result in significant venous edema and chronic lymphedema of the face and can be fatal in 10% of patients when performed simultaneously. At least one IJV should be preserved in bilateral procedures. If both IJVs are involved by disease, a staged neck dissection separated by at least 2 weeks should be performed to allow for collateral circulations to develop.

15. **What is a selective neck dissection (SND)?**
In an SND, an en bloc resection of one or more nodal groups is performed while preserving nonlymphatic structures. Only the nodal groups determined to be at highest risk for metastasis are removed, thus preserving functional and cosmetic structures within the neck.

16. **What are the indications for an SND?**
In previously untreated patients with SCCHN, the level of nodal metastasis occurs in a predictable pattern. This allows for the identification of highest-risk first-echelon lymph nodes for a variety of primary tumor sites (see Question 7). SND can be used for treatment in conjunction with resection of tumors with limited neck disease, for surgical staging of the neck in the clinically N0 neck, or to direct further adjuvant therapy if multiple nodes or the presence of extracapsular spread is found.

17. **What is the extent of SND in these primary SCCHN sites?**
    - Oral cavity: Levels I, II, III (supraomohyoid neck dissection)
    - Oropharynx, hypopharynx, larynx: Levels II-IV (lateral neck dissection)
    - Posterior scalp: Levels II-V, retroauricular, and suboccipital nodes (posterolateral neck dissection)
    - Preauricular, anterior scalp: Levels II-Va, parotid and facial nodes
    - Anterior and lateral face: Levels I-III, parotid and facial nodes
    - Thyroid, esophagus, advanced laryngeal tumor: Level VI (anterior or central neck dissection). Additional levels may also be dissected with advanced tumors.

18. **What is the role of lymphoscintigraphy in neck dissection?**
    The use of lymphoscintigraphy and sentinel lymph node biopsy (SNLB) in head and neck melanoma is well established and is a good predictor of disease-free survival with low false negative rates. In head and neck mucosal malignancies, SNLB can be used to (1) stage neck disease in clinically N0 necks; (2) identify lymphatic flows into atypical nodal basins that would not be addressed in classic SNDs; (3) determine lymphatic flow changes as a result of surgery and radiation that are at risk for metastasis from recurrent or residual disease. SNLB as a method for avoiding neck dissection is considered investigational and not widely accepted as standard of care.

19. **What are some complications after a neck dissection?**
    Chyle leak: Most commonly associated with a Level IV dissection. Occurs in 1% to 2% of neck dissections. Injury to the thoracic duct occurs as it enters the IJV laterally just superior to the junction of the IJV and subclavian vein. Daily output greater than 500 ml will require surgical exploration and ligation of the duct. Output of less than 500 ml may be managed conservatively with pressure dressing, low-fat diet, and wound drainage. Total parenteral nutrition may be considered in high-output leaks.
    Facial and cerebral edema: Associated with bilateral ligation of IJV and in patients with previous radiation therapy. This can be avoided by staged neck dissections and by preserving one or more external jugular veins. Cerebral edema resulting from IJV ligation can cause inappropriate secretions of antidiurectic hormone (SIADH). Intravenous fluids should be carefully administered in bilateral neck dissections where the IJV is ligated and serum and urine osmolarity carefully monitored perioperatively.
    Carotid rupture/blowout: This catastrophic complication is associated with salivary fistula, flap breakdown due to previous radiation, malnutrition, infection, and diabetes. Poorly placed and designed flap incisions can expose the carotid and increase risk of rupture. Placement of vascularized tissue over the carotid is indicated in cases of large salivary fistulas or carotid exposure.

20. **What is the difference between a salvage neck dissection and a planned neck dissection?**
    Salvage neck dissection is neck dissection that occurs in the setting of an incomplete response to organ preservation treatment (radiation or chemoradiation). Salvage neck dissection can occur immediately after chemoradiation or late for recurrent disease.
    Planned neck dissection refers to neck dissection that occurs early after chemoradiation as part of a planned treatment plan for large volume nodal disease (bulky N2b or N3 disease) regardless of the response to chemoradiation. The rationale behind planned neck dissection is that large pretreatment nodes may contain nests of viable SCC cells that can become the focus of recurrent disease.

21. **Types of neck dissection after chemoradiation or radiation therapy.**
    Neck dissection after chemoradiation falls into one of three categories:
    1. **Failure at the primary site:** Neck dissection is performed at the same time as salvage surgery for the primary site. Usually done regardless of nodal status at completion of treatment.
    2. **Salvage neck dissection:** Neck dissection is performed only if there is persistent nodal disease after treatment. Assessment of nodal disease is performed 8 to 10 weeks post-treatment using PET scan or CT and MRI.
    3. **Planned neck dissection:** Some surgeons will recommend a planned neck dissection for high volume nodal disease (N3) regardless of response to therapy. In low volume nodal disease (N1 or N2), surgery is performed only if there is persistent nodal disease at post-treatment assessment at 8 to 10 weeks.

CONTROVERSIES

22. **Fine needle aspiration (FNA) versus open biopsy (excisional or incisional) of suspected cervical lymph nodes.**
    An open biopsy may not increase rates of local recurrence, complications, and distant metastasis as previously believed, as long as adequate treatment is started in a timely fashion. But with FNA approaching 99% in sensitivity and specificity for SCC, the need for an open biopsy should be limited to those nodes suspected of having lymphoma. Neck dissection in a field that has been violated by an open biopsy may require resection of structures that normally would have been spared in SND, resulting in greater functional and cosmetic deficits to the patient. For this reason alone, an open biopsy should never be used as a first-line diagnostic procedure in SCC of the head and neck.

23. **Surgical treatment of the clinically negative (N0) neck.**
    The rationale for operating on the N0 neck includes: (1) decreasing locoregional recurrence; (2) decreasing risk of distant metastasis; (3) improved overall survival benefit; and (4) pathologic staging of regional lymph nodes. While most trials have not supported any overall survival benefits of electively treating the N0 neck over close clinical observation, many institutions continue to support elective treatment when the risk of occult metastasis is greater than 15%. SND encompassing the highest risk nodal basins is favored over MRND in elective treatment of the N0 neck.

24. **Should a carotid artery involved by tumor be sacrificed in neck dissection?**
    This is one of the most controversial issues in neck dissection. Opponents point to the relatively high rates of mortality (30%) and CNS complication (45%) with carotid resection with only 15% of patients alive and free of disease at 1 year despite carotid sacrifice. Proponents argue that with improved methods for assessing collateral circulation through the circle of Willis (endovascular balloon occlusion testing, xenon inhalation CT scan, intraarterial xenon, PET scan), a planned ligation and reconstruction of the carotid artery can result in acceptable CNS complications (12%) and improved 1-year disease-free survival rates (45%). Others have demonstrated a 22% 2-year disease-free survival. Some surgeons advocate peeling gross residual tumor off of the carotid artery as a compromise between these two approaches. A frank discussion with the patient as well as thorough preoperative testing should be performed in any cases where carotid artery resection is contemplated.

25. **Are MRND and SND comparable in controlling locoregional disease?**
    Most studies to date support SND for both N0 and N+ neck disease in selected patients. The locoregional control rates for SND are comparable to MRND for N0 (5% recurrence) and N+ (10% recurrence) disease, especially when postoperative radiotherapy is added to groups with multiple positive nodes or nodes with extracapsular spread (ECS). Regional control rates of more than 94% are seen in large multi-institutional studies looking at the efficacy of SND in clinically N+ disease in SCCHN.

26. **Should SND or MRND be performed after chemoradiation?**
    In the past, most surgeons advocated MRND after radiation or chemoradiation in order to encompass all five nodal levels in salvage or planned surgery. Current data, however, suggest that for some N1 and even N2 disease, SND may be as effective as MRND in locoregional control after therapy. Even in those patients with bulky N2 or N3 disease before treatment, very few had recurrences outside of Levels II to IV, suggesting that Level V dissection may be unnecessary in a majority of salvage neck dissections. One notable exception is the posterior scalp in which Level V is a first echelon lymph node basin. For most other primary head and neck sites, SND is likely more than adequate for salvage neck dissection unless there is fixation or infiltration of surrounding tissue by nodal metastasis.

BIBLIOGRAPHY

Bocca E, Pignataro O, Oldini C, et al: Functional neck dissection: an evaluation and review of 843 cases, *Laryngoscope* 94:942–945, 1984.

Collins SL: Controversies in management of cancer of the neck. In Thawley SE, et al, editors: *Comprehensive Management of Head and Neck Tumors*, ed 2, Philadelphia, 1999, WB Saunders, pp 1479–1563.

Deschler DG, Day T, editors: *TNM Staging of Head and Neck Cancer and Neck Dissection Classification*, ed 3, Alexandria, 2008, American Academy of Otolaryngology-Head and Neck Surgery Foundation, Inc.

Gavilan C, Gavilan J: Five-year results of functional neck dissection for cancer of the larynx, *Arch Otolaryngol Head Neck Surg* 115:1193–1196, 1989.
Lindberg R: Distribution of cervical lymph node metastases from squamous cell carcinoma of the upper respiratory and digestive tracts, *Cancer* 29:1446–1449, 1972.
Martin H: The treatment of cervical metastatic cancer, *Ann Surg* 114:972–985, 1941.
Robbins KT, Shaha AR, Medina JE, et al: Consensus statement of the classification and terminology of neck dissection, *Arch Otolaryngol Head Neck Surg* 134:536–538, 2008.
Shah JP: Patterns of cervical lymph node metastasis from squamous cell carcinomas of the upper aerodigestive tract, *Am J Surg* 160:405–409, 1990.
Snyderman CH, D'Amico F: Outcome of carotid artery resection for neoplastic disease: A meta-analysis, *Am J Otolaryngol* 13:373–380, 1992.

CHAPTER 17

VASCULAR TUMORS OF THE HEAD AND NECK

Matthew Old, MD, FACS

KEY POINTS

1. Most paragangliomas are nonfunctional, although suspected sympathetic symptoms (flushing, palpatations, sweating) should be evaluated thoroughly, particularly if the patient is to undergo surgery.
2. Treatment involves surgery, observation, or radiation depending on patient factors, growth rate, and suspicion for malignancy.
3. The natural history of a hemangioma is rapid development and then involution, so a conservative approach is recommended for most of these lesions unless significant airway involvement is present.

Pearls

1. Carotid body tumors are the most common head and neck paragangliomas.
2. Carotid body paragangliomas present as a pulsatile neck mass that have characteristic CT, MRI, or angiography findings of splaying of the external and internal carotids (Lyre's sign).
3. Familial paragangliomas constitute between 10% and 28% of cases with the remainder being sporadic. Multicentricity is present in 10% of sporadic cases versus 30% to 40% in familial situations.
4. Familial parangliomas are inherited in an autosomal dominant fashion with genomic imprinting. Fifty percent of the offspring of carrier males will develop paragangliomas. Females can inherit the trait (and develop paragangliomas) but will pass it along silently.
5. A teenage male with unilateral nasal obstruction, epistaxis, and a bluish mass filling the nasal cavity is the typical presentation of a juvenile nasopharyngeal angiofibroma.

QUESTIONS

1. **What are paragangliomas? From what tissues are they derived?**
Paragangliomas are benign or malignant vascular soft tissue tumors that arise anywhere paraganglia that have a neural crest origin are present. Paraganglia are present in the vascular adventitia or intraneuronally, releasing catecholamines and neurotransmitters. Most degenerate after birth but some persist, primarily along the autonomic nervous system.

2. **What are the commonly used and confusing names for paragangliomas?**
These tumors have various terminologies such as chemodectoma, nonchromaffin paragangliomas, carotid body tumors, and glomus tumors. Due to the physiologic function of the carotid body as a chemoreceptor, carotid body tumors are known as chemodectomas. *Chemodectoma* only applies to carotid body paragangliomas as the carotid body and aortic body are the only paraganglia that act as chemoreceptors. *Nonchromaffin* refers to the histologic staining that distinguishes all paragangliomas from the chromaffin-reacting tissue of the adrenal medulla. *Glomus* is the most frequently misused term in the literature as it is technically a term for a histologically different benign cutaneous tumor. The WHO has designated these paragangliomas by their location (i.e., carotid, vagal, jugular, and tympanic paragangliomas).

3. **Where are paragangliomas commonly found?**
The most comon site is the adrenal medulla (pheochromcytoma) with 90%, followed by abdominal (8.5%), thoracic (1.2%), and then head and neck (0.3%). The carotid body bifurcation (carotid body tumor) is the most common location of a head and neck paraganglioma. Jugular paragangliomas (glomus jugulare) is the next most common head and neck, followed by paragangliomas on the promontory of the middle ear (glomus tympanicum) and vagal paragangliomas. Rare locations can include the larynx, thyroid, paranasal sinuses or any other structures that harbor paraganglia.

4. **How do paragangliomas present?**
Most paragangliomas are discovered incidentally on imaging. Carotid body tumors typically present with a pulsatile neck mass that is mobile in the horizontal direction but not vertically. The growth rate is estimated at 0.5 cm per year. Tympanic paragangliomas are found on otoscopy as a bluish mass behind the eardrum. Because of their location in the temporal bone, the presenting symptoms can include pulsatile tinnitus and cranial nerve involvement (IX, X, and XI), if large.

5. **Is a tympanic paraganglioma (glomus tympanicum) the same as a jugular paraganglioma?**
No. Tympanic paragangliomas arise in the middle ear on the promontory of the cochlea. The morbidity associated with surgical resection is minimal. They present with pulsatile tinnitus, conductive hearing loss, and/or a blue mass behind the tympanic membrane on examination. Jugular tumors arise from paraganglionic tissue in the jugular bulb. Their site of origin is in the temporal bone, and their growth creates a great deal of bony destruction. Tumors of the jugular foramen put the IX, X, and XI nerves at risk, and resection in this region involves a combined skull base procedure and can result in significant cranial nerve related morbidity.

6. **What is the most important aspect of working up a paraganglioma patient?**
It is important to gather a thorough history to assure there are no signs of a functional tumor (flushing, heat intolerance, palpitations, etc.). If there are, evaluate urinary metanephrines and vanillylmandelic acid (VMA) and serum catecholimines, and strongly consider an endocrinology referral if positive. Functional tumors are rare and only comprise approximately 1% to 3% of paragangiolmas in the head and neck. The next most important aspect is the physical examination, which should include a comprehensive cranial nerve examination.

7. **What is the ideal imaging for paragangliomas?**
A computed tomographic scan with contrast or magnetic resonance imaging with gadolinium (and CT/MR angiography if needed) will often provide the diagnosis and superior anatomic extent. Vascular flow voids are often demonstrated on imaging, which strongly predict a paraganglioma. Ultrasonography may be helpful on intial examination to determine the difference between a vascular tumor and lymph node. Angiography was very common prior to CT or MR angiography technology but is now reserved for preoperative embolization if the surgeon desires. The classic angiography of a carotid body paraganglioma is splaying of the internal and external carotid artery at the bifurcation (Lyre's sign) (Figure 17-1).

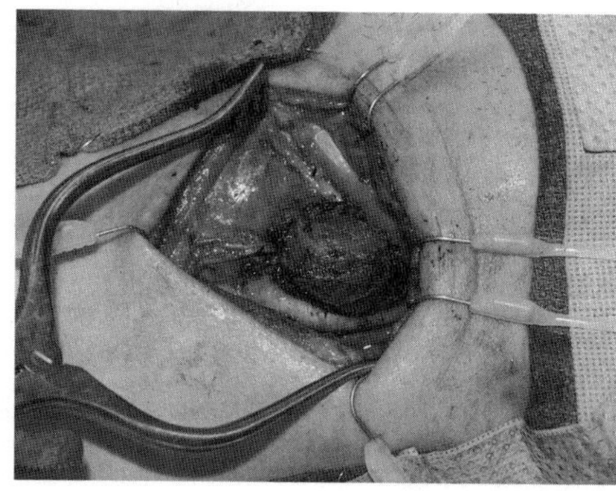

Figure 17-1. Carotid body paraganglioma during dissection. Note internal carotid posterior and hypoglossal superior.

8. **What is the inheritance pattern of familial paragangliomas?**
Although most paragangliomas are sporadic in nature, up to 30% are familial. A higher incidence of multicentric tumors exists in patients with the familial pattern (30% to 40% versus 10% in sporadic paragangliomas). Familial parangliomas are inherited in an autosomal dominant fashion with genomic imprinting. Fifty percent of the offspring of males with the gene develop paragangliomas, but when transmitted by the mother the gene is swiched off and the offspring will not exhibit the disease. The primary gene (PGL1) codes for the succinate dehydrogenase complex; malignant paragangliomas are more common with SDHB patients.

9. **Discuss the treatment options for paragangliomas.**
Options for treatment inlude surgery, observation, and radiation, depending on the patient-oriented factors, growth rate, malignancy potential, and multicentricity. Tumors often remain stable for many years or grow very slowly, so observation may be reasonable in some. Classically, surgery remained the mainstay of treatment, and it is the only way to fully eradicate a tumor. However, over the years a more conservative approach based primarily on patient factors (age, comorbidities, cranial nerve deficits, growth rates) has been taken due to the potential for surgical morbidity in certain cases (jugular or vagal paragangliomas, bilateral carotid body tumors).

10. **What is the classic histology of a paraganglioma?**
There are three types of cells: capillaries, chief cells (Type I), and sustentacular cells (Type II). The pattern in which these cells are arranged is termed Zellballen. These tumors are highly vascular and are of neural crest in origin.

11. **Can malignant potential of a paraganglioma be determined on histologic analysis of the primary tumor?**
No. Paragangliomas have a low potential for malignancy and the only method to determine malignancy is the presence of tumor in the lymph nodes or distant metastases. Vagal paragangliomas have the highest malignant potential (16%) compared to carotid body (6%) and jugulotympanic (4%) tumors.

12. **Discuss the management of jugular paraganglioma.**
Jugular paragangliomas typically arise in the temporal bone and are usually associated with significant bone destruction. They typically involve structures of the jugular foramen (cranial nerves IX, X, and XI). Surgical resection involves radical skull base surgery and frequent compromise of these cranial nerves. Preoperative cranial nerve examination is critical because surgery can result in aspiration, dysphagia, and possible facial nerve injury; such risks make radiotherapy an attractive alternative. However, for younger patients and those whose cranial nerves have already been compromised by the tumor, compensation often will have happened preoperatively. These patients do much better with surgery than those whose cranial nerves are normal. With modern skull base techniques, total resection with excellent rehabilitation of the patient is possible; however, radiation should be strongly considered based on patient-oriented factors.

13. **What can happen if bilateral carotid body (or one vagal and one carotid body tumor on opposite sides) tumors are excised (Figure 17-2)?**
Bilateral denervation of the carotid bodies results in severe paroxysms of hyper- and hypotension and is termed baroreflex failure. These are managed in the perioperative period with sodium nitroprusside, clonidine, phenoxybesamine, and antianxiety medications (anxiety can exacerbate fluctuations). Compensation can occur but the rate and timing of this is variable. In these situations, unilateral radiation or observation should be considered for at least one of the tumors.

14. **What is the role of radiation therapy in the management of paragangliomas?**
Improved techniques and more experience with radiating paragangliomas have demonstrated a 90% control rate of benign tumors, defined as cessation of growth or regression. It is extremely rare for tumors to completely resolve. With newer techniques and doses of 45 gy for standard fractionation typically given, complications are rare. Nevertheless, most individuals still prefer surgical excision of lesions.

15. **A 12-year-old boy presents with a history of unilateral nasal obstruction and heavy episodes of epistaxis. Physical examination reveals a large, purplish mass filling the nasopharynx. Should you biopsy this mass?**
No. Your next step should be a contrast CT to evaluate for a likely juvenile nasopharyngeal angiofibroma, which occurs exclusively in males, often presenting with nasal congestion, unilateral

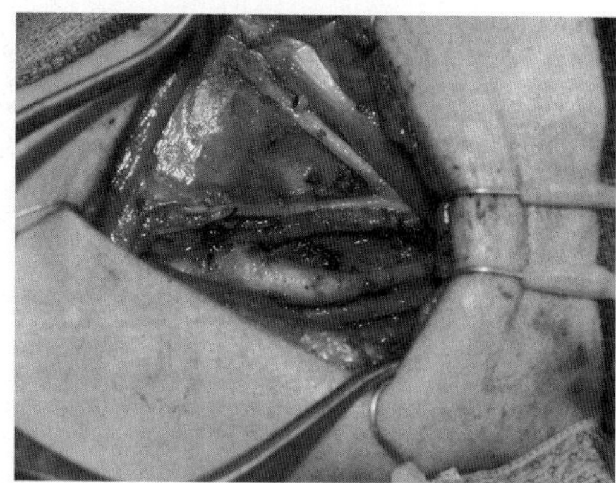

Figure 17-2. Post removal of carotid body tumor. Note splaying of carotids, ansa hypoglossal and hypoglossal nerve just underneath the digastrics.The vagus nerve is posterior to the internal carotid.

nasal obstruction, epistaxis, and sometimes anosmia. These tumors are hormonally responsive and usually occur during adolescence. Although they are histologically benign, they may be locally invasive and have the potential to extend intracranially. Treatment involves surgery, with or without preoperative embolization. Radiation therapy is reserved for unresectable cases. These vascular tumors are associated with a high recurrence rate if not excised fully, but eventually regress once the patient reaches adulthood.

16. **An infant develops a rapidly enlarging hemangioma on her cheek. What is the appropriate treatment?**
Counsel on the natural history of these lesions and try to avoid surgery. Hemangiomas are the most common head and neck tumors in children. They are more frequently found in females than males (3:1). The typical history is a period of rapid enlargement followed by gradual involution. Fifty percent have involuted by the age of 5 years, and 70% by age 7.

17. **A child with a large facial hemangioma develops a coagulopathy. What is this entity? How is it managed?**
This is a disseminated intravascular coagulation–like syndrome with platelet trapping in the tumor and is termed Kasabach-Merritt syndrome. It is treated by transfusion of clotting factors and platelets as necessary, in addition to addressing the responsible lesion.

18. **A child with a facial hemangioma presents with stridor. What is your presumed diagnosis and next steps?**
Subglottic or other airway hemangioma. Direct laryngoscopy and bronchoscopy is warranted with the possibility for a tracheostomy if the airway is severely compromised. Hemangiomas may occur in the airway as well as on the skin. About 50% of children with subglottic hemangiomas also have cutaneous lesions. Medical therapy may consist of steroids and/or beta-blockers.

19. **A young male presents with a port-wine stain of the right face. What is your diagnosis?**
Sturge-Weber syndrome. This is a congenital syndrome of unknown etiology charaterized by port-wine nevi in the distribution of the first and second trigeminal branches as well as angioma of the cerebral leptomeninges. It is important to have neurology and ophthalmology evaluations and imaging of the brain, as this syndrome can involve seizures, brain calcifications, and ophthalmologic findings. Port-wine stains can be managed with laser therapy.

20. **What types of lasers are used to treat cutaneous vascular lesions?**
The laser best suited for cutaneous vascular lesions is currently the pulsed-dye laser. It is excellent for port-wine stains. Argon and potassium titanyl phosphate (KTP) lasers have wavelengths specific for hemoglobin, which enhances their ability to treat such lesions. Yttrium-aluminum-garnet (YAG) lasers (and also argon lasers) have been associated with the involution and arrest of growth of hemangiomas, although a conservative approach is usually preferable for these lesions.

Bibliography

Barnes L, Everson J, Reichart P, et al, editors: *World Health Organization Classification of Tumours: Pathology and Genetics of Tumours of the Head and Neck*, Lyon, 2005, IARC.

Burnichon N, Rohmer V, Amar L, et al: The succinate dehydrogenase genetic testing in a large prospective series of patients with paragangliomas, *J Clin Endocrin Metab* 94(8):2817–2827, 2009.

Chino JP, Sampson JH, Tucci DL, et al: Paraganglioma of the head and neck: long-term local control with radiotherapy, *Am J Clin Oncol* 32(3):304–307, 2009.

Martin TPC, Irving RM, Maher ER: The genetics of paragangliomas: a review, *Clin Otolaryngol* 32:7–11, 2007.

Mendenhall WM, Hinerman RW, Amdur RJ, et al: Treatment of paragangliomas with radiation therapy, *Otolaryngol Clin North Am* 34(5):1007–1020, 2001.

Netterville JL, Reilly KM, Rovertson D, et al: Carotid body tumors. A review of 30 patients with 46 tumors, *Laryngoscope* 105:115–126, 1995.

Netterville JL, Jackson CG, Miller FR, et al: Vagal paraganglioma: a review of 46 patients treated during a 20-year period, *Arch Otolaryngol Head Neck* 124:1133–1140, 1998.

Old MO, Netterville JL: Paragangliomas of the Head and Neck. In Bernier J, editor: *Head and Neck Cancer: Multimodality Management*, New York, 2011, Springer.

Powell J: Update on hemangiomas and vascular malformations, *Curr Opin Pediatr* 11:457–463, 1999.

Sevilla MA, Hermsen MA, Weiss MM, et al: Chromosomal changes in sporadic and familial head and neck paragangliomas, *Oto Head and Neck Surg* 140:724–729, 2009.

CHAPTER 18

SINONASAL TUMORS

Jon Mallen-St. Clair, MD, PhD and Jeffrey D. Suh, MD

KEY POINTS

1. Sinonasal tumors are rare and account for 3% of upper aerodigestive tract cancers.
2. Squamous cell carcinoma is the most common sinonasal malignancy.
3. Occupational exposures are the main risk factors for sinonasal malignancies. Risk factors for adenocarcinoma are wood dust exposure and leather working.
4. Sinonasal malignancies typically present at a late stage because diagnosis is delayed due to nonspecific clinical presentation, which often mimics benign conditions.
5. Surgery followed by radiation therapy is the mainstay of treatment for sinonasal malignancies. For both benign and malignant tumors, obtaining clear margins is critical to reduce the risk of local recurrence. The best approach (endoscopic versus open) depends on a variety of factors including tumor location, type, size, and surgeon comfort.

Pearls

1. Ohngren's line is an imaginary line drawn from the medial canthus to the angle of the mandible. The significance of this marker is that maxillary sinus tumors that are located above this line on presentation are associated with a poor prognosis and tend to spread superiorly and posteriorly, and are more prone to perineural invasion and skull base invasion.
2. Adenocarcinoma is associated with exposure to wood and leather dust. Squamous cell carcinoma is associated with exposure to chromium, nickel, mustard gas, and aflatoxin.
3. The classic radiographic findings for JNA are expansion of the PPF on axial view (Holman-Miller sign), widening of the sphenopalatine and vidian foramina, and bony destruction of the pterygoid process.

QUESTIONS

GENERAL/EPIDEMIOLOGY

1. What are the important epidemiologic aspects of sinonasal cancer?
   Sinonasal cancer is rare, accounting for only 3% of upper aerodigestive tract malignancies. There are varied histologic subtypes of sinonasal cancer, which at least in part explains the diverse behavior and presentation of these tumors. Sinonasal malignancies tend to be diagnosed in the fifth and sixth decades of life. The disease is most common in Caucasians, and men are affected at twice the rate of women. A number of occupational exposures are associated with these cancers, including industrial fumes, nickel, leather, and wood dust (more details later in this chapter). There is also a higher rate of sinonasal cancers in cigarette smokers and heavy alcohol users. The 5-year survival for all nasal and paranasal malignancy is 40%, although this varies based on the histopathology of the tumor.

2. Is there a difference in rates of malignancy between tumors found in the nasal cavity and paranasal sinuses?
   Tumors of the nasal cavity are more likely to be benign than tumors found in the paranasal sinuses. Tumors of the nasal cavity are approximately equally split between benign and malignant neoplasms. The most common benign tumor of the nasal cavity is inverted papilloma (IP), the majority of which arise along the lateral nasal wall. The most common malignant tumor of the nasal cavity is squamous cell carcinoma (SCC). Tumors of the paranasal sinuses are more likely to be malignant than benign, with SCC also representing the majority of these tumors.

3. **What are the most common presenting symptoms of sinonasal tumors? What symptoms are particularly concerning for malignancy?**
Unilateral nasal symptoms are the most common presenting symptoms of sinonasal tumors, including obstruction, discharge, congestion, and epistaxis. These symptoms are often overlooked because they can mimic chronic sinusitis or allergies. However, persistent or worsening unilateral nasal symptoms or development of orbital symptoms, such as vision loss, tearing (epiphora), diplopia, or exophthalmos warrant a detailed examination.
Paresthesia or pain along V2 (maxillary nerve), cheek swelling, and numbness of the face or palate would be unusual for sinusitis, and are symptoms that are concerning for malignancy. Cavernous sinus invasion by sphenoid tumors can lead to dysfunction of cranial nerves III, IV, V1, V2, and VI. Thus, the most important indicators of malignancy include cranial neuropathies and orbital complications.

Benign Sinonasal Tumors

4. **What are the different types of nasal papillomas?**
Nasal papillomas are characterized based on their histologic appearance.
- **Exophytic (fungiform) papilloma:** The most common subtype, accounting for 50% of nasal papillomas. These papillomas typically arise from the nasal septum and resemble papillomas found in other locations on the body in terms of histopathology. In contrast to the other types of nasal papillomas, the exophytic papilloma does not have malignant potential.
- **Inverted (endophytic) papilloma:** These arise from Schneiderian mucosa, most commonly located on the lateral nasal wall or maxillary sinus, however any paranasal sinus can be involved (Figure 18-1). These papillomas account for 47% of nasal papillomas, and are associated with high rates of recurrence if not completely resected. Inverted papillomas are associated with an 8% to 10% chance of malignant transformation to squamous cell carcinoma. Inverted papilloma is associated with HPV infection.
- **Oncocytic (cylindrical) papilloma:** Oncocytic papillomas usually arise from the lateral nasal wall and are the rarest of the three papillomas types, accounting for only 3% of nasal papillomas. These tumors are thought to have rare malignant potential, usually reported to be between 4% and 17% (Figure 18-1).

5. **What is the standard treatment for inverting papilloma?**
Complete surgical resection with clear margins is the treatment of choice for all sinonasal papillomas. Identification and removal of the tumor site of attachment (origin) gives the highest chance of cure. Radiation with or without chemotherapy is reserved for tumors with malignant transformation.
Traditional open surgery utilizes a lateral rhinotomy or midface degloving to provide access into the nasal cavity for tumor removal. Endoscopic or endoscopic-assisted approaches have largely

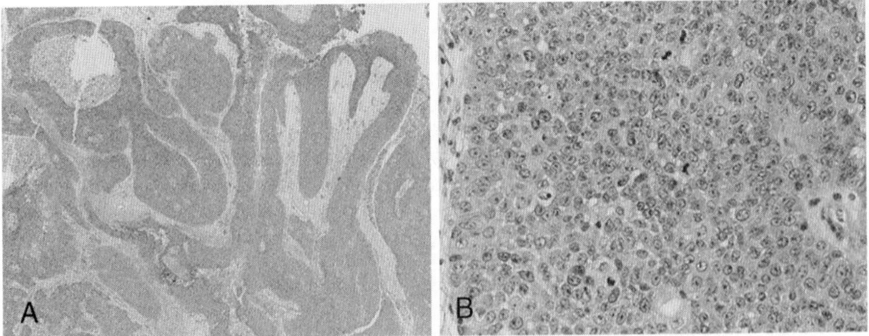

Figure 18-1. **A**. Hematoxylin and eosin (H&E) stain 4×: Epithelial proliferation demonstrating an endophytic growth pattern characteristic of Schneiderian papilloma, inverted type. **B**. H&E 40×: The epithelial proliferation exhibits a disorganized architecture and the epithelial cells demonstrate frank atypical features including marked pleomorphism, increased nuclear to cytoplasmic ratio, prominent nucleoli, increased mitotic activity, and atypical mitotic figures indicative of severe dysplasia.

replaced open approaches for most IPs, and have reduced the tumor recurrence rate from 20% to 12%.

6. **What is a juvenile nasopharyngeal angiofibroma (JNA)?**
JNA is a benign but aggressive vascular tumor. They are seen exclusively in adolescent males. These tumors are slow growing, locally invasive, and do not metastasize. However, these tumors can be quite large at presentation, and can involve the intracranial cavity, orbit, pterygopalatine fossa, or infratemporal fossa. JNAs often present with unilateral, recurrent epistaxis. CT/MRI adding angiography can be helpful to visualize the vascularity of the tumor and confirm the diagnosis. Biopsy carries a high risk of hemorrhage and is not recommended.

7. **What is Fisch's classification system for JNA?**
Fisch I: Limited to nasal cavity
Fisch II: Extends to pterygomaxillary fossa or sinuses with bony destruction
Fisch III: Invades orbit, infratemporal fossa, or parasellar area
Fisch IV: Extends to cavernous sinus, optic chiasm, or pituitary fossa

8. **What is the treatment of JNA?**
Tumors are typically embolized prior to surgical removal to reduce intraoperative bleeding. Endoscopic techniques are typically used for Fisch I and II, whereas more advanced lesions may require a craniofacial or endoscopic-assisted resection. Radiation therapy may be used for unresectable tumors.

9. **What other benign tumors are found in the nasal cavity? What are the unique features of these tumors?**
   - **Osteomas** are the most common benign sinonasal tumors and are slow growing tumors of mature bone. Multiple osteomas can be associated with Gardner's syndrome. These are most often incidentally discovered on CT scans of the sinus, although they can cause symptoms by obstruction of normal sinus drainage or through direct mass effect. The most common location of osteomas in the paranasal sinuses is in the frontal sinuses, with over 80% presenting in this location.
   - **Hemangiomas** are rare and most often present on the septum or inferior turbinate.
   - **Pyogenic granulomas** are benign, friable polypoid lesions often found on the septum that can be caused by irritation, physical trauma, and hormonal factors. There is a female predilection and increased incidence during the first trimester of pregnancy.
   - **Hemangiopericytomas** are vascular tumors derived from pericyte cells (Zimmerman pericytes) that surround capillaries and postcapillary venules; they account for about 1% of all vascular tumors. Hemangiopericytomas are usually well-differentiated tumors with a low potential for recurrence with complete resection. The treatment of choice is surgical resection.
   - **Salivary gland tumors** arising from minor salivary glands in the sinuses are rare. The most common is pleomorphic adenoma.
   - **Chordomas**—benign, locally aggressive tumors arising from notochord—are usually found in the clivus, and often present with cranial nerve palsy.

Malignant Sinonasal Tumors

10. **Describe the epidemiology of sinonasal malignancy.**
Sinonasal malignancies are rare and represent 3% of head and neck malignancies, typically presenting in the fifth to sixth decade of life.

11. **What are the most common pathological types of sinonasal malignancy?**
Squamous cell carcinoma and adenocarcinoma are the most common histologic subtypes. Others include esthesioneuroblastoma, adenoid cystic, mucoepidermoid, mucosal melanoma, sinonasal undifferentiated carcinoma, sarcoma, and lymphoma.

12. **What are the distinctive features of the following malignant sinonasal tumors?**
   - **Squamous Cell Carcinoma:** Most common sinonasal malignancy, representing approximately 80% of these tumors.
   - **Adenocarcinoma:** Presents most commonly in the ethmoid sinuses, with increased incidence in wood and leather workers.

- **Sinonasal Undifferentiated Carcinoma (SNUC):** These tumors typically arise near the olfactory groove. These tumors portend a very poor prognosis because they are rapidly progressive, cause extensive local tissue destruction, and commonly metastasize.
- **Esthesioneuroblastoma:** These tumors arise from olfactory epithelium and show bimodal distribution in teenage and the elderly populations. They frequently involve the skull base and orbit. There are two staging systems for these tumors: Kadish and Dulguerov-Calcaterra.
  - Kadish
    A: Tumors confined to the nasal cavity
    B: Tumor in nasal cavity with extension to the paranasal sinuses
    C: Tumor extending to the orbit, skull base, brain, or with distant metastasis
  - Dulguerov-Calcaterra
    T1: Tumor involving the nasal cavity or paranasal sinuses (excluding sphenoid or superior ethmoid air cells)
    T2: Tumor involving the nasal cavity or paranasal sinuses including the sphenoid, or with extension to the cribiform plate
    T3: Extension to orbit or anterior cranial fossa
    T4: Extension to the brain
- **Mucoepidermoid:** Salivary gland tumors that rarely present in the nasal cavity.
- **Adenoid Cystic Carcinoma:** Characterized by insidious growth, distant metastasis, and perineural invasion. Long-term surveillance is important due to a higher risk of late tumor recurrence.

13. Are there occupational exposures that increase the risk of certain sinonasal tumors?

Adenocarcinoma is associated with exposure to wood and leather dust, as well as organic solvents. Squamous cell carcinoma is associated with exposure to chromium, nickel, mustard gas, and aflatoxin. Exposure to tobacco smoke, alcohol, and salted or smoked foods increases the risk of all types of sinonasal malignancy.

14. What is the most common sinonasal tumor in the pediatric population?

Sinonasal tumors are rare in the pediatric population. Sarcomas represent approximately 75% of sinonasal malignancies in this demographic.

15. What is the prognosis of sinonasal malignancy?

Five-year survival has been reported ranging from 20% to 50%, but this can vary based on location and histology. Tumors in the maxillary sinus located superior to Ohngren's line (a line drawn from the medial canthus to the angle of the mandible) are associated with poorer survival (see Question 25 for more details).

16. What are the subsites of sinonasal malignancy?

- **Paranasal sinuses:** Each sinus can be involved with a tumor. The maxillary sinus is the most common subsite (70%), followed by the ethmoid sinus (20%), sphenoid sinus (3%), and frontal sinus (less than 1%).
- **Nasal cavity:** Second most common subsite overall, however, more associated with benign tumors.

Sinonasal malignancy may also spread into the anterior cranial fossa via frontal and ethmoid sinuses, the middle cranial fossa via the sphenoid sinus, pterygopalatine fossa, infratemporal fossa, and orbital cavity.

17. What are the treatment modalities for sinonasal malignancy, and what are limitations of adjuvant treatments?

Surgical resection is the mainstay of therapy for early stage disease. Radiation therapy is given postoperatively based on tumor histology (high-grade tumors), positive margins, or if there is evidence of perineural invasion. Chemotherapy is also considered in advanced disease or when there are metastases. Radiation therapy is limited by close proximity to the orbit and brain. Unresectable tumors can be managed with chemoradiation.

18. What are contraindications for surgery?

Sisson outlined four factors that make sinonasal tumors inoperable.

1. Significant involvement of brain parenchyma (superior extension)
2. Invasion of prevertebral fascia (posterior extension)

3. Invasion into the cavernous sinus (lateral extension)
4. Involvement of the bilateral orbits or optic chiasm

19. **What are the benefits of proton therapy in the treatment of sinonasal malignancy?**
Sinonasal tumors may be difficult to treat with conventional radiotherapy protocols given the proximity of multiple sensitive organs in the vicinity, including the optic nerves, orbit, and brain. Proton therapy has a potential advantage over conventional electron or photon based therapy, as it has a finite penetration range, and it is easier to contour a uniform dose to a target tumor volume. It has been applied in multiple situations in which tumors are in close proximity to vital organs. Several case series have indicated improved tumor control with decreased complication rates when comparing proton therapy to conventional radiotherapy in the treatment of esthesioblastoma and skull base chordomas. Despite these early successes, clinical trials directly comparing conventional treatment to proton therapy have not been performed to date.

20. **What is the nodal drainage pattern of sinonasal malignancy? How is the neck typically treated?**
The nodal drainage pathway depends on the subsite. The anterior nasal cavity follows an anterior drainage pathway to the perifacial and Level IA/IB nodes. In contrast, the middle and posterior nasal cavity as well as the paranasal sinuses drain into the retropharyngeal and upper jugulodigastric nodes with a relatively low rate of occult neck metastasis (<10%). When tumors invade the orbit, they may also drain to periparotid lymph nodes. In accordance with this information, the N0 neck is typically not treated with an elective neck dissection. Clinical nodal disease, on the other hand, is a grim prognostic indicator and should be addressed with a neck dissection and postoperative radiation.

Surgical and Anatomic Correlates

21. **What are symptoms associated with orbital invasion and what are the indications for orbital exenteration?**
Orbital invasion is associated with rapidly progressive symptoms, including diplopia, proptosis, worsening acuity, lid edema, chemosis, and epiphora. Orbital exenteration is indicated for tumors located within the orbital apex, or demonstrated erosion of the orbital bone with invasion through the periorbita (periosteum of the orbit) and into the extraocular muscles. However, the prognosis for these patients is poor even after orbital exenteration, so palliative measures can also be considered.

22. **What are the surgical approaches used to treat sinonasal malignancies?**
    - Endoscopic approach: Previously limited to benign tumors, now increasingly used in malignant disease and advanced disease. Advantages of the endoscopic approach include decreased morbidity, no external incisions, shorter hospitalizations, and improved visualization of structures and margins.
    - Transfacial open approaches
        - Lateral rhinotomy: The incision begins at medial brow and extends along the lateral nasal side wall, around the alar cartilage to the philtrum and through the lip. This is the classic approach to a medial maxillectomy providing access to the maxillary sinus, medial orbital wall, nasal cavity, ethmoid and sphenoid sinuses (Figure 18-2). Lip split is performed to improve exposure of the hard palate. Can be combined with a sublabial or transpalatal approach for tumors involving the floor of nose or inferior portion of maxilla.
        - Weber-Ferguson: Lateral rhinotomy approach in combination with a lip splitting incision that extends sublabially. A subciliary/transconjunctival incision is also made which provides improved access to the maxilla for a total maxillectomy.
        - Midface degloving: Involves gingivobuccal incisions as well as bilateral intercartilaginous incisions. The advantage of this approach is avoiding an external scar, and adequate visualization of the inferior and medial maxillary walls.
        - Facial translocation: Involves extensive facial flaps with sacrifice of the frontal branch of the facial nerve. The approach affords wide exposure of the skull base, infratemporal fossa, and pterygopalatine fossa.
        - Infratemporal approach: Access though a preauricular or postauricular incision that extends coronally. High risk of damage to the frontal branch of the facial nerve.

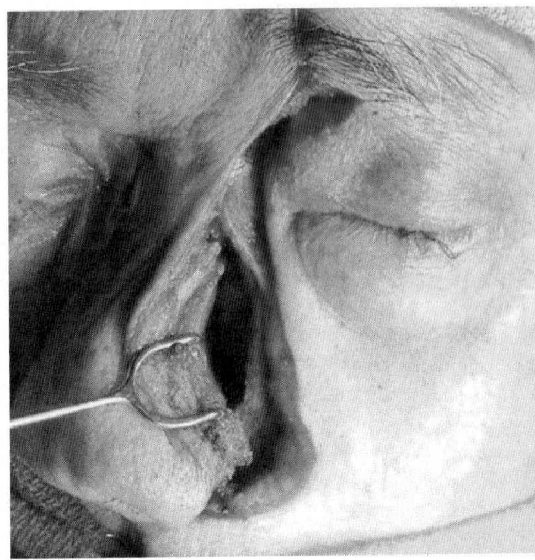

Figure 18-2. Lateral rhinotomy incision used to gain access to the nasal cavity and paranasal sinuses.

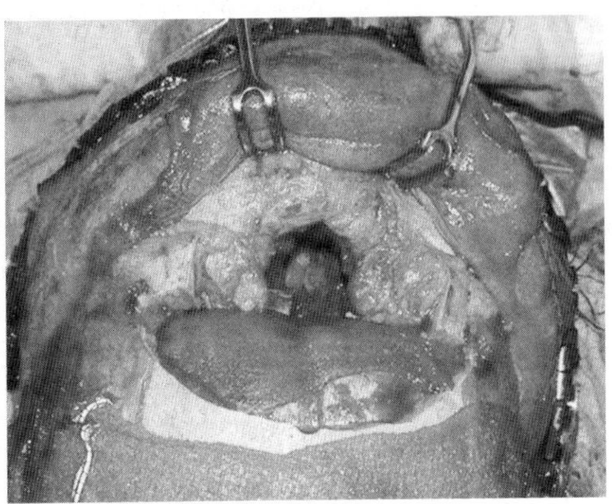

Figure 18-3. Coronal incision and frontal craniotomy used as part of the craniofacial resection. The cribiform plate has been removed and the frontal lobe is exposed.

- Craniofacial resection: Combined approach from above and below. Involves en bloc tumor removal of the anterior cranial base including the dura, cribiform plate, and ethmoid sinuses (Figure 18-3).

23. What are the anatomic boundaries of the different types of maxillectomies? What are the indications for these surgeries?
    - **Medial maxillectomy:** Removal of lateral nasal wall and medial maxilla, with or without sphenoethmoidectomy. May be performed endoscopically or open. This technique is commonly utilized for tumors in the maxillary sinus.
    - **Inferior maxillectomy:** Involves removal of the inferior portion of the maxillary sinus. Indicated for tumors involving the maxillary alveolar process or limited hard palate lesions.
    - **Total maxillectomy:** Includes en bloc removal of the entire maxilla. Indicated for tumors involving the maxillary antrum.
    - **Radical maxillectomy:** Total maxillectomy with orbital exenteration (Figure 18-4).

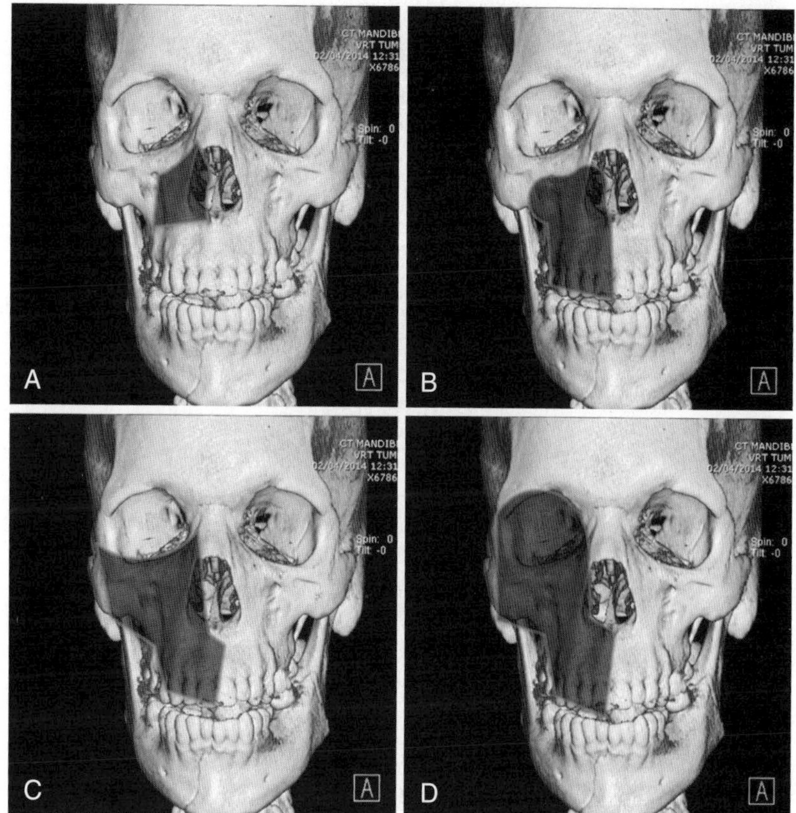

Figure 18-4. Illustration of maxillectomy defects. Medial maxillectomy **(A)**, inferior maxillectomy **(B)**, total maxillectomy **(C)**, radical maxillectomy **(D)**.

24. **What are the most common surgical complications?**
Complications can usually be predicted based on the origin of the tumor. The general complications that can occur after any sinonasal tumor removal are bleeding, postoperative infection, and smell loss. Intracranial complications can include meningitis, CSF leak, and tension pneumocephalus. Orbital complications include hematoma, emphysema, optic nerve injury, epiphora from injury to the nasolacrimal duct, and diplopia from injury to any of the extraocular muscles. Cranial nerve injuries can also occur to cranial nerves III, IV, V1, V2, and VI (see Question 3).

Anatomic Correlates

25. **What is Ohngren's line? What is the importance of this anatomic marker?**
Ohngren's line (Figure 18-5) is an imaginary line drawn from the medial canthus to the angle of the mandible. The significance of this marker is that maxillary sinus tumors that are located above this line on presentation are associated with a poor prognosis, tend to spread superiorly and posteriorly, and are more prone to perineural invasion and skull base invasion.

26. **What is the pterygopalatine fossa? What important structures are located in this space?**
The pterygopalatine fossa (PPF) is a pyramidal space located below the apex of the orbit.
    - Boundaries: Superiorly, apex of the orbit; anteriorly, the posterior wall of the maxillary sinus; posteriorly, the pterygoid plates. It opens laterally into the infratemporal fossa.

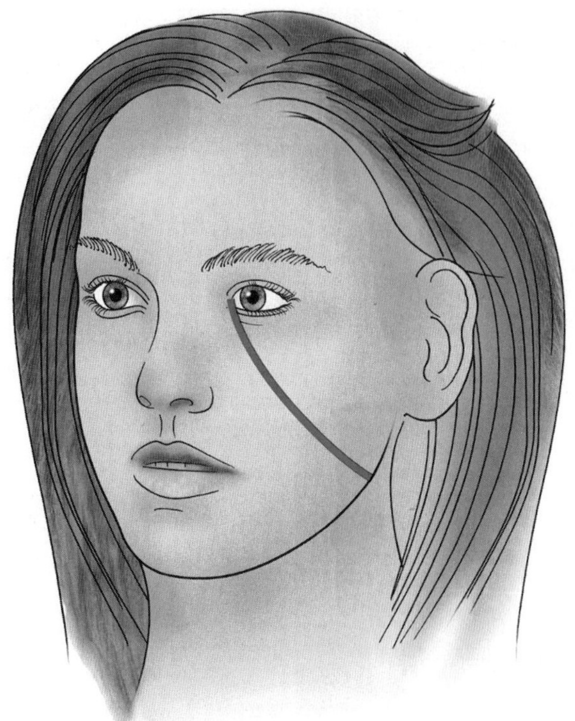

Figure 18-5. Ohngren's Line. Tumors located superior to this line are associated with a worse prognosis given the proximity to the skull base.

- Contents: Fat, foramen rotundum (contains the maxillary nerve, V2), vidian nerve, pterygopalatine ganglion and nerve, lesser and greater palatine nerves, and the internal maxillary artery.

27. What is the infratemporal fossa and what important structures are located in this space?
    - Boundaries: Anteriorly bounded by the maxilla, posteriorly bounded by the glenoid fossa and mandible. Medially bounded by the lateral pterygoid plates. Connects to the PPF via the pterygomaxillary fissure.
    - Contents: Pterygoid muscles and venous plexus, foramen ovale and V3, foramen spinosum, internal maxillary artery

28. What subsite of paranasal cancer is associated with more frequent injuries to cranial nerves?
    The sphenoid sinus, given its proximity to the cavernous sinus and optic nerve. Contents of the cavernous sinus include the internal carotid artery and CNs III, IV, V1, V2, and VI. The abducens nerve is located most medially in the cavernous sinus, and is usually affected first from sphenoid sinus tumors spreading to the cavernous sinus.

29. What is cavernous sinus syndrome?
    Cavernous sinus syndrome (CSS) is characterized by ophthalmoplegia caused by compression of CN III/IV and VI. It is also characterized by numbness in the distribution of V1 and V2, and potentially an ipsilateral Horner's syndrome. A complete lesion results in a fixed dilated pupil and hypesthesia of V1/V2. This can be caused by mass effect from a skull base tumor or secondary to thrombosis from a retrograde spreading infection.

BIBLIOGRAPHY

Batsakis JG: Pathology consultation: Nasal papillomas, *Ann Otol Rhinol Laryngol* 90(2):190–191, 1981.

Bhattacharyya N: Cancer of the nasal cavity: Survival and factors influencing prognosis, *Arch Otolaryngol Head Neck Surg* 128(9):1079–1083, 2002.

Busquets JM, Hwang PH: Endoscopic resection of sinonasal inverted papilloma: A meta-analysis, *Otolaryngol Head Neck Surg* 134(3):476–482, 2006.

Caplan LS, Hall I, Levine RS, et al: Preventable risk factors for nasal cancer, *Ann Epidemiol* 10(3):186–191, 2000.

Igaki H, Tokuuye K, Okumura T, et al: Clinical results of proton beam therapy for skull base chordoma, *Int J Radiat Oncol Biol Phys* 60(4):1120–1126, 2004.

Leong SC: A systematic review of surgical outcomes for advanced juvenile nasopharyngeal angiofibroma with intracranial involvement, *Laryngoscope* 123(5):1125–1131, 2013.

Nishimura H, Ogino T, Kawashima M, et al: Proton-beam therapy for olfactory neuroblastoma, *Int J Radiat Oncol Biol Phys* 68(3):758–762, 2007.

Reder LS, Kokot N: Management of the neck in sinonasal malignancy. In Chiu AG, Ramakrishnan VR, Suh JD, editors: *Sinonasal Tumors*, New Delhi, India, 2012, Jaypee Brothers Medical Publishers, pp 142–144.

Rokade A, Sama A: Update on management of frontal sinus osteomas, *Curr Opin Otolaryngol Head Neck Surg* 20(1): 40–44, 2012.

Suh JD, Ramakrishnan VR, Chi JJ, et al: Outcomes and complications of endoscopic approaches for malignancies of the paranasal sinuses and anterior skull base, *Ann Otol Rhinol Laryngol* 122(1):54–59, 2013.

Vorasubin N, Vira D, Suh JD, et al: Schneiderian papillomas: comparative review of exophytic, oncocytic, and inverted types, *Am J Rhinol Allergy* 27(4):287–292, 2013.

Weymuller EA, Davis GA: Malignancies of the paranasal sinus. In Flint P, Haughey B, Lund V, et al, editors: *Cummings Otolaryngology: Head and Neck Surgery*, ed 5, Philadelphia, PA, 2010, Mosby Elsevier, pp 1636–1642.

Zevallos JP, Jain KS, Roberts D, et al: Sinonasal malignancies in children: a 10-year, single-institutional review, *Laryngoscope* 121(9):2001–2003, 2011.

Zheng W, McLaughlin JK, Chow WH, et al: Risk factors for cancers of the nasal cavity and paranasal sinuses among white men in the United States, *Am J Epidemiol* 138(11):965–972, 1993.

CHAPTER 19

SKULL BASE SURGERY

William C. Yao, MD, Jeffrey D. Suh, MD and Vijay R. Ramakrishnan, MD

KEY POINTS

1. Proper selection of the surgical approach requires thorough evaluation to meet the surgical goals, while attempting to minimize injury to adjacent neurovascular structures.
2. A multidisciplinary team is helpful in the management of skull base tumors, including an otolaryngologist, neurosurgeon, neuroradiologist, neuropathologist, radiation oncologist, and medical oncologist.
3. The nasoseptal flap is a popular method of reconstruction that can provide reliable closure for large defects.
4. If there is a CSF leak following a repair, consider conservative management with a lumbar drain if the leak is small and the repair is sound. In addition, recognize the potential need for early intervention for continued leaks due to risk of postoperative meningitis.
5. Clinically significant pneumocephalus should be addressed with conservative measures and evacuation to prevent major neurologic compromise.
6. Endoscopic skull base surgery has a learning curve for both the otolaryngologist and neurosurgeon. It is best to begin with simple cases, or those in which the endoscope is used as an adjunct to an open approach.

Pearls

1. A Weber-Ferguson incision consists of a lip splitting extension of a lateral rhinotomy and a subciliary incision extended to the lateral canthus.
2. CN VI is the most medial nerve in the cavernous sinus, and is the most commonly injured.
3. CN III, IV, V1, V2, VI, internal carotid artery and venous channels are present in the cavernous sinus.
4. The vidian nerve consists of parasympathetic and sympathetic fibers from the greater petrosal nerve and deep petrosal nerve. The canal lies medial to the foramen rotundum. The maxillary branch of the trigeminal nerve runs through the foramen rotundum.
5. CSF production is approximately 20 ml/hr.
6. The crista ethmoidalis is a reliable landmark for endoscopically locating the sphenopalatine artery.

QUESTIONS

BASICS

1. What are the compartments of the skull base?
The skull base is separated into three compartments, or fossae: anterior, middle, and posterior. The anterior compartment extends from the frontal sinus to the anterior clinoid process and planum sphenoidale (sphenoid roof). The middle cranial fossa extends from the greater wing of the sphenoid to the clivus, including the sella turcica. The posterior fossa consists of the occiput and begins from the basal aspect of the occipital bone (Figure 19-1).

2. What are the most common pathologies in which skull base surgery (SBS) is performed?
Benign sinonasal pathologies include inverted papilloma, juvenile nasal angiofibroma, fibrous dysplasia, and osteoma. Common intracranial skull base tumors include pituitary tumor,

craniopharyngioma, and meningioma. Sinonasal malignancies include olfactory neuroblastoma (esthesioneuroblastoma), sinonasal undifferentiated carcinoma (SNUC), squamous cell carcinoma, adenocarcinoma, and melanoma.

3. **How can the skull base be accessed?**
The skull base can be accessed using open, endoscopic, microscopic, or combined open-endoscopic approaches. The goal of any approach is to provide the best visualization and exposure to surrounding neurovascular structures and the tumors.

4. **What types of approaches are used to access the skull base?**

Table 19-1. Open Approaches to the Skull Base

Anterior Skull Base	Middle Skull Base
Subfrontal approach Transfrontal sinus—osteoplastic flap Frontotemporal—orbitozygomatic Transmaxillary sinus Transfacial LeFort osteotomy Facial translocation Lateral infratemporal fossa approach Fisch type approaches Type A: Anterior transposition of CN VII Type B: Sigmoid to petrous tip Type C: Extended approach to include cavernous sinus	In addition to the anterior skull base approaches: Transoral Trans-septal Palatal split Mandibular split Middle cranial fossa subtemporal **Posterior Skull Base** Transoral approach Palatal split Translabyrinthine approach Retrosigmoid Suboccipital

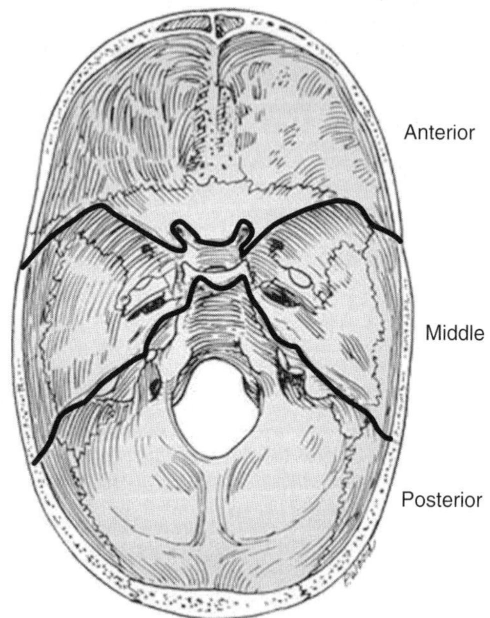

Figure 19-1. An axial section of the skull base. Dark lines separate the three skull base compartments: anterior, middle and posterior. *(Image edited from Flint PW: Cummings Otolaryngology: Head and Neck Surgery, 2010, Philadelphia. Mosby Elsevier.)*

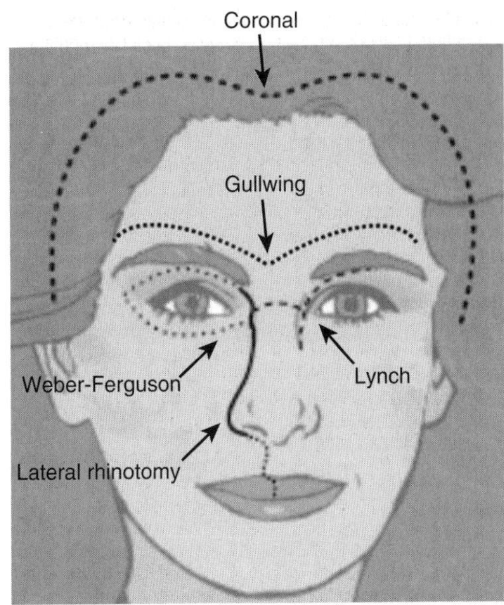

Figure 19-2. Image depicting various external incisions that will allow access to the skull base.

5. **What incisions may be used to access the anterior skull base?**
   Open approaches to the anterior fossa may use the coronal, lid crease, brow, gullwing, Lynch (medial orbital), lateral rhinotomy, Weber-Ferguson, or midface degloving incisions (Figure 19-2).

6. **What tests and examinations are helpful prior to resecting a skull base malignancy?**
   For surgical planning, basic laboratory studies including CBC, BMP, and coagulation studies should be obtained as well as imaging of the primary site (fine cut CT and MRI). Other labs may be obtained depending on tumor type (e.g., for pituitary tumor: ACTH, PRL, LH/FSH, GH, TRH) and location (arteriography). If indicated, a thorough evaluation for distant metastases should be performed.

7. **What imaging studies should be obtained?**
   Fine cut CT scans (≈1mm section) should be obtained for evaluation of bony anatomy of the skull base; the use of contrast may be helpful in defining the lesion and nearby vasculature. MRI with and without contrast is useful to delineate the lesion from surrounding structures, help create a radiologic differential diagnosis, and evaluate for soft tissue invasion and perineural spread. CT, MR, or fused CT-MR images are helpful for intraoperative image guidance. PET scans can be used to rule out distant metastases.

8. **What is endoscopic skull base surgery (ESBS)?**
   Endoscopic skull base surgery is an extension of endoscopic sinus surgery. The endoscope is used to improve visualization, illumination, and may obviate the need for facial incisions such as a lateral rhinotomy. Recent reports have demonstrated that endoscopic resections of skull base tumors may yield similar oncologic results to traditional open approaches in appropriately selected cases.

9. **When is an endoscopic skull base approach appropriate?**
   Potential indications for endoscopic transnasal skull base surgery are increasing. The areas accessible via endoscopic endonasal approaches include the entirety of the anterior skull base, much of the middle cranial fossa, and portions of the posterior fossa. ESBS performed through small incisions is leading to minimally invasive lateral approaches and neurosurgical approaches as well.

10. **What are the advantages of an endoscopic skull base approach?**
    Compared to open surgery, the endoscopic approach allows for more direct visualization with less manipulation of the surrounding soft tissues. This may allow for a more precise resection of the

lesion due to better visualization, and minimal manipulation of nearby neurovascular structures. Compared to the traditional microscopic view, endoscopes give a dynamic operative view with the added ability to see around corners using angled endoscopes. ESBS can avoid scars, decrease hospital stays, and cause less postoperative pain.

11. **What are the limitations of endoscopic skull base surgery?**
Not all areas of the skull base can be visualized and safely instrumented via a transnasal endoscopic route. Malignancy involving the orbit and facial skin are considered contraindications to endoscopic skull base surgery. As a general rule, the endoscopic approach should not compromise the ability to achieve the appropriate oncologic resection, and crossing major neurovascular structures is not suggested.

12. **In what situations should adjuvant radiotherapy and/or chemotherapy be considered?**
The primary modality of treatment for the majority of skull base malignancy is surgical resection. There are some exceptions to the rule (e.g., lymphoma and plasmacytoma). Adjuvant radiotherapy is considered when there is a high propensity of tumor recurrence, which includes presence of perineural invasion, high-grade tumor, and close or positive margins. Chemotherapy can be considered for induction therapy and for metastatic disease, or may be used as adjuvant therapy for chemosensitive histologies. Radiation therapy may have a role in the management of certain benign skull base pathologies, such as meningioma, schwannoma, vascular tumors, and chordoma.

13. **What is stereotactic radiosurgery?**
Stereotactic radiosurgery utilizes ionizing radiation to treat well-defined targets with high accuracy and precision. This can be applied to areas with adjacent critical neurovascular structures such as in the skull base. It is most often used for pituitary adenoma, schwannoma, meningioma, AV malformations, and metastases.

14. **Where is CSF produced and absorbed?**
CSF is produced by the choroid plexus in the lateral ventricles, and is reabsorbed into the dural venous sinuses through the arachnoid villi. Total CSF volume is approximately 150 ml. An adult produces approximately 20 ml/hr and 550 ml/day. Normal adult intracranial pressure ranges from 10 to 20 cm H_20.

15. **What are the three layers of the meninges?**
The dura mater, arachnoid, and pia mater. The dura mater is separated into the superficial layer and the meningeal layers.

16. **Describe the segments of the carotid artery.**
The internal carotid artery can be separated into seven anatomic segments: C1 cervical, C2 petrous, C3 lacerum, C4 cavernous, C5 clinoid, C6 ophthalmic, and C7 communicating. A mnemonic for remembering branches in the skull is **P**lease **L**et **C**hildren **C**onsume **O**ur **C**andy (Figure 19-3).

APPROACH

17. **How are approaches classified in endoscopic transnasal skull base surgery?**
Approaches to the ventral skull base are classified according to their location in the sagittal or coronal plane (Table 19-2 and Figures 19-4 and 19-5).

18. **What is the crista ethmoidalis?**
The crista ethmoidalis is a bony landmark located just anterior to the sphenopalatine foramen.

19. **How can the lateral aspect of the sphenoid sinus be accessed?**
The lateral recess of a pneumatized sphenoid sinus can be accessed by the use of angled instruments following a wide sphenoidotomy, or through the transpterygoid approach through the posterior wall of the maxillary sinus and pterygopalatine fossa.

20. **What is the vidian canal?**
The vidian canal runs through the inferolateral aspect of the sphenoid sinus, transmitting the vidian nerve and an arterial branch from the internal carotid artery. It can be used as a surgical landmark for finding the internal carotid artery (Figure 19-6).

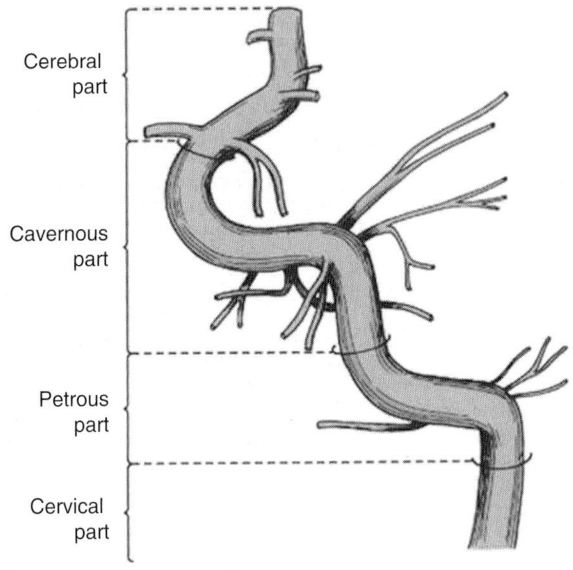

Figure 19-3. Image of the internal carotid artery traversing through the skull base. *(Image from Myers, EN: Operative Otolaryngology: Head and Neck Surgery, 2 ed, Philadelphia, 2008, Elsevier.)*

Table 19-2. Endonasal Approaches to the Ventral Skull Base

Sagittal Plane
Transfrontal
Transcribriform
Transplanum/tuberculum
Transsellar
Transclival
Transodontoid

Coronal
Anterior Coronal Plane
- Supraorbital
- Transorbital

Middle Coronal Plane
- Medial petrous apex
- Petroclival approach
- Quadrangular space
- Cavernous sinus
- Transpterygoid/Infratemporal approach

Posterior Coronal Plane
- Infrapetrous
- Transcondylar
- Transhypoglossal
- Parapharyngeal space
    - Medial (Jugular foramen)
    - Lateral

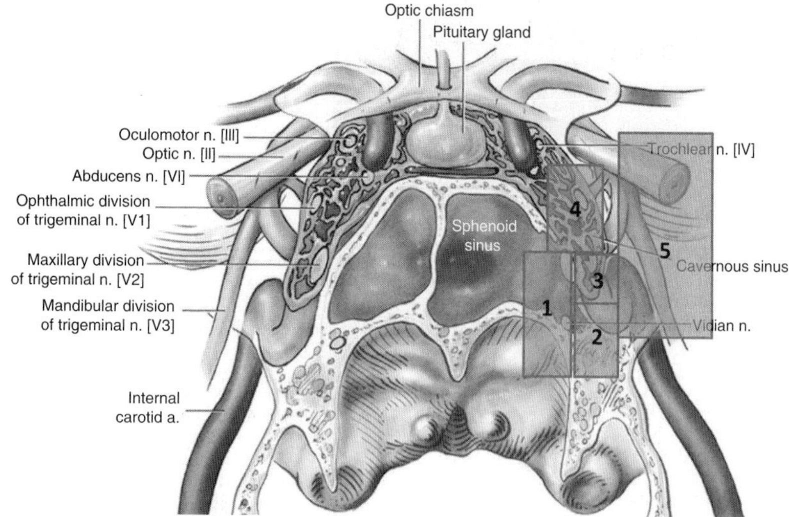

Figure 19-4. Schematic description of the endonasal surgical approaches in the coronal plane. [1] Medial petrous apex, [2] Petroclival, [3] Quadrangular space, [4] Superior cavernous sinus, [5] Transpterygoid/Infratemporal approach. *(Image edited from Palmer JN: Atlas of Endoscopic Sinus and Skull Base Surgery. 2013, Philadelphia, Saunders Elsevier.)*

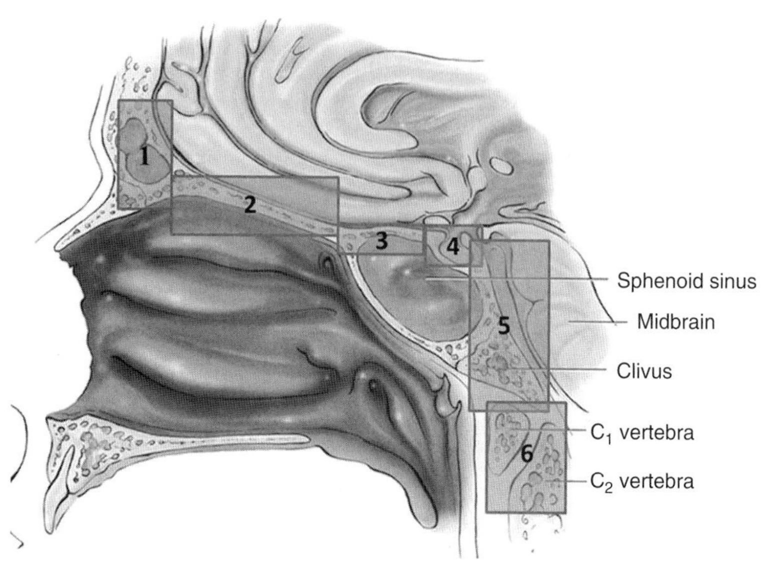

Figure 19-5. Schematic description of the endonasal surgical approaches in the sagittal plane. [1] Transfrontal, [2] transcribiform, [3] transplanum, [4] transsphenoid, [5] transclival, [6] transodontoid. *(Image edited from Palmer JN. Atlas of Endoscopic Sinus and Skull Base Surgery. 2013, Philadelphia, Saunders Elsevier.)*

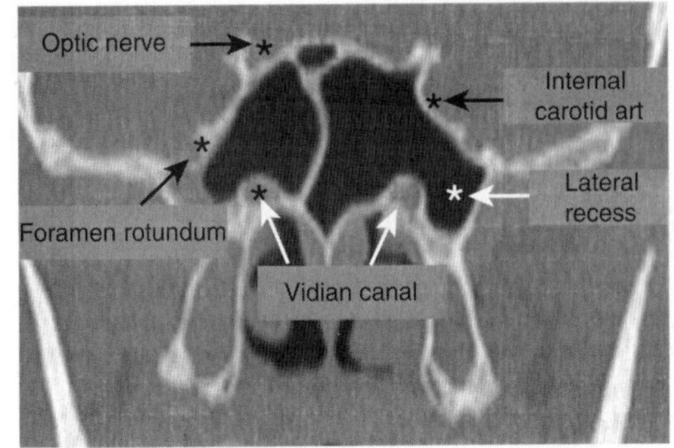

Figure 19-6. Coronal section of the sphenoid bone. The white arrow represents the vidian canal. The black stars are labeled accordingly. The white * depicts the lateral recess of the sphenoid bone.

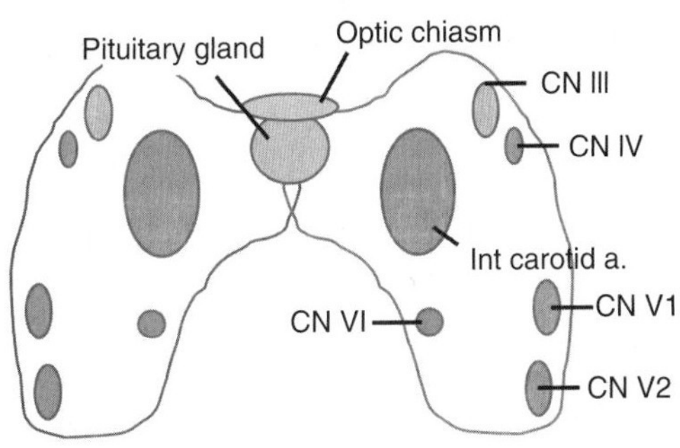

Figure 19-7. Coronal diagram of the cavernous sinus.

21. **What structures are present in the cavernous sinus?**
    Within the cavernous sinus lie cranial nerves III, IV, and VI as well as the ophthalmic/maxillary branch of the trigeminal nerve (CN V1 + V2) and the carotid artery. CN VI is the most medial and therefore the most commonly injured (Figure 19-7).

Reconstruction

22. **How is a skull base defect reconstructed?**
    The skull base defect can be repaired in layers using autologous or synthetic materials. The dural layer can be reconstructed using temporalis fascia or fascia lata, or allogeneic materials. The bony defect may be reconstructed with cartilage or bone from the septum, turbinate, or split calvarial grafts, if desired. The mucosal surface may be repaired with free mucosal grafts, fascia, autologous fat, or pedicled rotational flaps (i.e., nasoseptal flap). If the need arises, external approaches utilizing the pericranium may also be considered. Packing material, tissue glues or direct suture techniques may be used to fix graft materials in place.

23. **Describe the nasoseptal flap.**
    The nasoseptal flap is the workhorse pedicled mucosal flap based off of the posterior septal branch of the sphenopalatine artery. Its size can be customized, and its wide arc of rotation makes it versatile.

24. **What is a free mucosal transfer?**
    A free mucosal transfer utilizes a mucosal graft harvested from another area in the nasal cavity, similar to a skin graft. Common sites of graft harvest include the inferior or middle turbinates, septum, or nasal floor.

25. **What free flaps are preferred for reconstruction of larger defects?**
    Common flap options include anterolateral thigh, radial forearm, latissimus dorsi, and rectus myocutaneous flaps. If an osseocutaneous flap is required, options include a free fibula flap and scapular flap.

Complications

26. **What are the complications of skull base surgery?**
Common complications from open skull base surgery include anosmia and associated taste dysfunction, poor aesthetic results, and neurologic complications such as cranial nerve injury or those secondary to brain retraction. Major skull base surgery complications include CSF rhinorrhea, meningitis, intracranial hemorrhage, orbital complications such as diplopia or vision loss, vascular injury, stroke, and death.
Complications from endoscopic approaches are similar to those from the open approach, however there is improved cosmesis and less brain retraction. The most common complications are hyposmia and associated taste disturbance, epistaxis, and prolonged local wound healing.

27. **What are the rates of complications of open and endoscopic skull base surgery?**
There is a 5% to 20% rate of surgical complications and 8% to 40% rate of medical complications. Several studies now demonstrate that both medical and surgical complications are more frequent and severe with open approaches compared to endoscopic approaches.

28. **What are signs of failure in reconstruction?**
Symptoms include clear rhinorrhea and constant postnasal drip. Other signs may include meningitis, severe headaches, seizures, and worsening pneumocephalus.

29. **If a CSF leak is identified, what nonoperative management options exist?**
If the defect is small and there is confidence in the original reconstruction, conservative management with bed rest, stool softeners, and lumbar drainage can be considered. Antibiotics are sometimes administered for meningitis prophylaxis. Medications may be prescribed to decrease CSF production (acetazolamide, furosemide, digoxin) or decrease ICP (corticosteroids).

30. **What causes postoperative pneumocephalus?**
Nearly all patients undergoing skull base surgery will have some degree of postoperative pneumocephalus on initial imaging. Significant pneumocephalus is reported in 5% to 10% of patients when a ball valve action occurs along the reconstruction, either from increased negative pressure from the intracranial side (excessive CSF drainage from lumbar drain) or increased extracranial pressure (coughing, nose-blowing, CPAP use).

31. **What are the consequences of a pneumocephalus?**
Patients with pneumocephalus may present with headaches, dizziness, nausea and vomiting, seizures, depressed neurologic status, or neurologic symptoms from mass effects on nearby structures.

32. **What is the treatment of symptomatic pneumocephalus?**
Nasal packing should be removed and the lumbar drain should be clamped. If severe, emergent drainage with needle aspiration should be performed if the area is safely accessible. The reconstruction may need to undergo revision, or in refractory cases airway diversion (tracheotomy) can be considered.

Controversies

33. **Oncologic outcomes for endoscopic versus open surgery for malignancies.**
Endoscopic management of skull base tumors appears to have similar outcomes to open approaches in properly selected cases. True en bloc resection does not appear necessary to achieve good oncologic outcomes. The surgeon must evaluate whether complete tumor resection with negative margins can be accomplished through an endoscopic approach.

34. **What is the role of lumbar drains?**
Lumbar drains can decrease intracranial pressure and thereby reduce the pressure applied to the skull base reconstruction; however, they may be associated with significant morbidity and potential for complications. The use of lumbar drain primarily following a repair varies from different surgeons, and should not be universally utilized in a routine fashion. When used, the duration of drainage is also up to surgeon discretion.

35. **Best type of reconstruction.**
Most reconstructive methods appear to have similar efficacy, and therefore there is no universal "best type of reconstruction." In general, small defects (<1cm) can be closed in a single layer, and

multilayer repair is preferred for larger defects. Some surgeons prefer to use a rigid layer of bone or cartilage to reconstruct the skull base, although this is not required. Vascularized mucosal tissue (e.g., nasoseptal flap) has been demonstrated to improve repair results for larger defects; however, single layer nonvascularized tissue can also be successful in this setting.

36. **Use of perioperative antibiotics.**
    Postoperative antibiotics are an important consideration for skull base surgery because of the temporary connection between the intracranial space and external world. Rates of postoperative wound infection following ESBS are approximately 2%, and appear to be higher in open skull base surgery. Broad coverage with IV cephalosporins with or without vancomycin (or oral amoxicillin/clavulanate) is most often recommended. Studies are lacking to support the use of prolonged postoperative antibiotics, although most surgeons prefer to use systemic or topical antibiotics in some form after surgery.

Bibliography

Bleier BS: Comprehensive techniques in CSF leak repair and skull base reconstruction, *Adv Oto Rhino Laryngol* 74: 1–11, 2013.

Bolger WE, Borgie RC, Melder P: The role of the crista ethmoidalis in endoscopic sphenopalatine artery ligation, *Am J Rhinol* 13(2):81–86, 1999.

Kennedy DW, Hwang PH: *Rhinology: Disease of the Nose, Sinuses and Skull Base*, New York, 2012, Thieme.

Lund VJ, Stammberger H, Nicolai P, et al: European position paper on endoscopic management of tumours of the nose, paranasal sinuses and skull base, *Rhinol Suppl* 1(22):1–143, 2010.

Myers EN: *Operative Otolaryngology: Head and Neck Surgery*, ed 2, Philadelphia, 2008, Elsevier.

Teknos TN, Smith JC, Day TA, et al: Microvascular free tissue transfer in reconstructing skull base defects: lessons learned, *Laryngoscope* 112(10):1871–1876, 2002.

Timperley DG, Banks C, Robinson D, et al: Lateral frontal sinus access in endoscopic skull base surgery, *Int Forum All Rhinol* 1(4):290–295, 2011.

Schirmer CM, Heilman CB, Bhardwaj A, et al: Pneumocephalus: case illustrations and review, *Neurocrit Care* 13(1): 152–158, 2010.

Simmen DB, Raghavan U, Briner HR, et al: The anatomy of the sphenopalatine artery for the endoscopic sinus surgeon, *Am J Rhinol* 20(5):502–505, 2006.

Suh JD, Ramakrishnan VR, Chi JJ, et al: Outcomes and complications of endoscopic approaches for malignancies of the paranasal sinuses and anterior skull base, *Ann Otol Rhinol Laryngol* 122(1):54–59, 2013.

Wormald PJ: *Endoscopic Sinus Surgery: Anatomy, Three-Dimensional Reconstruction, and Surgical Technique*, ed 3, New York, 2013, Thieme.

CHAPTER 20

HEMATOLOGIC MALIGNANCY

Vignesh Narayanan, MD and Daniel A. Pollyea, MD, MS

KEY POINTS

1. Painless lymph node enlargement is the most common head and neck manifestation of lymphoma.
2. Hematologic malignancies can involve extranodal tissues of the paranasal sinuses, salivary glands, and thyroid.
3. "B" symptoms include fevers, weight loss, and night sweats. They are associated with poor prognosis.
4. Antibiotics are not useful in the majority of patients with painless lymphadenopathy.
5. Excisional lymph node biopsy is the preferred means of obtaining tissue diagnosis in suspected cases of lymphoma, although flow cytometry from FNA specimens may be diagnostic in some cases.
6. Severe oral mucositis is a dreaded complication of some intensive chemotherapy regimens and hematopoietic stem cell transplantation.
7. Ototoxicity from chemotherapeutic agents may be irreversible.
8. Anosmia and dysguesia due to chemotherapy can contribute to cancer-related cachexia.

Pearls

1. Lymphomatous nodes are "rubbery" in consistency.
2. Mediastinal adenopathy can cause hoarseness due to recurrent laryngeal nerve compression.
3. Sore throat can be the earliest symptom of severe neutropenia.
4. Use of ice chips in the mouth during chemotherapy can prevent mucositis by causing vasoconstriction, and rinsing the mouth with buffered saline can treat mucositis.

QUESTIONS

Classification, History, and Exam

1. **What are the broad classes of hematologic malignancies?**
   Hematologic malignancies encompass leukemias, lymphomas, and multiple myeloma. The leukemias are either acute or chronic and classified based on myeloid or lymphoid lineage. The lymphomas are further categorized as B-cell (Hodgkin's and non-Hodgkin's) or T-cell neoplasms.

2. **What are the head and neck manifestations of hematologic malignancies?**
   This can be broadly divided into nodal and extranodal manifestations.
   - **Nodal:** Cervical lymphadenopathy is one of the commonest presentations of lymphomas and is also seen in chronic lymphocytic leukemia (CLL). Involvement of the Waldeyer's ring is also frequently encountered.
   - **Extranodal:** Involvement of the lymphoid tissues in the salivary glands, thyroid, and paranasal sinuses may present as masses in these regions. Endemic Burkitt's lymphoma has a distinct propensity to present as masses of the facial bones. Extramedullary plasmacytomas can originate in the sinonasal tissues. Mediastinal lymphadenopathy could cause compression of the superior vena cava and resultant facial plethora. Other presentations are summarized in Table 20-1.

3. **In a patient with cervical lymphadenopathy, what features should alert the clinician to the possibility of lymphoma?**
   (1) Unexplained fevers with temperature above 38° C during the previous month, (2) unintentional weight loss of at least 10% of body weight during the previous six months, and (3) drenching night

Table 20-1. ENT Manifestations of Hematologic Malignancies

I. Nodal	Lymphadenopathy Involvement of Waldeyer's ring
II. Extranodal	Nasal obstruction Paranasal sinus involvement Facial bone erosion Thyroid infiltration Salivary gland involvement
III. Vascular	Superior vena cava (SVC) syndrome
IV. Neurologic	Cranial nerve palsy (if CNS involvement) Mental nerve involvement Recurrent laryngeal nerve palsy
VI. Cytopenias	Anemia: mucosal pallor Thrombocytopenia: epistaxis, mucosal petechiae, purpura Neutropenia: sore throat

sweats during the previous month are the classically designated "B" symptoms and portend a poor prognosis. Although nonspecific, approximately 25% of patients with Hodgkin's lymphoma and up to 40% of patients with non-Hodgkin's lymphoma present with "B" symptoms. Additional suggestive features include fatigue, and for Hodgkin's, pruritus and pain after alcohol consumption.

4. **What are the physical exam characteristics of lymphadenopathy in lymphomas?**
On palpation, lymphomatous nodes have a typical "rubbery" firm consistency, as compared to the stony hard lymphadenopathy in metastatic solid tumors. Lymphoma involved nodes are nontender, and could be matted and fixed to underlying structures.

5. **What is lethal midline granuloma?**
This term is used to describe an aggressive form of extranodal natural-killer/T-cell lymphoma mediated by Epstein-Barr virus infection. It is common in East Asia and Latin America. Patients present with destructive masses involving the nasal cavity, sinuses, or palate, sometimes with extension into the upper airway and Waldeyer's ring. Biopsy of these lesions usually reveals extensive necrosis with lymphomatous infiltration and vascular invasion. Localized disease is responsive to concurrent chemo-radiotherapy, but advanced stage disease is rapidly fatal despite treatment.

Diagnosis

6. **Should patients with cervical lymphadenopathy be given a trial of empiric antibiotics?**
Empiric antibiotics are generally not useful due to the multitude of possible etiologies and could result in delay of diagnosis. There is insufficient data to support this practice. Biopsy of suspicious lymph nodes should be performed without delay.

7. **What are the indications for cervical lymph node biopsy in suspected lymphomas?**
Typically, lymph nodes that are larger than 2 cm in diameter or 2.25 cm^2 (with bi-perpendicular diameter of 1.5×1.5 cm) are associated with a higher diagnostic yield. Persistent lymphadenopathy for more than 4 to 6 weeks and progressive increase in size are other indications.

8. **What is the importance of performing an excisional lymph node biopsy in suspected lymphomas?**
Excisional biopsy is preferred because it ensures adequate quantity of tissue to perform various histologic, immunologic, and molecular biological tests. It also permits careful examination of the

entire lymph node architecture including normal and abnormal zones and capsular integrity. This is crucial for precise classification of the subtype of lymphoma.

9. **What is the role of core biopsy and fine needle aspiration of suspicious lymph nodes?**
   In situations where excisional lymph node biopsy is fraught with risks due to unfavorable location, or there is a suspicion of squamous cell carcinoma, fine needle aspiration can be utilized as a first step in establishing a diagnosis; however, if lymphoma cells are present, an excisional biopsy may still be indicated.

10. **What blood tests are indicated in patients with suspected hematologic malignancies?**
    A complete blood count with differential counts, peripheral blood smear evaluation, erythrocyte sedimentation rate, coagulation profile (PT/INR and PTT), comprehensive metabolic panel, and serum lactate dehydrogenase (LDH) levels are useful basic tests in patients with suspected hematologic malignancies. Evaluation of HIV status, viral hepatitis panel, and uric acid levels might also be warranted.

Complications of Treatment

11. **Name some of the early ENT indicators of complications from treatment of hematologic malignancies.**
    Sore throat is one of the earliest manifestations of agranulocytosis. Mucosal pallor results from severe anemia due to myelosuppression. Epistaxis and palatal petechiae might indicate thrombocytopenia due to chemotherapy.

12. **What toxicities pertaining to the head and neck result from the treatment of hematologic malignancies?**
    Ototoxicity, radiation induced xerostomia, hypothyroidism, fibrosis of neck muscles, carotid injury, and second malignancies are some complications to be aware of. Chronic graft versus host disease after hematopoietic stem cell transplant can cause severe xerostomia as well.

13. **Can treatment of hematologic malignancies cause ototoxicity?**
    Yes. Cisplatin, vinblastine, nitrogen mustard, arsenic trioxide, and bleomycin have been implicated in the development of hearing loss. It is usually dose dependent and symptoms vary from mild tinnitus to high-frequency sensorineural hearing loss and permanent vestibulo-cochlear damage.

14. **Which agents used in the treatment of hematologic malignancies cause impaired sense of smell?**
    Anosmia and hyposmia have been described in patients treated with cytosine arabinoside and methotrexate, which cause mucosal cell death and impaired mucosal cell regrowth respectively. Bleomycin and cisplatin can also cause significant dysguesia and even aguesia.

15. **What is mucositis and how is it graded?**
    Mucositis is a term used to describe inflammation and loss of mucosal integrity of the gastrointestinal tract. Mucositis is a common complication in patients undergoing hematologic stem cell transplant, especially with conditioning regimens that use high-dose melphalan and radiation. The mouth and oropharynx are frequently involved, and clinical manifestations range from mild pain that does not limit oral intake to severe ulcerations that could result in profound weight loss and even death (Table 20-2).

16. **What is the pathogenesis of mucositis?**
    Chemotherapy and radiation result in DNA damage mediated by reactive oxygen species. This results in the release of proinflammatory cytokines that cause tissue damage and ulceration. Secondary colonization by bacteria, fungi or viruses results in severe manifestations that can be life-threatening (Table 20-3).

17. **Describe the management of mucositis.**
    Preventive measures: (1) oral hygiene; (2) cryotherapy during infusion (ice chips swished around the mouth for 30 minutes) can cause vasoconstriction and reduced drug concentration in oropharyngeal mucosa; (3) calcium phosphate rinse (Caphosol® artificial saliva); (4) intravenous glutamine; and (5) keratinocyte growth factor.

Table 20-2. Grades of Oral Mucositis

Grade 1	Asymptomatic or mild symptoms; no intervention required
Grade 2	Moderate pain, not interfering with oral intake. Dietary modifications required
Grade 3	Severe pain, interfering with oral intake
Grade 4	Life-threatening, requires urgent intervention
Grade 5	Death

Table 20-3. Adverse Effects Due to Treatment of Hematologic Malignancies

TOXICITY	IMPLICATED DRUGS
Ototoxicity	Cisplatin, vinblastine, bleomycin, nitrogen mustard, arsenic trioxide
Hyposmia/anosmia	Cytosine arabinoside, methotrexate
Dysguesia/aguesia	Cisplatin, methotrexate, melphalan
Oral mucositis	Bleomycin, cytarabine, doxorubicin, etoposide, methotrexate, radiation

Treatment of established mucositis: (1) Salt and baking soda rinse every 4 hours, prepared by adding one teaspoon of baking soda and one half teaspoon of salt to a quart of water; (2) "magic mouthwash" rinses that include equal parts of viscous lidocaine, diphenhydramine, sodium bicarbonate, and magnesium aluminum hydroxide; and (3) systemic analgesics.

Bibliography

Ackerman BH, Kasbekar N: Disturbances of taste and smell induced by drugs, *Pharmacother* 17(3):482–496, 1997.

Amador-Ortiz C, Chen L, Hassan A, et al: Combined core needle biopsy and fine-needle aspiration with ancillary studies correlate highly with traditional techniques in the diagnosis of nodal-based lymphoma, *Am J Clin Pathol* 135(4):516, 2011.

Anderson T, Chabner BA, Young RC, et al: Malignant lymphoma: the histology and staging of 473 patients at the National Cancer Institute, *Cancer* 50(12):2699, 1982.

Common terminology criteria for adverse events (CTCAE) Version 4.0. Available at: http://evs.nci.nih.gov/ftp1/CTCAE/CTCAE_4.03_2010-06-14_QuickReference_5x7.pdf. Accessed February 2013.

Kwong YL: The diagnosis and management of extranodal NK/T-cell lymphoma, nasal-type and aggressive NK-cell leukemia, *J Clin Exp Hematop* 51(1):21, 2011.

Lister TA, Crowther D, Sutcliffe SB, et al: Report of a committee convened to discuss the evaluation and staging of patients with Hodgkin's disease: Cotswolds meeting, *J Clin Oncol* 7(11):1630, 1989.

Orient JM: Sapira's art and science of bedside diagnosis. In *Examination of Lymph Nodes*, ed 3, Philadelphia, 2005, Lippincott Williams & Wilkins, p 165.

Swerdlow SH, Campo E, Harris NL, et al, editors: *World Health Organization Classification of Tumours of Haematopoietic and Lymphoid Tissues*, Lyon, 2008, IARC Press.

Suzuki R: NK/T-cell lymphomas: pathobiology, prognosis and treatment paradigm, *Curr Oncol Rep* 14(5):395–402, 2012.

Worthington HV, Clarkson JE, Bryan G, et al: Interventions for preventing oral mucositis for patients with cancer receiving treatment, *Cochrane Database Syst Rev* 13(4):CD000978, 2011.

RADIATION AND SYSTEMIC THERAPY FOR HEAD AND NECK CANCER

Timothy V. Waxweiler, MD and Sana D. Karam, MD, PhD

CHAPTER 21

KEY POINTS

1. Radiation therapy (RT) uses ionizing radiation to locally treat cancers while systemic therapy uses cytotoxic chemotherapy or molecularly targeted biologics to systemically treat cancers.
2. Compared to surgery, radiation can offer a curable alternative for treatment of head and neck cancers with the sometimes added benefit of organ preservation.
3. Prompt dental evaluation with necessary tooth extractions and optimal lifetime dental hygiene are critical for all head and neck cancer patients who may receive radiation to minimize the risk of long-term osteoradionecrosis.
4. In the combined setting, chemotherapy primarily acts to potentiate the effects of RT to improve local tumor control.
5. Cisplatin is the standard of care for systemic therapy for head and neck cancer with concurrent radiation, although the final choice of systemic therapy is at the discretion of the medical oncologist.

Pearls

1. Postoperative chemoradiation is indicated for positive margins or nodal extracapsular extension.
2. Definitive head and neck (HN) cancer radiation doses generally range from 66 to 70 Gray (Gy).
3. Definitive radiation is an effective treatment alternative for nonmelanomatous skin lesions.
4. The likelihood of long-term complications depends on the total dose of radiation delivered, the dose per fraction, the time frame over which it was given, and the anatomic sites included within the radiation fields.
5. Induction chemotherapy has not been shown to improve disease control or overall survival.

QUESTIONS

1. **What is radiation therapy (RT) and what are the common techniques used in treating cancers of the head and neck (HN)?**
Radiotherapy, also called radiation therapy, is the localized treatment of cancer and other diseases with ionizing radiation. Ionizing radiation induces mitotic cell death via damage to DNA through a variety of atomic interactions including free radical generation and direct DNA strand breaks. The primary goal of all RT is to maximize cell kill of the target (e.g., cancer cells) while minimizing damage to healthy normal tissues. Radiation is most commonly delivered by an external source (i.e., external beam radiotherapy [EBRT]) using electrons, photons, protons, and other heavy particles, but may also be administered by temporarily or permanently placing radioactive sources into a patient's body (i.e., brachytherapy). Patients are not radioactive when treated with EBRT. The most frequently used modern EBRT techniques for treatment of head and neck cancers are three-dimensional conformal radiotherapy (3DCRT) and the more complex method of intensity modulated radiotherapy (IMRT). Varying dose rates/energies, multiple beam angles/arcs, and dynamic multileaf collimator shapes combine to optimize delivery of the radiation. Image-guided radiotherapy (IGRT) uses imaging capabilities on the treatment machine (e.g., X-rays and cone-beam CT scans) to verify

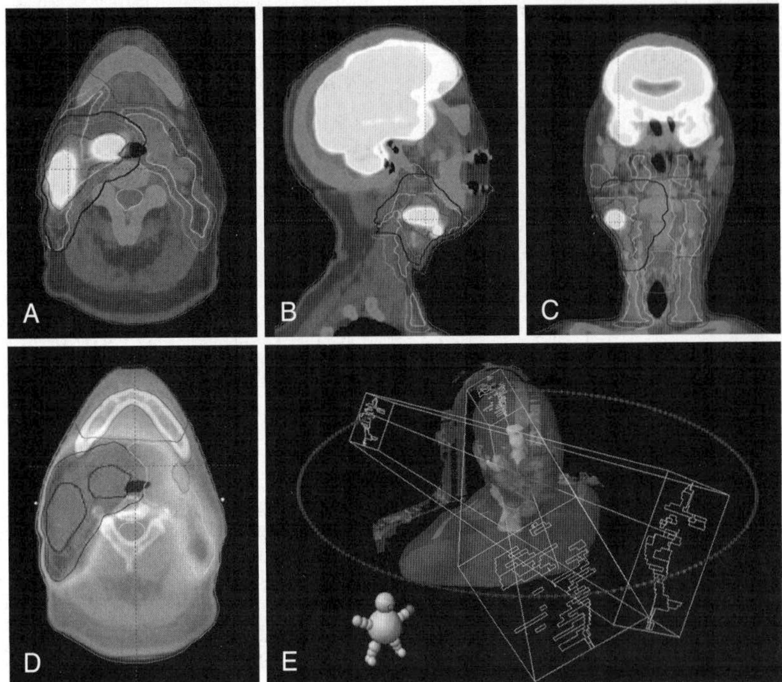

Figure 21-1. Overview of planning volumes drawn on CT images with PET fusion (**A–C**), visualization of expected dose delivery with inner circles being the highest dose (**D**), and 3D visualization of beam arcs and shapes with respect to patient (**E**).

patient setup. Stereotactic body RT (SBRT) is an additional technique often used in the palliative or re-irradiation setting that delivers high doses of radiation in five or fewer treatments (Figure 21-1).

2. **Who should evaluate a patient prior to initiating RT with or without systemic therapy?**

Patients undergoing radiation treatment for head and neck cancers require timely coordination and support from a multitude of care providers. Multidisciplinary evaluation and tumor board discussion of a patient's case can be critical for providing optimal care. The following specialists will often be involved:

- **Radiation oncologist:** A formal H&P evaluation and review of all available imaging is necessary to determine the appropriate radiation targets, dosing, and schedule.
- **Medical oncologist:** A formal medical oncology evaluation is recommended for any patient that may be a candidate for systemic therapies.
- **Dentist or oral surgeon:** Any patient who may receive radiation in the region of the mandible, maxilla, or teeth should receive a formal evaluation and any necessary dental work (e.g., extraction of unhealthy teeth, fillings, fluoride trays) prior to initiating RT. Most institutions require a minimum of 2 to 4 weeks healing prior to starting radiation. A delay in the dental evaluation is one of the most common yet significant causes of delay in initiating RT. For patients with clearly unhealthy teeth who undergo initial surgical resection, teeth extractions are often performed by the otolaryngologist in anticipation of adjuvant RT.
- **Nutritionist:** Regular assessments of nutritional status for HN cancer patients before, during, and after RT and systemic therapy are critical. Nutritionists can also provide teaching and support for patients with feeding tubes.
- **Speech and swallow therapy:** A baseline evaluation is recommended for patients with current or anticipated speech or swallowing problems.

- **Pathology, radiology, and otolaryngologist:** Involvement is recommended to help with RT planning.
- **Additional consultants:** May include interventional radiology, audiology, ophthalmology, neurosurgery, plastic surgery, physical medicine and rehabilitation, social work, addiction services, and palliative care.

3. Beyond initial multidisciplinary consultations, what are the specific steps necessary for a patient with head and neck cancer to receive radiation?

- **CT simulation:** Planning, or simulation, CT scans are performed in the radiation oncology department at which time immobilization devices customized to the patient are made including a thermoplastic molded mask, a mouth piece, and a head rest. MRI, PET/CT, and additional scans may be performed to assist with both staging and treatment planning. Whenever possible, patients should receive these additional scans in the radiation treatment position using their mask, mouth piece, and head rest to assist with immobilization. Having similar positions between all imaging modalities optimizes the accuracy of image fusions used for target delineation planning software (Figure 21-1).
- **Drawing volumes:** The radiation oncologist will then use planning software to outline gross tumor, areas of potential microscopic disease, and normal tissues. This process is known as "drawing volumes," often takes several hours, and may involve more than twenty distinct volumes or structures.
- **Planning:** A dosimetrist, physicist, and the radiation oncologist then work together to create the optimal plan for delivering the radiation to the target while restricting the dose to normal tissues. These plans are often reviewed by multiple people and run through quality assurance checks on the treatment machine.
- **Treatment:** Radiation treatment for HN cancer patients often involves once daily radiation for 6 to 7 weeks with weekly check-up appointments with the radiation oncologist to evaluate and treat toxicities.

4. How do radiation and surgery compare to each other?

Both RT and surgery are local therapies. Definitive RT strives for organ preservation to maintain critical functions such as swallowing, normal speech, and airway protection, and attempting to maximize quality of life in patients that might otherwise undergo significantly morbid surgeries. Additionally, RT is typically delivered daily Monday through Friday over 6 to 8 weeks on an outpatient basis without need of anesthesia, making it an ideal modality for poor surgical candidates. This protracted time commitment can be problematic for noncompliant or elderly patients and those living great distances from a radiation oncology facility. Surgery is advantageous in providing a one-time procedure and optimal pathologic assessment of primary tumors and nodal disease. While acute side effects of surgery occur primarily in the immediate postoperative time frame, acute RT toxicities typically build up gradually throughout the course of treatment. Extent of disease and involvement of critical structures limits both surgeons in their ability to achieve complete resection of disease and radiation oncologists in their ability to treat these disease sites to full definitive doses. Both specialties must balance aggressive treatment with acute and long-term local toxicities.

5. What are the general doses used in RT for HN cancers?

A Gray (Gy) represents one joule per kilogram and is the standard unit of absorbed dose used in clinical radiation oncology. A variety of doses and fractionation schedules are used in treating HN cancers. In the typical daily radiation setting, daily doses of 180 to 225 cGy (1.8 to 2.25 Gy) are used. General, non–site specific total doses vary based on the setting (definitive RT to gross disease ≈66 to 70 Gy; high-risk elective neck coverage ≈60 Gy; low-risk elective neck ≈54 Gy; and postoperative RT ≈66 Gy).

6. Who cannot be treated with RT?

Patients who should not receive radiation are those with collagen-vascular diseases, other hypersensitivity conditions (e.g., ataxia-telangiectasia), pregnant women particularly in the first two trimesters, and those who would exceed maximum safe cumulative doses of RT to critical structures. Some patients can be retreated, usually with a lower dose, after time has elapsed since the previous treatment. Additionally, disorders of DNA repair and conditions (e.g., Li-Fraumeni syndrome and xeroderma pigmentosum) put patients at high risk for radiation induced secondary cancers.

7. **What is systemic therapy and how does it work both with and without radiation?**
Chemotherapy and biologics are the two main groups of systemic therapies. These treatments deliver cytotoxic drugs or molecularly targeted therapeutic agents that travel through the bloodstream with the goal of treating cancer cells throughout the body. Cytotoxic drugs interfere with DNA replication, microtubule formation, and other cellular processes to impair mitosis and/or induce apoptosis. While these agents tend to primarily damage cells with high mitotic rates (e.g., cancer, mucosal tissues, and bone marrow), they are fairly indiscriminate. Biologics, in turn, typically employ antibodies to specifically target proteins ubiquitous among a clonal cancer cell population such as a surface antigen and/or components critical to a cancer signaling pathway. Often times concurrent chemoradiation (CRT) or radiation with targeted therapies provides a synergistic effect allowing improved tumor control. The systemic therapy can put cancer cells into a radiosensitive state by manipulation of the proliferative pathways.

8. **What are the most common systemic agents used in treatment of nonmetastatic HN cancers and their associated toxicities?**
Cisplatin is the most commonly used systemic therapy in both the induction and concurrent setting. For concurrent chemoradiation, high-dose cisplatin is given weekly or every 3 weeks. Systemic agents most often used for treatment of nonmetastatic head and neck cancers, along with their main adverse effects are reported in Table 21-1.

9. **How is systemic therapy used in the treatment of head and neck cancers?**
Systemic therapy may be administered in the following settings with different goals:
   - **Neoadjuvant or induction:** Given prior to definitive treatment (i.e., surgery or radiation) to decrease the size/extent of cancer to allow for less extensive local treatment, and in some cases allow for organ preservation.
   - **Adjuvant:** Given after definitive treatment with hopes of decreasing recurrence either locally or distally (not currently standard of care in HN cancers)
   - **Concomitant or concurrent with radiation:** Used to augment the efficacy of radiation via radiosensitization. In this setting, the systemic therapy is not thought to significantly improve control of undetectable metastatic disease.
   - **Metastatic:** Primarily used to prolong disease control and palliate symptoms.

10. **Who should receive induction therapy?**
Multiple randomized trials have demonstrated no significant benefits of induction chemotherapy prior to definitive treatment of SCC of the head and neck. Some evidence exists for a reduction of distant metastases and improved organ preservation in hypopharynx and nasopharynx cancers, but the role of induction chemotherapy remains controversial. Currently, induction chemotherapy should be considered only in clinical trials or in select conditions (e.g., upper airway obstruction or dental abscesses) due to delays in initiation of definitive concurrent chemoradiation. Multidisciplinary tumor board review and treatment at experienced tertiary care centers are highly recommended when considering induction therapy.

Table 21-1. Common Systemic Agents Used in HN Cancer Treatments and Their Associated Toxicities

AGENT	NOTABLE TOXICITIES
Cisplatin	Hearing loss, renal failure, peripheral neuropathy, electrolyte abnormalities, GI toxicity
Carboplatin	Electrolyte abnormalities, myelosuppression
5-Fluorouracil	Mucositis, hand-foot syndrome, photosensitivity, maculopapular rash
Paclitaxel	Peripheral neuropathy, arthralgia, myalgia
Docetaxel	Peripheral neuropathy, edema, asthenia
Cetuximab	Acneiform rash, dermatitis, hypomagnesemia, neutropenia

NOTE: Additional side effects seen in many of these agents include myelosuppression, diarrhea, nausea/vomiting, alopecia, and hypersensitivity reactions.

11. **What is the role of cetuximab in treating HN cancers?**
Cetuximab is a monoclonal antibody that targets the extracellular domain of endothelial growth factor receptor (EGFR). EGFR is frequently mutated and/or overexpressed in HN cancers. While cisplatin remains the gold standard systemic therapy in concurrent chemoradiation setting, cetuximab is an FDA approved alternative with a different side effect profile making it a suitable alternative in select situations (e.g., following a cisplatin based induction regimen).

12. **Which tumors can be definitively treated with radiation as the sole treatment modality and when should concurrent systemic therapy be added?**
Surgery is often preferred in the setting where complete resection with sufficient margins can be expected without causing significant morbidity; however, nearly all early stage head and neck cancers that are T1 to T2 and N0-1 are candidates for definitive RT alone. These include primary tumors of the tongue, tonsil, larynx, and hypopharynx. Exceptions include cancers of the nasopharynx, in which external beam RT is the standard treatment regardless of T or N stage. Tumors of the salivary glands and floor of the mouth are generally managed primarily with surgery, even if diagnosed at an early stage.
Concurrent systemic therapy should be added to radiation for more advanced (e.g., T3–T4, N2–N3) head and neck tumors. Multiple randomized trials and meta-analyses have shown an absolute survival benefit in this setting.

13. **What are the standard indications for adjuvant RT and/or systemic therapy after surgical resection of a SCC head and neck tumor?**
Positive margins, T3–4 tumors, multiple or bulky positive lymph nodes, nodal extracapsular extension (ECE), perineural invasion (PNI), lymphovascular invasion (LVI), or nodal disease in levels IV or V. Additionally, oral cavity cancers with depth of invasion greater than 2 mm or close margins should receive adjuvant radiation. In most cases, patients with recurrent disease treated with salvage surgery should be offered adjuvant radiation therapy when feasible.

14. **What are the standard indications for concurrent chemotherapy with RT after surgical resection of an SCC head and neck tumor?**
The addition of concurrent chemotherapy to adjuvant radiation is typically recommended for patients with positive margins or ECE. Two major randomized trials (i.e., RTOG 95-01 and EORTC 22931) have examined adjuvant radiation with or without concomitant cisplatin with results showing local control, disease-free survival, and possibly overall survival benefits when using combined modality treatment.

15. **What are the indications for adjuvant RT after surgical resection for salivary gland tumors?**
For salivary gland tumors, adjuvant RT should be offered to patients with close or positive margins, pT3–4 tumors, intermediate/high grade, adenoid cystic carcinoma histology, bone invasion, PNI, LVI, and pathologic node positive disease. The addition of concurrent chemotherapy may be considered on a case by case basis and is the subject of multiple ongoing trials. For salivary gland tumors, postoperative radiation also improves overall survival in addition to local regional control in patients with high-grade histology or locally advanced tumors.

16. **What is the recommended time between surgery and initiation of adjuvant RT for most HN cancers?**
Generally 4 to 6 weeks is recommended because there is a direct correlation between the time to initiation of postoperative RT and tumor control outcomes, but patients must be well healed before starting radiation. Several studies have validated the importance of a timely "package time" being ≈13 weeks from date of surgery to completion of adjuvant radiation. Delays or breaks in treatment are associated with poor outcomes for two primary reasons: (1) HN cancers exhibit accelerated repopulation and (2) an inherent bias exists in that patients with advanced disease tolerate treatment poorly and require these delays and breaks.

17. **When delivering RT for an HN cancer of unknown primary, which areas should be treated?**
Possible primary mucosal sites that commonly metastasize, including the nasopharynx and oropharynx, and bilateral neck (unilateral coverage is controversial). The larynx, hypopharynx, and oral cavity may be treated if the patient is suspected to be at high risk in those areas.

18. Does HPV status, p16 status, or any other molecular markers affect the recommended doses for RT?
No. Currently no molecular markers support escalation or de-escalation of the standard recommendations for radiation dosing. While HPV(+) and p16(+) oropharynx patients have better outcomes, and retrospective data shows favorable outcomes with dose de-escalation, no level 1 evidence exists for de-escalation. Treatment deintensification is an active area of research.

19. Which head and neck skin cancer patients should be considered for definitive radiation?
Patients with large lesions that would require significant morbid surgeries, those with lesions of the central face or other locations for which surgery would result in significant cosmetic defects (e.g., nasal ala), and nonsurgical candidates.

20. What are the indications for adjuvant therapy after surgical resection for head and neck skin cancers?
Perineural invasion, positive surgical margins, parotid invasion, or an ear primary with high-risk features (i.e., depth of invasion >2 mm, Clark's level ≥IV, poor differentiation).

21. What features of a primary skin cancer warrant elective nodal irradiation?
Multiple positive lymph nodes (>3), extracapsular extension, large tumors (>4 cm), deep invasion of underlying structures (e.g., cartilage), or cancer of the ear, particularly preauricular.

22. What are the common acute adverse effects of RT to the head and neck region and how are they managed?
The acute side effects of RT usually appear in weeks 2 to 3, gradually progress through the week after the last radiation treatment, and resolve within 4 to 6 weeks after completion. Toxicities are often worse with concurrent systemic therapy. Optimal supportive management is necessary to avoid treatment breaks which have been proven to decrease treatment efficacy. Supportive treatments for the most common symptoms include the following:

- Fatigue: An active exercise regimen and general healthy lifestyle practices, psychostimulants, and antidepressants
- Skin reactions: Nonperfumed moisturizers and humectants
- Mucositis, dysphagia, odynophagia: Dietary modifications, green tea, Manuka honey, liquid lidocaine, benadryl, antacids, NSAIDs, narcotics, sucralfate, steroids, and optimal hydration/nutrition support which sometimes includes feeding tube placement
- Xerostomia: Mouth rinses (including combinations of water, baking soda, salt, hydrogen peroxide), biotin, pilocarpine, prophylactic amifostene, and optimal oral hygiene

Depending on the site receiving radiation, hoarseness, otitis media, dry eyes, conjunctivitis/keratitis, sinonasal congestion, and epistaxis may also occur.

23. Why is hydration/nutrition important for patients receiving radiation and/or systemic therapies for head and neck tumors?
Most of these patients are nutritionally depleted due to the morbidity of the tumor itself. Mucositis, nausea, vomiting, and anorexia from multimodality treatments add to the nutritional depletion, compounding the weight loss. Poor nutrition or hydration may lead to hospitalization and treatment breaks. In addition, patients that lose significant amounts of weight may not align correctly in their positioning masks for radiation which can require replanning with treatment breaks. Treatment breaks, while sometimes necessary, decrease cure rates and should be avoided when at all possible. Enteral gastrostomy feedings are often used when patients receive bilateral neck radiation to support nutrition and hydration.

24. What are the potential long-term complications of RT?
Serious radiation complications are unusual (with an incidence of less than 10%) but are difficult to manage when they occur. The likelihood of a given patient developing long-term complications depends on the total dose of radiation delivered, the dose per fraction, the time frame over which it was given, and the anatomic sites included within the radiation portal. In general, the risk increases with increasing doses delivered over shorter time periods to greater volumes of tissue. Complications include xerostomia, skin changes, hypothyroidism, osteoradionecrosis, bone exposure, laryngeal edema with voice changes, esophageal stenosis, vision/hearing deficits, fibrosis including trismus, and induction of secondary cancers. Xerostomia is one of the most common and

bothersome long-term side effects of head and neck irradiation. When possible, attempts should be made to minimize doses to parotid and submandibular glands without sacrificing tumor coverage. Dry mouth also causes an increased risk of developing dental carries with subsequent increased risk for osteoradionecrosis.

25. **What is the benefit of intensity-modulated radiotherapy (IMRT) in treating HN cancers?**
IMRT has become the standard RT technique for head and neck cancers in the past 15 years and multiple trials have shown an ability to achieve similar rates of local control while lowering the incidence of acute and long-term toxicities by decreasing radiation dose to critical organs (e.g., salivary glands for xerostomia, constrictor muscles for dysphagia).

26. **When should a neck dissection be performed after definitive RT?**
Patients with clinical or radiographic residual gross nodal disease or initially bulky nodal disease should be considered for post-RT neck dissection. A balance is necessary as tumors can take weeks to months to respond to radiation therapy yet fibrosis can develop in a similar time frame, which can make surgery difficult. The response to radiation treatment is generally assessed by PET/CT at 12 weeks post-treatment.

27. **When should re-irradiation be considered?**
Recurrent disease, when the patient is not eligible for salvage surgery or with post salvage surgery high-risk features, may be considered for re-irradiation. In the re-irradiation setting, the risks for both acute and long term toxicities are increased. Stereotactic body radiotherapy (SBRT) is one technique under investigation for use in the re-irradiation setting as a means of delivering highly conformal high-dose radiation to areas of relapse while sparing normal tissues.

Bibliography

Bonner JA, Harari PM, Giralt J, et al: Radiotherapy plus cetuximab for locoregionally advanced head and neck cancer: 5-year survival data from a phase 3 randomized trial, and relation between cetuximab-induced rash and survival, *Lancet Oncol* 11(1):21, 2010.

Cooper JS, Zhang Q, Pajak TF, et al: Long-term follow-up of the RTOG 9501/intergroup phase III trial: postoperative concurrent radiation therapy and chemotherapy in high-risk squamous cell carcinoma of the head and neck, *Int J Radiat Oncol Biol Phys* 84(5):1198–1205, 2012.

Mahmood U, Koshy M, Goloubeva O, et al: Adjuvant radiation therapy for high-grade and/or locally advanced major salivary gland tumors, *Arch Otolaryngol Head Neck Surg* 137(10):1025, 2011.

NCCN Clinical Practice Guidelines in Oncology: Head and Neck Cancers Version 2. 2013. Available from http://www.nccn.org/professionals/physician_gls/pdf/head-and-neck.pdf.

Pignon JP, le Maître A, Maillard E, et al: Meta-analysis of chemotherapy in head and neck cancer (MACH-NC): an update on 93 randomised trials and 17,346 patients, *Radiother Oncol* 92(1):4, 2009.

Terhaard CH, Lubsen H, Rasch CR, et al: The role of radiotherapy in the treatment of malignant salivary gland tumors, *Int J Radiat Oncol Biol Phys* 61(1):103, 2005.

III

ALLERGY AND RHINOLOGY

SINONASAL ANATOMY AND EMBRYOLOGY WITH RADIOLOGY CORRELATES

Richard R. Orlandi, MD and Jeremiah A. Alt, MD, PhD

CHAPTER 22

KEY POINTS

1. Embryologic patterns of pneumatization of the frontal and sphenoid sinuses help one to understand the anatomic variations that may be seen in these sinuses.
2. While there can be great variation in sinus anatomy, the drainage patterns of the sinuses are fairly constant. Understand the relationships of the frontal, sphenoid, and maxillary sinus drainage pathways.
3. Knowledge of the arterial blood supply to the nose and sinuses facilitates understanding how to avoid and treat bleeding during and following sinus surgery.
4. Diseases of the paranasal sinuses can extend hematogenously or directly into adjacent structures in the head. An understanding of how these may manifest clinically is critical to early detection and treatment.

Pearls

1. The paranasal sinuses form as evaginations from the nasal cavity. The ethmoid and maxillary sinuses are present at birth, and all of the sinuses continue to develop postnatally with the sphenoid and frontal developing last.
2. The osteomeatal unit (OMU) is a functional anatomic unit. Obstruction in this area can lead to anterior ethmoid and maxillary sinusitis, and possibly frontal sinusitis.
3. CT with triplanar reconstruction is the preferred method for evaluating the sinuses radiographically.
4. Sinus disease can spread via vascular channels into the intracranial cavity and orbit.

QUESTIONS

1. **Describe the septum and the turbinates.**
   The nasal septum is the midline partition that separates the left and right sides of the nasal cavity. It is made of the quadrangular cartilage, perpendicular plate of the ethmoid bone, vomer, and maxillary crest. There are three paired turbinates, or *concha*, on each side. The middle and superior turbinates are part of the ethmoid bone, whereas the inferior turbinate is its own bone.

2. **Define the paranasal sinuses.**
   The paranasal sinuses are pneumatized areas of the facial and skull base bones. They communicate with the nasal cavity through small ostia, allowing air exchange and drainage of secreted mucus.

3. **What epithelium lines the paranasal sinuses?**
   The sinuses are lined by pseudostratified ciliated columnar or respiratory epithelium. The cilia beat in a coordinated fashion to transport mucus from the point of its secretion in the sinus toward its natural ostium. From there, the cilia within the nasal cavity move the secretions toward the nasopharynx.

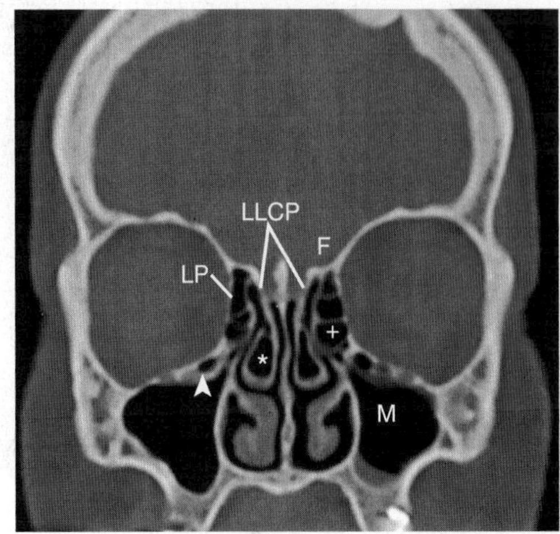

Figure 22-1. Coronal computed tomography (CT) scan image in a bone window algorithm showing pneumatization in the head of the middle turbinate (*), also called a concha bullosa. Infraorbital ethmoid air cells (Haller cells) are seen as pneumatized air cells off the inferior orbital floor (arrow). This can narrow the drainage of the maxillary sinus (M). The lateral wall of the ethmoid cavity is the lamina papyracea (LP). The olfactory cleft and lateral lamella of the cribriform plate (LLCP) is depicted. Note the relationship of the LLCP with the insertion of the basal lamella of the middle turbinate, as well as the fovea ethmoidalis (F) laterally. The LLCP is commonly asymmetric. This asymmetric anatomic variation should be recognized on presurgical planning to prevent iatrogenic cerebrospinal fluid leaks. The ethmoid bulla is seen adjacent to the LP (+).

4. **What is the function of the paranasal sinuses?**
   The short answer is that the function is unknown. A number of theories exist about the possible function of the sinuses, including lightening of the skull, enhancing vocal resonance, absorption of mechanical force during trauma in order to protect the eyes and brain, and production of or reservoir for nitric oxide, a postulated aerocrine substance that may regulate pulmonary function. All of these theories have evidence for and against them.

5. **Where is the maxillary sinus located?**
   The maxillary sinus is located within the body of the maxilla. Medially it is bounded by the lateral nasal wall, superiorly by the floor of the orbit (containing the infraorbital nerve and artery), posteriorly by the pterygopalatine and infratemporal fossae, and inferiorly by the alveolar process and hard palate. The maxillary tooth roots commonly reach to the floor of the maxillary sinus (Figure 22-1).

6. **Where are the ethmoid sinuses located?**
   The ethmoid sinuses form a honeycomb-like series of cells medial to the orbits and inferior to the anterior cranial base. They are functionally divided into the anterior and posterior ethmoid cells by a portion of the middle turbinate called the basal lamella. The anterior cells are bounded medially by the middle turbinate and drain into the middle meatus. The posterior ethmoid cells are bounded medially by the superior turbinate and drain into the superior meatus. The ethmoid cells are bounded laterally by the lamina papyracea of the orbit. Posterior to the posterior ethmoid cells is the sphenoid bone containing the sphenoid sinus. The nasal cavity is inferior to the ethmoid air cells and the frontal bone is superior. As the ethmoid cells form embryologically, they expand into the frontal bone superiorly and make shallow depressions in it, called fovea ethmoidales. The frontal bone abuts the cribriform plate of the ethmoid medially and a small portion of the cribriform plate sits superior to the ethmoid cells. This area tends to be very thin and easily punctured during sinus surgery, which can lead to a cerebrospinal fluid leak.

7. **Where is the sphenoid sinus located?**
   The sphenoid sinus pneumatizes the sphenoid bone and is posterior to the ethmoid sinus. The sella turcica and pituitary gland lie superior to the sphenoid sinus. Within the lateral wall of the sphenoid

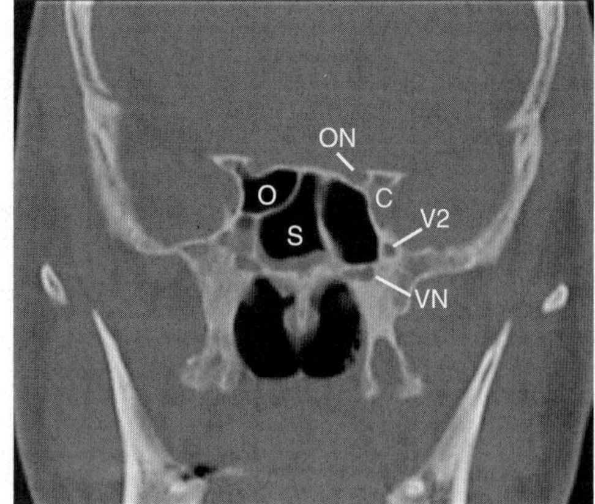

Figure 22-2. Coronal computed tomography (CT) scan in a bone window algorithm showing a right sphenoethmoidal air cell (Onodi cell) which is located superior and lateral to the sphenoid sinus (S). The optic nerve (ON) and carotid artery (C) are seen as bony protrusions in the sphenoethmoidal air cell (O) rather than the sphenoid sinus. The vidian nerve (VN) and the maxillary division of the trigeminal nerve (V2) can be seen inferior and laterally.

sinus is the venous cavernous sinus, containing the internal carotid artery. The optic nerve also lies within the lateral wall of the sphenoid sinus. Posterior to the sphenoid sinus is the posterior cranial fossa (Figure 22-2). The sphenoid sinus can pneumatize laterally into the pterygoid region of the sphenoid and thus lie inferior to the temporal lobes of the brain.

8. **Where is the frontal sinus located?**
The frontal sinuses are air spaces within the frontal bones. The frontal bone thus has an anterior and posterior wall. The anterior wall lies deep to the forehead skin. The frontal lobes of the brain lie posterior to the frontal sinus. Inferiorly the frontal sinuses lie adjacent to the orbits laterally and the anterior ethmoid sinuses medially.

9. **At what point during gestation do the sinuses begin to develop?**
The sinuses begin to form in the third fetal month but only the ethmoid and maxillary sinuses are present at birth. They form as evaginations from the developing nasal cavity that invade into the surrounding bones.

10. **Do the sinuses continue to develop postnatally?**
Yes. The maxillary sinus continues to grow in size as the face grows overall. The maxillary sinus enlarges significantly again after eruption of the permanent dentition. The ethmoid sinuses continue to develop postnatally until about age 12. The frontal sinus pneumatizes slowly postnatally, rarely reaching any significant size during the first decade of life. Thereafter, it rapidly pneumatizes into the frontal bone reaching its final size near the end of the second decade of life. Likewise, the sphenoid sinus develops little until about age 7, after which it rapidly pneumatizes and reaches its final size during adolescence (Figure 22-3).

11. **How are the sinuses evaluated radiographically?**
The advent of high-resolution thin cut multiplanar computed tomography (CT) has dramatically improved the assessment of the complex anatomy of the paranasal sinuses. Early CTs used direct acquisition of coronal and axial images. Direct acquisition in the axial plane with reconstruction in the coronal and sagittal planes is now commonplace. Such triplanar imaging allows for study of complex anatomic relationships throughout the paranasal sinuses and cranial base. Of the three views, the coronal images can be considered the most useful because they closely resemble the surgeons' endoscopic surgical view. Inflammation of the sinuses is seen on CT as thickening of the mucoperiosteum of the paranasal sinuses.
Plain radiographs of the sinuses are rarely used due to the lack of anatomic detail seen with CT imaging. MRIs can augment CTs by providing soft tissue analysis, as when secretions cannot be differentiated from a neoplasm. Due to the lack of bony detail, they are not commonly used for standard sinus evaluations.

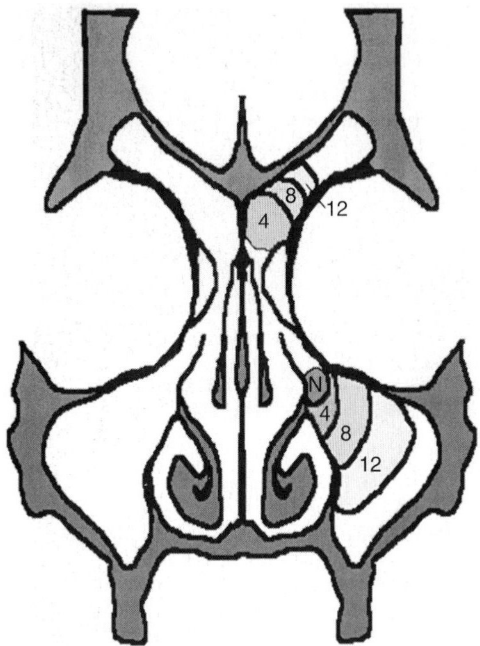

Figure 22-3. Coronal representation of the development of the frontal and maxillary sinus. The frontal sinus begins to develop at the age of 4 years and does not fully mature until after the age of 12 years. The newborn (N) has a small maxillary sinus that continues to expand in a lateral inferior direction, reaching adult pneumatization after 12 years of age.

12. **What is the osteomeatal unit and what structures make up this area?**
The osteomeatal unit (OMU) is a functional anatomic area within the middle meatus comprised of:
    - Ethmoid bulla
    - Uncinate process
    - Ethmoid infundibulum
    - Hiatus semilunaris

    The OMU is the common drainage pathway of the anterior ethmoid and maxillary sinuses. Depending on the superior attachment of the uncinate process, it may also drain the frontal sinus. Inflammation within the OMU may lead to obstruction of and inflammation within these draining sinuses.

13. **What is the ethmoid bulla?**
The ethmoid bulla is the most consistent and typically largest anterior ethmoid cell. Its lateral wall is the lamina papyracea. It usually has a rounded shape anteriorly, running parallel to the uncinate process (see Figure 22-1).

14. **What is an uncinate process?**
The term *uncinate process* means "hook-shaped" bone. It is a crescent- or hook-shaped fold of bone that sweeps from superior to posterior just anterior to the ethmoid bulla within the anterior ethmoid sinuses. The uncinate process and anterior face of the bulla tend to run parallel to each other, forming a small gap called the hiatus semilunaris. The uncinate process is attached to the lateral wall of the nose and has a free edge posteriorly. It therefore forms a trough-shaped space that runs from superior to posterior within the anterior ethmoid sinuses. This space is called the *ethmoid infundibulum.*

15. **What is the difference between the hiatus semilunaris and the ethmoid infundibulum?**
The hiatus semilunaris is a two-dimensional gap (*hiatus* means "gap") between the ethmoid bulla and the uncinate process. The ethmoid infundibulum is a three-dimensional trough between the uncinate process and lateral nasal wall/lamina papyracea. Surgically, the ethmoid infundibulum can

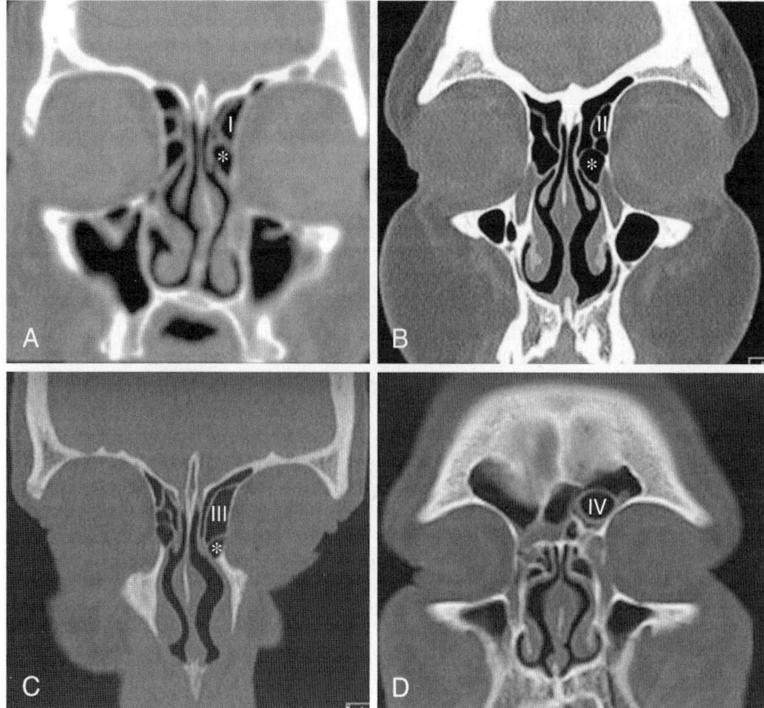

Figure 22-4. Computed tomography (CT) images in bone window algorithms demonstrating types of frontal cells (Kuhn Classification I-IV): **A**, Type I cell directly above the agger nasi cell (*). **B**, Type II cell, **C**, Type III Kuhn cell. The coronal CT imaging shows bilateral Kuhn Type III frontal air cells. **D**, Type IV Kuhn frontal cell is isolated within the left frontal sinus.

be accessed through the hiatus semilunaris. In other words, the trough is reached through the semilunar gap.

16. **What is the agger nasi?**
The term agger nasi means "nasal mound" and refers to the area in the lateral wall of the nasal cavity that projects medially, just superior to the middle turbinate's anterior superior attachment. It is commonly pneumatized, forming an agger nasi cell (Figure 22-4).

17. **How do the sinuses drain into the nasal cavity?**
Each sinus communicates with the nasal cavity through an ostium. The size of the ostia vary but are generally 1 to 3 mm in size. Each ethmoid cell has a variably placed ostium. The anterior ethmoid cells as a group drain into the middle meatus and the posterior ethmoid cells drain collectively into the superior meatus.

The frontal, sphenoid, and maxillary sinuses have more reliably defined drainage patterns.

- The maxillary sinus ostium drains into a structure called the ethmoid infundibulum. From there it drains into the middle meatus of the nasal cavity.
- The frontal sinus may also drain into the ethmoid infundibulum of the anterior ethmoid sinus. If, however, the uncinate process attaches to the lamina papyracea, the frontal sinus will bypass the ethmoid infundibulum and drain directly into the middle meatus.
- The sphenoid sinus ostium drains into the sphenoethmoidal recess, between the superior turbinate and the nasal septum.

Once the secretions have reached the nasal cavity, they are carried into the nasopharynx and then pass into the digestive system, where they and whatever debris they carry are destroyed.

18. What variations are seen in the anatomy of the ethmoid sinuses?

Infraorbital ethmoid air cells (Haller cells) may be present laterally within the ethmoid sinus, adjacent to the inferior orbital floor and at the medial extent of the roof of the maxillary sinus. These cells are important to identify because they have the potential to narrow the ethmoid infundibulum and maxillary sinus drainage. The coronal CT is the best view for diagnosing these air cells (see Figure 22-1).

The term *concha bullosa* is used to describe pneumatization of the middle turbinate. A concha bullosa of the middle turbinate can narrow the OMU by compressing the uncinate process laterally (see Figure 22-1).

19. What variations are seen in the anatomy of the sphenoid sinus?

Sphenoethmoidal cells (Onodi cells) are posterior ethmoid cells that pneumatize into the sphenoid bone. This cell can extend superiorly, posterior and laterally and therefore have an intimate relationship with the optic nerve and carotid artery in its lateral wall. The sphenoethmoidal cell is best visualized on the coronal CT views with the appearance of a horizontal split of the sphenoid sinus. However, the coronal, sagittal, and axial views should be reviewed to clarify if the origin of the cell is from the posterior ethmoids rather than the sphenoid, which is medial and inferior (see Figure 22-2).

20. What structures make up the frontal recess?

The frontal outflow tract does not form a true duct but rather an hourglass shaped space formed by a number of variable structures surrounding it. Generally these boundary structures are:

- Agger nasi cell anteriorly
- Middle turbinate medially
- Anterior fossa cranial base posterior-superiorly
- Lamina papyracea laterally
- Ethmoid bulla posterior-inferiorly

21. What are frontal cells?

The pattern of pneumatization within the ethmoid sinuses is highly variable from individual to individual. Sometimes ethmoid or other air cells can be present superiorly within the frontal sinus drainage. They have been grouped into four principal types or patterns (see Figure 22-4):

- Type 1: A single ethmoid cell resting immediately superior to the agger nasi cell
- Type 2: More than one ethmoid sitting atop the agger nasi cell
- Type 3: A significantly pneumatized ethmoid cell that extends beyond the frontal recess into the frontal sinus
- Type 4: An air cell that is isolated within the frontal sinus

All of these types of cells can narrow the frontal sinus drainage.

22. Explain the concepts of functional endoscopic sinus surgery (FESS).

Functional endoscopic sinus surgery stresses restoring the normal drainage ("function") of the sinuses through their natural ostia. Part or all of the ethmoid partitions may be removed to promote drainage of the ethmoid cells. The ostia of the affected frontal, sphenoid, or maxillary sinuses may then be widened to promote their drainage into the nasal cavity. The remaining mucosa is maximally preserved to restore normal mucociliary clearance. Previous to FESS, mucosa was thought to be irreversibly diseased and was therefore removed. This removal destroyed the normal mucociliary clearance, leading to dysfunctional sinuses that depended on gravity to drain.

23. Describe the blood supply to the nose and paranasal sinuses.

The nose and ethmoid sinuses are principally supplied by three arteries whose branches form anastomoses with one another:

- The anterior and posterior ethmoid arteries are branches of the ophthalmic artery, which branches from the internal carotid artery. They arise in the orbit and pass into the roof of the ethmoid sinuses through foramina in the lamina papyracea. They supply much of the ethmoid sinuses and the superior nasal septum.
- The sphenopalatine artery is a terminal branch of the internal maxillary artery, which arises from the external carotid artery. It has two principal branches, one of which passes just inferior to the sphenoid sinus ostium and supplies the posterior nasal septum. A second branch enters into the middle turbinate. Smaller branches supply the nasal floor and inferior turbinate.

- The frontal, maxillary, and sphenoid sinuses are supplied by small arteries that perforate their bony walls.

24. **Describe the venous drainage of the nose and paranasal sinuses.**
The venous drainage of the nose and sinuses passes into venous sinuses in the pterygopalatine fossa, which then communicate with the venous cavernous sinus lateral to the sphenoid sinus. Some of the venous drainage can pass through the lamina papyracea.

The frontal sinus drains intracranially through small veins that perforate the posterior table of the frontal bone.

Infection in the sinuses can pass into the orbit or cranial cavity through these venous drainage pathways.

25. **Name and describe the lamellas that originate from the bony ridges (ethmoturbinals) in the lateral nasal wall during embryologic development.**
    - First lamella is made up of both an ascending and descending portion and becomes the agger nasi cell and the uncinate process respectively.
    - Second lamella becomes the bulla ethmoidalis.
    - Third lamella becomes the basal lamella of the middle turbinate. It provides a clear distinction between the anterior and posterior ethmoid air cells.
    - Fourth lamella becomes the superior turbinate.
    - Fifth lamella is more varied but arises from the fusion of the fifth and sixth ethmoturbinals to become the supreme turbinate (if one is present).

26. **What areas of a CT scan should be specifically evaluated prior to sinus surgery?**
Inflammation within the sinuses is assessed by examining the scan for any mucosal thickening. The frontal, anterior ethmoid, posterior ethmoid, maxillary, and sphenoid sinuses and OMU are assessed bilaterally. Anatomic variants that may contribute to obstruction or that may impact surgery are noted.

The following areas can be involved in potential complications and should be investigated during the planning stages of surgery:
    - Lamina papyracea integrity
    - Cribriform plate anatomy—specifically, the depth of the olfactory fossa and the symmetry between the two sides
    - Ethmoid skull base integrity
    - Anterior ethmoid artery location—does it run along the skull base or does it run in a more inferiorly-positioned bony mesentery?
    - Sphenoethmoidal (Onodi) cell presence
    - Optic nerve anatomy—covered by bone or dehiscent?
    - Internal carotid anatomy—covered by bone or dehiscent?

CONTROVERSIES

27. **How much does anatomy contribute to rhinosinusitis?**
Chronic rhinosinusitis is an inflammatory process that involves edema within the paranasal sinuses and nasal cavity. Its etiology remains elusive and is likely multifactorial. Anatomic variations may play a role in some cases, but overall the impact appears to be small. Simple correction of sinus anatomic issues without attention to accompanying mucosal inflammation only occasionally resolves chronic rhinosinusitis.

Recurrent acute rhinosinusitis is a less common form of sinus inflammation. Recent studies have implicated narrowing of the ethmoid infundibulum as a possible risk factor for this condition.

28. **In performing functional endoscopic sinus surgery, how large should the surgeon make the surgical ostia?**
Promoting sinus drainage and ventilation through the natural ostia of the sinuses forms the foundation of surgical treatment of rhinosinusitis. Exactly how large to make the ostia, or to enlarge them at all, remains controversial decades after the development of endoscopic sinus techniques. On one end of the spectrum is removal of the uncinate process alone to open the ethmoid infundibulum without enlarging the maxillary ostium. Similarly, the ostia can be dilated with medialization of a preserved uncinate using balloon dilation techniques. The sphenoid and frontal

sinus ostia can be addressed similarly. At the other end of the spectrum is the creation of maximally enlarged ostia to their anatomic limits.

Chronic rhinosinusitis exists in a variety of manifestations, ranging from simple OMU obstruction to extensive eosinophilic polyposis. Some surgeons take the pragmatic position of "small holes for small disease, big holes for big disease."

Inasmuch as little evidence exists to guide the surgeon in resolving this controversy, rigid adherence to any dogma is likely inadvisable.

BIBLIOGRAPHY

Deutshmann MW, Yeung J, Bosch M, et al: Radiologic reporting for paranasal sinus computed tomography: a multi-institutional review of content and consistency, *Laryngoscope* 123:1100–1105, 2013.

Stammberger H: *Functional Endoscopic Sinus Surgery*, Philadelphia, 1991, B.C. Decker.

Stammberger HR, Kennedy DW: Paranasal sinuses: anatomic terminology and nomenclature, *Ann Otol Rhinol Laryngol Suppl* 167:7–16, 1995.

Wise S, DelGaudio J, Orlandi RR: Sinonasal anatomy and development. In Kennedy DW, Hwang PH, editors: *Rhinology: Diseases of the Nose, Sinuses, and Skull Base*, Philadelphia, 2012, Thieme.

CHAPTER 23

EPISTAXIS

Alexander Connelly, MD and Vijay R. Ramakrishnan, MD

KEY POINTS

1. Anterior epistaxis is most common, and most often originates from Little's area in Kiesselbach's plexus, whereas posterior bleeds commonly originate from the sphenopalatine artery distribution.
2. The most important evaluation of a patient with epistaxis is a rough gauge of epistaxis severity, and if needed, ABCs and vital signs. This plays the key initial role in evaluation and planning.
3. There are a number of modifiable factors that should be kept in mind in the treatment of epistaxis, such as current medications, home/work environment, and indoor humidity at place of residence, with many conservative measures that can be employed prior to surgical options in nonurgent cases.
4. In cases of repeated epistaxis without an identified cause, conditions such as coagulopathy, vascular abnormality, drug use, hereditary disorders, inflammatory and autoimmune conditions need to be further explored.
5. When considering intervention for posterior epistaxis, SPA ligation is a more efficacious and cost-effective means of controlling epistaxis compared to posterior packing and hospitalization or embolization, although embolization may be preferred in the poor surgical candidate.

Pearls

1. Wegener granulomatosis, now referred to as granulomatosis with polyangiitis (GPA), affects the upper airway, kidneys, and lungs, and can present to the otolaryngologist as epistaxis, hearing loss, or subglottic stenosis.
2. Conditions to be considered in a patient with refractory epistaxis associated with thrombocytopenia include: massive hemorrhage, disseminated intravascular coagulation (and associated underlying medical issues such as sepsis), thrombotic microangiopathy, heparin or other drug-induced thrombocytopenia, idiopathic thrombocytopenic purpura, and bone marrow suppression.
3. A patient who requires posterior nasal packing should be admitted to the hospital and placed on telemetry and continuous pulse oximetry.
4. In general, endoscopic sphenopalatine artery ligation for posterior epistaxis is both more effective and more cost-beneficial than arterial embolization.
5. A teenage male presenting with unilateral nasal obstruction and epistaxis should raise suspicion for juvenile nasopharyngeal angiofibroma (JNA). JNA is a rare, highly vascularized benign tumor that originates near the medial pterygopalatine fossa (PPF). Diagnosis is made by classic history and radiology (widening of the PPF and anterior bowing of the posterior maxillary sinus wall, or Holman-Miller sign); biopsy should be avoided due to risk of hemorrhage.

QUESTIONS

1. **Discuss the epidemiology of epistaxis.**
   Epistaxis commonly occurs in all age groups with a bimodal distribution in the young and the elderly. The vast majority of episodes are benign and self-limited. Epistaxis can be broadly categorized into childhood versus adult epistaxis, or primary versus secondary epistaxis, which is important for diagnostic and therapeutic decision-making.

2. **What blood vessels supply the nasal mucosa?**
   The anterior and posterior ethmoid arteries supply the superior nasal cavity and septum; they arise from the ophthalmic branch of the internal carotid artery. The sphenopalatine artery is the terminal branch of the internal maxillary artery (from the external carotid circulation), and supplies the

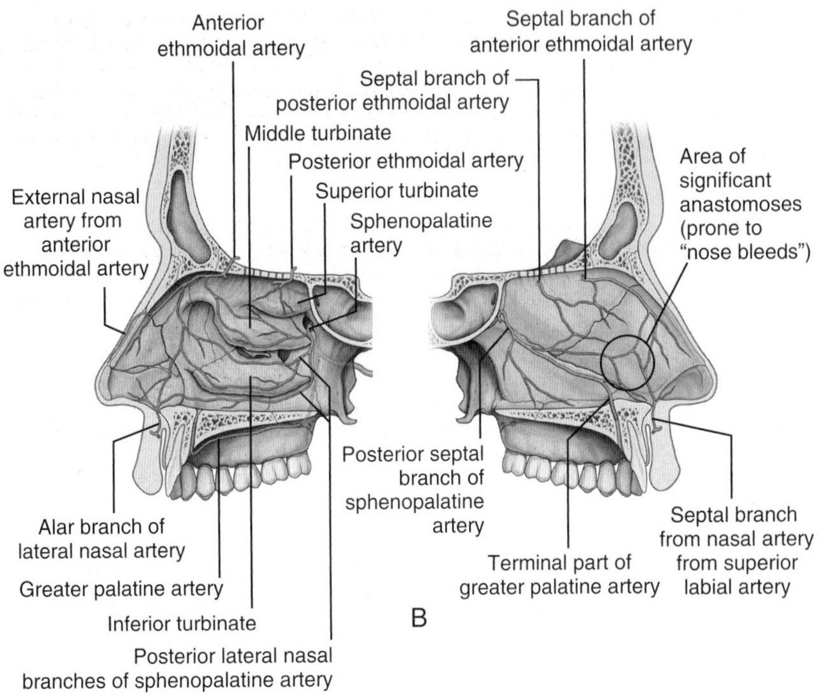

Figure 23-1. Arterial supply of the nasal cavities. **A**, Lateral wall of the right nasal cavity. **B**, Septum (medial wall of right nasal cavity). *(From Drake RL, Vogl AW, Mitchel AWM: Gray's Anatomy for Students, 2 ed, St Louis, 2009, Elsevier.)*

posterior lateral nasal wall and nasal cavity. The facial artery, also from the external carotid distrubition, provides additional supply to the anterior nasal cavity (Figure 23-1).

3. **What is Kiesselbach's plexus? What is Woodruff's plexus? Where are they located?**
Kiesselbach's plexus is a confluence of vessels arising from both the internal and external carotid artery systems. It supplies an area on the anterior-inferior nasal septum known as Little's area, the most common site for epistaxis.
Woodruff's plexus is a plexus of thin-walled veins located posteriorly in the inferior meatus. This area was previously thought to be arterial and also thought to be a main contributor to posterior bleeds, but this does not appear to be the case.

4. **What is meant by "anterior" and "posterior" epistaxis?**
The majority of bleeds (90% to 95%) originate anteriorly; many of the anterior bleeds occur in Little's area within Kiesselbach's plexus. Occurring much more often than posterior bleeds because of their location (nose picking/local trauma, dryness), anterior bleeds are easily accessible and managed with conservative measures such as moisturization, pressure, decongestion, or topical cautery. Posterior bleeds are generally from the distribution of the sphenopalatine artery. The exact focus of origin is more challenging to identify, and these bleeds are therefore more likely to require nasal packing as part of intervention.

5. **What should be included in the history evaluation of a patient with new-onset epistaxis?**
In the emergent setting, emphasis should be placed on managing airway, breathing, and circulation, with volume replacement as needed with crystalloid +/– blood products as needed, and a focused

history to expedite locating the source by nasal endoscopy and controlling hemorrhage. In the nonemergent setting, a careful and thorough history and physical exam can be obtained. The history should include timing, frequency, sidedness, and severity of epistaxis (which can be quantified by volume of observed blood or number of tissues), exploring predisposing conditions such as trauma, recent surgery, coagulopathy, cancer, medications and illicit drug use, contributory chronic medical issues, and current symptoms indicative of blood loss such as lightheadedness or dyspnea. Family history of bleeding disorder or epistaxis is worthy of inquiry, as well.

6. **What are the initial measures utilized to control mild epistaxis?**
(1) Instruct the patient to gently blow the nose. This removes blood/clots. (2) Intranasal administration of nasal decongestant spray such as oxymetazoline (a selective alpha-1 agonist/partial alpha-2 agonist). (3) Instruct the patient to pinch the nasal alae against the septum to apply hemostatic pressure, and hold for 10 to 15 minutes, or longer if needed. (4) Place a cold compress over the bridge of the nose, if available.

7. **Why is it helpful to have the patient lean forward in addition to the measures suggested in the previous question?**
Having the head tilted posteriorly may result in posterior drainage of blood, increasing the potential for bloody aspiration and/or gastric irritation with resultant bloody emesis. Additionally, having the blood fall back into the throat and be swallowed makes it difficult to quantify the amount of bleeding.

8. **What are the key components of the initial physical examination for an epistaxis patient?**
Initial physical evaluation should include ensuring patency of the airway, appropriate breathing and circulation (ABCs), obtaining vital signs, and checking mental status. Check for signs of shock (anxiety, cool/clammy skin, oliguria or anuria, weakness, pallor, diaphoresis, altered mentation), and signs of coagulopathy, such as petechiae or purpura.

9. **How is the nose examined in the epistaxis evaluation?**
Anesthesia can be provided by using anesthetic/analgesic-soaked topical sprays or cotton strips, with preparations such as 2% lidocaine or 4% cocaine. Oxymetazoline can also be given for its vasoconstrictive action; phenylephrine spray may alternatively be used. The patient may expectorate blood/clots as tolerated to better visualize the nasal cavity, and maintain the sniffing position.
A nasal speculum should be used initially, and suction can be used to help remove blood and clots. Inspect relevant anatomic locations such as Kiesselbach's plexus, septum, and turbinates. In addition to bleeding, the clinician can discover ulcerations, excoriations, and erosion of the mucosa. This will be sufficient for most anterior bleeds, but may not be for many posterior bleeds. Endoscopy should be utilized if the source of bleeding is not clear on anterior rhinoscopy, posterior epistaxis is suspected on history, conservative measures have not been successful, or a tumor or lesion is suspected on history.

10. **Should you obtain bloodwork in the above evaluation?**
It is not currently recommended to obtain routine CBC or coagulation studies in the initial assessment, unless the history is suggestive of significant blood loss, repeated large episodes, suspicion of coagulopathy, or current use of anticoagulant medication.

11. **What is primary versus secondary epistaxis? After determining if the bleed is primary or secondary in nature, how should you proceed?**
Primary (idiopathic) epistaxis is a spontaneous bleed without any identified precipitant, while those with an identified cause are termed secondary. Primary epistaxis with an identified source, especially when anterior, should be treated with direct therapy measures such as topical emollients, application of topical hemostatic agents, and/or focal cauterization if necessary. Posterior primary bleeds can be treated with nasal packing, chemical and/or electrocautery, arterial ligation or embolization.
In secondary epistaxis, the underlying disorder needs to be addressed in addition to resuscitative efforts and local modalities. Common causes of secondary epistaxis include liver disease, hematologic disorders (e.g., leukemia), anticoagulant medications such as warfarin or antiplatelet agents (see Controversies section for further discussion). Other causes of secondary epistaxis include trauma, recent surgery, hereditary disorders, and neoplasms.

12. **Describe the treatment of epistaxis in the pediatric population.**
In children with recurrent epistaxis, a recommended treatment option is antiseptic cream (chlorhexidine/neomycin). Unilateral cauterization with silver nitrate also seems to be safe and effective. It is rare for children to require surgical intervention.

13. **Describe the placement of an anterior nasal pack.**
Anterior packing can be performed with either gauze or nasal tampons that expand with the addition of saline. A nasal tampon is placed by first applying topical anesthetic/analgesic intranasally, and coating the pack with antibiotic ointment (this serves as both lubrication and possibly prevention of toxic shock syndrome), sliding the tampon into place, and expanding with saline application. Balloon/merocel combinations have also been utilized, and are another effective method for temporary epistaxis control. Petroleum-impregnated gauze can also be used with antibiotic ointment, placed intranasally with bayonet forceps and layered top to bottom/back to front until tamponade is achieved.
Other custom-fashioned hemostatic packs can be used in similar fashion, such as an absorbable gelatin sponge wrapped in oxydized cellulose dressing.

14. **How is silver nitrate chemical cautery applied?**
Bleeding must be of minimal severity for silver nitrate to be successful, and ideally unilateral to avoid bilateral cauterization which can carry a risk of septal perforation. The mucosa needs to be relatively dry for the silver nitrate to take effect, so topical decongestant and pressure is applied first to slow bleeding. The silver nitrate stick should be focally placed at the origin of the bleed, holding the tip of the applicator stick against the mucosa until the mucosa becomes gray, working from the periphery to the center of the bleeding site; it should not take any longer than 10 seconds until graying occurs. Silver nitrate works by cauterizing superficial blood vessels in the nose. Topical saline or decongestant is applied to halt the chemical reaction once the desired effect is achieved.

15. **Describe the placement of posterior packs and their associated complications.**
A posterior pack can be performed with insertion of a cotton pack or Foley catheter. A small red rubber tube is carefully inserted in the nose, passed through the oropharynx, and the end is retrieved through the mouth using a ring forceps. On the oral end of the tube, a cotton pack is attached with silk ties. The tube is gently pulled anterio-inferiorly from the nasal side until the pack passes through the oropharynx to a resting place in the nasopharynx and posterior choana. The anterior nasal cavity may be packed subsequently, and the tube is fastened externally while care is taken not to exert excessive pressure on the nasal ala. The patient should be admitted for telemetry and pulse oximetry, and antibiotic therapy.
Potential complications include pain, discomfort, respiratory difficulty (including aspiration of the packing material), infection (as well as toxic shock syndrome, sinusitis from blocking outflow tracts), alar/septal necrosis, and pharyngeal fibrosis/stenosis. Supplemental oxygen may be required; telemetry monitoring is required given the risk of arrhythmia and syncope.

16. **What are surgical interventions for persistent epistaxis?**
Endoscopic diathermy, laser photocoagulation, septal surgery, arterial ligation, and embolization can be used for persistent bleeding. Endoscopic sphenopalatine artery ligation or even internal maxillary artery ligation is now frequently used in the management of posterior epistaxis. In the past, the transantral approach was used but is associated with avoidable complications such as oroantral fistula and dysesthesia. Endoscopic sphenopalatine artery ligation has been highly successful as well as cost-saving for overall hospitalization when compared to nasal packing or embolization.

17. **How do SPA ligation and embolization compare in the management of epistaxis?**
Embolization results in almost twice the hospital cost compared to that of surgical ligation, and does not carry the same effectiveness in bleeding control. Although it carries a low risk of major complication, embolization may be a nice alternative in patients who cannot tolerate general anesthesia or are otherwise not good surgical candidates.

18. **List a broad differential for new-onset nasal bleeding.**
- Environmental: Cold air/dry air can be compounded by central heating systems for rooms that are not humidified (dryness results in mucosal irritation)

- Trauma: Most commonly digital trauma (nose picking), but can also be from other local trauma/facial trauma, foreign body, surgery
- Inflammatory (exacerbated by upper respiratory infections, sinusitis, environmental or other allergies, drugs/chemicals) or autoimmune
- Medications: Antiplatelet agents or anticoagulants, nasal sprays
- Vascular: Arterial aneurysm or pseudoaneurysm
- Congenital/Developmental: Septal abnormality such as deviation or perforation
- Genetic: Osler-Weber-Rendu syndrome/hereditary hemorrhagic telangiectasia (HHT)
- Systemic disorders: Arteriosclerosis, hypertension, blood dyscrasias (von Willebrand, paraneoplastic effects, liver disease, hemophilias, thrombocytopenia)
- Neoplastic: Benign or malignant processes

19. **What are some medications, including complementary and alternative medicines, that may contribute to epistaxis?**
Aspirin, clopidogrel, warfarin or other forms of anticoagulation; intranasal steroids; nasal cannula oxygen; chemotherapy. Herbal medicines that confer antiplatelet effects or affect the liver's CYP3A4 enzymes, including fish oil, evening primrose, garlic, cranberry juice, vitamin E, echinacea, ginseng, St. John's wort, ginkgo biloba, ginger, kava, and saw palmetto.

20. **What is Osler-Weber-Rendu syndrome/hereditary hemorrhagic telangiectasia (HHT)?**
HHT is an autosomal dominant disorder characterized by vascular malformations that does not manifest at birth but rather as one ages. Diagnostic criteria include spontaneous/recurrent epistaxis, mucocutaneous telangiectasias, visceral involvement (e.g., hepatic, pulmonary, cerebral, gastrointestial arteriovenous malformations), and an affected first-degree relative (known as Curacao criteria). Generally, epistaxis is the first manifestation of the disease, occurring during childhood. Epistaxis management includes utilization of topical emollients, topical cautery or packing in acute events, laser photocoagulation or oblation of lesions, septodermoplasty, or nasal closure in extreme cases. Newer experimental therapies including antiangiogenic medications and sclerotherapy are being investigated.

21. **A patient presents with epistaxis from a nasal mucosal ulcer. What is the differential diagnosis? Describe the workup.**
Nasal cavity ulcerations should be treated conservatively and worked up if they do not spontaneously resolve, or when suspicion for underlying tumor is present (pain, numbness, smoking history). Epistaxis may be the first sign of malignancy, granulomatosis with polyangiitis, sarcoidosis, lupus, syphilis, leprosy, tuberculosis, and occupational irritants.
Nasal biopsies should always be performed when a malignancy is suspected, and when an underlying autoimmune disorder is suspected. Recent studies have suggested that biopsies to rule out autoimmune disease are not mandatory in the absence of any nasal or systematic signs of vasculitis, and with negative c-ANCA and ACE test results.

CONTROVERSIES

22. **What is the recommended medical management for an epistaxis patient currently on anticoagulation for cardiac disease?**
    1. Obtain a complete blood count including platelets, +PT/INR if taking warfarin, for all patients.
    2. If the patient has a metal heart valve, INR dictates warfarin administration (if overanticoagulated, hold until INR is therapeutic; if INR is therapeutic, continue current regimen).
    3. If life-threatening bleeding occurs in a patient with a metal heart valve, care planning should be discussed with the cardiologist prior to discontinuing aspirin if a coronary stent is in place, as platelet transfusions may be utilized.
    4. For all other patients (without metal heart valve), aspirin or clopidogrel should be continued, but if a life-threatening bleed occurs discussion with the cardiologist about the utility of platelet transfusion should also occur.
    5. These patients should also continue warfarin if therapeutic and have it withheld if overanticoagulated.

23. **What is the role of antibiotic prophylaxis with nasal packing?**
It is controversial whether or not to administer systemic antibiotics prophylactically for prevention of toxic shock syndrome in patients who undergo nasal packing. Toxic shock syndrome is an extremely rare complication and as a result, appropriate studies are lacking. Although controversial, antibiotic administration with nasal packing is commonly performed. If used, the antibiotic chosen should have staphylococcal coverage (e.g., amoxicillin-clavulanate).

24. **What is the link between hypertension and epistaxis?**
Several case series demonstrate a relationship between hypertension and epistaxis, although population-based studies have not confirmed this relationship. Even if not a causative factor, elevated blood pressure may be associated with patient anxiety surrounding epistaxis and intervention, and may slow resolution. The best approach is to offer reassurance and treat the hypertension if possible, as this may worsen the epistaxis if left untreated.

Bibliography

Biswas D, Mal RK: Are systemic prophylactic antibiotics indicated with anterior nasal packing for spontaneous epistaxis?, *Acta Otolaryngol* 129(2):179, 2009.

Chiu TW, Shaw-Dunn J, McGarry GW: Woodruff's plexus, *J Laryngol Otol* 122(10):1074–1077, 2008.

Current Opinion in Otolaryngology & Head and Neck Surgery: Issue 19(1):P 30-35, 2011.

Douglas R, Wormald PJ: Update on epistaxis, *Curr Opin Otolaryngol Head Neck Surg* 15(3):180–183, 2007.

French A: Case 2: A teenage boy with epistaxis, *Paediatr Child Health* 14(2):99–102, 2009.

Moore KL, Dalley AF, Agur AM: *Clinically Oriented Anatomy*, ed 6, Philadelphia, 2010, Lippincott Williams & Wilkins, p 959.

Riviello RJ: Otolaryngologic procedures. In *Clinical Procedures in Emergency Medicine*, ed 4, Philadelphia, 2004, WB Saunders, p 1300.

Shakeel M, Trinidade A, Iddamalgoda T, et al: Routine clotting screen has no role in the management of epistaxis: reiterating the point, *Eur Arch Otorhinolaryngol* 267(10):1641–1644, 2010.

Soyka MB, Nikolaou G, Rufibach K, et al: On the effectiveness of treatment options in epistaxis: an analysis of 678 interventions, *Rhinology* 49(4):474–478, 2011.

Villwock JA, Jones K: Recent trends in epistaxis management in the United States: 2008–2010, *JAMA Otolaryngol Head Neck Surg* 139(12):1279–1284, 2013.

Walker FDL, Rutter C, McGarry GW: The use of anticoagulants in epistaxis patients, *Rhinology* 46(346), 2008.

Wax MK, American Academy of Otolaryngology: *Primary Care Otolaryngology*, ed 3, Alexandria, VA, 2011, Head and Neck Surgery Foundation.

www.uptodate.com/contents/contents/approach-to-the-adult-with-epistaxis?source=search_result&search=epistaxis&selectedTitle=1%7E150.

CHAPTER 24

RHINITIS

Lindsay K. Finkas, MD and Rohit K. Katial, MD, FAAAAI, FACP

KEY POINTS

1. Allergic rhinitis can present with seasonal or perennial symptoms.
2. β2 transferrin present on nasal discharge indicates CSF leak.
3. Rhinitis medicamentosa is associated with use of over-the-counter intranasal decongestants that contain α-adrenergic compounds for more than 3 to 5 days.
4. Allergen immunotherapy is the only disease-modifying treatment available for allergic rhinitis.

Pearls

1. There is a strong overlap of asthma and allergic nasal disease in patients.
2. Smoking and work exposures can trigger nonallergic rhinitis.
3. Surgery is reserved for refractory cases of rhinitis that have failed medical management.
4. Skin testing is rarely associated with anaphylaxis and is a relative contraindication in pregnant patients.

QUESTIONS

1. **What is rhinitis?**
   Rhinitis is tissue inflammation and nasal hyperfunction that leads to nasal congestion, obstruction, rhinorrhea, nasal itching, and/or sneezing. Although rhinitis is generally not life-threatening, it is associated with significant loss of productivity and decreased quality of life.

2. **How is rhinitis classified?**
   Rhinitis may be classified into structural, noninflammatory, and inflammatory etiologies. Noninflammatory causes of rhinitis include nonallergic rhinitis, gustatory rhinitis, hormone induced rhinitis, atrophic rhinitis, CSF leak, and drug induced rhinitis. Inflammatory rhinitis includes allergic rhinitis, infectious rhinitis, nonallergic rhinitis with eosinophilia, nasal polyps, and rhinitis associated with systemic disease.

3. **What are structural causes of rhinitis?**
   Concha bullosa, nasal polyps, septal deviation, adenoid enlargement, sinonasal tumors, and nasal foreign bodies can cause rhinitis. Nasal foreign body is a more common finding in the pediatric population. Nasal polyps are both structural and inflammatory in nature, with associated obstructive nasal symptoms, and may be accompanied by asthma or aspirin exacerbated respiratory disease.

4. **How does one distinguish clear rhinorrhea of rhinitis from CSF leak?**
CSF leak presents with clear rhinorrhea and oftentimes has a unilateral presentation. There is generally a history of preceding trauma though CSF leak can be spontaneous or idiopathic. Approximately 70% to 80% of CSF rhinorrhea is attributed to accidental trauma. If there is any doubt about a diagnosis CSF leak, qualitative β2-transferrin of nasal discharge is checked. β2 transferrin is found only in the CSF and its presence in nasal discharge therefore indicates CSF leak.

5. **What is non-allergic rhinitis with eosinophilia (NARES) and how is it differentiated from allergic rhinitis?**
NARES is a perennial cause of rhinitis and common symptoms include congestion and clear nasal discharge. Nasal cytology demonstrates increased levels of eosinophils similar to allergic rhinitis, though these patients do not have sensitization on skin prick testing or specific IgE blood tests.

6. **What is rhinitis medicamentosa and how is it treated?**
Rhinitis medicamentosa is rebound congestion that occurs with long-term use of intranasal decongestants that contain α-adrenergic compounds such as phenylephrine, oxymetolazine, or xylometolazine. Rebound effect is due to downregulation of α-adrenergic receptors as well as desensitization. Nasal sprays containing these medications should be limited to 3 to 5 days of use to avoid the rebound effect. Treatment of rhinitis medicamentosa involves weaning the intranasal decongestant spray, the addition of intranasal corticosteroids, and in some cases systemic corticosteroids. In refractory cases, inferior turbinate reduction may be needed.

7. **What is hormonal rhinitis?**
Hormonal rhinitis is most often seen in pregnant women and about 20% to 30% of pregnant women will develop rhinitis of pregnancy. It is felt that rhinitis of pregnancy is due to changes in estrogen and progesterone though the mechanism remains undetermined. Symptoms generally resolve within 2 weeks after delivery. Hypothyroidism has also been implicated as a potential cause of chronic rhinitis.

8. **What is atrophic rhinitis?**
Atrophic rhinitis is characterized by nasal dryness and congestion. Symptoms of atrophic rhinitis include crusting, purulent nasal discharge, nasal obstruction, and halitosis. This form of rhinitis typically presents in middle-aged populations. The cause of primary atrophic rhinitis is unknown and it is uncommon in North America, but has increased prevalence in areas with warm temperatures. Secondary atrophic rhinitis is seen in individuals who have undergone multiple aggressive sinonasal surgeries, but is also associated with trauma and granulomatous diseases. Secondary atrophic rhinitis is typically seen in an older population.

9. **What is work-related rhinitis?**
Work-related rhinitis is rhinitis that is associated with environmental exposures. Occupational rhinitis has a prevalence of approximately 5% to 15% worldwide. The rhinitis may be allergic or nonallergic and is further divided based on the substance causing the symptoms. Provoking substances may be irritants, corrosives or immunogens. Irritants include perfumes, paints, dust, and smoke. Corrosive rhinitis is associated with high levels of exposure to chemicals such as chlorine, sulfur dioxide, and ammonia. Immunologic exposure results in an IgE mediated response and include animal danders and grains. To diagnose work-related rhinitis it is helpful to have patients keep a diary of the timing of their symptoms.

10. **What is gustatory rhinitis?**
Gustatory rhinitis is a noninflammatory rhinitis that presents with symptoms of rhinorrhea and/or postnasal drip following eating. It is more common with spicy or hot foods and is also more common in the elderly. Current prevalence is unknown and the mechanism is thought to be due to parasympathetic activation.

11. **What are the common drugs associated with rhinitis?**
Angiotensin-converting enzyme inhibitors, β-adrenergic blockers, amiloride, hydralazine, many psychotropic medications, and phosphdiesterase-5 inhibitors.

12. **What are "allergic salute," "allergic shiners," and "allergic gape"?**
Patients (particularly children) with persistent rhinorrhea often wipe the nose in an upward direction with the palm of the hand, which has been referred to as the allergic salute. Consequently, these patients may have a horizontal crease in the skin of the lower nose by the tip. Also, patients with allergic rhinitis can have darkened areas under their eyes, which are referred to as allergic shiners which are caused by swelling and congestion of small blood vessels beneath the skin. The allergic gape is a characteristic open mouth from nasal obstruction causing mouth breathing.

13. **How can allergic rhinitis be differentiated from other causes of rhinitis?**
Generally seasonal allergic rhinitis has a seasonal variation and symptoms cease after the first frost. Physical exam findings suggestive of allergic rhinitis include pale, boggy nasal turbinates, allergic shiners, and allergic salute. Skin testing and specific IgE testing are also useful to differentiate allergic from nonallergic rhinitis. Nasal cytology may also be performed; however, this is not commonly used. Specific allergen challenges have also been utilized in research settings.

14. **How is allergic rhinitis classified?**
Allergic rhinitis is classified based on severity and frequency. Intermittent allergic rhinitis has symptoms on fewer than 4 days per week or for less than 4 weeks. Persistent allergic rhinitis is symptoms that occur for more than 4 days per week or more than 4 weeks. Severity is divided into mild and moderate/severe. Mild disease has normal sleep and no impairment of daily activities, sports, and leisure. Mild disease does not interfere with school and work. Moderate to severe disease must have at least one of the following present: sleep disturbance; impairment of daily activities, leisure, and/or sport; impairment of school or work; or troublesome symptoms.

15. **What is the pathophysiology of allergic rhinitis?**
Allergens in the nasal mucosa are phagocytized by antigen presenting cells that present antigens to CD4 lymphocytes. Presentation to CD4 T-cells involves peptide presentation via the MCH class II complex. CD4+ T-cells then differentiate into a TH2 subset, where IL-4, IL-5, and IL-13 mediate eosinophil recruitment and survival. IL-4 and IL-13 are also necessary to promote the secretion of IgE from B-cells. The allergic response involves an early and late phase. Early phase reactions occur within minutes of exposure to the allergen and are due to release of preformed mediators in mast cells and basophils that are primed with IgE. Specific allergen binding promotes release of these mediators including histamine, tryptase prostaglandin D2, leukotriene C4, leukotriene B4, major basic protein, and platelet-activating factor. This results in symptoms of pruritus, sneezing, congestion, and rhinorrhea. Late phase reactions occur hours after allergen exposure and peak at 6 hours following exposure. Late reaction symptoms are primarily nasal congestion. Late phase reactions involve cellular infiltration and recruitment to the nasal mucosa and involve eosinophils, neutrophils, monocytes, and basophils, leading to longer-standing inflammation (Figure 24-1).

16. **Identify the classic seasons in which particular pollens are present.**
- Tree: Spring
- Grass: Spring/Summer
- Weeds: Summer/Fall

17. **What are perennial allergens?**
Perennial allergens include animal dander (cat, dog), dust mites, cockroaches, and molds.

18. **What is the role of surgery in treatment of rhinitis?**
Surgery is used in those with significant structural disease such as septal deviation and nasal polyps. Turbinate reduction may be considered in patients refractory to medical therapies.

19. **What are general classes of medications available in the treatment of rhinitis?**
Corticosteroids, both topical and systemic, are effective therapy for treatment of both inflammatory and noninflammatory causes of rhinitis. Topical and oral antihistamines are also available

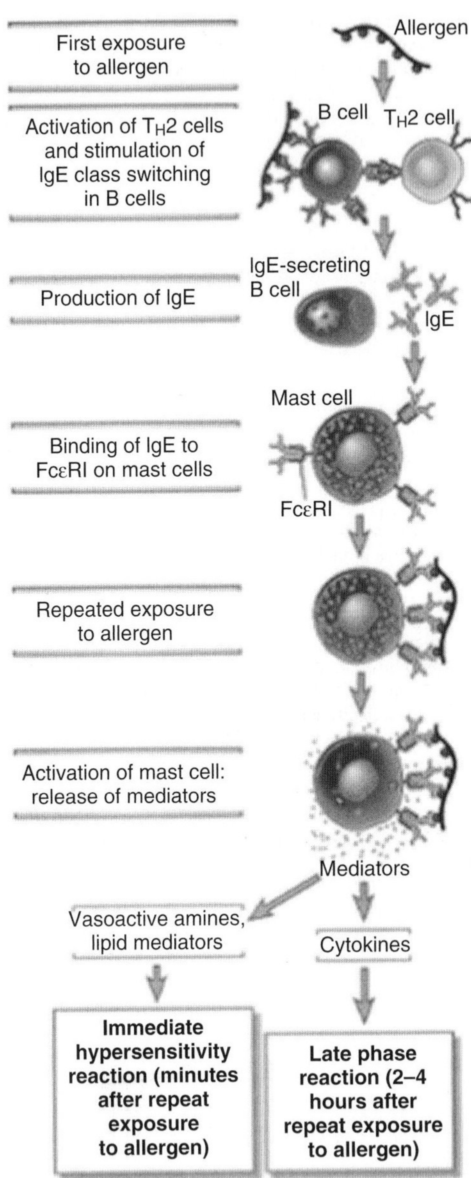

Figure 24-1. Immediate hypersensitivity diseases are initiated by the introduction of an allergen, which stimulates T_H2 reactions and IgE production. IgE sensitizes mast cells by binding to FcεRI, and subsequent exposure to the allergen activates the mast cells to secrete the mediators responsible for the pathologic reactions of immediate hypersensitivity. *(From Abbas A, Lichtman, Pillai S: IgE-dependent immune responses and allergic disease. In Cellular and Molecular Immunology. Elsevier Saunders, 2012, p. 425–444.)*

Table 24-1. Medication Class and Effectiveness in Treating Symptoms of Rhinitis

DRUG CLASS	RHINORRHEA	NASAL ITCH	SNEEZING	CONGESTION	OCULAR SYMPTOMS
Nasal Steroids	+	+	+	+	–/+
Oral Antihistamines	+	+	+	–	+
Intranasal Antihistamines	+	+	+	+	+
Decongestants (oral and nasal)	–	–	–	+	–
Antileukotrienes	+	–/+	+	–/+	–/+
Chromones	–/+	–/+	–/+	–/+	–
Nasal Anticholinergic	+	–	–	–	–

+ is effective, – is not effective and –/+ is possibly effective.

treatments. Intranasal anticholinergics are useful for rhinorrhea. Topical chromones that work as mast cell stabilizers and antileukotrienes may also be used in allergic rhinitis. Topical and oral decongestants are also available for temporary treatment of rhinitis over the counter, but have significant side effects if used extensively. See Table 24-1.

20. **What are the disadvantages of oral decongestants?**
Oral decongestants are associated with tachycardia and elevated blood pressure and should be avoided in hypertensive patients. Additional adverse effects include tremor, insomnia, dizziness, and irritability.

21. **What are common side effects of intranasal steroids?**
Intranasal steroids may cause dryness, epistaxis, nasal irritation or stinging, or rarely septal perforation. Caution should also be taken in using intranasal steroids in patients with increased intraocular pressure.

22. **What is unique about treatment with allergy immunotherapy?**
Immunotherapy is the only disease-modifying treatment available and is effective in treatment of allergic rhinitis. Allergy immunotherapy results in an initial increase in IgE followed by a slow decrease in specific IgE. This is followed by an increase in allergen-specific IgG. It is also believed that treatment with allergy immunotherapy results in a shift from a Th2 response to a Th1 mediated response, as well as induction of T regulatory cells. The effects may also be long lasting after discontinuing treatment.

Bibliography

Abbas A, Lichtman A, Pillai S: IgE-dependent immune responses and allergic disease. In *Cellular and Molecular Immunology*, Philadelphia, 2012, Elsevier Saunders, pp 425–444.

Allen MW, Schwartz DL, Rana V, et al: Long-term radiotherapy outcomes for nasal cavity and septal cancers, *Int J Radiat Oncol Biol Phys* 71:401, 2008.

Bernstein JA: Characterizing rhinitis subtypes, *Am J Rhinol Allergy* 27(6):457–460, 2013.

Corren J, Fauad MB, Pawankar R: Allergic and nonallergic rhinits. In Franklin Adkinson N Jr, et al, editors: *Middleton's Allergy: Principles and Practice*, ed 8, Philadelphia, 2014, Elsevier Saunders, pp 664–684.

Durham SR, Walker SM, Varga EM, et al: Long-term clinical efficacy of grass-pollen immunotherapy, *N Engl J Med* 341(7):468–475, 1999.

Gautrin D, Desrosiers M, Castano R: Occupational rhinitis, *Curr Opin Allergy Clin Immunol* 6:77, 2006.

Greiner AN, Hellings PW, Rotiroti G, et al: Allergic rhinitis, *Lancet* 378:2112, 2011.

Kerr JT, Chu FW, Bayles SW: Cerebrospinal fluid rhinorrhea: diagnosis and management, *Otolaryngol Clin North Am* 38(4):597–611, 2005.

Meltzer EO, Bukstein DA: The economic impact of allergic rhinitis and current guidelines for treatment, *Ann Allergy Asthma Immunol* 106(2 Suppl):S12–S16, 2011.

Wallace DV, Dykewicz MS, Bernstein DI, et al: The diagnosis and management of rhinitis: an updated practice parameter, *J Allergy Clin Immunol* 122:S1, 2008.

ACUTE RHINOSINUSITIS AND INFECTIOUS COMPLICATIONS

Jeffrey Chain, MD

CHAPTER 25

KEY POINTS

1. Antibiotics are frequently administered for acute rhinosinusitis, but guidelines supporting appropriate use should be followed.
2. Infectious complications of rhinosinusitis are rare, but can include orbital and intracranial spread.
3. Acute invasive fungal sinusitis must be suspected in diabetic or immunocompromised patients with acute, rapidly progressive disease.

Pearls

1. Viruses are usually responsible for the symptoms in acute rhinosinusitis, not bacteria.
2. Know the Chandler classification for orbital infection: I, preseptal cellulitis; II, orbital cellulitis; III, subperiosteal abscess; IV, orbital abscess; V, cavernous sinus thrombosis.
3. Acute infectious complications of the frontal lobe may result from spread of infection through venous channels directly communicating from the frontal sinus.

QUESTIONS

1. How is acute rhinosinusitis defined?
   Acute rhinosinusitis is symptomatic inflammation of the nasal and paranasal sinus mucosa for up to 4 weeks. The most common causes of this condition are viral and bacterial infections. Recurrent acute rhinosinusitis (RARS) is defined as four or more episodes of ABRS per year without persistent symptoms between episodes.

2. What is the pathophysiology of acute rhinosinusitis?
   Inflammation of the nasal and paranasal sinus mucosa with subsequent edema is the initiating factor in this disease. Most often, this inflammation is caused by viral URI and/or allergic rhinitis. This edema can cause obstruction of normal sinus drainage, impaired mucociliary clearance and altered local immune system function. These changes create an ideal environment for pathogen colonization and growth.

3. How common is acute rhinosinusitis?
   Rhinosinusitis is a major burden on the healthcare system with 13.4% of adults diagnosed with RS annually. The incidence tends to be higher for women (almost two-fold), and adults aged 45 to 74 years are most commonly affected. ARS is the fifth leading indication for antibiotic prescriptions; 21% of antibiotics prescribed for adults are for ARS.

4. How common are infectious complications of acute rhinosinusitis?
   Infectious complications of ARS are extremely rare in immunocompetent individuals with a rate of less than 0.01% per episode of ARS in children, and even less in adults. In immunocompromised patients (diabetes mellitus, HIV positive, immunosuppressed due to chemotherapy) the complication rate is likely higher.

5. **How can the clinician differentiate viral rhinosinusitis (VRS) from acute bacterial rhinosinusitis (ABRS)?**
   Specific signs and symptoms and their timing are the most important history items in diagnosing ABRS. Symptoms required to diagnose ABRS are purulent rhinorrhea, nasal obstruction, and facial pressure or pain. Occasionally fever and hyposmia are considered as "major" symptoms required for the diagnosis. The following are considered "minor" symptoms: cough (more common in children), malaise, maxillary tooth pain, and ear fullness or pressure. The generally accepted time course for ABRS is persistent symptoms for at least 10 days (but less than 12 weeks) or worsening symptoms after 5 days that were initially improving ("double-sickening" or "worsening course"). Also warranting consideration of ABRS are patients with severe symptoms lasting 3 to 4 days that include high fever (>39° C) and purulent nasal discharge or facial pain.

6. **What bacteria are the most common pathogens in ABRS?**
   Understanding the bacteriology of ARS is paramount to choosing the most effective antibiotic regimen to treat the disease. *Streptococcus pneumoniae, Haemophilus influenzae,* and *Moraxella catarrhalis* (more common in children) are generally accepted as the most common pathogens in this disease. *Streptococcus pyogenes, Staphylococcus aureus,* gram-negative bacilli, and anaerobes are less common.

7. **What is the relevance of antibiotic resistant organisms and vaccination in ABRS?**
   H. influenzae (30%) and *M. catarrhalis* (90%) have an increasing prevalence of beta-lactamase producing organisms. *S. pneumoniae* prevalence seems to be decreasing due to pneumococcal vaccination. However, its resistance to penicillin and macrolides is approximately 30%. Knowledge of regional antibiotic resistance is important to help guide therapy.

8. **What are the goals of treatment of ABRS?**
   In treating ABRS, the clinician's primary goals are attempting to decrease the duration and severity of symptoms, prevent infectious complications, prevent progression to chronic rhinosinusitis (CRS), and restore the patient's quality of life. Secondary goals include minimizing side effects of medications and unnecessary antibiotics that could promote resistant organisms.

9. **When should antibiotics be prescribed for ABRS?**
   Studies in both adult and pediatric patients confirm that patients with ABRS treated with antibiotics experience more rapid resolution of symptoms when compared with placebo. If stringent criteria are used for establishing the diagnosis, empiric antimicrobial therapy should be started as soon as the diagnosis of ABRS is made. Another option of "watchful waiting" or "observation" has been described, when antibiotics are withheld unless the patient does not improve with symptomatic management. Some studies cite a 60% to 70% chance of spontaneous improvement in patients with ABRS by 7 to 12 days, which supports the "watchful waiting" approach.

10. **Which antibiotic should be prescribed for ABRS?**
    In both children and adults, amoxicillin or amoxicillin-clavulanate is recommended as initial empiric antimicrobial therapy. The preference for amoxicillin-clavulanate is due to increasing prevalence of beta-lactamase producing *H. influenzae* and *M. catarrhalis* since the use of pneumococcal vaccine. High-dose amoxicillin-clavulanate (90 mg/kg/day PO BID or 2 grams PO BID) is recommended in communities with high prevalence of penicillin-nonsusceptible *S. pneumoniae* or in high-risk patient populations for antibiotic resistance. Second-line antibiotics include macrolides (clarithromycin or azithromycin), trimethoprim-sulfamethoxazole (TMP-SMX), doxycycline, second or third generation cephalosporins (cefpodoxime, cefixime, cefdinir), clindamycin, and respiratory fluroquinolones (levofloxacin or moxifloxacin). Macrolides have an approximately 30% rate of resistance to *S. pneumoniae.* TMP-SMX has a 30% to 40% resistance to both *S. pneumoniae* and *H. influenzae.* Doxycycline can be used only in adults due to risk of staining teeth in children younger than 8 years old. In children, ceftriaxone single dose (50 mg/kg IV or IM) followed by an oral second or third generation cephalosporin is an option. Due to variable rates of resistance among *S. pneumoniae,* oral cephalosporins are recommended in combination with clindamycin.

11. **How long should antibiotics be prescribed and when should empiric antibiotics be changed if ineffective?**
    The optimal duration of antibiotic treatment is controversial. New guidelines recommend empiric antibiotics for 5 to 10 days in adults (termed "short-term" antibiotics) and 10 to 14 days in children

for uncomplicated ABRS. Other studies done in ABRS require patients to complete a 2 week course of antibiotic. If symptoms worsen after 48 to 72 hours or fail to improve after 3 to 7 days, patients should be evaluated for resistant pathogens or a noninfectious etiology.

12. **What other treatments, in addition to antibiotics, should be considered in ARS?**
Nasal saline irrigations and intranasal corticosteroids are usually the most commonly recommended adjuvant treatments for ARS. Topical or oral decongestants, antihistamines, and mucolytics are also commonly recommended. Some type of analgesia, usually initially in the form of acetaminophen and ibuprofen, should also be considered.

13. **What tests can be performed to help diagnose ABRS?**
The diagnosis of ABRS is made on history, especially in the outpatient clinic setting. Computed tomography (CT) of the paranasal sinuses is nonspecific and generally is not indicated in uncomplicated ABRS. Studies indicate that during uncomplicated viral URI, the majority of patients will have significant abnormalities seen on imaging. Culture from the sinus cavity recovering greater than 10^4 colony forming units (CFU) per mL is the gold standard for the diagnosis of ABRS. Due to issues of patient discomfort, time, and cost, endoscopic guided cultures of the middle meatus have been used as a surrogate for direct sinus cultures.

14. **When is testing appropriate in patients with ABRS?**
CT or MRI should be reserved for patients with RARS (more than four episodes per year), severe cases, or when suppurative complications are suspected. CT is generally the preferred initial modality and is superior for defining the bony anatomy of the paranasal sinuses. Contrast should be used if intraorbital or intracranial abscess is suspected. MRI with gadolinium is recommended if the clinician suspects central nervous system complications of ABRS. Endoscopic culture of the middle meatus can be very helpful, especially in patients at high risk for antibiotic resistance (age younger than 2 or older than 65, daycare, prior antibiotics within past month, recent hospitalization, comorbidities, immunosuppression). Sometimes an allergy/immunology evaluation can also be helpful in patients with RARS to identify concurrent predisposing factors causing mucosal inflammation.

15. **What are the suppurative complications of ABRS?**
Sequelae of ABRS can be divided into intraorbital and intracranial complications. The most common complication is orbital involvement and is due to ethmoid sinusitis. The second most common infectious complication is meningitis, usually due to sphenoid sinusitis. The third most common complications are epidural (Figure 25-1) or subdural abscesses due to frontal sinusitis. Brain

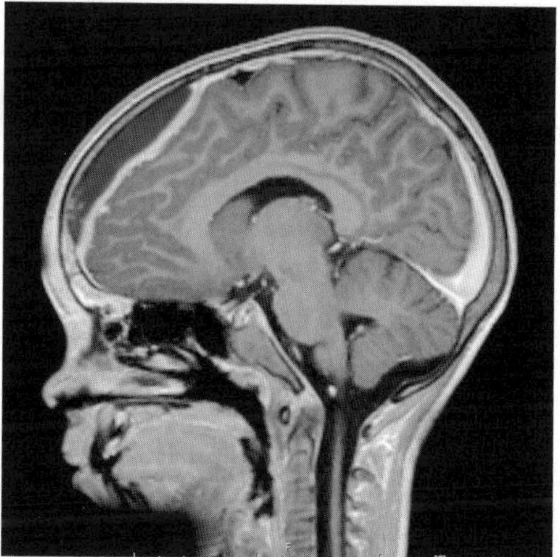

Figure 25-1. Large epidural abscess in MRI in 7-year-old with frontal sinusitis.

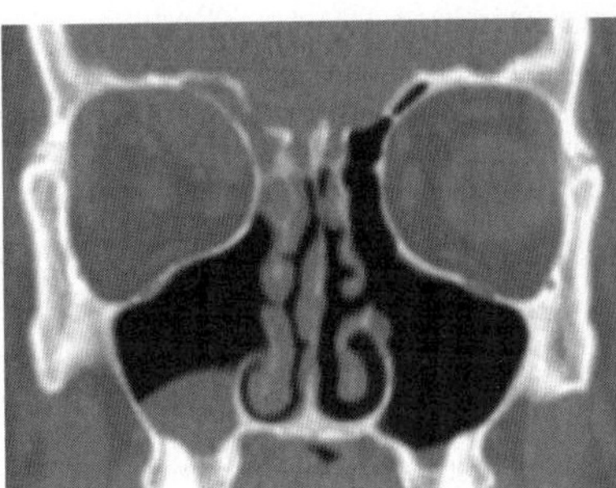
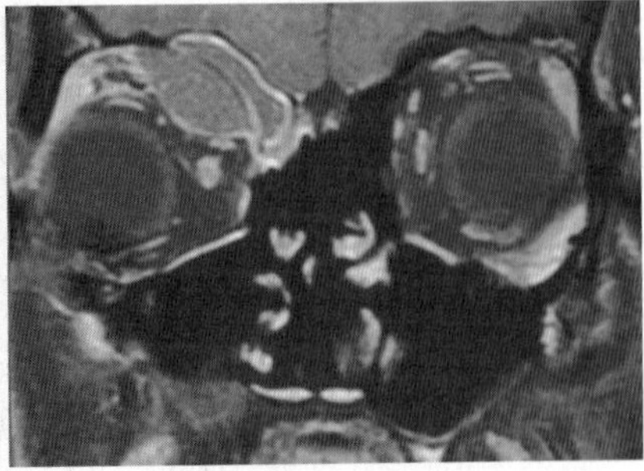

Figure 25-2. Right subperiosteal abscess of the orbit. Note the sinus disease in the right frontal sinus.

abscesses, venous thrombosis, mucocele or mucopyocele, and "Pott's puffy tumor" (osteomyelitis of the frontal bone) are also possible complications.

16. **How are orbital complications of ABRS classified?**
The Chandler classification, published in 1970, is still used to classify orbital complications of ABRS. Stage 1 is *preseptal cellulitis* and is thought to be due to impaired venous outflow from sinusitis and edema. The next stage is *orbital cellulitis* which causes impaired extraocular movements, proptosis, and chemosis. The third stage is a *subperiosteal abscess* in which pus accumulates between the lamina papyracea and the medial periorbita (Figure 25-2). Visual acuity can be impaired and the globe can become inferolaterally displaced. Stage 4 is *orbital abscess,* usually accompanied by severe visual impairment and complete ophthalmoplegia. The last stage is *cavernous sinus thrombosis* characterized by bilateral ocular symptoms among other central nervous system signs and symptoms.

17. **Is surgery required for subperiosteal orbital abscesses in children?**
Generally, small (<0.5 to 1 mL in volume) medially located abscesses without a decrease in visual acuity or systemic involvement can be managed medically. These patients require ophthalmologic evaluation and surgery is indicated if there is failure to improve within 24 to 48 hours, decreasing visual acuity, and/or progressive systemic involvement. Generally, ethmoidectomy and drainage of the abscess is the surgery of choice.

18. **How are intracranial complications of ABRS managed?**
Management of these complicated problems generally requires collaboration with a neurosurgeon and an infectious disease specialist. Broad-spectrum antibiotics with adequate penetration through the blood–brain barrier are required. Systemic steroids may be temporarily used to decrease inflammation. Usually the sinuses that harbor the infection require endoscopic surgical drainage. Also, surgery may be required to drain intracranial abscesses if they develop. For patients with thrombosis, anticoagulants are usually prescribed. Frequently these patients require intensive care unit monitoring.

19. **What is the role of fungi in acute rhinosinusitis?**
Fungal infections can cause rhinosinusitis in one of three ways. *Allergic fungal rhinosinusitis* occurs when atopic patients inhale fungi causing type I Ig-E mediated hypersensitivity and mucosal inflammation. Diagnosis is made in patients with nasal polyposis and allergies with presence of allergic mucin containing eosinophils, Charcot-Leyden crystals, and possibly fungal hyphae. *Fungus ball* or *mycetoma* is a noninvasive fungal infection usually occurring in nonatopic immunocompetent patients. *Invasive fungal sinusitis* occurs in immunocompromised patients and involves invasion of blood vessels and bony/soft tissue erosion. While all fungal ARS episodes are generally treated surgically to remove the fungal organism, *invasive fungal sinusitis* requires aggressive surgical debridement and systemic antifungal therapy due to its high morbidity and mortality (Figure 25-3).

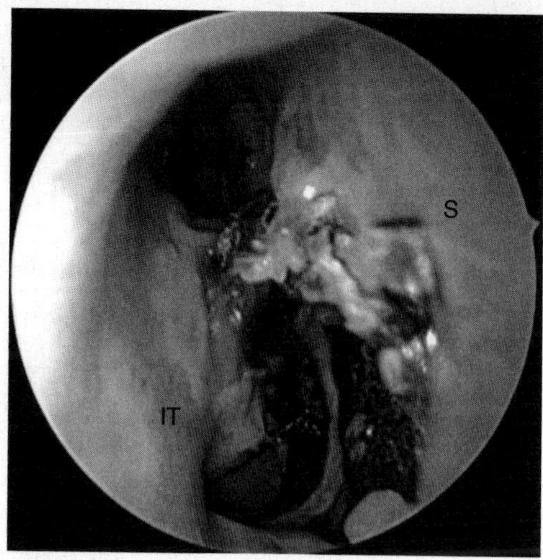

Figure 25-3. Rigid nasal endoscopy of the right nasal cavity in a patient with invasive fungal sinusitis. MT, middle turbinate; IT, inferior turbinate; S, septum.

Bibliography

Chow AW, Benninger MS, Brook I, et al: IDSA clinical practice guideline for acute bacterial rhinosinusitis in children and adults, *Clin Infect Dis* 54(8):e72–e112, 2012.

Coenraad S, Buwalda J: Surgical or medical management of subperiosteal orbital abscess in children: a critical appraisal of the literature, *Rhinology* 47(1):18–23, 2009.

Fokkens WJ, Lund VJ, Mullol J, et al: European position paper on rhinosinusitis and nasal polyps 2012, *Rhinology* 50(S23):1–298, 2012.

Meltzer EO, Hamilos DL, Hadley JA, et al: Rhinosinusitis: Developing guidance for clinical trials, *Otolaryngol Head Neck Surg* 135(5):S31–S80, 2006.

Rosenfeld RM, Andes D, Bhattacharyya N, et al: Clinical practice guidelines: Adult sinusitis, *Otolaryngol Head Neck Surg* 137(3):S1–S31, 2007.

Rosenfeld RM, Singer M, Jones S: Systematic review of antimicrobial therapy in patients with acute rhinosinusitis, *Otolaryngol Head Neck Surg* 137(3):S32–S45, 2007.

Sinus and Allergy Health Partnership: Antimicrobial treatment guidelines for acute bacterial rhinosinusitis, *Otolaryngol Head Neck Surg* 130(1):S1–S45, 2004.

Wald ER, Applegate KE, Bordley C, et al: Clinical practice guideline for the diagnosis and management of acute bacterial sinusitis in children aged 1 to 18 years, *Pediatrics* 132(1):e262–e280, 2013.

CHAPTER 26

CHRONIC RHINOSINUSITIS

Leah J. Hauser, MD and Todd T. Kingdom, MD

KEY POINTS

1. Chronic rhinosinusitis (CRS) in both adults and children is defined based on specific guidelines including both subjective and objective criteria.
2. CRS is a multifactorial inflammatory process characterized by a dysfunctonal local host–environment interaction.
3. Medical management of CRS involves agents that target the inflammatory process in addition to antibiotics, most importantly saline nasal rinses and topical corticosteroids.
4. The effectiveness of surgical management in the CRS patient that has failed medical therapy has been established.

Pearls

1. There is an important association between the presence of asthma, CRS, airway inflammation, and nasal polyposis. Added to this is an increased incidence of aspirin exacerbated respiratory disease (AERD).
2. The importance of bacteria (and all microbes) in the etiology of CRS and the role of antibiotics in its management remains poorly defined and understood.
3. Surgery in patients that have failed medical therapy has an important role in the management of CRS.

QUESTIONS

1. **Define chronic rhinosinusitis (CRS).**
   CRS is chronic inflammation of the mucosal lining of the paranasal sinuses that persists for at least 12 weeks. Clinically, rhinosinusitis is defined by clinical symptoms (subjective) plus suggestive endoscopic and/or CT changes (objective).
2. **What are the symptoms associated with CRS in adults and children?**
   The most common symptoms include nasal congestion or blockage, nasal discharge (either anterior or posterior), facial pain and pressure, and reduction in sense of smell. Other symptoms that may be associated are cough, headache, throat discomfort, laryngeal irritation, hoarseness, halitosis, ear pressure, dental pain, and malaise. In general, the same symptoms are seen with acute and chronic rhinosinusitis, but the symptom pattern and chronicity are different.
3. **What are the endoscopic and CT findings that are typical with CRS?**
   Endoscopic signs include nasal polyps (Figure 26-1), mucopurulent discharge (primarily from the middle meatus) (Figure 26-2), and mucosal edema (also primarily in the middle meatus). CT findings include mucosal thickening of the paranasal sinuses and osteomeatal complex and fluid or debris in the paranasal sinuses (opacification) (Figure 26-3).
4. **How is CRS diagnosed in adults?**
   As stated earlier, the diagnosis of CRS is based on both subjective and objective criteria (Table 26-1).
5. **How is CRS diagnosed in children?**
   The diagnostic criteria in children are very similar to criteria in adults, however, cough is accepted as a symptom of CRS in the pediatric population. In addition, CT scans are ordered less frequently due to concern for unnecessary radiation exposure (Table 26-2).

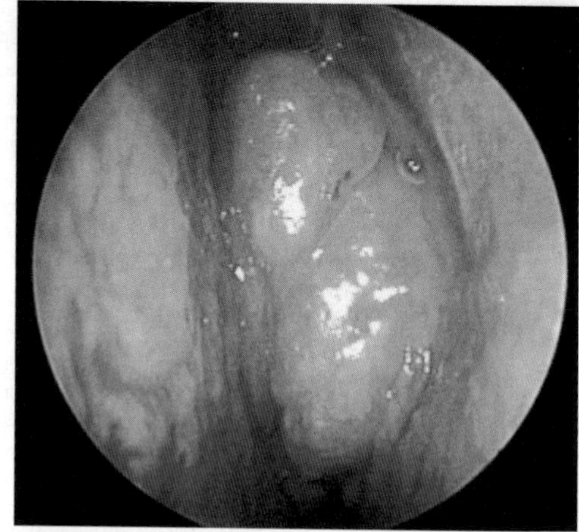

Figure 26-1. Nasal endoscopy, left nasal cavity. Nasal polyps arising from middle meatus.

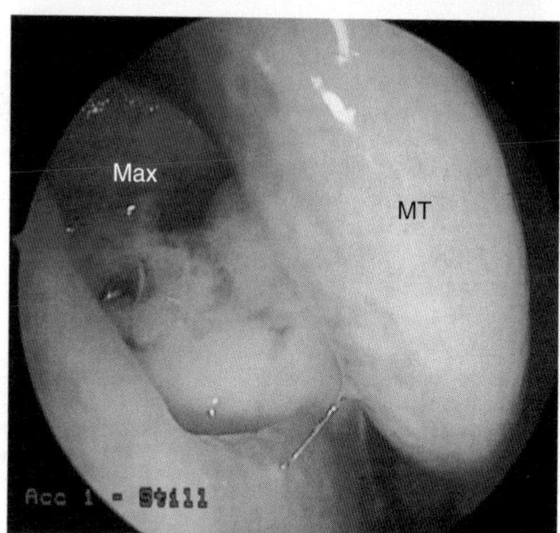

Figure 26-2. Nasal endoscopy, right nasal cavity showing purulent secretions pooling in right maxillary sinus. *MT* = middle turbinate, *Max* = maxillary sinus.

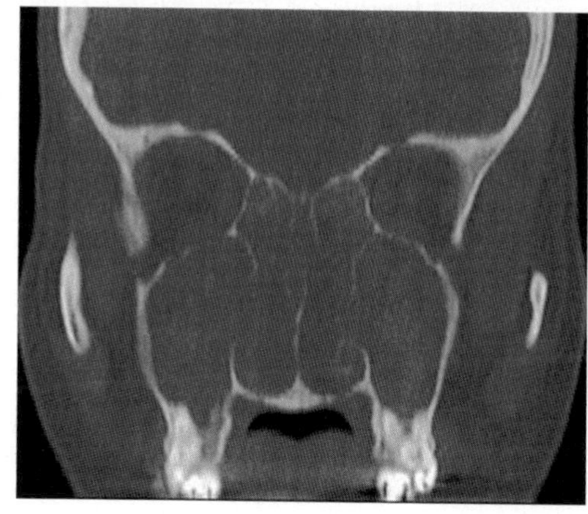

Figure 26-3. Coronal noncontrast CT scan showing opacification of all paranasal sinuses.

Table 26-1. Diagnosis of CRS in Adults

Subjective	
≥12 weeks of 2 or more symptoms:	
Either	• Nasal blockage/obstruction/congestion *OR* • Anterior nasal discharge/Posterior nasal drip
+/–	Facial pain/pressure
+/–	Reduction or loss of sense of smell
Objective	
Either endoscopic signs and/or CT changes	
Endoscopic signs	• Nasal polyps • Mucopurulent discharge • Mucosal edema
CT changes	• Obstruction of the osteomeatal complex • Mucosal thickening or opacification of the paranasal sinuses

Source: Data from the European Position Paper on Rhinosinusitis. Rhinology 2012 was used to create this table.

Table 26-2. Diagnosis of CRS in Children

Subjective	
≥12 weeks of 2 or more symptoms:	
Either	• Nasal blockage/obstruction/congestion *OR* • Anterior nasal discharge/Posterior nasal drip
+/–	Facial pain/pressure
+/–	Cough
Objective	
Either endoscopic signs and/or CT changes	
Endoscopic signs	• Nasal polyps • Mucopurulent discharge • Mucosal edema
CT changes	• Obstruction of the osteomeatal complex • Mucosal thickening or opacification of the paranasal sinuses

Source: Data from the European Position Paper on Rhinosinusitis. Rhinology 2012 was used to create this table.

6. **How common is CRS?**
   Based on a National Health Interview Survery, about 13% of the U.S. population report that they suffer from "sinusitis." However, it has been shown that the incidence of physician-diagnosed CRS is only about 1% of the population. Therefore, many patients have symptoms they attribute to CRS, which are actually due to other causes, most commonly allergic rhinitis and chronic headaches. CRS has a significant negative quality of life impact, as patients report higher measures of bodily pain and lower social functioning than patients with chronic back pain, COPD, and CHF.

7. **Describe the pathophysiology of CRS.**
   The cause of CRS continues to be a topic of much research and debate; however, in general it is a multifactorial inflammatory process characterized by a dysfunctional local host–environment interaction. Possible contributing factors include abnormal host production of pro- and anti-inflammatory cytokines (as is seen with nasal polyps), eosinophilic tissue infiltration, defects in sinonasal epithelial mechanical barrier or immune response, defects in ciliary function, allergies, and

asthma. Genetic factors may also be important and include primary immunodeficiencies and cystic fibrosis. The role of bacteria in the development of CRS continues to be unclear, but it is widely accepted that bacteria do contribute to initiation or propagation of the inflammatory response in some way. The makeup of the bacterial community (microbiome), biofilm production, presence of intracellular or intramucosal bacteria, and *Staphylococcal* superantigens are all currently being studied to determine their association with CRS. It is now believed that bacteria likely are an important disease modifier.

Perhaps the two most important potential triggers underlying sinusitis are upper respiratory viral infection and upper airway inflammation from other causes. These factors may include allergy (atopy), environmental hypersensitivities, mucociliary dysfunction (primary and acquired), anatomic relationships (septal deviation, nasal polyposis), immunodeficiencies, and fungal hypersensitivities. In general, the end result of this inflammatory process is mucosal edema. Similar to acute sinusitis, this may lead to obstruction of the drainage routes of the sinuses, causing stasis of secretions and an overall physiologic change in the sinus cavity.

8. **Which sinus is most often involved in CRS?**
In contrast to acute sinusitis, the anterior ethmoid sinuses are the most commonly affected in CRS, followed by maxillary, posterior ethmoid, sphenoid, and then frontal sinuses.

9. **What inflammatory pathways are characteristic of CRS?**
There are multiple inflammatory markers that are characteristic of CRS. In general, CRS with nasal polyps (CRSwNP) is separated from CRS without NP (CRSsNP) in terms of inflammatory pathways; however, both show an increase in proinflammatory leukotrienes and a decrease in anti-inflammatory prostaglandins. CRSwNP is characterized by an increase in serum and tissue eosinophilia and the Th2-mediated pathway (including IL-4, IL-5, and IL-13), while CRSsNP is characterized by a predominance of Th1-mediated pathway, fibrosis, and high levels of TGF-β. Those patients with asthma have increased tissue eosinophilia and predominance of Th2-mediated inflammation similar to those with CRSwNP. It appears, however, that eosinophilic inflammation is important in most forms of CRS.

10. **Which organisms are associated with CRS?**
The same organisms found in acute disease are also prevalent in CRS, but coagulase-negative *Staphylococcus* species, *S. aureus*, *Pseudomonas aeruginosa*, gram-negative rods, and anaerobes are more frequently associated with CRS. Generally speaking, gram-negative rods and staphylococcal species become more important pathogens in CRS.

11. **What is the relationship between allergy and CRS?**
Atopy and allergies lead to the elaboration of multiple early- and late-phase inflammatory mediators, many of which are also active in CRS. Theoretically, active allergies would contribute to nasal inflammation and therefore could be a disease modifier in CRS; however, this has been extensively studied and only about half of these studies have been able to find an association between the two. Therefore, the role of allergy in CRS remains controversial and not completely defined. In general, patients with allergy symptoms should be tested and treated and this can also be considered for those with recalcitrant CRS.

12. **How does fungus play a role in CRS?**
The role of fungus in CRS continues to be an area of active research. *Allergic fungal rhinosinusitis* (AFRS) and *fungus ball* (mycetoma) represent two subsets of CRS in which fungus plays a role. Both are found in immunocompetent patients in contrast to acute invasive fungal sinusitis.

Diagnostic criteria of *AFRS* include nasal polyposis, computed tomographic (CT) scan with evidence of hyperdense sinus infiltrates or calcifications, eosinophilic mucin, and noninvasive fungal identification by culture or histopathology. These patients tend to have significant burden of polyps and over a prolonged period of time the thick, eosinophilic mucin can act as a benign soft tissue denisty in the paranasal sinuses with possible expansion into nearby structures, including the orbit and cranium. Treatment is with a combination of medical and surgical therapy, similar to other cases of chronic sinusitis. Neither systemic or topical antifungal therapy has been shown to improve treatment outcomes in this population.

A *fungus ball* (mycetoma) is a collection of inspissated fungal debris and mucus in an isolated paranasal sinus. Symptoms are similar to CRS or patients can occasionally be asymptomatic. The maxillary sinus is the most common location. Characteristic CT appearance is a heterogeneous hyperdensity within a sinus with microcalcifications. Intraoperatively, fungal balls appearing as a mass of thick, crumbly debris and fungal hyphae are often appreciable. Treatment is endoscopic removal, and antifungal medications are not typically required.

13. **What is the association of asthma with CRS?**
As the upper and lower airways (nose and bronchi) are connected anatomically and both lined by pseudo-stratified respiratory epithelium, they are often affected by similar disease processes and this is seen specifically in CRS and asthma. Asthma is present in up to 50% of patients with CRS without nasal polyps; this figure rises to 80% in the setting of CRS with nasal polyps. Both diseases can have similar inflammatory pathways, specifically eosinophilia and Th2-mediated inflammation. In general, aggressive management of CRS improves asthma symptoms. This association has lead to the "single airway" concept for this patient group.

14. **What is aspirin exacerbated respiratory disease (AERD)?**
Aspirin exacerbated respiratory disease (AERD) is a subset of CRS characterized by nasal polyps, aspirin sensitivity, asthma, and eosinophilic CRS. Previously known as Samter's triad, AERD is now the more accepted term for this important condition. This triad, or more accurately tetrad, is present in approximately 10% to 25% of patients with CRSwNP and 25% to 40% of patients with CRSwNP and asthma. These patients are thought to have a dysfunction in the arachidonic acid metabolism pathway, with a resultant increase in the proinflammatory leukotrienes and a decrease in the anti-inflammatory prostaglandins both in serum and respiratory mucosa. Bronchospasm, mucosal edema and an influx of eosinophils results when exposed to aspirin or nonsteroidal anti-inflammatory medications. These patients also tend to have more severe polyposis than others with CRSwNP. In addition to standard treatment for CRSwNP, aspirin desensitization is often a therapeutic option.

15. **What is cystic fibrosis and how is it associated with CRS?**
Cystic fibrosis (CF) is an autosomal recessive genetic disorder of the cystic fibrosis transmembrane regulator gene (CFTR). A defective chloride channel results in thick secretions and impaired mucociliary function. Manifestations include chronic pulmonary disease, pancreatic insufficiency, and CRS (with or without NPs). CF patients often have severe sinus disease requiring multiple surgeries and maximal medical therapy. Exacerbations of lung and sinus disease are often concurrent and similar to asthma. Treatment of sinus exacerbation (including surgery) can improve lung symptoms. CRS can be the presenting symptom in some patients who are heterozygous for a CFTR mutation.

16. **How does the management of CRS differ from the management of ABRS?**
The medical management of CRS differs from ABRS in that (1) the role of chronic inflammation is greater, (2) the bacterial pathogens may differ, and (3) the duration of therapy is typically longer. In addition, surgical management is a consideration in select cases of CRS refractory to medical treatment.

17. **Discuss the role of anti-inflammatory agents in the treatment of CRS.**
The majority of medical management of chronic rhinosinusitis is directed at controlling the inflammatory component of the disease and is often more important than antimicrobial treatment. Key treatment options include nasal saline rinses, prolonged intranasal steroids, systemic steroids, leukotriene modifiers, asthma management, and immunotherapy for allergic disease. The length and type of therapy will depend on clinical symptoms and objective findings, stage of disease, and suspected underlying triggers.

18. **Describe the role of antimicrobial treatment in CRS.**
The incidence of *S. aureus, Staphylococcus epidermidis, P. aeruginosa*, and other gram-negative organisms appears to be higher in CRS than in ABRS. This presents a problem in many cases due to reduced antibiotic sensitivities for these organisms. The end result may be a limited number of oral antibiotic options, potentially increasing the need for alternative delivery options (e.g., topical). In cases where bacterial infection is suspected to be a major factor, the typical approach will be culture-directed antibiotic therapy for a period of 3 to 6 weeks. Duration of therapy will be dependent on patient symptoms, repeat culture data, nasal endoscopy, and CT findings. There is little current evidence, unfortunately, defining or supporting the routine use of antibiotics in the treatment of CRS. The precise role of bacteria in CRS remains poorly defined.

19. **What is the role of surgical intervention in CRS?**
Surgery is a key component and an important consideration in the comprehensive management of CRS. Endoscopic sinus surgery (ESS) is indicated for disease that is unresponsive to medical management. The goal of surgery is to facilitate the natural drainage of the sinuses, eradicate pathogenic bacteria, and remove nasal polyps or other mucosal disease. Generally speaking, surgery is not a cure for CRS but an adjunctive treatment option for select patients. Medical management remains the primary option and is effective in the majority of patients. Recent outcomes data has demonstrated significant improvement in CRS patients that underwent ESS following failed medical therapy. In fact, data showed greater improvement in the surgical group when compared to a patient cohort that continued with medical therapy.

Bibliography

Fokkens WJ, Lund VJ, Mullol J, et al: European position paper on rhinosinusitis and nasal polyps 2012, *Rhinol Suppl* 23:1–298, 2012.
Giklick RE, Metson R: The health impact of chronic sinusitis in patients seeking otolaryngologic care, *Otolaryngol Head Neck Surg* 113(1):104–109, 1995.
Kim JK, Kountakis SE: The prevalence of Samter's Triad in patients undergoing functional endoscopic sinus surgery, *Ear Nose Throat J* 86(7):396–399, 2007.
Nicolai P, Lombardi D, Tomenzoli D, et al: Fungus ball of the paranasal sinuses: Experience in 160 patients treated with endoscopic sugery, *Laryngoscope* 119(11):2275–2279, 2009.
Rosenfeld RM, Andes D, Bhattacharyya N, et al: Clinical practice guideline: Adult sinusitis, *Otolaryngol Head Neck Surg* 137:S1–S31, 2007.
Sacks PL, Harvey RJ, Rimmer J, et al: Antifungal therapy in the treatment of chronic rhinosinusitis: a meta-analysis, *Am J Rhinol Allergy* 26(2):141–147, 2012.
Soler ZM, Oyer SL, Kern RC, et al: Antimicrobials and chronic rhinosinusitis with or without polyposis in adults: an evidence-based review with recommendations, *Int Forum Allergy Rhinol* 3(1):31–47, 2013.
Smith TL, Kern RC, Palmer JN, et al: Medical therapy vs surgery for chronic rhinosinusitis: a prospective, multi-institutional study, *Int Forum Allergy Rhinol* 1(4):235–241, 2011.
Smith TL, Kern RC, Palmer JN, et al: Medical therapy vs surgery for chronic rhinosinusitis: a prospective, multi-institutional study with 1-year follow up, *Int Forum Allergy Rhinol* 3:4–9, 2013.
Soler ZM, Wittenberg E, Schlosser RJ, et al: Health state utility values in patients undergoing endoscopic sinus surgery, *Laryngoscope* 121:2672–2678, 2011.
Tan BK, Chandra RK, Pollak J, et al: Incidence and associated premorbid diagnoses of patients with chronic rhinosinusitis, *J Allergy Clin Immunol* 131(5):1350–1360, 2013.
Wilson KF, McMains C, Orlandi RR: The association between allergy and chronic rhinosinusitis with and without nasal polyps: an evidence-based review with recommendations, *Int Forum Allergy Rhinol* 4:93–103, 2014.

CHAPTER 27

SEPTOPLASTY AND TURBINATE SURGERY

Jeevan B. Ramakrishnan, MD

KEY POINTS

1. The various approaches to septoplasty include endonasal (Killian, hemitransfixion, transfixion incisions), open, endoscopic, and endoscopic assisted.
2. During septoplasty, care should be taken to leave at least a 1.5 cm strut of dorsal and caudal septal cartilage during resection to avoid postoperative loss of nasal tip support and saddle nose deformity.
3. Prior to completion of a septoplasty, five areas of the septum should be checked to ensure there is no further obstruction that needs to be addressed: the dorsal septum, caudal septum, middle septum, maxillary crest, and posterior/bony septum. The insertion points of the middle turbinates into the lateral nasal walls should be readily visible with anterior rhinoscopy or nasal endoscopy.
4. During septoplasty, repairing rents, or tears, in the mucosal flaps and replacing the previously excised cartilage into the mucoperichondrial pocket can help to decrease the risk of septal perforation postoperatively.
5. Medications used during nasal surgery are potentially dangerous if used improperly. Safe use of these medications requires familiarity with their pharmacology, dosing, and management of complications.

Pearls

1. The major nasal tip support mechanisms include the attachments between the septum, lower lateral cartilages, and upper lateral cartilages. The minor tip support mechanisms include the interdomal ligament, the dorsal septum, the membranous septum, the sesamoid complex, the skin and subcutaneous tissue of the nasal tip, and the maxillary spine.
2. The blood supply to the inferior turbinate is from a branch of the posterior lateral nasal artery.
3. How is the nose anomalous in a patient with unilateral cleft lip/palate? The ipsilateral lower lateral cartilage is displaced inferiorly, posteriorly, and laterally. The nasal tip, caudal septum, and columella are displaced toward the non-cleft side. The bony septum is deviated toward the cleft side.
4. The nasal cycle refers to the cyclic nature of blood flow distribution within the nasal cavity. About every 4 hours, blood flow increases on one side of the nasal cavity relative to the other side. Normally this occurs imperceptibly. Sometimes patients will have bilateral alternating nasal congestion related to this if there is associated septal deviation and/or turbinate hypertrophy.
5. Septal perforation and saddle nose deformity are the most common complications of an untreated septal hematoma.
6. During nasal surgery, a medication is injected intranasally. Almost immediately, the patient becomes severely hypertensive and tachycardic. It is discovered that oxymetazoline was accidentally injected instead of a local anesthetic. What should be the next step? Intravascular injection of oxymetazoline causes stimulation of alpha 1 receptors resulting in vasoconstriction, hypertension, and tachycardia. Initial treatment should include administration of an alpha blocker, such as phentolamine, followed by other resuscitative therapies.
7. Toxic shock syndrome is a rare complication of *S. aureus* infection characterized by high fever, rash, hypotension, vomiting, diarrhea, and multiorgan failure. Treatment consists of removal of the nasal packing, IV antibiotics, and supportive/resusitative care.

QUESTIONS

1. **What is the clinical presentation of a patient with a deviated nasal septum and when should surgical correction be considered?**
   Nasal septal deviations can be congenital, developmental, or secondary to nasal trauma. About 50% of the general population are thought to have some deviation in their nasal septum, and most of these are asymptomatic. Symptomatic patients will often present with nasal congestion, and can also present with nasal drainage, decreased sense of smell, difficulty sleeping, dryness, and pain. If the deviation is severe, it can impinge on the turbinates, lateral nasal wall, and middle meatus, and can predispose patients to recurrent and/or chronic sinusitis. Surgical correction should be considered in appropriate patients with chronic symptoms related to a deviated nasal septum that are significantly affecting their quality of life.

2. **What are the various approaches to the nasal septum when performing a septoplasty?**
   Typically, a septoplasty is performed through an endonasal approach. Unilateral incisions are made just pass the mucocutaneous junction, known as a Killian incision, or more anterior at the mucocutaneous junction, known as a hemitransfixion incision. The latter type of incision allows better access to the caudal septum, compared to a Killian incision, and allows for elevation of bilateral mucoperichondrial flaps if needed. A full transfixion incision is one that is made at the mucocutaneous junction on one side and is extended through to the contralateral mucocutaneous junction. Again, this type of incision allows for access to the caudal septum, columella, and medial crura. The hemi- and full transfixion incisions can cause disruption of the septo-columellar ligamentous tissue, and can theoretically lead to loss of nasal tip support. Finally, complete access to the entire septum can be achieved via a degloving, or external rhinoplasty, approach if more advanced maneuvers are required for addressing abnormalities of the dorsal and/or caudal septum (Figure 27-1).

3. **What is an endoscopic septoplasty?**
   Most otolaryngologists perform a septoplasty using a headlight and direct vision for visualization of the surgical field. Many otolaryngologists are now using the endoscope for enhanced visualization. Advantages of this approach include magnification of the surgical field, improved ergonomics, improved access and visualization for the posterior nasal cavity, and the potential for more limited dissection in certain cases. Disadvantages include a potential inability to adequately address severe deviations of the anterior and caudal septum. Since the endoscope is often used through incisions that are traditionally used for headlight visualization, a more accurate term for this procedure may be endoscopic assisted septoplasty.

4. **What are the steps for performing a typical septoplasty?**
   1. Decongest nasal cavities with topical oxymetazoline spray. Inject lidocaine mixed with epinephrine into the septum bilaterally in a subperichondrial plane.
   2. Make incision near the caudal septum. Elevate flap in the subperichondrial plane using broad, sweeping movements with the elevator. The elevation is carried posteriorly as required (Figure 27-2).
   3. Disarticulate septal cartilage from the bony septum, and resect bony septum as required.
   4. Resect septal cartilage as required, taking care to leave dorsal and caudal struts with a width of at least 1 to 1.5 cm for proper support of the nasal tip and dorsum.
   5. Repair any tears in the mucosal flaps primarily if possible with dissolvable suture.
   6. Consider replacing the previously excised cartilage into the mucoperichondrial pocket to decrease the risk of septal perforation, taking care not to cause further obstruction of the nasal cavity by doing so. Also consider documenting the precise amount of cartilage excised or remaining in the operative note, in case revision surgery is ever needed.
   7. The mucosal incision is then closed with absorbable suture. At this point, the septum can be quilted with absorbable suture and/or splints can be placed.

5. **What is a typical postoperative course after septoplasty/turbinate surgery?**
   Most patients are discharged home after surgery. Some patients are kept overnight for observation if there is concern for complications or significant sleep apnea. Recovery can take anywhere from several days to several weeks. During this time, patients will usually have nasal congestion, moderate nasal and midfacial pain, mild intermittent bloody nasal drainage, and generalized fatigue.

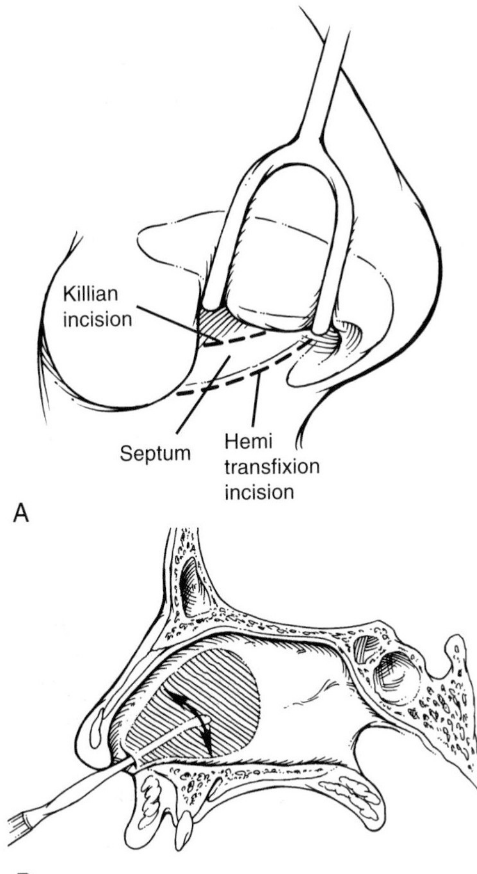

Figure 27-1. A, B. Various approaches to the nasal septum when performing a septoplasty. *(From Cummings C, Flint P, Harker L. Cummings Otolaryngology Head & Neck Surgery, 4th ed. 2005. 1001–1027.)*

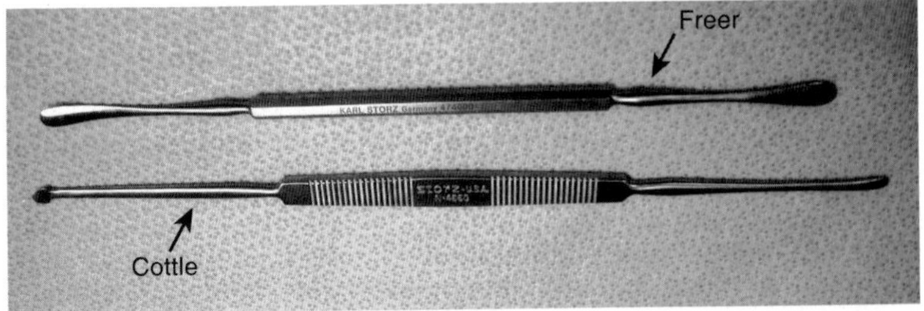

Figure 27-2. Tools to perform a typical septoplasty.

Patients may also have nausea, difficulty sleeping, and dry mouth. Antibiotics, analgesics, and antiemetics are typically prescribed. Patients are instructed to moisten the nasal cavities with saline frequently and to keep the head elevated. Patients should plan on taking at least a week off of work or school before returning. Light activities are permitted during the first week after surgery, and full activities can gradually be resumed after 1 to 2 weeks. Patients are seen for follow-up 1 to 2 weeks after surgery. Complete healing of the mucosa usually occurs at 3 to 4 weeks after surgery.

6. **What are the possible risks involved with septoplasty/turbinate surgery?**
Risks of surgery should be discussed with patients preoperatively as part of the informed consent process. These include infection, excessive bleeding, nasal dryness/crusting, persistent nasal congestion, septal hematoma/abscess, septal perforation, scarring, alteration of sense of smell/taste, numbness, CSF leak, cosmetic deformity, complications of anesthesia, and need for further surgery.

7. **What is the anatomy of the inferior turbinate?**
The inferior concha is its own bone, which attaches to the medial maxilla. The medial submucosal tissue is made mostly of venous channels and erectile tissue, whereas the lateral submucosal tissue is mostly glandular. Hasner's valve, a flap of tissue at the nasolacrimal duct orifice, opens into the inferior meatus.

8. **What are the topical medications typically used during septoplasty/turbinate surgery?**
Oxymetazoline and phenylephrine are medications that are commonly applied topically to the nasal cavities as decongestants. Topical epinephrine can also be used if desired. These medications work as α-1 receptor agonists, causing vasoconstriction and decongestion of the nasal mucosa, resulting in decreased systemic absorption of local anesthetics, improved visualization, working space, and hemostasis. Topical cocaine is less commonly used nowadays, but is also a very effective decongestant and anesthetic. These can be applied preoperatively and/or intraoperatively as needed. Care should be taken to only use these medications topically, and not accidentally inject them intravascularly. This can cause immediate and life-threatening hypertension, tachycardia, and arrythmias, and could lead to myocardial infarction or stroke.

9. **What anesthetics are used during septoplasty/turbinate surgery? Can surgery be performed under local anesthesia?**
In the past, nasal surgery was commonly performed under local anesthesia with light sedation. Currently, most nasal surgery is performed under general anesthesia for improved patient comfort. During surgery, a local anesthetic mixed with dilute epinephrine is injected into the submucosal septum/turbinates. This results in hydrodissection of the injected plane, assisting with ease of surgical dissection, improved hemostasis as a result of vasoconstriction caused by the dilute epinephrine, and helps with pain control in the immediate postoperative period.

Local anesthetics are divided into amides and esters. Amides are metabolized in the liver, and esters are metabolized in both the liver and plasma. Lidocaine and bupivicaine (amides) are the most common local anesthetics used during nasal surgery. The maximum dose of lidocaine is 4 mg/kg (with epi 7.5 mg/kg), and the maximum dose of bupivicaine is 3 mg/kg. The maximum dose of cocaine (ester) is 2 to 3 mg/kg or 200 mg. Signs of adverse reactions to local anesthetics should be recognized and treated promptly if needed. Signs of epiniphrine toxicity include restlessness, anxiety, a sense of impending doom, headache, palpitations, repiratory distress, hypertension, and tachycardia. Allergic reactions are extremely rare and are usually attributed to the preservatives in the anesthetic. True allergic reactions are almost always caused by the ester anesthetics. Signs can range from a simple rash to anaphylaxis. Finally, local anesthetics administered in toxic doses can result in a progression from CNS and cardiovascular excitation to depression. First, the patient may show anxiety, disorientation, rambling speech, seizures, tachycardia, hypertension, vomiting, and sweating. This is followed by loss of consciousness, apnea, bradycardia, hypotension, and cardiovascular collapse. Treatment should consist of supportive care, including supplemental O_2, airway support, IV fluids, and appropriate supportive medications, which may include antiseizure medications or benzodiazepines.

10. **What is a unique adverse reaction to toxic doses of prilocaine and benzocaine?**
The max dose of benzocaine is 200 mg, and the max dose of prilocaine is 7 mg/kg. Above these doses, methemoglobinemia can occur, resulting in hypoxia, shortness of breath, cyanosis, mental status changes, and headaches. Severe cases can result in arrhythmias, seizures, coma, and death. Pulse oximetry is inaccurate in assessing oxygenation with this condition. Treatment includes supplemental O_2 and a slow IV infusion of 1 to 2 mg/kg of 1% methylene blue.

11. **What are some techniques that help with hemostasis during and after septoplasty/turbinate surgery?**
Hemostasis is important during nasal surgery to ensure proper visualization, which allows for a more thorough and complete procedure. It is also important after surgery to decrease the risk for

hemorrhage, and to improve the patient's comfort and postoperative experience. Hemostasis starts preoperatively by reviewing the patient's medications, and stopping anticoagulants, NSAIDs, vitamins, and herbal supplements 1 to 2 weeks prior to surgery. Restarting these meds postoperatively should be delayed for 1 to 2 weeks if possible, but may need to be restarted sooner, depending on the patient's comorbidities. Mucosal inflammation is treated preoperatively with topical nasal steroids, antihistamines, oral steroids, and antibiotics as indicated. On the day of surgery, topical decongestants are applied just prior to surgery and/or during surgery. Local anesthetics mixed with dilute epinephrine are injected into the septum and turbinates, resulting in further vasoconstriction. The patient is then positioned with the head elevated 30 degrees, decreasing venous congestion. Careful surgical technique with minimization of mucosal trauma is a must. Finally, dissolvable or nondissolvable nasal packing can be placed in the nasal cavities at the end of the procedure, but these have not been shown to significantly reduce rates of hemorrhage.

12. **What is the clinical presentation of a patient with turbinate hypertrophy and when should surgery be considered?**
Patients with turbinate hypertrophy usually present with chronic complaints of nasal congestion, and can also have symptoms of nasal drainage, facial pressure, ear fullness, and sleeping difficulty. The congestion is often described as bilateral, alternating from side to side, worse during sleep in a supine position, and improved in the upright position, with exposure to steam (e.g., in the shower), with exercise, and with use of decongestants. A history of allergies is common. Surgery should be considered when symptoms related to turbinate hypertrophy are significantly affecting quality of life despite medical treatments, including nasal steroids, antihistamines, nasal saline, and decongestants.

13. **How is turbinate surgery performed?**
Once the appropriate candidate is identified, surgery can be performed under local or general anesthesia. The surgery is often performed in conjunction with a septoplasty and is usually directed toward the inferior turbinates. The goal of surgery is to reduce the size of the turbinate, thereby improving the nasal airway, without sacrificing function. There are a wide variety of techniques for turbinate reduction, and this is best accomplished by a submucous resection of soft tissue and/or bone, thereby preserving the overlying functional mucosa as much as possible. Some of the various techniques that have been described include (full/partial) turbinate resection, laser cautery, electrocautery (monopolar or bipolar), cryotherapy, coblation, radiofrequency ablation, submucosal resection, and lateral outfracture.

14. **What is empty nose syndrome?**
Also called ozena or chronic atrophic rhinitis, empty nose syndrome is an uncommon condition in which the patient experiences chronic symptoms of nasal congestion despite a widely patent nasal airway. Additional symptoms can include dryness, crusting, bleeding, drainage, and pain. Typically, patients have a history of prior nasal surgery. On exam, the turbinates have been resected, and there may be a septal perforation. It is thought that the severe distortion of intranasal anatomy results in decreased sensation of normal airflow, thereby resulting in a subjective sensation of congestion. Treatment options are limited, and include nasal saline, topical ointments, and antibiotics when indicated. Surgical augmentation of the inferolateral nasal wall has been reported with some success. The best strategy is avoidance of this complication with careful preoperative planning and proper surgical technique.

15. **When is middle turbinate surgery indicated?**
The middle turbinate is an important intranasal structure that facilitates humidification, normal airflow, proper sinus drainage, and olfaction. Unlike the inferior turbinates, middle turbinates do not commonly develop mucosal or submucosal hypertrophy, and do not fluctuate as much in size with changes in blood flow. As a result, middle turbinate surgery is less common. In some cases, the middle turbinate can have a concha bullosa, which is an air-filled cell of thin bone, causing it to be much larger than normal. This can contribute to symptoms of nasal obstruction, deviation of the septum, and impair mucociliary drainage of the sinuses. In cases of severe nasal polyps, the middle turbinate can develop polypoid degeneration. In these cases, reduction of the middle turbinate can be considered.

16. **What is the nasal valve?**
The nasal valve refers to the narrowest area in the anterior nasal cavity through which air flows. Abnormalities of the nasal valve result in symptoms of nasal obstruction. The valve has both internal

and external components. The internal nasal valve refers to the area of the nasal cavity bounded by the septum, head of the inferior turbinate, and upper lateral cartilage. The external nasal valve refers to the area bounded by the columella, lateral crus of the lower lateral cartilage, and nasal ala. The area between the internal and external valves is referred to as the intervalve area.

17. How is the nasal valve evaluated?
When evaluating a patient with symptoms of nasal congestion, the external nose and nasal valve should be examined along with the intranasal anatomy. The nasal dorsum, nasal sidewalls, nasal tip, nasal alae, and columella are examined from an anterior view, profile view, and base view at rest and during inspiration. The Cottle maneuver is performed by displacing the cheek laterally. The modified Cottle maneuver is performed by supporting the lateral nasal wall intranasally with a cotton tip applicator or ear curette during inspiration. In patients with abnormalities of the nasal valve, these maneuvers will result in marked improvement in nasal breathing. Abnormalties of the nasal valve are important to detect preoperatively, as they can cause persistent symptoms of nasal obstruction after septoplasty/turbinate surgery.

18. What is nasal valve collapse?
Nasal valve collapse refers to nasal obstruction caused by an abnormality of the nasal valve. This can be congenital or acquired from prior surgery, trauma, or facial paralysis. Symptoms of congestion are usually constant, improved with use of Breathe Right nasal strips or lateral displacement of the cheeks, and worse with exercise. "Collapse" can be either static or dynamic depending on the patient's anatomy.

19. How is nasal valve collapse treated?
Nonsurgical treatment options include use of Breathe Right nasal strips or disposable intranasal stent devices. There are a wide variety of surgical treatment options depending on what is found on physical exam. These include placement of spreader grafts, flaring sutures, butterfly graft, batten grafts, lateral crural strut grafts, alar rim grafts, and bone anchored suture techniques to name a few. Surgery can be performed via a closed or open approach. Cartilage grafts are harvested from the septum, ear, or rib.

20. What is the clincal presentation and treatment for a septal hematoma/abscess?
This condition can occur as a result of recent nasal surgery or nasal trauma. Symptoms include acute onset of severe nasal congestion, pain, swelling, and possibly fever. Exam shows occlusion of one or both nasal cavities by fluctuance of the septum. Treatment is immediate incision and drainage of the fluid collection under local or general anesthesia and placement of nasal splints for 1 week to prevent recurrence. Delay in treatment could result in necrosis of septal cartilage, septal perforation, and saddle nose deformity.

21. What is the clinical presentation and treatment of a septal perforation?
Septal perforations can cause symptoms including a whistling sound with respiration, dryness, crusting, bleeding, pain, congestion, and drainage, or may be asymptomatic. The differential includes prior surgery, trauma, drug use (nasal sprays, recreational), vasculitis, atypical infection, granulomatous disease, or malignancy. On exam, the size and location of the perforation should be noted. Nonsurgical treatment options include nasal saline and topical ointment. Surgical treatment options include placement of a silastic septal button or surgical repair. Perforations 5 mm or less can be repaired primarily with placement of an interpositional graft via an endonasal approach. For perforations 5 mm to 2 cm, an open approach should be considered, and local mucosal flaps will be needed. Perforations greater than 2 cm are more difficult to successfully repair. Surgery is contraindicated in patients actively abusing cocaine, or with active infectious, inflammatory or malignant disease.

22. What is the clinical presentation and treatment of saddle nose deformity?
Patients with saddle nose deformity present with a depression or concavity involving the dorsum of the middle third of those. This is typically caused by prior nasal trauma or overly aggressive nasal surgery during dorsal hump reduction, or from overresection of the dorsal septal strut during septoplasty. Surgical correction is performed using an open approach for exposure of the nasal dorsum. The deficient area is then augmented with either conchal (ear) or rib cartilage using an onlay graft technique.

23. **What is toxic shock syndrome?**
Toxic shock syndrome is a rare complication of *S. aureus* infection. The TSST-1 toxin produced by the bacteria causes high fever, rash, hypotension, vomiting, diarrhea, and multiorgan failure. This has rarely been associated with nasal packing. As a result, patients with nasal packing or splints are typically covered with antistaphylococcal antibiotics. Treatment includes removal of the nasal packing, IV antibiotics, and supportive/resuscitative care.

24. **What considerations are involved in revision nasal surgery?**
About 5% to 10% of patients have persistent or recurrent symptoms of nasal congestion after nasal surgery. A careful history and exam should be performed, and a CT scan should be considered to evaluate for sinus disease. The prior operative notes should be reviewed if possible, and the full differential for nasal congestion should be considered in the assessment. If revision surgery is considered, surgical options include revision septoplasty for persistent deviation, revision turbinate reduction for recurrent hypertrophy, and nasal valve surgery. An open approach may be needed for modification of the remaining septal struts, placement of cartilage grafts, or nasal valve surgery.

25. **What are some limitations to the endonasal approach for septoplasty?**
The endonasal approach to septoplasty refers to making a Killian or transfixion incision to access the septal cartilage and bone. This approach allows limited access to and manipulation of the dorsal septum, septal angle, caudal septum, and nasal spine. Deviation from the midline in these areas is a common cause for failure of primary septoplasty. If deviation is noted in one or more of these areas, an open approach to the septum should be considered for adequate exposure. Deviation of the dorsal septum and septal angle can be corrected by conservative shaving and (extended) spreader grafts. A deviation of the posterior septal angle can be corrected by conservative shaving and/or repositioning of the cartilage on the nasal spine. A deviation in the caudal septum can be corrected with a septal batten graft, repositioning, tongue in groove technique, caudal septal extension graft, or other modifications.

26. **Is nasal surgery safe to perform in children?**
The nasal septum is important in development of the infantile nose into the adult nose. Therefore, with few exceptions, septoplasty is usually not performed until at least 16 years of age when the development of the nose is typically complete. Turbinate surgery can be safely performed in young children if needed, but should be done conservatively to minimize the risk of long-term complications.

CONTROVERSIES

27. **What is Sluder's neuralgia?**
This is an antiquated term now referred to as sphenopalatine ganglion neuralgia or contact point headache. Symptoms include midfacial pain that is typically unilateral and localized. Decongestants sometimes provide symptom relief, while other medications typically do not. Exam and CT scan may show a deviated septum impinging into a turbinate and/or lateral nasal wall with no significant sinus disease. The pain may be exacerbated by manipulation of the septal deviation and relieved with application of topical anesthetic. Some consider this a structural problem and recommend septoplasty for treatment, while others consider this a neurologic condition requiring medical treatment.

28. **Should the middle turbinate be preserved at all costs during nasal/sinus surgery?**
Prevailing opinion discourages resection of the middle turbinate in order to preserve its functions of humidification, mucociliary clearance, olfaction, and as an important surgical landmark. In certain cases, some argue that it is beneficial to resect the middle turbinate, such as a large middle turbinate concha bullosa and severe polypoid degeneration. Advantages to resection include improved access to the sinuses postoperatively for surveillance, instrumentation, and penetration of topical irrigations. Recent studies have shown no significant differences between patients with and without middle turbinate resections.

29. **Are the placement of nasal splints necessary after nasal surgery?**
Traditionally, splints have been placed as dressing/packing in the nasal cavities after nasal surgery, especially septoplasty. This serves to eliminate dead space between the mucosal flaps, prevent

septal hematoma, enhance healing of the mucosa, and prevent synechiae formation. When aggressive maneuvers have been performed to correct a severe deviation, splints can also serve to stabilize the remaining septal cartilage. The splints are usually removed about 1 week after surgery. The placements of splints can result in discomfort after surgery and potentially be a source of infection. Recent studies have shown that patients who did not have splints placed after septal surgery had similar success and complication rates compared to those who had splints placed, suggesting splints may not be necessary at all.

30. **Is nasal surgery effective for treatment of snoring and/or obstructive sleep apnea?**
The importance of nasal breathing in normal sleep is well known. However, recent studies have shown that, in general, nasal surgery does not seem to significantly improve snoring or sleep apnea objectively. These same studies did show improvement in subjective sleep symptoms, quality of life, and CPAP compliance, so there seems to be a role for nasal surgery in patients with sleep disordered breathing. The effect of nasal surgery on snoring and sleep quality can be assessed preoperatively by asking the patient to use Breathe Right nasal strips and/or use topical decongestants for a few nights at bedtime. If snoring and/or sleep quality is significantly improved, then nasal surgery is more likely to help, and vice versa.

Bibliography

Ballert J, Park S: Functional rhinoplasty: Treatment of the dysfunctional nasal sidewall, *Facial Plast Surg* 22:49–54, 2006.

Cummings C, Flint P, Harker L: *Cummings Otolaryngology Head & Neck Surgery*, ed 4, Philadelphia, 2005, Elsevier Mosby, pp 1001–1027.

Kennedy D, Hwang P: *Rhinology Diseases of the Nose, Sinuses, and Skull Base*, New York, 2012, Thieme Medical Publishers.

Kridel R: Considerations in the etiology, treatment, and repair of septal perforations, *Facial Plast Surg Clin N Am* 12:435–450, 2004.

Lee KJ: *Essential Otolaryngology Head & Neck Surgery*, ed 8, New York, 2003, McGraw-Hill.

Passali F, Passali G, Damiani V, et al: Treatment of inferior turbinate hypertrophy: a randomized clinical trial, *Ann Otol Rhinol Laryngol* 112:683–688, 2003.

Soler Z, Hwang P, Mace J, et al: Outcomes after middle turbinate resection: revisiting a controversial topic, *Laryngoscope* 120(4):832–837, 2010.

CHAPTER 28

FUNCTIONAL ENDOSCOPIC SINUS SURGERY

Henry P. Barham, MD and Anne E. Getz, MD

KEY POINTS

1. The goals of sinus surgery include atraumatic surgical technique, mucosal preservation, and restoration of normal sinus physiology.
2. The most common major complications of sinus surgery include hemorrhage, intracranial injury/ CSF leak, and intraorbital injury.
3. Measures used to help improve visualization and decrease blood loss during sinus surgery include total intravenous anesthesia (TIVA), head of bed elevation >15 degrees, topical α1 blockers (epinephrine or oxymetazoline), and local infiltration of epinephrine.

Pearls

1. Know the Keros classification of olfactory fossa depth (Class I: 1 to 3 mm, Class II: 4 to 7 mm, Class III: 8 mm and greater)
2. The most common complication of sinus surgery is hemorrhage.

QUESTIONS

1. What is FESS?

Functional endoscopic sinus surgery. The goal of "functional" endoscopic sinus surgery is to correct underlying anatomic abnormalities or obstructions while preserving mucosa in order to restore mucociliary flow and normal sinus function. The term *functional* is directly related to techniques used to preserve the natural drainage pathway. The field of rhinology has undergone great advances in recent years with advances in imaging, endoscopic visualization, image guidance, and understanding of the anatomy and pathophysiology of rhinosinusitis.

2. What is the role of surgical intervention in rhinosinusitis?

Chronic rhinosinusitis is a medical disease in which surgery may play a role when medical therapy alone is not sufficient. Medical management is the primary, and often only treatment modality in the majority of patients. When medical therapy fails to control symptoms adequately, surgery may be indicated. In cases of chronic or recurrent sinusitis, surgical intervention should be directed at improving the natural drainage pathways of the sinuses. In cases of acute rhinosinusitis, surgical intervention is directed at decompression of the acutely infected sinus associated with possible complications, such as abscess formation.

3. What measures should be taken prior to surgical intervention for the treatment of rhinosinusitis?

A detailed history and physical examination should be performed on any patient to help determine which patients would potentially benefit from surgical intervention. Nasal endoscopy should be performed preoperatively to evalute the specific nasal anatomy along with assessment of the nasal mucosa. Fine cut computed tomography (CT) is an important objective measure performed to identify a patient's specific anatomy used in preparation for sinus surgery. Imaging should ideally be studied in triplanar (axial, coronal, and sagittal) orientation. As with any surgery, all preoperative medications (including over-the-counter medications) should be discussed with each patient to identify any medications that can increase the risk of bleeding.

4. What are the main goals of functional endoscopic sinus surgery?
   1. Thorough anatomic dissection of the paranasal sinuses to restore the normal drainage pathways. This dissection should be complete and mucosa sparing.
   2. Avoidance of complications. The paranasal sinuses reside in close proximity to critical structures including the orbit/eye, skull base, carotid artery, and optic nerve.

5. What are the most common causes of nasal airway obstruction and how are they addressed surgically?
   Deviated nasal septum and inferior turbinate hypertrophy are two of the most common causes of nasal airway obstruction that can be surgically corrected. Septoplasty is a procedure performed to straighten the deviated septum. Reduction and outfracture of the obstructing inferior turbinates are commonly performed to improve the nasal airway.

6. How should one proceed through dissection of the paranasal sinuses?
   Based on its anterior location, the maxillary sinus is often addressed first. Osteomeatal complex obstruction is addressed by performing a maxillary antrostomy. The natural ostium of the maxillary sinus is first exposed by removing the uncinate process. Once the natural ostium is identified, it is enlarged as indicated (this ostium is enlarged to include accessory ostia when present).

   The anterior ethmoid cells are then adressed by opening the ethmoid bulla. Once this has been completed, one may proceed anterior to posterior in an inferomedial direction. The basal lamella of the middle turbinate is then identified, which is the anatomic division between the anterior and posterior ethmoid sinuses. Proceeding posteriorly from the basal lamella, dissection is then carried posteriorly until the anterior face (rostrum) of the sphenoid sinus is encountered, marking the posterior limit of the posterior ethmoid sinus in the absence of an Onodi cell (posterior ethmoid cell pneumatizing superiorly to the sphenoid sinus).

   Medially, the superior turbinate can be used to identify the sphenoid os in the sphenoethmoidal recess. The sphenoethmoidal recess is located inferomedial to the superior turbinate in the vast majority of cases. If necessary, the inferior third of the superior turbinate may be removed to expose the sphenoid ostium. The sphenoid ostium should be enlarged inferiorly and medially to avoid injury to the skull base while avoiding the posterior septal artery (medial terminal branch of the sphenopalatine artery) inferiorly.

   The remaining ethmoid partitions are dissected in a posterior to anterior direction from the anterior face of the sphenoid sinus along the ethmoid skull base superiorly with the limits of dissection including the lamina papyracea laterally, middle turbinate medially, and frontal recess anteriorly.

7. How should one surgically address the frontal sinus?
   Endoscopic frontal sinusotomy has become the standard approach to treating rhinosinusitis involving the frontal recess and sinus. Recent advances in endoscopic visualization and angled instrumentation have improved the surgical treatment of frontal sinusitis. While commonly considered the most difficult sinus to address surgically because of the anterior and superior location, surrounding anatomy and associated risks, endoscopic surgery of the frontal sinus has become increasingly safe and successful. The successive approaches used to improve drainage of the frontal sinus include anterior ethmoidectomy, complete dissection of all anterior ethmoid and frontal cells within the frontal recess (also known as the Draf I procedure), widely opening the frontal ostium (Draf IIa), resection of the floor of the frontal sinus from the nasal septum medially to the lamina papyracea laterally (also known as the Draf IIb procedure), and connection of the two frontal sinuses from orbit to orbit with removal of each frontal sinus floor, inferior portion of the frontal intersinus septum, the superior part of the nasal septum (also known as the Draf III procedure, modified Lothrop, or transseptal frontal sinusotomy). External or open approaches may be used in select cases including a trephine, Lynch incision, or bicoronal flap with osteoplastic flap, which can be used for tumor removal, cranialization or obliteration procedure.

8. What is a common reason for surgical failure of the maxillary antrostomy?
   Failure to incorporate the true maxillary ostium located anterosuperiorally with the surgical antrostomy, resulting in two separate openings. This is a setup for recirculation of mucus from the natural ostium to the surgical ostium resulting in dysfunction and stasis of secretions within the maxillary sinus.

9. **What are the four lamellae that serve as anatomic landmarks to complete a sinus surgery?**
   - First lamella: Uncinate process
   - Second lamella: Ethmoid bulla
   - Third lamella: Basal lamella of the middle turbinate (horizontal component of the middle turbinate; this represents the anatomic division between anterior and posterior ethmoid air cells)
   - Fourth lamella: Superior turbinate

10. **What are common minor complications of sinus surgery?**
    Bleeding, hyposmia/anosmia, numbness, nasal obstruction, and adhesions. It is normal to have small amounts of bleeding after sinus surgery which rarely (less than 1%) requires intervention. Preoperative evaluation and discussion of all medications (prescription, over-the-counter, and supplements) known to cause increased bleeding and strict adherence to the principles of hemostasis can help minimize the bleeding risk. Hyposmia and rarely anosmia can occur. Although this is generally considered a minor complicaiton, it can be quite distressing to the patient. Care to avoid overdissection of the superior aspects of the middle and superior turbinates and mucosal stripping within the olfactory cleft can help prevent this. Infection, allergy, and the presence of nasal polyps can lead to impaired sense of smell postoperatively. An important point to discuss with patients is that decreased sense of smell preoperatively may or may not improve postoperatively. Numbness of the nose, upper lip, or central upper teeth can occur postoperatively but is usually self-limited. Nasal obstruction and pain are common self-limited minor complications. Postoperative crusting and adhesions may occur in both the nasal cavity and paranasal sinuses, which should be debrided during early postoperative visits to prevent mature scar formation and potential resultant dysfunction. This complication can be mitigated by performance of frequent postoperative saline irrigations by the patient and close endoscopic evaluation and debridement by the surgeon.

11. **What are the major complications of sinus surgery?**
    Orbital injury, intracanial injury, and hemorrhage. The medial orbital wall, or lamina papyracea, is the lateral boundary of the ethmoid sinus. This close proximity of the orbit to the paranasal sinuses makes orbital injury an inherent risk. The lamina papyracea separating the ethmoid sinuses from the orbit is one of the thinnest bones in the human body. Transgression of this bone and bleeding into the bony orbit can cause complications ranging from periorbital ecchymosis and emphysema to orbital hematoma and blindness. Anisocoria, ophthalmoplegia, and proptosis are ominous signs demanding prompt action. In cases of increased orbital pressure, steroids, mannitol, and/or orbital decompression via lateral canthotomy and cantholysis or endoscopic decompression should be performed immediately to relieve the pressure and preserve vision. Damage to the extraocular muscles, most commonly the medial rectus, can occur, leading to permanent diplopia. Overly aggressive anterior dissection of the maxillary antrostomy can result in injury to the nasolacrimal system. Injury to the lacrimal system can result in epiphora or recurrent dacryocystitis, and may require correctional surgery.

    Intracranial complications can occur because of the proximity of the skull base to the frontal, ethmoid, and sphenoid sinuses. The bone separating the paranasal sinus from the intracranial cavity is also very thin, on the order of millimeters. Injury most commonly occurs at the cribriform plate and roof of the ethmoid sinus where the bone is thinnest. Complications associated with intracranial entry include CSF leak, meningitis, carotid artery injury, tension pneumocephalus, and direct brain injury. Intracranial entry should be identified immediately and repaired.

    Injury to the ethmoidal, sphenopalatine, or internal carotid arteries (ICA) can result in major hemmorhage. In the case of ICA injury, stroke and death are possible. Direct endoscopic repair of an ICA injury is technically difficult given the high-flow bleeding and difficult visualization. Management typically involves aggressive packing to tamponade the hemorrhage, and transfer to interventional radiology for possible ICA embolization. Injury to the anterior ethmoidal arteries along the skull base can result in intracranial hemorrhage as well as intraorbital hematoma and resultant blindness. The internal maxillary artery courses behind the posterior wall of the maxillary sinus within the pterygopalatine fossa. Its terminal branch, the sphenopalatine artery, exits into the nose through the sphenopalatine foramen into the inferior portion of the basal lamella of the middle turbinate. Injury to the artery can result in significant epistaxis.

12. **What does IGS stand for and what are the indications for use?**
Image guided surgery (IGS) is a computerized navigation system that tracks surgical instruments in space using a patient's preoperative CT (or MRI) scan and displays the instrument location in a triplanar (axial, coronal, and sagittal) fashion. Indications include: nasal polyps, revision sinus surgery, frontal or sphenoid surgery, orbital surgery, surgery for skull base disorder, or CSF leak. IGS is never a substitute for the surgeon's anatomic knowledge.

13. **What type of general anesthesia has been shown to improve visualization in sinus surgery?**
Total intravenous anesthesia (TIVA). TIVA has been shown to improve the surgical field visualization by correlating decreased heart rate and improved surgical field visualization with decreased blood loss. A lower heart rate has the added benefit of lower mean arterial pressures, avoidance of excess fluid shifts, and lower central venous pressures. Avoidance of inhalational anesthetics prevents the peripheral vasodilation that accompanies these agents.

14. **How does patient positioning affect visualization?**
Elevation of the patient's head, or reverse Trendelenberg positioning, has been shown to improve the surgical field visualization.

15. **How do topical medications affect sinus surgery?**
Nasal pledgets soaked in oxymetazoline, neosynephrine or epinephrine (1:1000) can be placed into the nasal cavity to cause vasoconstriction and help improve generalized mucosal oozing. They carry a low complication rate (0.001%) but should be used with caution in pediatric patients and patients with cardiovascular risks or hypertension.

16. **What local injections can be used in sinus surgery?**
Local vasoconstrictive/anesthetic injections are important for decreasing blood loss and optimizing visualization. Anterior injection into the lateral nasal wall at the insertion of the root of the middle turbinate is effective in anterior hemostasis during surgery of the maxillary, anterior ethmoid, and frontal sinuses. Posterior injection on the region of the sphenopalatine foramen or transoral injection into the greater palatine foramen is effective for posterior hemostasis during surgery of the posterior ethmoid and sphenoid sinuses. Typically 1% lidocaine with 1:100K or 1:200K epinephrine is used.

17. **What is the most important factor in preventing major complications during endoscopic sinus surgery?**
Thorough knowledge of the anatomy is paramount in prevention of major surgical complication. Meticulous and detailed review of the patient's CT imaging preoperatively is an absolute requirement prior to surgery.

18. **What is the incidence of major complications in endoscopic sinus surgery?**
The overall major complication rate is estimated to be less than 1%.

19. **What are important anatomic factors to consider while reviewing a CT scan of the sinuses prior to surgery to avoid complications?**
First, one should always verify the correct patient and left/right orientation of the scan. Verify the integrity of the lamina papyracea and confirm there is no dehiscence. Pay attention to the height of the maxillary sinus relative to the height of the ethmoid sinuses. Tall maxillary sinuses result in relatively short ethmoid height and may disorient the surgeon as the skull base may be lower than anticipated. Assess the configuration of the skull base in terms of height, slope, symmetry, and depth of the cribriform plate. Assess the position of the anterior ethmoidal artery, and if it is within the bony skull base or running below the bony skull base (higher risk for injury). Verify the integrity of the bony skull base and note if there are any areas of dehiscence. Within the sphenoid sinus, inspect the bone of the optic and carotid canals. These can often be partially dehiscent, placing these structures at greater risk.

20. **What radiologic staging system is used to assess the ethmoid skull base?**
The Keros classification is a method of classifying the depth of the olfactory fossa (Figure 28-1). The depth of the olfactory fossa is determined by the height of the cribriform plate and is staged into three categories; Type 1 has a depth of 1 to 3 mm (26% of the population), Type 2 has a depth of 4 to 7 mm (73% of the population), and Type 3 has a depth of 8 to 16 mm (1% of the population).

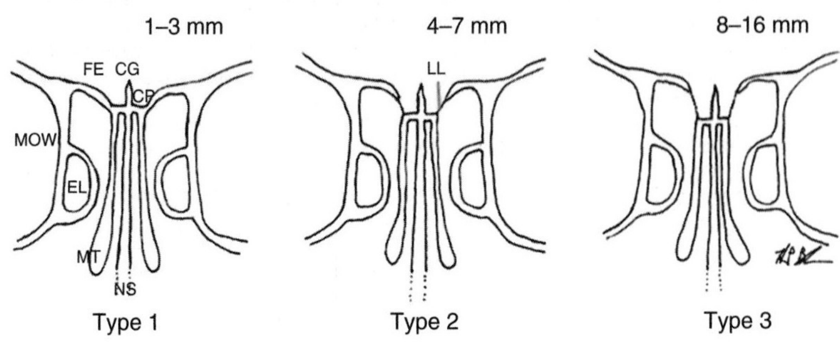

Figure 28-1. Keros classification of depth of olfactory fossa.

21. What is a Caldwell-Luc procedure?
    This procedure was designed to treat the "irreversibly diseased" maxillary sinus by removing mucosa and creating a gravity-dependent drainage. The maxillary sinus is opened through a sublabial approach, sinus mucosa is removed, and a large inferior meatal antrostomy is created. This technique is rarely used in the era of endoscopic functional sinus surgery.

Bibliography

Ahn H, Chung S, Dhong H, et al: Comparison of surgical conditions during propofol or sevoflurane anaesthesia for endoscopic sinus surgery, *Br J Anaesth* 100:50–54, 2008.

Fraire ME, Sanchez-Vallecillo MV, Zernotti ME, et al: Effect of premedication with systemic steroids on surgical field bleeding and visibility during nasosinusal endoscopic surgery, *Acta Otorrinolaringol Esp* 64(2):133–139, 2013.

Hathorn IF, et al: Comparing the reverse Trendelenburg and horizontal position for endoscopic sinus surgery: a randomized controlled trial, *Otolaryngol Head Neck Surg* 148(2):308–313, 2013.

Higgins TS, Hwang PH, Kingdom TT, et al: Systematic review of topical vasoconstrictors in endoscopic sinus surgery, *Laryngoscope* 121:422–432, 2011.

Khosla AJ, Pernas FG, Maeso PA: Meta-analysis and literature review of techniques to achieve hemostasis in endoscopic sinus surgery, *Int Forum Allergy Rhinol* 3(6):482–487, 2013.

Krings JG, Kallogjeri D, Wineland A, et al: Complications of primary and revision functional endoscopic sinus surgery for chronic rhinosinusitis, *Laryngoscope* 124(4):838–845, 2014.

Ramakrishnan VR, Kingdom TT, Nayak JV, et al: Nationwide incidence of major complications in endoscopic sinus surgery, *Int Forum Allergy Rhinol* 2(1):34–39, 2012.

Senior BA, Kennedy DW, Tanabodee J, et al: Long-term results of functional endoscopic sinus surgery, *Laryngoscope* 108:151–157, 1998.

Stankiewicz JA: Complications of endoscopic sinus surgery, *Otolaryngol Clin North Am* 22:749–758, 1989.

Timperley D, Sacks R, Parkinson RJ, et al: Perioperative and intraoperative maneuvers to optimize surgical outcomes in skull base surgery, *Otolaryngol Clin North Am* 43:699–730, 2010.

CHAPTER 29

CEREBROSPINAL FLUID LEAKS AND ENCEPHALOCELES

Henry P. Barham, MD and Anne E. Getz, MD

KEY POINTS

1. Trauma is the most common cause of cerebrospinal fluid (CSF) leaks.
2. Endoscopic repair of CSF leaks is effective and offers decreased morbidity compared to open approaches.
3. Meticulous technique is key to success in repair of skull base defects.
4. Materials used and procedures employed are less important than the quality of the repair.

Pearls

1. The lateral lamella of cribriform is the most common site of iatrogenic CSF leak during functional endoscopic sinus surgery (FESS).
2. Conservative management is often the first step in managing CSF leaks resulting from acute trauma.
3. Spontaneous CSF leaks are likely associated with idiopathic intracranial hypertension.

1. What are the most common causes of CSF leaks?

- Trauma
  - Nonsurgical: Most common etiology (70% to 80%). One percent to 3% of acute head injuries result in a CSF leak. Seventy percent of leaks close spontaneously with observation and conservative management which may include bed rest, head of bed elevation, and lumbar drainage. Overall, there is a 30% to 40% risk of meningitis with conservative treatment.
  - Surgical (planned and unplanned):
    - FESS (<1% incidence of CSF leak): Most common site of skull base injury is the lateral lamella of the cribriform plate. The posterior ethmoid skull base is at greater risk when the maxillary sinus is highly pneumatized in the superior-inferior dimension, which creates a relatively decreased posterior ethmoid height (Figure 29-1).
    - Neurologic Surgery: Transsphenoidal approach for sellar and suprasellar lesions (0.5% to 15% incidence of CSF leak)
- Neoplasm: Mechanisms include direct tumor invasion and/or mass effect leading to intracranial hypertension.
- Congenital: Failure of closure of developmental spaces with resultant herniation of intracranial contents. Foramen cecum is the most common location (50%).
- Spontaneous: Often the result of idiopathic intracranial hypertension (IIH) resulting from decreased CSF reabsorption. Patient characteristics and symptoms often include middle-age, obesity, female, pressure-type headaches, pulsatile tinnitus, and balance dysfunction.

2. What is empty sella syndrome and how is it treated?

Empty sella syndrome is a radiographic appearance of CSF-filled sella due to flattening of the pituitary gland (Figure 29-2). The pituitary gland is an endocrine gland that resides in the sella turcica and functions to control other endocrine glands (adrenal glands, thyroid, ovaries, testicles) by secretion of controlling hormones. Empty sella syndrome can be seen in IIH, which typically affects obese women. Patients typically will present with headaches, pulsatile tinnitus, and diplopia. A hallmark physical exam finding is bilateral optic disc edema secondary to increased intracranial

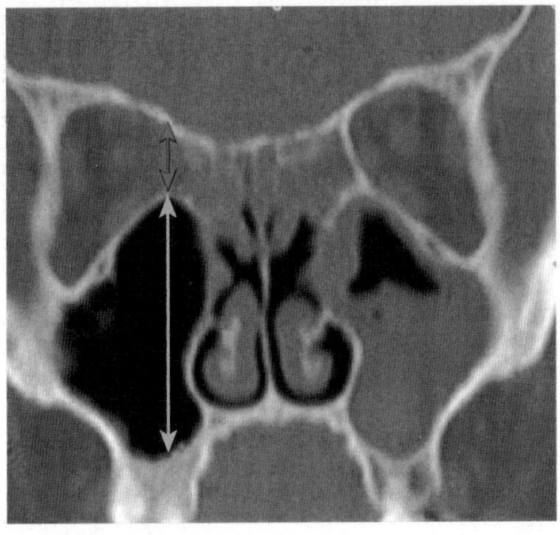

Figure 29-1. A relatively short height of the ethmoid sinus *(top arrow)* as a result of a highly pneumatized, tall maxillary sinus *(bottom arrow)*.

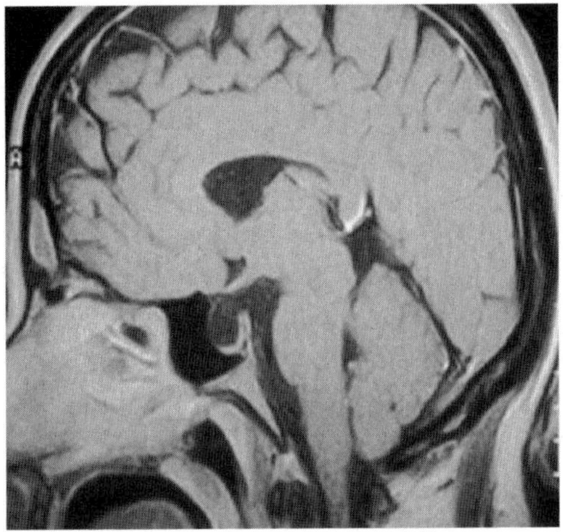

Figure 29-2. Sagittal MRI of an "empty" sella turcica filled with CSF.

pressure (ICP). Treatment is focused on decreasing ICP with pharmacologic therapy consisting of acetazolamide and furosemide to lower ICP, and headache management, which may include amitriptyline and propranolol. In severe cases with vision problems, surgical intervention may be required, including optic nerve decompression or CSF shunting. Empty sella syndrome can be seen in conjunction with spontaneous CSF leaks.

3. What is an encephalocele?
An encephalocele is herniation of neural tissue through a defect in the skull base (Figures 29-3 and 29-4) and is defined by the type of tissue that herniates through the defect. A meningocele contains herniated meninges, a menigoencephalocele contains herniated brain matter and meninges, and a meningoencephalocystocele is made up of herniated brain matter and meninges that communicate with a cerebral ventricle.

4. Where do encephaloceles occur?
Encephaloceles can occur in both the skull and spinal column. Twenty percent occur within the cranium and 15% of these are associated with the nasal cavity. Nasal encephaloceles are divided

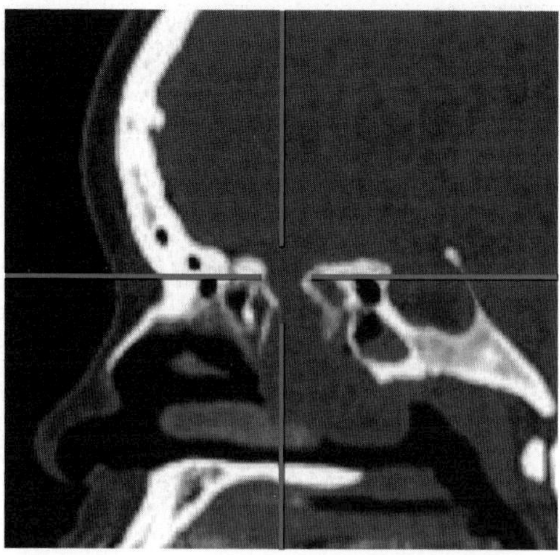

Figure 29-3. Large encephalocele of the ethmoid skull base. Crosshairs localize the bony skull base defect.

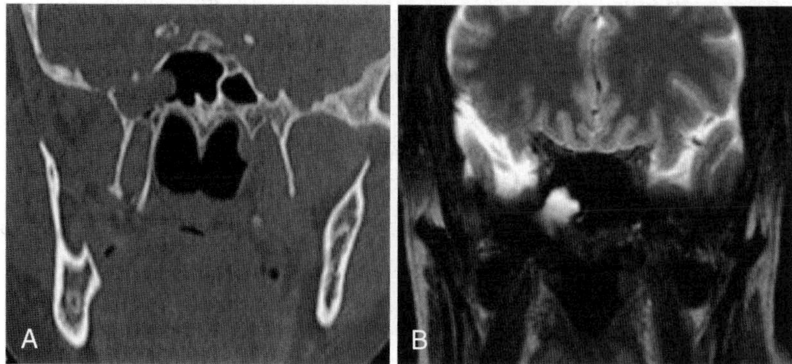

Figure 29-4. CT **(A)** and MRI **(B)** of meningocele protruding into lateral recess of right sphenoid sinus.

into two types: sincipital and basal. Sincipital (anterior and superior) encephaloceles make up approximately 60% of nasal encephaloceles and typically present as a soft compressible mass over the glabella. Basal encephaloceles occur through the skull base more posteriorly and make up approximately 40% of nasal encephaloceles. They may remain hidden for many years because they are located more posteriorly than the sincipital type.

5. **How is an encephalocele diagnosed?**
   Patients will often present with rhinorrhea or recurrent meningitis and may have a broad nasal dorsum or hypertelorism. Encephaloceles may characteristically transilluminate, expand with the Valsalva maneuver, and demonstrate a positive Furstenberg sign (enlargement with compression of internal jugular veins). Radiologic imaging including computed tomography (CT) and magnetic resonance imaging (MRI) may be used to evaluate the size and location of encephaloceles (see Figures 29-3 and 29-4).

6. **Describe the physiology of CSF production.**
   CSF is produced by the choroid plexus of the lateral, third and fourth ventricles at a rate of 0.35 mL/min (20 mL/hr or 350 to 500 mL/d) in the normal physiologic states. The total volume of

circulating CSF is 90 to 150 mL. The entire volume of CSF turns over three to five times per day. Typical intracranial pressure is 5 to 15 cm H_2O and is considered elevated when it is greater than 15 cm H_2O.

7. **What is the most common complaint in patients presenting with concern for a CSF leak?**
Clear rhinorrhea that is unilateral, watery, and salty to taste is the most common complaint in CSF leaks. It may run out of the nose in more anterior leaks, or down the back of the throat in more posterior leaks. The drainage can be exacerbated by the Dandy maneuver, which entails tilting the head forward into a chin-tuck position and straining.

8. **What laboratory tests can be performed to diagnose a CSF leak?**
The most sensitive and specific test is qualitative β_2-transferrin evaluation of the nasal drainage. β_2-transferrin is detected in few fluids in the body including CSF, perilymph, and aqueous humor. Only 0.2 mL is needed for an adequate specimen. β_2-transferrin has a sensitivity of 97% and specificity of 93%. False positive results can occur with abnormal transferrin metabolism from chronic liver disease, glycogen metabolic disease, and carcinomas; therefore, results should be verified with a negative serum β_2-transferrin. β-trace protein is a newer laboratory test with higher sensitivity and specificity which offers faster results than β_2-transferrin, however it is not universally available.

9. **Describe the radiologic evaluation of a patient with CSF rhinorrhea.**
The radiologic evaluation of a CSF leak can be extensive and often begins with a fine cut maxillofacial CT scan to demonstrate bony abnormalities such as defects and fractures. CT is the mainstay for radiologic workup of CSF rhinorrhea with a sensitivity of 92% and a specificity of 92% to 96%. If the initial imaging does not show an obvious abnormality but suspicion is still high, a CT cisternogram may be useful. This study entails injection of radiopaque material through a lumbar drain into the intrathecal space to help delineate the CSF leak. Presence of contrast within the nasal space or paranasal sinuses indicates a CSF leak. CT cisternography has a sensitivity of 92% with an active leak to 40% with an intermittent leak. MRI cisternography (T2 weighted fast-spin protocol) can be helpful in cases of neoplasm, meningoencephalocele, encephalocele, and in patients with an iodine allergy.

10. **Describe the workup of suspected CSF rhinorrhea.**
    - If β_2-transferrin or β-trace protein is positive, obtain a fine cut maxillofacial CT scan to assess for source.
    - If β_2-transferrin or β-trace protein is negative, and clinical suspicion is low, workup is complete. If clinical suspicion remains high, evaluate with maxillofacial CT.
    - If a single, small (less than 1 cm) bony defect is present on the CT in a patient with normal intracranial pressure, conservative therapy may be attempted. If the bony defect is greater than 1 cm, or if the patient has elevated intracranial pressure and a high-pressure leak, surgical management is recommended.
    - If more than one bony defect is seen on CT imaging, cisternography can be helpful in determining which site(s) is/are leaking.
    - If no bony defect is detected on maxillofacial CT, repeat β_2-transferrin or β-trace protein may be sent. If positive, CT or MRI cisternogram is recommended. If negative, and clinical suspicion is high, surgical exploration is indicated, possibly with utilization of intrathecal fluorescein.
    - If a bony defect is present on CT with associated soft tissue mass, MRI or MRI cisternogram is recommended to further evaluate the characteristic of the soft tissue mass, which may represent a meningocele or other neoplasm.

11. **What does conservative therapy for CSF leaks entail?**
In patients who have a traumatic leak and normal CSF pressure, conservative treatment consists of bed rest with head of bed elevation and lumbar drainage of CSF for 5 to 10 days. With conservative management, there is a reported risk ranging from 7% to 30% of ascending meningitis. The incidence of spontaneous resolution with conservative management is reported to be 70%.

12. **Should antibiotics be used in patients with known CSF rhinorrhea?**
The general consensus among practicing otolaryngologist is that antibiotics should not be used for conservative management unless there is a very large defect with comminuted bone of the skull

base as a simple CSF leak carries a 7% infection rate (meningitis, intracranial abscess, cellulitis/abscess, and osteomyelitis) and prophylactic antibiotics have not been shown to decrease the risk of infection. After endoscopic repair, antibiotics are generally recommended for 24-48 hours including Cefazolin (1gm q8), Vancomycin (1gm q12), or Clindamycin (600mg q8). This is done to cover possible contamination at the time of surgery in a non-sterile field with concomitant sealing of the sterile to non-sterile flushing of an active leak.

13. **How has surgical management of CSF leaks improved with the use of endoscopic surgery?**
Advancements in the endoscopic surgical repair of CSF leaks and encephaloceles have resulted from improvements in instrumentation, visualization, access, and technique. Improved diagnostic imaging and surgical navigation have also improved management. Advancements in endoscopic reconstructive techniques of the skull base including utilization of local vascularized flaps have improved success rates with endoscopic approaches.

14. **Describe the use of intrathecal fluorescein in the surgical repair of CSF leaks.**
Its advantages include the ability to stain defects that may be more difficult to identify clinically, through the visible dye of CSF to a light green color. The surgeon can also use it to confirm a water-tight repair. It carries a 0% false positive rate. Its disadvantages include a moderate false negative result. It requires a lumbar puncture, and the use of fluorescein intrathecally is not FDA-approved. Rare complications including seizures (0.3%) and death have been reported; however, these have more commonly been associated with administration through a suboccipital puncture. If used to help localize a CSF leak it should be used with caution and should be dosed as 0.05 to 0.1 mL per 10 kg body weight up to maximum 0.1 mL 10% fluorescein. This is mixed in 10 mL of preservative-free normal saline or CSF. The surgeon should inject slowly (over 5 to 10 min) without paralytics in the anesthetic regimen to assess for seizure activity. Fluorescein should be avoided in patients with abnormal renal function.

15. **What are the goals of skull base reconstruction?**
The primary goal in endoscopic repair of CSF leaks and skull base reconstruction is to definitively identify all leaks in order to completely reconstruct all defects. After identifying the leak or leaks, the goals of reconstruction are creation of a safe barrier with separation of intracranial and sinonasal spaces and elimination of any dead space. As with any surgical intervention, meticulous surgical technique is paramount for success.

16. **What can be used to reconstruct the skull base?**
A reconstructive ladder should be used to help determine the type of repair performed.
For simple, small (less than 1 cm) defects, a fat plug harvested from the earlobe or abdomen can be used to plug the defect. The next option includes a simple overlay graft harvested from the nasal floor mucosa, turbinate mucosa, or nasal septum. If a more complex, larger reconstruction is in order, a composite (underlay and overlay) graft can be used consisting of an intracranial underlay of bone or cartilage from nasal septum, auricular cartilage or turbinate bone, and an overlay graft of mucosa (free or pedicled) as above. Local pedicled flaps should include the nasoseptal flap, which is supplied by the posterior nasal septal artery, a terminal branch of the sphenopalatine artery. Additional grafts that can be useful in larger defects include temporal fascia or tensor fascia lata grafts. These grafts are often bolstered in the sinonasal cavity with abdominal fat, a nasoseptal flap or both. In complex situations of extensive defects or poor local tissue, such as in chemoradiated patients, a craniotomy with pericranial flap or free flap reconstruction of the skull base may be necessary.

17. **What are the reported outcomes of endoscopic repair of CSF leaks?**
A multitude of studies over the past 20 years have shown high success rates of primary repair around 90%, and secondary repair around 97%. These success rates compare favorably to traditional craniotomy approaches with reported success rates between 70% and 80% that carry a higher morbidity profile.

BIBLIOGRAPHY

Bernal-Sprekelsen M, Alobid I, Mullol J, et al: Closure of cerebrospinal fluid leaks prevents ascending bacterial meningitis, *Rhinology* 43(4):277–281, 2005.

Brown SM, Anand VK, Tabaee A, et al: Role of perioperative antibiotics in endoscopic skull base surgery, *Laryngoscope* 117(9):1528–1532, 2007.
Hegazy HM, et al: Transnasal endoscopic repair of cerebrospinal fluid rhinorrhea: a meta-analysis, *Laryngoscope* 110(7):1166–1172, 2000.
Lanza DC, O'Brien DA, Kennedy DW: Endoscopic repair of cerebrospinal fistulae and encephaloceles, *Laryngoscope* 106(9 Pt 1):1119–1125, 1996.
Lund V, et al: European position paper on endoscopic management of tumours of the nose, paranasal sinuses and skull base, *Rhinol Suppl* 1(22):1–143, 2010.
May M, Levine HL, Mester SJ, et al: Complications of ESS: analysis of 2,018 patients, *Laryngoscope* 104:1080–1083, 1994.
Mincy J: Posttraumatic cerebrospinal fluid fistula of the frontal fossa, *J Trauma* 6(5):618–622, 1966.
Schlosser RJ, Bolger WE: Nasal cerebrospinal fluid leaks, *J Otolaryngol Suppl* 1:S28–S37, 2002.
Suwanwela C, Suwanwela N: A morphological classification of sincipital encephalomeningoceles, *J Neurosurg* 36: 201–211, 1972.
Wolf G, et al: Endoscopic detection of cerebral spinal fistulas with a fluorescence technique. Report of experiences with over 925 cases, *Laryngorhinootogie* 76(10):588–594, 1997.
Zweig JL, et al: Endoscopic repair of cerebrospinal fluid leaks to the sinonasal tract: predictors of success, *Otolaryngol Head Neck Surg* 123(3):195–201, 2000.

ORBITAL SURGERY

Henry P. Barham, MD and Todd T. Kingdom, MD

CHAPTER 30

KEY POINTS

1. Endoscopic sinus surgical techniques have advanced to include the treatment of select orbital pathology due to the close proximity of the orbit to the paranasal sinuses, advances in surgical instrumentation, and a working relationship with ophthalmologists.
2. Endoscopic approaches to the orbit require a deep knowledge and an accurate intraoperative identification of orbital anatomy.
3. Excess tearing (epiphora) can result from hypersecretion or failure of drainage (nasolacrimal system obstruction). Endoscopic dacryocystorhinostomy (DCR) is the preferred treatment for nasolacrimal duct obstruction.
4. Thyroid eye disease (TED) is the most common extrathyroidal manifestation of Graves' disease and is the leading cause of proptosis in adults. Endoscopic orbital decompression is often an important treatment approach to these patients.
5. Traumatic optic neuropathy is categorized as direct or indirect, and surgical intervention appears to be of limited benefit.

Pearls

1. Thyroid eye disease results from autoimmune inflammation of muscle and fat, where the TSH receptor is the autoantigen.
2. Dacryocystorhinostomy is an effective surgical management for nasolacrimal duct obstruction.
3. The medial rectus, superior rectus, inferior rectus, and inferior oblique muscles are innervated by cranial nerve III. The superior oblique muscle is innervated by cranial nerve IV. The lateral rectus muscle is innervated by cranial nerve VI.
4. The anterior and posterior ethmoid arteries are distal branches of the internal carotid circulation.

QUESTIONS

1. **Describe the important bony anatomy of the orbit.**
   The orbit is a pyramidal shaped space that is made up of seven bones: frontal, zygomatic, ethmoid, lacrimal, maxillary, sphenoid, and palatine (Figure 30-1). The medial walls of each orbit lie parallel to each other and the lateral walls lie 45 degrees to the ipsilateral medial wall and 90 degrees to the contralateral lateral wall. The orbital walls are lined by periosteum referred to as *periorbita.*

2. **What bones make up each wall of the orbit?**
   The roof of the orbit is made up of the frontal bone and lesser wing of the sphenoid. The floor of the orbit is made up of the maxillary, palatine, and zygomatic bones. The medial wall of the orbit is made up of the ethmoid, lacrimal, maxillary, and sphenoid bones. The lateral wall of the orbit is made up of the zygomatic bone and greater wing of the sphenoid.

3. **What are the dimensions of the orbit in adults?**
   The pyramidal shaped orbit has a typical volume of 30 mL. The entrance height is 35 mm and the entrance width is 40 mm. The width of the orbit is greatest 1 cm posterior to the entrance of the orbit which corresponds to the equator of the globe. The medial wall length is 45 mm.

4. **What are the orbital foramina and what structures are contained within them?**
   The *optic foramen* passes through the lesser wing of the sphenoid extending from the middle cranial fossa to the orbital apex and contains the optic nerve, ophthalmic artery, and sympathetic fibers

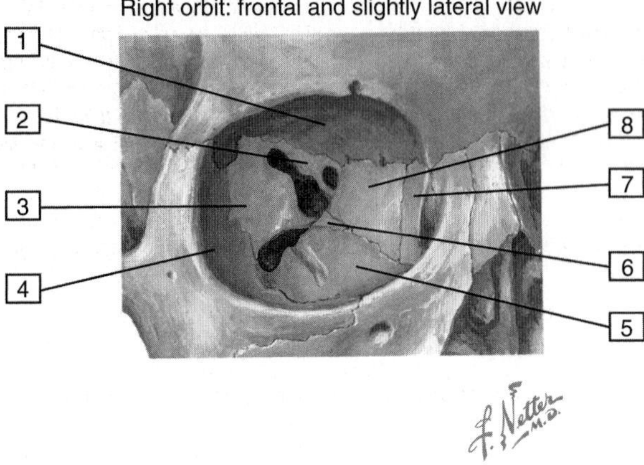

1. Frontal bone
2. Lesser wing of the sphenoid
3. Greater wing of the sphenoid
4. Zygomatic bone
5. Maxillary bone
6. Palatine bone
7. Lacrimal bone
8. Ethmoid bone

Bones creating the orbital margin include:
- Frontal
- Zygomatic
- Maxilla

Walls of the orbit

Superior	Frontal (orbital plate) Lesser wing of sphenoid
Inferior	Maxilla Zygomatic Palatine (orbital process)
Medial	Ethmoid (lamina papyracea) Lacrimal Sphenoid Maxilla
Lateral	Zygomatic Greater wing of sphenoid

Figure 30-1. Bony anatomy of the orbit. *(From Gentile MA, Tellington AJ, Burke WJ, et al: Management of midface maxillofacial trauma. Atlas Oral Maxillofacial Surgery Clini 21(1): 69–95, 2013.)*

from the carotid plexus. The *supraorbital foramen* is located at the medial third of the superior margin of the orbital rim and contains the supraorbital nerve, artery, and vein. The *anterior ethmoidal foramen* is located at the frontoethmoidal suture 24-mm posterior to the orbital rim and contains the anterior ethmoidal vessels and nerve. The *posterior ethmoidal foramen* is located 12 mm posterior to the anterior ethmoidal foramen at the junction of the medial wall and orbital roof and contains the posterior ethmoidal vessels and nerve. The 24/12/6 rule is a nice reference to help remember foramina locations in the orbit, which stands for anterior ethmoid artery (24 mm), posterior ethmoid artery (12 mm), and optic nerve (6 mm) in sequential measurements from the posterior lacrimal crest. The *zygomaticotemporal* and *zygomaticofacial foramina* are located within the lateral wall of the orbit and transmit branches of the zygomatic nerve and artery.

5. **What are the orbital fissures and what structures are contained within them?**
   The *superior orbital fissure* is 22 mm in length and lies inferior and lateral to the optic foramen. It is formed by the greater and lesser wing of the sphenoid and is divided into superior and inferior parts by the lateral rectus. The superior part contains the frontal and lacrimal branches of cranial nerve V1 and cranial nerve IV. The inferior part contains the superior and inferior divisions of cranial nerve III, the nasociliary branch of V1, cranial nerve VI, the superior ophthalmic vein, and the sympathetic nerve plexus. The *inferior orbital fissure* lies between the lateral wall and orbital floor (runs deep to the orbital floor) and contains branches of cranial nerve V2 and the inferior ophthalmic vein (Figure 30-2).

6. **What are the extraocular muscles and where are they located?**
   There are six extraocular muscles (Figure 30-3) within each orbit that control movement of the globe: medial rectus, lateral rectus, inferior rectus, superior rectus, superior oblique, and inferior oblique. With the inferior oblique as the exception, all extraocular muscles originate at the orbital apex. The four rectus muscles originate from the annulus of Zinn (a tendinous ring that encircles the inferior portion of the superior orbital fissure and optic foramen) and insert onto the anterior portion of the globe. The superior oblique travels from the orbital apex to the trochlea and makes a sharp turn (54 degrees) to insert on the globe. The inferior oblique travels from a shallow depression in the

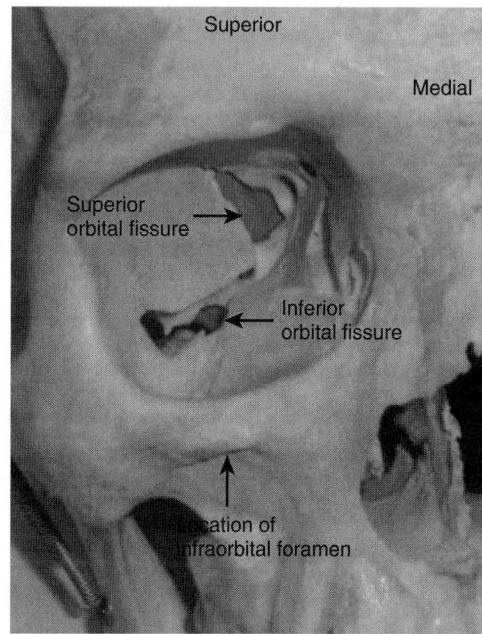

Figure 30-2. An anterior view of the orbit on a dry skull. Foramina, or openings in the bone, can be seen. The superior orbital fissure is found at the orbital apex. The inferior orbital fissure is found on the orbital floor. The optic foramen is found on the superior-medial wall. *(From Anderson BC, McLoon LK: Cranial nerves and autonomic innervation in the orbit. In Dartt DA (ed.): Encyclopedia of the Eye, Oxford, 2010, Academic Press, p. 537–548.)*

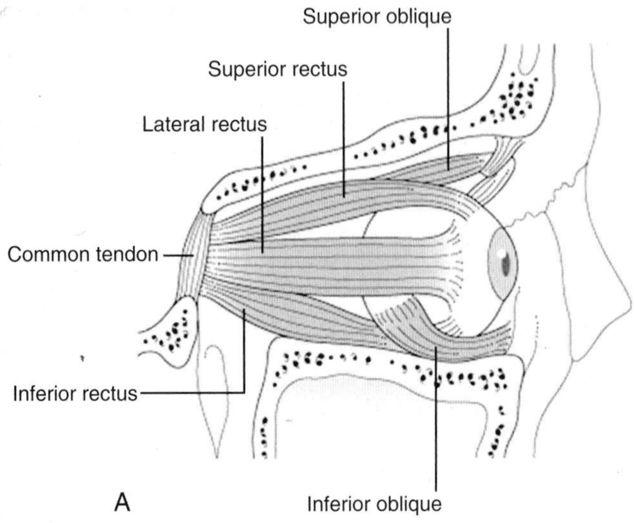

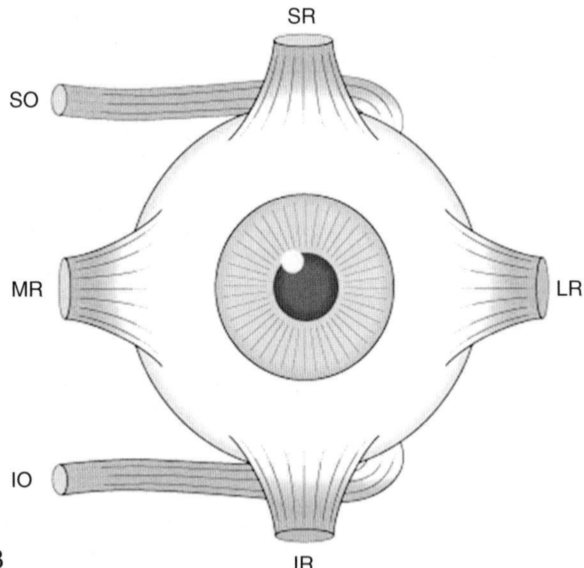

Figure 30-3. Schematic diagrams depicting the extraocular muscles from a lateral (**A**) and cut anterior (**B**) view. SO, superior oblique; IO, inferior oblique; MR, medial rectus; LR, lateral rectus; SR, superior rectus; IR, inferior rectus. In the lateral view (**A**), the muscles are depicted attached to the common tendon. *(From Carreiro JE: Ophthalmology. In Carreiro JE (ed.): An Osteopathic Approach to Children, 2 ed, Edinburgh, 2009, Churchill Livingstone, p. 197–214.)*

orbital plate of the maxillary bone, inferior to the lacrimal fossa, posteriorly laterally and sup insert on the globe.

7. **Describe the innervation of the extraocular muscles.**
The medial rectus, superior rectus, inferior rectus, and inferior oblique muscles are innervated by cranial nerve III. The superior oblique muscle is innervated by cranial nerve IV. The lateral rectus muscle is innervated by cranial nerve VI. The blood supply to the extraocular muscles is provided by the inferior and superior muscular branches of the ophthalmic artery, lacrimal artery, and infraorbital artery.

8. **Describe the vasculature to the orbit.**
The arterial supply to the orbit is from the internal carotid artery via the ophthalmic branch with contributions from the external carotid artery system (superficial facial artery). The branches of the ophthalmic artery include the central retinal, the lateral and medial posterior ciliary, the lacrimal, muscular, supraorbital, anterior and posterior ethmoidals, supratrochlear, nasofrontal, and dorsonasal arteries. The lacrimal artery forms an anastomosis with the external carotid system via the transverse facial and superficial temporal arteries. Medially, the dorsonasal arteries anastomose with the external carotid system via the angular arteries. The maxillary artery contributes via its infraorbital branch.
The venous drainage of the orbit is from the superior and inferior ophthalmic veins. The inferior ophthalmic vein originates from a plexus of vessels in the inferior orbit, joins the pterygoid plexus, and terminates at the superior ophthalmic vein to enter the cavernous sinus. The superior ophthalmic vein originates at the superior medial orbit and crosses midorbit below the superior rectus muscle. The lacrimal vein joins the superior ophthalmic vein prior to exiting the orbit to enter the cavernous sinus.

9. **Describe the anatomy of the lacrimal system.**
The lacrimal gland, which is responsible for reflex tearing, is found within the lacrimal fossa in the orbital portion of the frontal bone. The gland is divided into the palpebral lobe and the orbital lobe by the lateral horn of the levator aponeurosis. Eight to twelve lacrimal gland ductules empty into the superior lateral conjunctival fornix. The accessory lacrimal glands (glands of Wolfring and Krause), which are responsible for basal tearing, are located in the eyelid. The lacrimal papillae are located medially on the posterior edge of the upper and lower eyelids and lead to the lacrimal canaliculi. The lacrimal canaliculi (superior and inferior) lead to the lacrimal sac within the lacrimal fossa, most often (>90%) forming a single common canaliculus prior to entering the sac. The valve of Rosenmuller is located at the medial end of the common canaliculus and prevents tear reflux. The nasolacrimal duct forms (exits) at the inferior portion of the lacrimal sac and lies within the bony nasolacrimal canal. The nasolacrimal duct drains into the inferior meatus of the nose beneath the inferior turbinate through the valve of Hasner.

10. **What is a dacryocystorhinostomy (DCR)?**
DCR is a surgical procedure involving fistulization of the lacrimal sac into the nasal cavity. The procedure can be performed through an external incision or endoscopically through the nose.

11. **What are the advantages of endoscopic DCR?**
With the advances in endoscopic visualization and the development of improved instrumentation, endoscopic DCR has shown success rates (80% to 100%) that are similar to traditional external techniques. The advantages of endoscopic approaches include the absence of external skin incision and resultant scar, the preservation of the orbicularis oris pump mechanism, decreased disruption of the medial canthal anatomy, decreased intraoperative bleeding, and the abilty to address contributing nasal cavity or paranasal sinus abnormalities.

12. **What are the indications of endoscopic DCR?**
Excess tearing (*epiphora*) can result from hypersecretion (lacrimation) or failure of drainage. Bothersome epiphora due to nasolacrimal duct obstruction is the primary indication for DCR. Other causes include recurrent dacryocystitis, dacryolithiasis, tumors of the lacrimal system, nasal pathology, or anatomic abnormalities that obstruct the drainage pathway. Nasolacrimal duct obstruction often presents with epiphora or infection and can be confirmed via several diagnostic tests including the dye disappearance test, lacrimal system irrigation or probing, scintigraphy, and contrast dacryocystography.

riorly to

...rform an endoscopic DCR?

...i is similar to performing endoscopic sinus surgery. Important landmarks ... line (corresponds to the suture line between the frontal process of the maxilla ...), which serves as a landmark for the lacrimal sac, the uncinate process, and ...nt of the middle turbinate. A sickle knife is used to create a mucosal flap on ... over the lacrimal sac, which may be debulked or trimmed. The lacrimal bone and frontal process of the maxilla are removed to expose the medial portion of the lacrimal sac. The sac is incised and marsupialized into the nasal cavity, and silicone lacrimal intubation stents may be placed.

14. **What is the leading cause of proptosis in adults?**
Thyroid eye disease (TED or Graves' opthalmopathy) is the most common extrathyroidal manifestation of Graves' disease and is the leading cause of proptosis in adults. It is considered an autoimmune process with thyroid stimulating hormone (TSH) receptor as the likely autoantigen in both the thyroid gland and orbit. Fibroblasts and adipocytes act as effector cells, inducing a complex cytokine-mediated immunologic response marked by tissue inflammation and hypertrophy.

15. **What is the typical presentation of thyroid eye disease?**
Patients will often complain of blurry vision, foreign body sensation, photophobia, tearing, diplopia, dull pain, and discomfort. Clinical features include eyelid retraction (90% of patients), periorbital soft tissue swelling, lid lag, lagophthalmos, conjunctival injection, exposure keratopathy, restrictive myopathy, exophthalmos, and optic neuropathy. Imaging usually reveals fusiform enlargement of the extraocular muscles. MRI is more sensitive than CT for showing optic nerve compression at the orbital apex. Approximately 5% of patients will experience severe orbital inflammation and congestion resulting in compressive optic neuropathy, requiring urgent treatment.

16. **Describe the nonsurgical management of thyroid eye disease.**
In the majority of patients (80%) thyroid eye disease is self-limited, requiring only supportive care of ocular lubrication, cool compresses, and sunglasses to manage light sensitivity and glare. Medical treatment should center on correction of thyroid dysfunction because this may improve orbitopathy. The goal of medical therapy is to minimize the severity and shorten the duration of inflammation and associated fibrosis. Corticosteroids (oral or IV) are often prescribed for clinically active thyroid eye disease. Additional immunomodulators including azathioprine, cyclosporin, and IV immunoglobulin have been used in several small studies with mixed results. In selected patients, orbital radiation may be used to treat associated orbital inflammation and compressive optic neuropathy.

17. **What are the indications for surgical management of thyroid eye disease?**
Surgical intervention is indicated in cases of compressive optic neuropathy (CON), exposure keratopathy, and disfiguring proptosis. Diplopia is also a common clinical presentation for these patients. Multiple surgical approaches may be used to decompress the orbit including transcranial, transconjunctival/transcaruncular, transantral, and endonasal (endoscopic). The degree of exophthalmos recession achieved by decompression is related to the number of orbital walls decompressed. In cases of compressive optic neuropathy, decompression of the posterior aspect of the medial, inferior, and/or lateral walls of the orbit is essential. Surgical intervention is typically staged with orbital decompression first, followed by strabismus surgery, followed by eyelid surgery.

18. **How is an orbital decompression performed?**
Decompression of the medial wall is best performed through a transnasal endoscopic approach, though a medial transorbital approach may be used. The inferior orbital decompression is best approached via a transconjuctival technique with an extended lid incision to provide access to the lateral wall for additional decompression. Removal of orbital fat inferiorly and/or laterally is often performed to varying degress depending on the extent of reduction desired.

19. **Describe the anatomy of the optic nerve.**
The optic nerve is divided into four segments: intraocular, intraorbital, intracanalicular, and intracranial segments. The orbital segment of the optic nerve is 25 to 30 mm in length. The optic canal is formed by the two struts of the lesser wing of the sphenoid and contains both the optic nerve and ophthalmic artery. The optic nerve is a direct continuation of the brain and contains all three meningeal layers. The dural covering of the optic nerve is made up of two layers: an outer

layer arising at the orbital apex where the dura splits to form the optic nerve sheath and the periorbita, and an inner layer of arachnoid which is attached to the inner portion of the dural sheath.

20. When is endoscopic optic nerve decompression performed?
Traumatic optic neuropathy (TON) is the most common indication for optic nerve decompression. Improvements in endoscopic instrumentation and growing surgical experience have made endoscopic approach to the optic nerve possible. The endoscopic approach affords advantages over traditional external approaches including decreased morbidity, preservation of olfaction, faster recovery time, and more direct access to the relevant anatomy. Treatment for TON remains controversial due to limited evidence that surgical decompression is superior to medical managament or observation.

21. How is TON categorized?
TON is categorized as direct or indirect. Direct TON commonly occurs as a result of penetrating injury and involves the intraorbital portion of the nerve. Indirect TON occurs from blunt head trauma with or without a resulting fracture of the orbital canal. Visual loss in cases of indirect TON can result from neural edema, hematoma, bone fragment nerve compression, shearing nerve injury, vascular compromise or interuption of axonal transport. Optic nerve decompression is generally not indicated in direct TON but may be indicated in cases of indirect TON with hematoma, edema, or compression of the nerve within the bony canal.

22. How is TON managed?
There is no evidence-based consensus on management of TON and management should be determined on a case-by-case basis. Systemic corticosteroids and surgical decompression are currently considered the mainstays of treatment although neither has been shown to definitively improve outcomes. In patients with incomplete vision loss that fails to improve with systemic corticosteroids, surgical decompression is a reasonable treatment plan as studies have shown a potential benefit.

Bibliography

Durairaj VD: Clinical perspectives of thyroid eye disease, *Am J Med* 119(12):1027–1028, 2006.

Kennedy DW, Goodstein ML, Miller NR, et al: Endoscopic transnasal orbital decompression, *Arch Otolaryngol Head Neck Surg* 116(3):275–282, 1990.

Kikkawa DO, Pornpanich K, Cruz RC Jr, et al: Graded orbital decompression based on severity of proptosis, *Ophthalmology* 109(7):1219–1224, 2002.

Kingdom TT, Durairaj VD: Endoscopic Applications in orbital surgery. In Kennedy DW, Hwang PH, editors: *Rhinology: Diseases of the Nose, Sinuses, and Skull Base*, ed 1, New York, 2012, Thieme, pp 425–443.

Levin LA, Beck RW, Joseph MP, et al: The treatment of traumatic optic neuropathy: the International Optic Nerve Trauma Study, *Ophthalmology* 106(7):1268–1277, 1999.

Metson R, Dallow RL, Shore JW: Endoscopic orbital decompression, *Laryngoscope* 104(8 Pt 1):950–957, 1994.

Ramakrishnan VR, Hink EM, Durairaj VD, et al: Outcomes after endoscopic dacryocystorhinostomy without mucosal flap preservation, *Am J Rhinol* 21(6):753–757, 2007.

Tsirbas A, Davis G, Wormald PJ: Mechanical endonasal dacryocystorhinostomy versus external dacryocystorhinostomy, *Ophthal Plast Reconstr Surg* 20(1):50–56, 2004.

Wormald PJ, Kew J, Van Hasselt A: Intranasal anatomy of the nasolacrimal sac in endoscopic dacryocystorhinostomy, *Otolaryngol Head Neck Surg* 123(3):307–310, 2000.

IV

Otology and Audiology

OTOLOGY ANATOMY AND EMBRYOLOGY WITH RADIOLOGY CORRELATES

Renee Banakis Hartl, MD, AuD

CHAPTER 31

KEY POINTS

1. The ear is divided anatomically into the outer, middle, and inner ear. The outer ear begins at the auricle and ends at the tympanic membrane; the middle ear consists of the tympanic cavity, with the ossicular chain bridging the tympanic membrane to the cochlea; the inner ear contains the organs of hearing and balance, and the vestibulocochlear nerve (CN VIII).
2. The outer and middle ear structures are embryologically derived from the first and second branchial arches and the first branchial groove and pouch, while the bilateral otic placodes give rise to inner ear structures.
3. The end organ of hearing is the cochlea, which contains afferently innervated inner hair cells that are responsible for transduction of auditory information.
4. The three semicircular canals are oriented in distinct planes to detect changes in angular acceleration, while the utricle and saccule detect linear acceleration and are oriented in the horizontal and vertical planes, respectively.
5. Auditory information passes through the central nervous system via the following pathway: auditory nerve, cochlear nucleus, superior olivary complex, lateral lemniscus, inferior colliculi, medial geniculate body, and auditory cortex.

Pearls

1. Abnormalities of the external ear, including preauricular pits or tags, as well as malformations of the pinnae or ear canal, can be associated with congenital syndromes and may indicate the need for additional otologic and genetic workup.
2. The ossicles function to transform acoustic energy to overcome the impedance mismatch between the aerated external ear canal and the fluid-filled cochlea.
3. The cochlea is tonotopic, meaning specific areas of the cochlea are stimulated by specific tone frequencies. The physical properties of the cochlear basilar membrane (thick, stiff, narrow base and thin, flexible, wide apex) are responsible for its tonotopic properties.
4. The severity of cochlear deformities depends significantly on the gestational age of growth arrest or disruption.

QUESTIONS

1. Which structures comprise the outer ear?
The external ear is composed of the auricle and the external ear canal, terminating at the tympanic membrane (Figure 31-1). The lateral third of the canal is cartilaginous and has hair follicles, along with ceruminous and sebaceous glands. The medial two thirds of the canal is osseous and free of hairs and adnexal structures. The length of the external canal, about 2.5 cm in adults, gives it a resonance frequency of 3 to 4 kHz.

2. What are the hillocks of His? What structure do they ultimately form?
The hillocks are six small buds of mesenchyme surrounding the dorsal end of the first branchial cleft. Hillocks 1, 2, and 3 arise from the mandibular (or first) branchial arch, while 4, 5, and 6

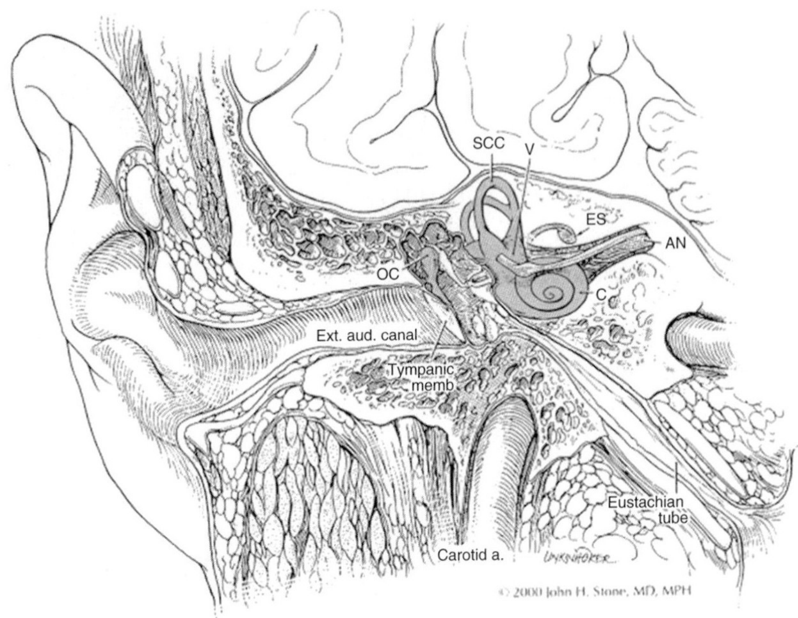

Figure 31-1. Anatomy of the ear. *(From Flint PW, et al: Cummings Otolaryngology: Head & Neck Surgery, 5th ed, Philadelphia, 2010, Mosby Elsevier, p. 1825.)*

develop from the hyoid (or second) arch. These mesenchymal structures ultimately rearrange to form the auricle. Though the exact embryology is controversial, it is classically taught that the first hillock forms the tragus, the second and third form the helix, the fourth and fifth develop into the antihelix, and the antitragus is formed from the sixth (Figure 31-2).

3. **What is the function of the auricle? How does its unique structure contribute to auditory function?**
   The cone-shaped auricle serves to collect and direct the sound down the ear canal toward the tympanic membrane. The shape of the auricle also creates small, unique, high-pitched frequency resonances that contribute to the ability to localize sound in vertical space.

4. **From which branchial structure does the external auditory canal develop?**
   The external auditory canal develops from the first (or mandibular) branchial groove.

5. **What are preauricular pits and tags? What is their clinical significance?**
   Preauricular pits and tags are benign malformations of the preauricular soft tissues. Pits are depressions in the skin located anterior to the ear canal. Epithelial mounds or pedunculated skin are known as preauricular tags. Structural abnormalities, including preauricular pits and tags, malformed pinnae, and stenotic or atretic ear canals, may indicate hearing loss and can be associated with congenital syndromes. Presence of these findings suggests the need for a thorough clinical exam for other congenital anomalies, audiometric evaluation, and possible genetic testing.

6. **Which congenital syndromes are associated with external ear abnormalities?**
   - **Treacher-Collins syndrome (mandibulofacial dysostosis):** Rare autosomal dominant condition with complete penetrance and variable expression consisting of downward-slanting palpebral fissures, auricular malformations with or without tags and preauricular blind fistulas, stenosis or atresia of the external ear canals, ossicular abnormalities, malar hypoplasia, flat nasal bridge, mandibular hypoplasia, cleft palate, and dental abnormalities.
   - **Goldenhar syndrome (Oculo-Auriculo-Vertebral syndrome):** Rare disorder of unknown inheritance pattern characterized by anomalous development of the first and second branchial

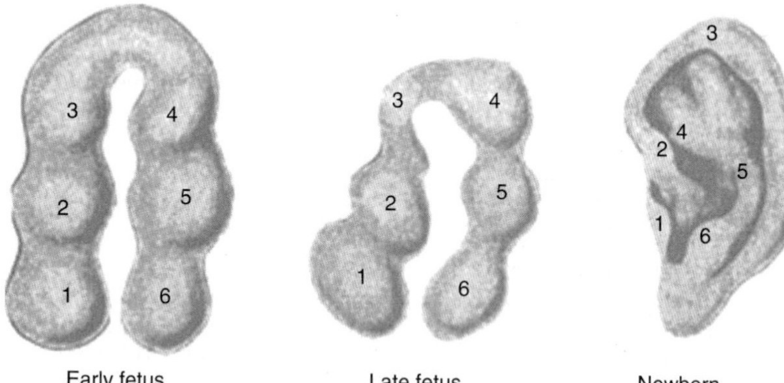

Figure 31-2. Auricular hillocks. By the fifth week of gestation, the area surrounding the first branchial groove becomes irregular, forming the six auricular hillocks of His. The following hillocks develop into the corresponding structures: 1—tragus, 2 and 3—helix, 4 and 5—antihelix, 6—antitragus. *(From Flint PW, et al: Cummings Otolaryngology: Head & Neck Surgery, 5th ed, Philadelphia, 2010, Mosby Elsevier, p. 2742.)*

arch, which often results in unilateral craniofacial malformations, including hemifacial microsomia, eye anomalies, strabismus, anotia, preauricular skin tags, and stenotic or atretic ear canals. It is also associated with severe scoliosis.

- **Branchio-oto-renal syndrome:** Rare autosomal dominant disorder that is characterized by hypoplastic or absent kidneys, preauricular pits or tags, middle ear malformation or absence, and branchial cleft cysts or fistulae.
- **CHARGE syndrome:** Rare syndrome with a cluster of associated malformations, including coloboma of the eye, heart defects, atresia of the choanae, retardation of growth/development, genital defects (hypogonadism), and ear anomalies (asymmetric pinnae with low-set, lop ears).
- **DiGeorge sequence:** 22q11 chromosomal deletion resulting in absence or hypoplasia of thymus and/or parathyroid glands with cardiovascular and craniofacial anomalies, including low-set ears, micrognathia, hypertelorism, short philtrum, cleft palate, and choanal atresia.
- **Crouzon syndrome:** Rare autosomal dominant syndrome characterized by premature skull bone fusion (craniosynostosis). Other physical features include exophthalmos, hypotelorism, strabismus, beak-shaped nose, hypoplastic maxilla, low-set ears, and ear canal stenosis or atresia.

7. Describe the middle ear. What structures can be found within the middle ear?
The middle ear is a 1 to 2 cm^3 air-filled cavity that houses the ossicles, the stapedius and tensor tympani muscles, and the chorda tympani nerve (containing taste fibers from the anterior two-thirds of the tongue and parasympathetic fibers to the submandibular and sublingual glands). The middle ear is bounded laterally by the tympanic membrane and medially by the lateral wall of the inner ear (otic capsule). It is continuous with the mastoid air cells via the antrum and the nasopharynx via the eustachian tube (see Figure 31-1).

8. What are the ossicles? What is their embryologic origin? What is their function?
The ossicular chain is composed of the malleus, incus, and stapes. The malleus attaches laterally to the tympanic membrane, the stapes couples medially to the inner ear via the oval window, and the incus bridges these two bones. The first branchial arch gives rise to the head and neck of the malleus and the body of the incus. The second branchial arch gives rise to the long process of the malleus, the long process of the incus, and the stapes suprastructure. The stapes footplate derives from both the second branchial arch and the otic capsule. The ossicles function to transform acoustic energy to overcome the impedance mismatch between the aerated external ear canal and the fluid-filled cochlea.

9. **What is unique about the embryologic derivatives of the tympanic membrane?**
The tympanic membrane consists of three layers, each of which is derived from a different germ layer. The outer epithelial layer derives from ectoderm, the middle fibrous layer derives from mesoderm, and the inner epithelial layer derives from endoderm. Neural crest–derived mesenchyme around the lateral margin of the membrane forms the tympanic annulus, which begins to ossify in the third month of gestation.

10. **Which muscles reside within the middle ear? Which cranial nerves innervate these muscles?**
The stapedius and the tensor tympani muscles can be found within the middle ear. The stapedius is innervated by the facial nerve (CN VII), and a branch of the mandibular division of the trigeminal nerve (CN V3) innervates the tensor tympani.

11. **What is the function of the stapedius and tensor tympani muscles?**
Contraction of both muscles can be induced with high-intensity acoustic stimuli, with a more pronounced effect at lower frequencies. When contracted, these muscles stiffen the ossicular chain, resulting in increased middle ear impedance and decreasing sound transmission to the inner ear. The exact function of this musculature remains somewhat controversial, though it has been proposed that these reflexes serve either as a mechanism for protection of the cochlea from intense sounds or to reduce intensity of low-frequency background noise to preserve higher-frequency speech information.

12. **Which structure provides aeration of the middle ear?**
The eustachian tube, by its connection to the nasopharynx, aerates and drains the middle ear. Its dysfunction can cause a plugged feeling or popping of the ear and is implicated in the pathophysiology of otitis media. The immature anatomy of the eustachian tube in children predisposes them to ear infections.

13. **Describe the temporal bone. Which important structures does it contain?**
The temporal bone is a pyramidal structure (apex pointing medially) that forms part of the base and lateral side of the skull. Its major divisions are the squamous, petrous, tympanic, and mastoid bone segments. It houses the hearing and vestibular organs. Parts of the carotid, jugular, and facial nerve course through it. It also includes the middle ear cavity and the mastoid air cells.

14. **Describe the tortuous path of the facial nerve through the temporal bone.**
After exiting the internal auditory canal, the facial nerve courses through the temporal bone via a z-shaped course in three divisions: the *labyrinthine*, the *tympanic*, and the *mastoid* segments (Figure 31-3). The labyrinthine segment begins as the nerve exits the internal auditory canal, traveling superior to the cochlea. Just lateral and superior to the cochlea, it angles sharply forward to reach the geniculate ganglion and then makes an acute posterior and slightly inferior turn. This "hairpin" bend is the first genu of the facial nerve. The tympanic segment extends from this point posteriorly and laterally along the medial wall of the tympanic cavity, above the oval window and below the bulge of the lateral semicircular canal, until reaching the pyramidal eminence. At this point, the nerve drops sharply inferiorly to form the second genu. The mastoid segment passes downward in the posterior wall of the tympanic cavity and the anterior wall of the mastoid to exit the base of the skull at the stylomastoid foramen.

15. **Why does complete radiologic evaluation of the facial nerve involve both CT and MRI studies?**
When evaluating the facial nerve for possible lesion, both a dedicated CT scan and an MRI are useful. A CT scan can demonstrate the integrity of the osseous facial nerve canal while an MRI can reveal enhancement of the facial nerve itself.

16. **Which structures comprise the inner ear?**
The osseous and membranous labyrinthine systems comprise the inner ear. The osseous labyrinth consists of a layer of dense bone, known as the otic capsule, and the enclosed perilymphatic space, which contains perilymph fluid. The membranous labyrinth system is embedded in the osseous labyrinth and consists of a series of continuous cavities filled with endolymph fluid. This system consists of the auditory end organ (cochlea), which is responsible for detection of sound, and the vestibular end organs (utricle, saccule, and semicircular canals), which sense linear and rotational acceleration.

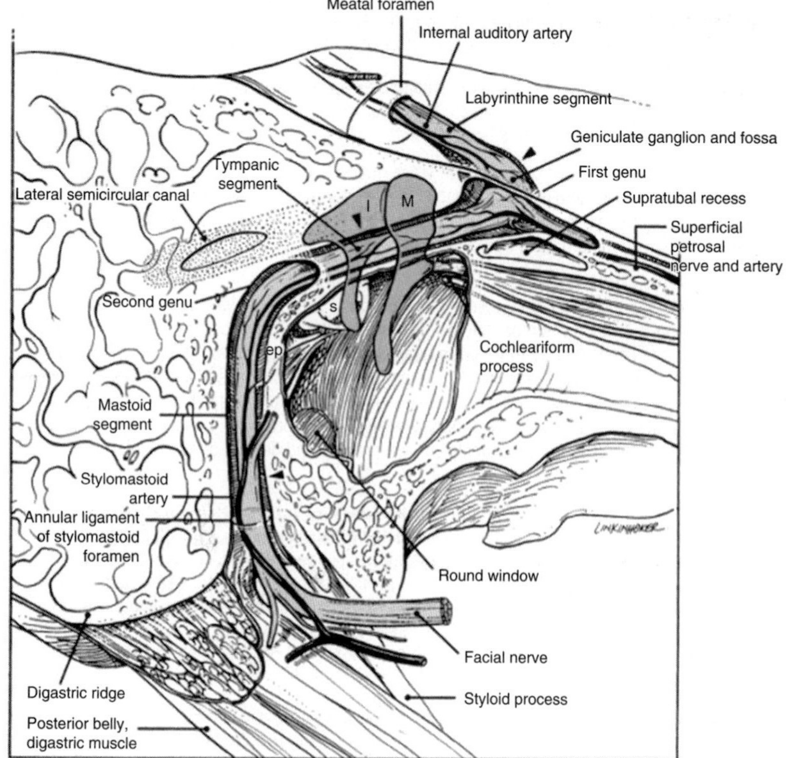

Figure 31-3. Anatomy of intratemporal facial nerve. *(From Flint PW, et al: Cummings Otolaryngology: Head & Neck Surgery, 5th ed, Philadelphia, 2010, Mosby Elsevier, p. 1826.)*

17. **What is endolymph? What is perilymph? How do they differ?**
Perilymph is the fluid contained within the osseous labyrinth that surrounds the membranous labyrinth. Endolymph is the fluid within the membranous labyrinth. Perilymph has an electrolyte composition similar to that of extracellular fluid (high in sodium, low in potassium) while the endolymph is high in potassium and low in sodium, similar to intracellular fluid. The difference in fluid characteristics sets up a large electrochemical gradient (about 80 to 100 mV) across the membranous labyrinth, which allows for transduction of acoustic energy into a neural impulse. This gradient (or endocochlear potential) is maintained by the stria vascularis, which resides on the outer wall of the membranous labyrinth in the cochlea.

18. **What is the basilar membrane? What unique physical properties does it have?**
The basilar membrane is the supporting structure on which the organ of Corti rests. The area below the basilar membrane contains perilymph while the organ of Corti above is bathed in endolymph. This membrane runs the length of the cochlea and its physical properties are responsible for the tonotopic frequency arrangement of the cochlea. The base of the basilar membrane is stiff, thick, and narrow, while the apex is wide, thin, and flexible.

19. **What is the "traveling wave"?**
G. von Bekesy is credited with describing the pattern of movement of the basilar membrane, or traveling wave, in response to sound. Each point on the basilar membrane moves at the same frequency as the acoustic stimulus; however, the amplitude and phase of the response varies considerably based on these physical properties. High frequencies cause the greatest physical

displacement of the basilar membrane near the base of the cochlea and the apex is the location of largest amplitude response to low frequencies.

20. **What is the organ of Corti?**
The organ of Corti contains the auditory receptor cells, called hair cells, and a host of other structural and supporting cells. The hair cells sit on the basilar membrane and are overlaid by the tectorial membrane. There are two types of hair cells in the cochlea: inner hair cells and outer hair cells.

21. **How does the innervation of inner and outer hair cells of the cochlea differ?**
Inner hair cells are predominantly afferently innervated. Afferent nerve fibers carry information from the hair cells to the brain. In contrast, outer hair cells are predominantly efferently innervated. Efferent fibers carry information from the brain to the hair cells.

22. **How are the cochlear hair cells stimulated?**
The hair cells are named for the presence of stereocilia, which are evaginations of the apical surface of the hair cell membrane that look like hair on the cell surface. The tectorial and basilar membranes are connected centrally. Sound moves these two structures differentially, causing a shear force that bends the stereocilia. Movement of the stereocilia opens and closes ion channels, producing a receptor potential in the inner hair cell. The receptor potential in turn releases neurotransmitters onto afferent nerve fibers, signaling to the brain the presence of a specific sound frequency. The specific hair cells stimulated by a given sound depend on the tonotopic map of the basilar membrane.

23. **What are the utricle and saccule? What are the semicircular canals?**
The utricle and saccule are vestibular organs that are responsible for detecting acceleration in a linear plane. The utricle detects horizontal accelerations and the saccule detects vertical accelerations, including gravitational force. The semicircular canals detect rotational or angular acceleration. There are three canals (lateral or horizontal, superior or anterior, and posterior), which are oriented in different planes. The vertical canals (superior and posterior) are oriented roughly at 45 degrees in relation to the sagittal plane, and the horizontal canal is tilted upward about 30 degrees anteriorly from the horizontal plane.

24. **From which embryonic structure does the labyrinthine membrane of the inner ear develop? From which germ layer is this structure derived?**
The structures of the inner ear and corresponding sensory innervation develop from bilateral otic placodes, which are ectodermal thickenings lateral to the rim of the neural tube. These placodes invaginate to become the otic pits and subsequently become enveloped by mesenchyme as vesicular structures known as otocysts. These bilateral otocysts will eventually differentiate into the membranous structures of the labyrinth. The otic capsule ossifies around the labyrinthine membrane between weeks 16 and 24 of gestation to form the bony labyrinth. Fetal hearing is possible about 2 to 3 months before birth because hair cell and auditory neural development are essentially complete by 26 to 28 weeks gestation.

25. **What types of defects can result from abnormal cochlear development? Which imaging modality is preferred to diagnose these defects?**
Inner ear malformations are described as being limited to the membranous labyrinth or involving both the osseous and membranous labyrinth. Dysplasia of the membranous labyrinth may be complete, limited to the cochlea and saccule, or involving only the basal turn of the cochlea. Membranous dysplasia is assumed to account for more than 90% of congenital deafness but can only be identified histopathologically. Only about 5% to 15% of congenitally deaf individuals have involvement of the otic capsule and thus show abnormality on imaging. These disorders include cochlear aplasia, cochlear hypoplasia, incomplete cochlear partition, and common cavity. The most severe agenesis is a complete aplasia of the entire osseous labyrinth (both cochlear and vestibular). Table 31-1 describes the osseous malformations in detail. High-resolution CT scan is the preferred imaging modality for diagnosing combined malformations of the osseous and membranous labyrinth.

26. **Which rare disorder of the semicircular canals is associated with an anomaly of the temporal bone? Which imaging modality is preferred for diagnosis?**
Superior canal dehiscence syndrome (SCDS) is characterized by conductive hearing loss, sound- or pressure-induced vertigo, and autophony resulting from absence of bone over the superior semicircular canal. The exact cause remains elusive, but dehiscent bone in SCDS has been

Table 31-1. Osseous Malformations of the Inner Ear

NAME	LOCATION	GESTATIONAL AGE OF DEVELOPMENT ARREST	APPEARANCE
Cochlear aplasia	Osseous and membranous labyrinth of cochlea	5th week	Only a vestibule and SCCs present
Cochlear hypoplasia	Osseous and membranous labyrinth of cochlea	6th week	Hypoplastic cochlea consisting of a single turn or less
Incomplete partition (Mondini)	Osseous and membranous labyrinth of cochlea	7th week	Cochlea with 1.5 turns, partially or completely lacks interscalar septum
Common cavity	Entire osseous and membranous labyrinth	4th week	Cochlea and vestibule are confluent, forming an ovoid cystic space without internal architecture
Complete labyrinthine aplasia (Michel)	Entire osseous and membranous labyrinth	Prior to 4th week	Complete absence of inner ear structures

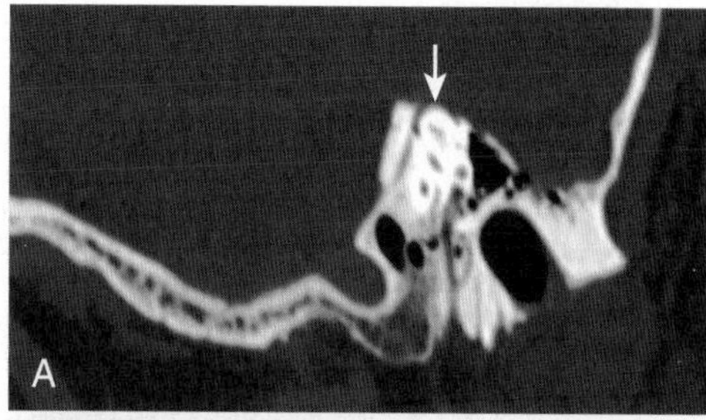

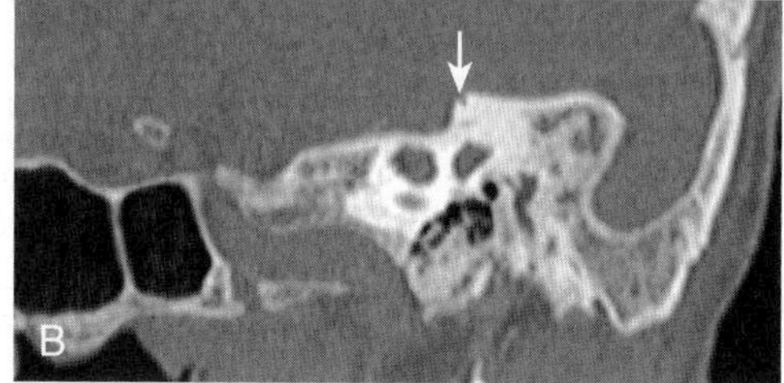

Figure 31-4. Superior canal dehiscence. CT scan of the temporal bone in the parallel plane (**A**) and perpendicular plane (**B**). Arrows demonstrate location of right superior canal dehiscence. *(From Elmali M, et al: Semicircular canal dehiscence: frequency and distribution on temporal bone CT and its relationship with the clinical outcomes. Eur J Radiol, 82(10):e607, 2013.)*

proposed to be related to incomplete ossification of the otic capsule, leading to either absent or thinned bone susceptible to trauma-related injury. High-resolution CT scan is the imaging study of choice in diagnosing SCDS (Figure 31-4).

27. **Which labyrinthine structure is thought to be a vestigial organ of hearing? Which electrophysiologic test is able to utilize this acoustic sensitivity?**
The saccule functions as an acoustic receptor in lower species that lack a cochlea. In humans, it has been shown to respond to auditory stimuli. One proposed theory to explain this sensitivity in

humans is that the saccule has retained acoustic sensitivity as a vestigial organ of hearing. The vestibular-evoked myogenic potential (or VEMP) is an electrophysiologic test used clinically to evaluate balance function that capitalizes on this retained ability.

28. **Describe the neural pathway of auditory information from the periphery to the brain.**
    After hair cells are stimulated, afferent neurons of CN VIII relay information to the cochlear nuclei. From there, stimuli travel to the superior olivary complexes, the lateral lemnisci, the inferior colliculi, and the medial geniculate bodies to the auditory cortex and association areas in the brain. Auditory information from each ear remains ipsilateral until the level of the superior olivary nucleus, at which point there is significant signal crossover. The afferent pathway of the stapedial reflex synapses at the superior olivary complex, resulting in a reflex response that can be measured bilaterally.

29. **Where is auditory information processed in the brain?**
    Auditory information is processed in the temporal cortex of the brain. The primary auditory cortex is located in the area known as Heschl's gyrus, on the superior surface of the temporal lobe close to the Sylvian fissure. This area is primarily responsible for integration and processing of auditory information and is arranged in a tonotopic fashion, with high frequencies represented medially and low frequencies represented laterally. The auditory association cortex is located lateral to the primary auditory cortex and is part of Wernicke's area, which is responsible for language reception.

BIBLIOGRAPHY

Bekesy GV: *Experiments in Hearing*, New York, 1960, McGraw-Hill.

Elmali M, Polat AV, Kucuk H, et al: Semicircular canal dehiscence: frequency and distribution on temporal bone CT and its relationship with the clinical outcomes, *Eur J Radiol* 82(10):e606–e609, 2013.

Flint PW, Haughey BH, Lund VJ, et al: *Cummings Otolaryngology: Head & Neck Surgery*, ed 5, Philadelphia, 2010, Mosby Elsevier.

Gorlin RJ, Toriello HV, Cohen MM: *Hereditary Hearing Loss and Its Syndromes*, New York, 1995, Oxford University Press.

Lalwani AK: *Current Diagnosis and Treatment in Otolaryngology—Head and Neck Surgery*, ed 3, New York, 2012, McGraw Hill Companies Inc.

Lee KJ: *Essential Otolaryngology: Head and Neck Surgery*, ed 8, New York, 2002, McGraw-Hill.

Mallo M: Embryological and genetic aspects of middle ear development, *Int J Dev Biol* 42:11–22, 1998.

Pasha R: *Otolaryngology Head and Neck Surgery, Clinical Reference Guide*, San Diego, 2000, Singular.

CHAPTER 32

HEARING LOSS AND OTOTOXICITY

Cristina Cabrera-Muffly, MD, FACS

KEY POINTS

1. When evaluating a patient with hearing loss, perform tuning fork tests (Weber and Rinne) to help determine the type of hearing loss. If this does not agree with the audiogram, discuss with the audiologist.
2. It is important to work up speech delay in children with audiometry and a comprehensive ear exam.
3. Medical clearance for hearing aids should be performed in every patient prior to hearing aid fitting. This includes a thorough history and physical exam to rule out other causes besides the most common presbycusis.
4. Common ototoxic medications include aminoglycoside antibiotics, platinum based chemotherapeutic medications, loop diuretics, and salicylates.
5. If a patient has prolonged unilateral otitis media with effusion, perform nasopharyngoscopy to rule out mass obstruction of the eustachian tube opening.

Pearls

1. Top causes of CHL
   - Cerumen impaction
   - Otitis media with effusion (most common cause in children)
   - Tympanic membrane perforation
   - Otosclerosis
2. Top causes of SNHL
   - Presbycusis
   - Noise exposure
   - Hereditary
3. Treatment for sudden SNHL
   - Confirm with audiogram
   - High-dose oral steroid burst and taper or transtympanic steroid injection
   - MRI IACs to evaluate for acoustic neuroma
4. When to get imaging for hearing loss
   - Temporal bone trauma
   - Suspected cholesteatoma
   - Suspected tumor (acoustic neuroma, glomus tumor, etc.)
   - Children (especially prior to any surgical intervention beyond PE tubes)
5. The most common radiographic finding in pediatric SNHL is enlarged vestibular aqueduct.

QUESTIONS

1. **What is sensorineural hearing loss (SNHL)?**
Sensorineural hearing loss is caused by inadequate sound processing by the end organ of hearing, the cochlea (*sensory*), or poor transmission by the eighth cranial nerve (*neural*) to the central nervous system. The function of the cochlea is to convert sound energy into electrical impulses that are then transmitted to the auditory centers in the brain. In sensorineural hearing loss, this pathway is disrupted.

2. **What is conductive hearing loss (CHL)?**
Conductive hearing loss is caused by impaired sound transmission to the inner ear. Abnormalities in the external canal, tympanic membrane, ossicles, and middle ear account for this type of hearing loss. The maximal amount of CHL is 60 decibels, and CHL over 50 decibels is most likely caused by ossicular chain pathology.

3. **What should your history include when evaluating hearing loss?**
When evaluating any type of hearing loss, it is important to ask about laterality, duration, progression, current severity, associated factors (such as otalgia, otorrhea, tinnitus, vertigo, and aural fullness), ototoxic medication use, head trauma, family history (to assess for genetic factors), autoimmune disease, and prior otologic surgery.

4. **What should your physical exam include when evaluating a patient with hearing loss?**
A complete head and neck exam should be performed, with a focus on the otologic and neurologic exams. The otologic exam should include examination of the pinna, external auditory canal, tympanic membrane, and middle ear. Tuning fork tests (Weber and Rinne) and pneumatic otoscopy should also be routinely performed.

5. **How can you differentiate between SNHL and CHL on an audiogram?**
The two main ways to differentiate between SNHL and CHL on an audiogram include the presence of an air–bone gap and abnormal tympanogram. An air–bone gap (Figure 32-1) is present during conductive or mixed (both SNHL and CHL) hearing losses, and is caused by differences in air-conducted and bone-conducted stimuli. During the vibratory portion of the audiogram, a patient with CHL will be better able to hear the stimulus because the transmission of sound through the mastoid bone is bypassing the site of blockage in the external or middle ear.
The tympanogram measures the compliance of the tympanic membrane. Increased compliance (type A_d) can indicate ossicular chain discontinuity, whereas decreased compliance (type A_s) can indicate otosclerosis, both of which can cause a conductive hearing loss. Poor compliance (type B) on a tympanogram can indicate a tympanic membrane perforation or middle ear effusion.

6. **What are the common causes of SNHL?**
The most common causes are presbycusis, noise exposure (i.e., machinery, artillery, loud music), and heredity. Less common causes are acoustic trauma, ototoxicity, sudden idiopathic hearing loss, autoimmune hearing loss, Meniere's disease, tumors, and infections (i.e., meningitis, viral labyrinthitis).

7. **What is presbycusis?**
Presbycusis is age-related hearing loss. This is the most common type of hearing loss in adults, encompassing the great majority of adult onset hearing loss. Presbycusis is bilateral, symmetric, slowly progressive high-frequency loss. Onset is in adults over 60 years, and the exact cause is unknown. Hearing aids are the most effective treatment.

8. **What guidelines are in place for newborn hearing screening?**
The U.S. federal government mandates newborn hearing screening, but programs are state regulated. The most commonly used test is otoacoustic emissions (OAE), which tests the outer hair cell response to acoustic stimulation. The other common test is auditory brainstem response (ABR), in which the eighth nerve and central nervous system produce sounds in response to an acoustic stimulation. In either case, if the test is abnormal, the newborn is referred for further testing.

9. **What is the incidence of congenital hearing loss?**
One to three infants per 1000.

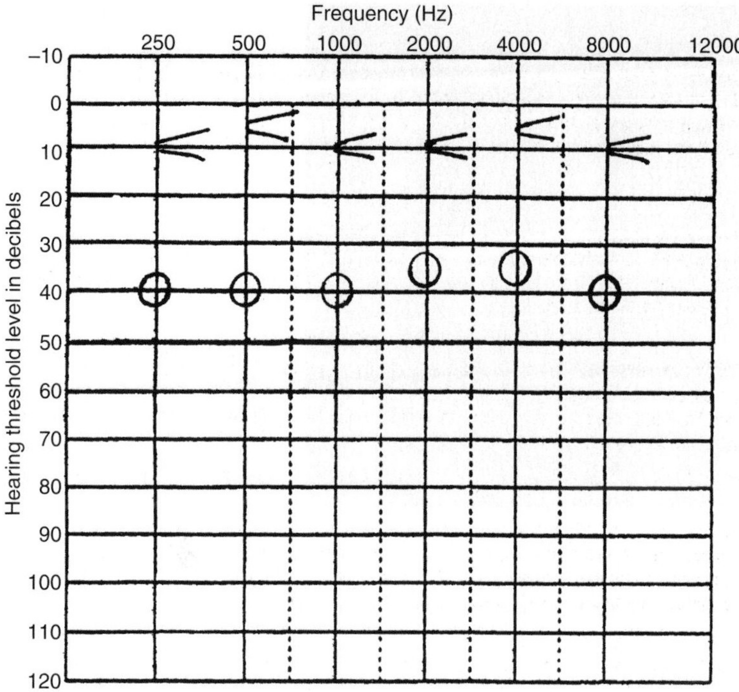

Figure 32-1. Audiogram demonstrating air–bone gap. *(From Jafek BW, Murrow BW: ENT Secrets, 3 ed. Philadelphia, Mosby, 2005.)*

10. What risk factors predispose children to hearing loss?

Risk factors that have been correlated with congenital hearing loss are (per Joint Committee on Infant Hearing):

- Family history of childhood onset permanent hearing loss
- In-utero infections (ToRCH = toxoplasmosis, other [syphilis, parvovirus, varicella], rubella, cytomegalovirus, herpes)
- Illness requiring NICU admission for more than 48 hours
- Craniofacial anomalies, especially involving the pinna or external auditory canal
- Characteristic signs of syndromes known to cause hearing loss

Other factors associated with increased rates of congenital hearing loss in the literature:

- Low birth weight (less than 1500 grams)
- Hypoxia
- Hyperbilirubinemia
- Low APGAR scores
- Head trauma
- Ototoxic medications

11. What are the developmental milestones for pediatric speech and hearing?

0 to 3 months: startled by loud sounds, calmed by familiar voices
6 months: localize sounds
9 months: respond to name and can mimic sounds
12 months: say first words
18 months: can follow simple commands
2 years: say 20 or more words and put together 2-word sentences

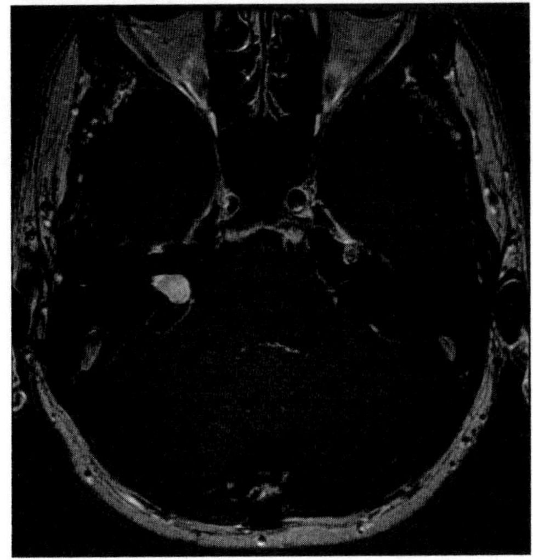

Figure 32-2. Imaging: acoustic neuroma T1-weighted axial MRI with contrast of a right sided acoustic neuroma. *(Courtesy of Stephen Cass, MD, Department of Otolaryngology, University of Colorado.)*

12. When should SNHL be evaluated with imaging?
    In children, MRIs or CT scans of the temporal bones are usually performed for all SNHL, although the majority of these scans will be normal. The most common finding in pediatric SNHL is enlarged vestibular aqueduct. In adults, MRI of the IACs with contrast is performed for asymmetric SNHL or sudden SNHL to evaluate for acoustic neuroma (Figure 32-2) and other cerebellopontine angle tumors.

13. What medications can cause ototoxicity?
    - Antibiotics (specifically aminoglycosides and vancomycin)
    - Chemotherapy drugs (cisplatin)
    - Loop diuretics (furosemide, ethacrynic acid)
    - NSAIDs and salicylates (aspirin)

14. How do ototoxic medications cause hearing loss?
    Aminoglycosides damage both vestibular and cochlear hair cells. Streptomycin and gentamycin affect vestibular function more than hearing function, and the opposite is true for neomycin and tobramycin. Vancomycin potentiates the ototoxic effect of aminoglycosides, but does not appear to be ototoxic alone. Cisplatin damages outer hair cells. Loop diuretics damage the stria vascularis (which maintains the endocochlear potential). NSAIDs and salicylates cause damage to the cochlea, only occurring with high doses, which is almost always completely reversible with discontinuation of the drug. Since most ototoxic medications are excreted by the renal system, renal impairment can lead to higher rates of ototoxicity.

15. How does ototoxicity present?
    The first symptom is usually tinnitus, followed by perception of hearing loss. Hearing loss is usually symmetric and affects the high frequencies first. With continued exposure, the lower frequencies are affected. The American Academy of Audiology recommends ototoxicity audiology protocols that include pure tone and DPOAE (a type of otoacoustic emission) testing at ultra-high frequencies (8 kHz to 20 kHz) because the earliest changes occur at frequencies greater than 8 kHz.

16. Which cause of SNHL is preventable?
    Noise exposure associated hearing loss is the only preventable cause of hearing loss. Common situations causing noise exposure hearing loss are exposure to industrial machinery, military or other exposure to gunfire, repeated loud music exposure, and acoustic trauma. Acoustic trauma is a single event of very loud noise that causes a permanent change in hearing (such as an explosion). Prevention includes both avoidance and use of hearing protection.

17. **What treatments are available for SNHL?**
Bilateral mild to severe SNHL is usually treated with hearing aids. Profound bilateral SNHL can be treated with a cochlear implant, which converts sound energy into electrical energy, directly stimulating the hearing nerve. Unilateral SNHL can be treated with a regular hearing aid, a contralateral routing of signals (CROS) hearing aid or a bone conduction implant. CROS hearing aids use the hearing aid on the poorer hearing ear as a microphone, transmitting the sound to the better hearing ear. A bone conduction implant is a hearing aid that turns sound energy into vibrational energy. An abutment is surgically implanted in the skull, to which the patient attaches a hearing aid. The vibration transmits through the skull to the better hearing ear. In cases of acoustic neuroma, surgery or radiation can sometimes improve hearing. For sudden idiopathic and immune-mediated SNHL, steroid therapy can be effective in improving the amount of hearing loss.

18. **What are the causes of sudden SNHL?**
Most cases of sudden SNHL are considered idiopathic because a cause is never identified. Sudden SNHL can rarely be caused by an acoustic neuroma, which is why an MRI of the internal auditory canals is recommended during workup. Other rare causes are syphilis, Lyme disease, vascular disease, or autoimmune disease.

19. **How should sudden SNHL be treated?**
The mainstay of therapy for sudden SNHL is steroids. This is usually given as an oral burst and taper of prednisone for 10 to 14 days, with a maximal dose of 60 milligrams daily. For patients who cannot tolerate oral steroids (for example, brittle diabetics or those in whom steroids exacerbate psychiatric disease), an alternative is transtympanic steroid injection. This procedure involves filling the middle ear space with a concentrated steroid solution. Antivirals are not recommended.

20. **Describe immune-mediated SNHL.**
Immune-mediated SNHL is usually bilateral and rapidly progressive. Many patients have roaring tinnitus. The most common treatment is high-dose steroid therapy, usually with a maximum dose of 60 milligrams for 4 weeks, followed by a taper. If the hearing loss returns after the steroids are weaned, other long-term immunosuppressant medications (such as methotrexate) may be used.

21. **What types of trauma can cause hearing loss?**
Acoustic trauma occurs due to exposure to a very loud noise. This can cause either a temporary threshold shift, which will resolve over time, or a permanent threshold shift, which does not resolve with time. Barometric trauma most commonly manifests as pain due to increased pressure in the middle ear which can lead, in severe cases, to tympanic membrane rupture. More rarely, pressure changes in the inner ear can lead to SNHL. Finally, head trauma can lead to either CHL or SNHL. Temporal bone fractures through the cochlea lead to SNHL, whereas fractures of the ossicles or tympanic membrane injury lead to CHL. Concussive injuries can also cause hearing loss, but this is less common.

22. **What are the common causes of CHL?**
The most common causes of CHL are cerumen impaction, foreign body in the canal, tympanic membrane perforation, middle ear effusion, and ossicular chain abnormalities (such as otosclerosis).

23. **What is otosclerosis?**
Otosclerosis is fixation of the stapes footplate in the oval window caused by abnormal remodeling of bone in this area. Otosclerosis causes either unilateral or bilateral conductive hearing loss that can have a Carhart notch pattern (artificial 10 to 15 decibel decrease in bone conduction at 2000 Hz). Many cases of otosclerosis are hereditary. Treatment includes either stapedectomy or a hearing aid.

24. **How much conductive hearing loss does ossicular chain disruption produce?**
While the amount of loss for other causes of CHL is variable, ossicular chain disruption usually causes a greater than 50 decibel hearing loss. “Maximal” CHL is 60 decibels.

25. **What is cholesteatoma?**
Cholesteatoma is accumulation of keratin debris in the middle ear or external auditory canal. If left untreated, the debris continues to accumulate and can cause erosion into surrounding tissues, leading to tympanic membrane perforation, damage to the ossicular chain, and even perilymphatic fistulas or tegmen defects. Cholesteatomas can become infected and can lead to recurrent otorrhea.

26. **When should nasopharyngoscopy be performed in the evaluation of CHL?**
Unilateral serous effusion lasting more than 3 months or without a preceding history of acute otitis media should be evaluated with a nasopharyngoscopy to assess for obstruction of the eustachian tube opening. Also, any serous effusion associated with recurrent epistaxis, headache, vision changes, or a painless neck mass should be evaluated with a nasopharyngoscopy to assess for nasopharyngeal carcinoma.

27. **When should CHL be evaluated with imaging?**
CHL after head trauma should be evaluated with temporal bone CT scan. Suspicion for cholesteatoma or middle ear mass (such as glomus tumor) should also be evaluated with a temporal bone CT. Prior to surgical correction of CHL in children, imaging is often performed to check for abnormalities of the inner ear such as enlarged vestibular aqueduct.

28. **What surgical therapies are used to address CHL?**
Perforated tympanic membrane can be repaired with tympanoplasty. Middle ear effusion can be treated by myringotomy with or without an ear tube. Stapedectomy can be done for otosclerosis, in which the stapes is replaced with a prosthesis. Cholesteatoma is treated with mastoidectomy to remove all of the squamous and keratinous debris. If the ossicular chain is disrupted, either a partial or total reconstruction prosthesis can be used to reconstruct the chain.

29. **What are the indications for placement of pressure equalization tubes in children?**
Per the 2013 clinical practice guidelines on tympanostomy tubes in children, tubes should be placed in children who have both persistent middle ear effusion for more than 3 months and documented evidence of hearing difficulty, vestibular problems, ear discomfort, or are at high risk for speech delay. Tubes should also be placed in children with recurrent acute otitis media if persistent effusion is present when the child is evaluated in the office.

30. **What is semicircular canal dehiscence and how does it cause hearing loss?**
This condition, also called labyrinthine fistula, can cause CHL by creating a third window into the inner ear (the first two are the oval and round windows). This is most commonly caused by a dehiscence of bone along the superior semicircular canal next to the dura. CHL occurs because sound energy is lost through the fistula. Tullio sign (dizziness or nystagmus after a loud sound) and Hennebert sign (dizziness or nystagmus after Valsalva maneuver or pneumatic otoscopy) are usually positive if a fistula is present.

Bibliography

Ashad S, Bojrab DI, Burgio DL, et al: Otology and neurotology. In Pasha R, editor: *Otolaryngology Head and Neck Surgery: Clinical Reference Guide*, San Diego, 2006, Plural Publishing, pp 295–390.

Brockenbrough JM, Rybak LP, Matz GJ: Ototoxicity. In Bailey B, editor: *Head and Neck Surgery—Otolaryngology.* Philadelphia, PA, 2001, pp 1893–1899.

Durrant JD, Campbell K, Fausti S, et al: *Ototoxicity Monitoring*, Washington, 2009, American Academy of Audiology.

Joint Committee on Infant Hearing; American Academy of Audiology: American Academy of Pediatrics; American Speech-Language-Hearing Association; Directors of Speech and Hearing Programs in State Health and Welfare Agencies: Year 2000 position statement: principles and guidelines for early hearing detection and intervention programs, *Pediatrics* 106(4):798–817, 2000.

Noise: American Speech-Language-Hearing Association, 2014. http://www.asha.org/public/hearing/Noise. Last accessed April 13, 2015.

Rosenfeld RM, Schwartz SR, Pynnonen MA, et al: Clinical practice guideline: tympanostomy tubes in children, *Otolaryngol Head Neck Surg* 149(1 Suppl):S1–S35, 2013.

Ryan AF, Harris JP, Keithley EM: Immune-mediated hearing loss: basic mechanisms and options for therapy, *Acta Otolaryngol Suppl* (548):38–43, 2002.

Stachler RJ, Chandrasekhar SS, Archer SM, et al: Clinical practice guideline: sudden hearing loss, *Otolaryngol Head Neck Surg* 146(3 Suppl):S1–S35, 2012.

EVALUATION OF HEARING

Sandra Abbott Gabbard, PhD, Stacy Claycomb, AuD and Kristin Uhler, PhD

CHAPTER 33

KEY POINTS

1. There are two major types of hearing loss—conductive and sensorineural—as well as mixed losses.
2. The patient's ability to understand speech is measured by the discrimination test.
3. The ABR tracks the electrical conductivity of the hearing signal up the brainstem.

Pearls

1. Decibel measurements of sound intensity are on a logarithmic scale.
2. Pure-tone average is the average air conduction hearing threshold at the frequencies associated with speech (500, 1000, and 2000 Hz)
3. Masking is the simultaneous presentation of sound to the *nontest* ear (to "mask" it) while actually testing the other ear with the stimulus.
4. A Stenger test can be performed to rule out malingering when there is at least a 20 dB difference between ears. A tone 10 dB above the threshold in the better ear is given while simultaneously presenting a tone 10 dB below the threshold in the poorer ear. The patient should respond if the hearing loss is geniune, but malingering patients will not respond and this is reported as a positive Stenger test.

QUESTIONS

1. **What questions do you ask of a patient presenting with hearing loss?**
As with any evaluation, it is important to first obtain a detailed history of the problem. Details such as onset, course since onset, ear(s) involved, excacerbating and relieving factors, and related symptoms are important. Also noted are the presence of tinnitus, vertigo, aural fullness, and ear pain. A detailed family, medical, and social history, including noise exposure, should be obtained to search for risk factors. Patients also should be asked about temporary or permanent functional changes involving other cranial nerves, in addition to a thorough cranial nerve examination. Recent trauma, either blunt or penetrating, may also produce hearing loss.

2. **Describe the two general types of hearing loss. How are they different?**
   1. Conductive hearing loss (CHL) results from any disruption in the passage of sound from the external ear to the oval window. Anatomically, this pathway includes the ear canal, tympanic membrane, and ossicles. Such a loss may be due to cerumen impaction, tympanic membrane perforation, foreign bodies, otitis media, or otosclerosis. Conductive losses are often correctable with medical or surgical treatment.
   2. Sensorineural hearing loss (SNHL) results from otologic abnormalities beyond the oval window. Such abnormalities may affect the sensory cells of the cochlea or the neural fibers of the eighth cranial nerve. Presbycusis, or hearing loss related to aging, is an example of an SNHL. Eighth cranial nerve tumors may also lead to such a loss. Sensorineural losses are generally permanent and are typically unmanagable medically. Hearing aids usually benefit these patients. Patients may also have a mixed hearing loss that combines both CHL and SNHL (e.g., resulting from chronic otitis media coexistent with cochlear damage) (Figure 33-1).

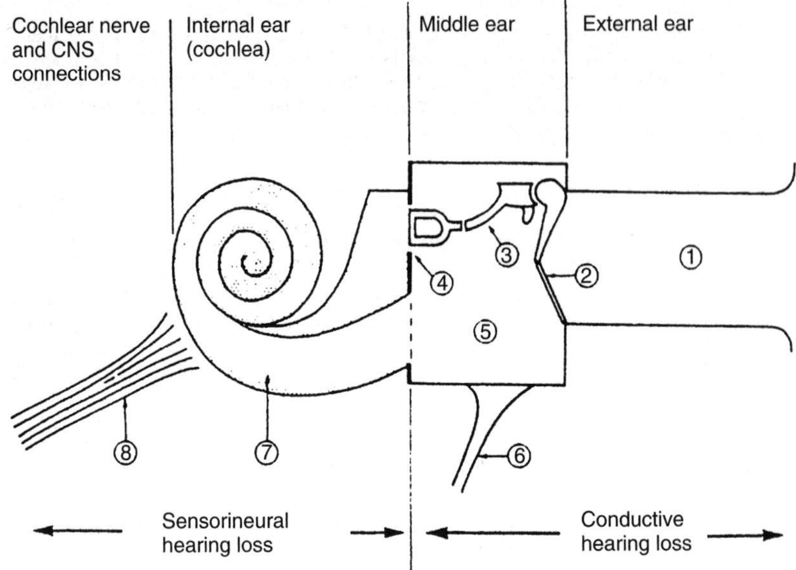

Figure 33-1. Conductive and sensorineural hearing loss. Examples: (1) wax, inflammatory swelling; (2) perforated eardrum; (3) necrosed or immobile ossicles; (4) stapes fixation by otosclerosis; (5) otitis media; (6) eustachian tube block; (7) sensory presbycusis, mumps, noise injury; (8) neural presbycusis, acoustic tumors. *(From Coleman BH: Diseases of the Nose, Throat, and Ear and Head and Neck. Edinburgh, 1992, Churchill Livingstone, p 106, with permission.)*

3. **What is the Weber tuning fork test? How is it performed and interpreted?**
   The Weber test is not a test of hearing, but it can provide information about the type of loss. In the Weber test a tuning fork is struck and its base is placed midline on the patient's skull. Commonly a 512 Hz and/or 1024 Hz (hertz or Hz: a unit of measure for cycles/second) tuning fork is used. The patient is first asked where the tone is perceived and next whether the tone is louder in one ear or the other. In CHL, the tone is louder and localizes to the poorer hearing or affected ear. In SNHL, the patient perceives the tone to be louder in the better hearing or unaffected ear. Patients with equal hearing or bilaterally symmetric hearing problems will localize the sound to the skull midline.

4. **What is the Rinne tuning fork test? How is it done?**
   The Rinne test is also used to differentiate between CHL and SNHL. The test is performed by alternately placing the prongs of a vibrating tuning fork at the patient's ear canal and the base of the tuning fork on the patient's mastoid bone. The patient is asked whether the tone is heard louder at the ear canal or on the mastoid. In the patient with normal hearing and normal middle ear status, the tuning fork is heard louder at the ear canal or equally loud in both positions. Similar findings are expected from a patient with SNHL. Patients with conductive loss, however, hear the tuning fork sound louder at the mastoid position (a negative Rinne test result, bone conduction is greater than air conduction). A negative test is obtained when the CHL is at least 25 decibels hearing level (dB HL).

5. **Describe the Schwabach's tuning fork test.**
   The Schwabach's test is a crude comparison of the patient's hearing to a presumed normal hearing person (the examiner) and does not replace a complete audiometric evaluation. The base of a vibrating tuning fork is placed on the patient's mastoid bone. When the tone decays to the point that the patient is unable to perceive it, the examiner quickly transfers the tuning fork to his or her own mastoid. If the examiner is able to hear the tone, the test indicates that the patient has an SNHL. The test result is then reported as "diminished," reflecting the patient's hearing status. This test, of course, requires that the examiner have normal hearing .

6. **Why are tuning fork tests performed?**
Tuning fork tests are done to primarily assist in evaluating the possible type of hearing loss (CHL versus SNHL). They contribute little to evaluating the presence or degree of hearing loss, which should be done with a complete audiometric evaluation. However, they can be useful in a situation where the patient would not tolerate complete audiometric testing, (e.g., a trauma patient in the ICU), or if audiometry is not available.

7. **How wide is the frequency range for normal hearing?**
The human ear can detect sound in the frequency range of 20 to 20,000 Hz. However, the typical adult can only detect frequencies between 200 and 10,000 Hz. The speech frequency spectrum ranges from 400 to 5000 Hz, and audiometric test procedures typically evaluate 250 to 8000 Hz.

8. **What is a decibel?**
A decibel is an arbitrary unit of measurement that is logarithmic in nature. Several decibel scales are used to measure sounds and hearing, and it is necessary to identify each reference scale when presenting a value in decibels. For example, hearing is measured on a biologic scale in decibels hearing level (dB HL), whereas environmental sounds are measured on a physical scale in decibels sound pressure level (dB SPL). The normal ear is not equally sensitive to all frequencies, and it is able to hear mid frequencies better than low and high frequencies. Normal hearing at 125 Hz is about 45 dB SPL, at 1000 Hz is about 7 dB SPL, and at 6000 Hz is about 16 dB SPL. A reference level of 0 dB HL represents normal hearing across the entire frequency spectrum.

9. **What is an audiogram?**
An audiogram is produced using a relative measure of the patient's hearing as compared with an established "normal" value (Figure 33-2). It is a graphic representation of auditory threshold responses that are obtained from testing a patient's hearing with pure-tone stimuli (Table 33-1). The parameters of the audiogram are frequency, as measured in cycles per second (Hz), and intensity,

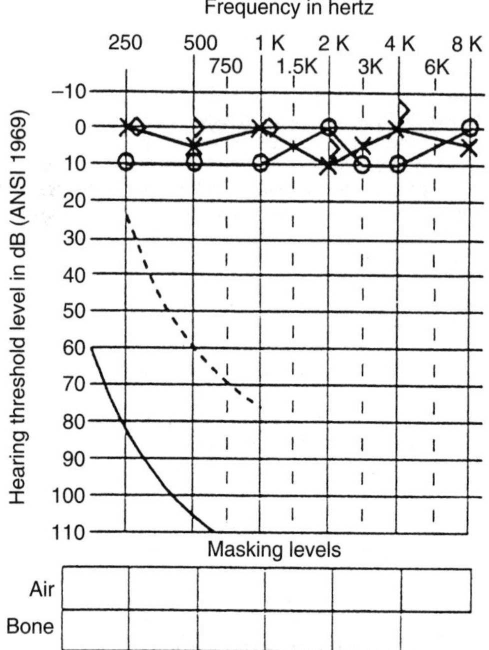

Figure 33-2. A normal audiogram. *(From Lee KJ: Essential Otolaryngology—Head and Neck Surgery, 5th ed, Norwalk, CT, 1995, Appleton & Lange, p 37, with permission.)*

Table 33-1. Commonly Used Audiogram Symbols

LEFT EAR	INTERPRETATION	RIGHT EAR
X	Unmasked air conduction	O
□	Masked air conduction	Δ
>	Unmasked conduction	<
]	Masked bone conduction	[
↘	No response	↙

Table 33-2. Hearing Threshholds

<20 dB HL	Normal hearing
20–40 dB HL	Mild hearing loss
40–60 dB HL	Moderate hearing loss
60–80 dB HL	Severe hearing loss
>80 dB HL	Profound hearing loss

as measured in dB HL. The typical audiogram is determined by establishing hearing thresholds for single-frequency sounds at 250, 500, 1000, 2000, 4000, and 8000 Hz; the primary speech thresholds are 500, 1000, and 2000 Hz. The interoctaves of 3000 and 6000 Hz are commonly measured as well.

10. **What is normal hearing?**
Practically speaking, normal adult hearing is represented as a general range between 0 and 20 dB HL. The measurement of hearing is based on threshold responses, with a threshold defined as that point at which a patient perceives a sound stimulus 50% of the time. Patients with hearing loss have audiograms with poorer thresholds (larger numbers in decibels) at the involved frequencies. This is generally considered to be >20 dB (Table 33-2).

11. **What is the pure-tone average?**
The pure-tone average (PTA) is an estimate of the patient's ability to hear within the speech frequencies. The value is calculated by averaging the air conduction hearing thresholds at 500, 1000, and 2000 Hz. For individuals with a precipitously sloping hearing loss, a Fletcher's average is commonly used, which is the average of the two best thresholds that are typically used to obtain the PTA.

12. **When an audiologist says that a hearing loss requires masking to verify, what does this mean?**
Loud sounds presented to the test ear can travel via bone conduction through the skull and be perceived in the opposite, nontest ear. This phenomenon, called crossover, can obscure measurement results in the test ear. Therefore, the nontested ear must be excluded from the test. Air conduction sounds can cross over when a difference of as little as 40 dB exists between the air conduction threshold of the test ear and the bone conduction threshold of the nontest ear. This may vary depending on head size and transducer used. Headphone crossover occurs at lower levels (40 to 60 dB) than insert earphones (70 to 90 dB). Bone conduction sounds may cross over when a difference as little as 0 dB exists between the bone conduction thresholds of the two ears. Masking is the simultaneous presentation of sound to the *nontest* ear while testing the other ear with the stimulus; this serves to prevent the nontest ear from interfering with true sound perception in the test ear.

13. **How does the audiologist distinguish between air and bone conduction deficits?**
In measurements of air conduction hearing thresholds, headphones or inserted ear phones deliver sound to the patient. If a hearing loss is noted on testing air conduction, bone conduction hearing

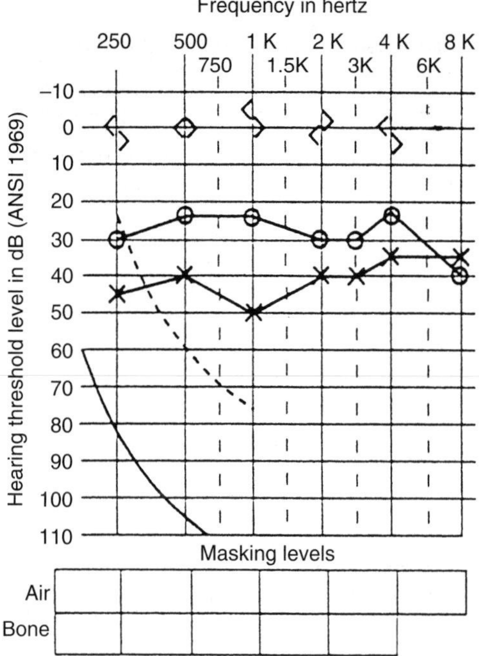

Figure 33-3. Air–bone gap typical of a conductive hearing loss. *(From Lee KJ: Essential Otolaryngology—Head and Neck Surgery, 5th ed, Norwalk, CT, 1995, Appleton & Lange, p 37, with permission.)*

thresholds are subsequently performed. Bone conduction is tested by placing a vibrating device (bone oscillator) behind the ear on the mastoid. The bone oscillator presents the sound to the inner ear, thus bypassing the middle ear system. Patients with SNHL have equal hearing thresholds by air and bone conduction measurements. Patients with CHL have normal cochlear function; therefore, they show normal hearing thresholds by bone conduction but poor hearing thresholds by air conduction.

14. **What do you look for on an audiogram to tell whether a hearing loss is sensorineural or conductive?**
Look for an air–bone gap. An air–bone gap is the difference in decibels between the hearing thresholds obtained using the insert earphones (air conduction) and those obtained using the bone oscillator (bone conduction). Significant air–bone gaps represent CHL (Figure 33-3). Because the patient hears better through bone conduction than with insert earphones/headphones, a gap exists between the two measurements. With normal hearing, the air and bone conduction thresholds are approximately equal (≤10 dB difference). With SNHL (Figure 33-4), the air and bone conduction thresholds are approximately equal but, overall, show a deficit (>10 dB). A conductive loss would result in a gap between a more normal bone conduction threshold, and the poorer air conduction threshold.

15. **What is the speech reception threshold (SRT) test?**
This test is performed to confirm the pure-tone threshold findings. The patient is familiarized with a specific set of bisyllablic words, known as spondees, which are then presented to the patient at decreasing intensities. Spondees are two-syllable compound words that are pronounced with equal emphasis on each syllable—for example, oatmeal, popcorn, and shipwreck. The SRT is the lowest intensity at which the patient correctly identifies the word in 50% of the presentations. The SRT should typically be within ±7 dB of the three-frequency pure-tone average or, for patients with a precipitously sloping hearing loss, the Fletcher's average.

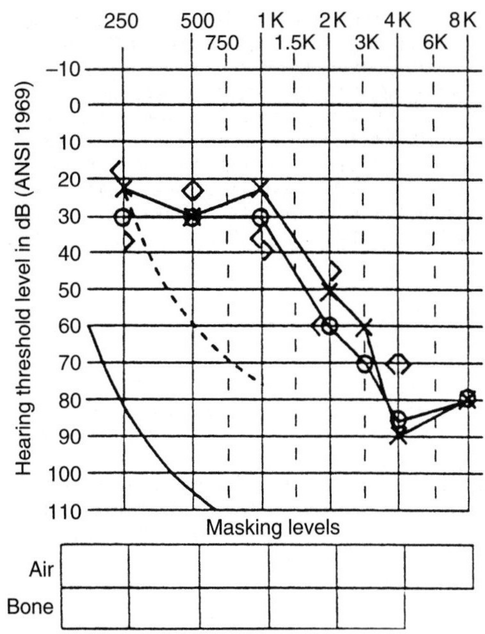

Figure 33-4. Audiogram showing sensorineural hearing loss. *(From Lee KJ: Essential Otolaryngology—Head and Neck Surgery, 5th ed, Norwalk, CT, 1995, Appleton & Lange, p 38, with permission.)*

16. **Describe the speech discrimination or recognition test.**
The purpose of the speech discrimination or recognition test in quiet is to assess the patient's understanding of speech when the loudness level is sufficient for the listener to perform maximally. A standardized list of single-syllable words are presented approximately 40 dB above the SRT or at the patient's most comfortable loudness level. The patient repeats each word, and the score is determined according to the percentage of words that are correctly identified. Good to excellent understanding is considered to result in scores between 80% to 100%; however, critical difference scores are dependent on the number of items in each list and test method. Recorded stimuli are considered to be the most generalizible between settings and sessions. While 25-word lists are generally the clinical standard, the critical difference scores or the test-reretest reliability can vary as much as 40%, with the most variability expected for poorer scores. Speech recognition can also be assessed with sentences in the presence of varying degrees of background noise. This application is typically used to estimate functional performance with and without hearing aids or cochlear implants.

17. **What do you do when the patient's tuning fork test results do not agree with the audiogram?**
Consider a number of factors. Has the audiometry equipment recently been producing questionable results? Do both headphones work? Is the examiner properly using the tuning forks? Is the examiner comfortable with the anatomy? Does the patient understand the instructions? Does the patient have a secondary gain? If available, old audiograms should be obtained for comparison. Most importantly, the inconsistency needs to be resolved.

18. **What is the immittance test battery?**
The immittance test battery is not a hearing test, but rather an electroacoustic testing procedure that is used to evaluate the status of the auditory system. The test battery typically includes tympanometry (a measurement of energy transmision through the middle ear) and ipsilateral and contralateral acoustic reflex measurements.

19. **How is the examiner's subjective evaluation of tympanic membrane mobility quantified objectively?**
Tympanometry can be thought of as electronic pneumatic otoscopy. Tympanometry is an objective test that measures the mobility, or compliance, of the tympanic membrane and the middle ear system. A seal is formed between the instrument probe and the external canal. Air pressure is manipulated into the space bound by the probe, the external ear canal, and the tympanic membrane. Tympanometry results are represented by air pressure/compliance graphs known as tympanograms. The compliance of the tympanic membrane is at its maximum when air pressure on both sides of the eardrum is equal. The peak air pressure of the tympanogram is equal to the patient's middle ear pressure. The range of normal middle ear pressures is between 0 and –150 mmH_2O and represents normal eustachian tube function. Middle ear pressures that are more negative than –150 mmH_2O are indicative of poor eustachian tube function.

20. **The chart of a patient says that she had a type B tympanogram on her last visit. What does this mean?**
Tympanograms are classified into five general configurations (Table 33-3).

21. **How can I tell whether a type B tympanogram results from fluid or a perforation?**
Look at the middle ear canal volume, normally recorded next to the tympanogram. This test is conducted with an immittance meter and measures the volume medial to a hermetically sealed probe. The result, typically reported in centimeters cubed (cm^3), is the absolute volume of the ear canal when the tympanic membrane is normal. However, in situations where the tympanic membrane is perforated, the measurement is quite large as the volume of the middle ear space is also included. Pressure equalization tubes will also result in a large volume measurements. Normal middle ear volumes for children range from about 0.5 to 1.0 cm^3, and normal middle ear volumes for adults are up to about 3 cm^3.

22. **What is the function of the stapedius muscle?**
The stapedius muscle, attached to the posterior crus of the stapes, contracts reflexively at the onset of a loud sound. The muscle contracts bilaterally, even when only one ear is stimulated. The stapedius muscle is thought to provide some protection to the inner ear in the presence of potentially damaging intense sound. The acoustic reflex causes immediate stiffening of the ossicles and increased compliance of the middle ear system and tympanic membrane. Testing the contraction of the stapedius muscle by measuring the compliance change of the tympanic membrane is known as the acoustic reflex, an important part of the immittance test battery.

23. **Describe the acoustic reflex neural pathways.**
The acoustic reflex has both an ipsilateral and contralateral pathway. The majority of neurons run through the ipsilateral pathway. The ipsilateral pathway begins at the cochlea and proceeds through the eighth nerve, cochlear nucleus, trapezoid body, superior olivary complex, and facial motor nucleus to the ipsilateral stapedial muscle. The contralateral pathway crosses the brain stem at the superior olivary complex to continue to the opposite cochlear nucleus, trapezoid body, contralateral olivary complex, motor nucleus of the facial nerve, and opposite stapedius muscle.

Table 33-3. Tympanogram Configurations

Type A	Normal middle ear function
Type A_S	Tympanic membrane is stiffer than normal (lower compliance) in the presence of normal middle ear pressures (e.g., otosclerosis).
Type A_d	Tympanic membrane is more flaccid than normal (higher compliance) in the presence of normal middle ear pressure (e.g., ossicular discontinuity).
Type B	Also known as a "flat" tympanogram, it shows no pressure peak and indicates nonmobility of the tympanic membrane (e.g., middle ear effusion or perforated tympanogram).
Type C	Tympanic membrane shows a peak in the negative pressure range (< –150 mm H_2O); indicates poor eustachian tube function.

24. **How is the acoustic reflex measured?**
The acoustic reflex is measured with the immittance meter. The change in compliance of the middle ear is caused by contraction of the stapedial reflex and is time-locked to the presence of a loud acoustic stimulus. The ipsilateral reflex is measured with the stimulus presented through a sealed probe. The contralateral reflex is measured through a probe on the opposite ear of the stimulus. Measurement of the acoustic reflex is a valuable technique that is used to determine the integrity of the neural pathways. It is also used to detect eighth nerve tumors, sensory cell impairment of the cochlea, and loudness intolerance for patients with SNHL.

25. **What is auditory brain stem response audiometry?**
Auditory brain stem response (ABR) is an objective, physiologic measurement of auditory neural function. This evoked potential can be useful as an assessment of audiologic or neurologic function. ABR recordings using clicks and frequency-specific tone bursts can be useful in predicting behavioral hearing thresholds in infants or young children, or in adults who cannot or will not give accurate behavioral results. By decreasing the amplitude of the stimulus, the peaks of the waveform will eventually disappear. The presence of neural tumors of the eighth cranial nerve, internal auditory meatus, and cerebellopontine angle often result in abnormal waveforms.

Accurate assessment requires that the patient is either asleep or in a quiet, relaxed state. The test is conducted using scalp electrodes to pick up the minute electroencephalographic activity created when sound travels through the auditory pathway listed below. A series of clicks or tone bursts is delivered to the patient through inserted earphones. When an acoustic signal stimulates the ear, it elicits, or "evokes," a series of small electrical events ("potentials") along the entire peripheral and central auditory pathway. This minute electrical activity is picked up by the electrodes, amplified, and averaged with a computer.

The electrical activity is displayed as a waveform with five latency-specific wave peaks. The latency of each wave peak corresponds to sites in the neural auditory pathway. In basic terms, each peak represents one anatomic structure in the auditory pathway. A tumor will slow the neural circuit and delay the waveform at the site of the lesion.

26. **How do you interpret an ABR?**
The mnemonic E COLI will help you to remember which structure corresponds to each waveform.

Wave I **E**ighth nerve action potential
Wave II **C**ochlear nucleus
Wave III **O**livary complex (superior)
Wave IV **L**ateral lemniscus
Wave V **I**nferior colliculus

Audiologists interpret the waveforms for proper identification and then compare them to clinical norms. Type, degree, and configuration of hearing loss can be estimated using ABR assessment. Additionally, click ABR is the gold standard for diagnosing auditory neuropathy, a less common disorder that is diagnosed by presence of a cochlear microphonic (outer hair cell function) with an absent wave I.

27. **What is auditory steady state response (ASSR)?**
ASSR is an evoked potential evaluation used to estimate hearing thresholds objectively. Unlike click ABR, which assesses the mid- to high-frequency region, ASSR uses frequency-specific tonal stimulus. It assesses whether the auditory response and neurologic integrity of the auditory system are phase locked to the stimulus. Because ASSR utilizes pure-tone stimuli,the presentation intensity can be louder than traditional ABR, and is a particularly important assessment tool in differentating severe and profound hearing loss. It cannot be used to assess neurologic function.

28. **What are otoacoustic emissions (OAEs)?**
OAEs are an objective measure that allows outer hair cell function of the cochlea to be assessed. Evoked OAEs are low-level sounds produced by the cochlea following acoustic stimulation. Transient evoked otoacoustic emissions (TEOAEs) and distortion product otoacoustic emissions (DPOAEs) are two types of OAEs used clinically. OAEs are present in patients with auditory neuropathy because OAEs are not a measure of neural function.

29. **What is pseudohypacusis (also known as nonorganic hearing loss)?**
A number of factors may lead a person to feign a hearing loss that does not exist or exaggerate an existing hearing loss. While it is beyond the scope of this chapter to discuss some potential reasons, such as monetary gain or psychological reasons, certain outcome measures obtained from the audiogram can indicate pseudohypacusis. Based on the cross-check principle (Jerger and Hayes, 1976) all components of the audiogram should be consistent. Specifically, there should be good PTA-SRT/SAT agreement and there should be good test-retest reliability. Additionally, in a patient presenting with a unilateral hearing loss the audiologist should notice a shadow curve, meaning that once the stimulus in the poorer ear is increased to a certain loudness level (40 to 70 dB, depending on frequency and air conduction transducer) the energy would cross over to the better ear and the patient would begin to respond. However, patients who are malingering would not respond even when it becomes audible in the contralateral ear. The same is true for bone conduction, which has an interaural attenuation of 0 dB; if it is placed on the "poor" ear they will likely not respond. Another way to quantify if hearing loss truly exists when patients are feigning a unilateral loss is the Stenger test. The Stenger test can be done when there is at least a 20 dB difference between ears. It is conducted at any frequency where the difference between ears is ≥20 dB HL by presenting a tone 10 dB above the threshold in the better ear while simultaneously presenting a tone 10 dB HL below the threshold in the poorer ear. The patient should respond if the hearing loss is geniune. However, patients with nonorganic hearing loss will not respond, and this will be reported as a positive Stenger test. Additional measures discussed above (ABR and OAE) can assist in teasing out presence or absence of hearing loss.

CONTROVERSY

30. **When should a primary care physician be concerned about a patient's hearing complaint?**
Always. All patients who suspect hearing loss or who report difficulty with speech understanding need further evaluation. Often, patients with conductive hearing problems may be successfully treated by medical or surgical means. Patients with SNHL need to be medically evaluated prior to audiologic fitting with hearing aids. Patients with a history of sudden-onset hearing loss, trauma, infection associated with the loss, or asymmetric hearing loss should be given thorough hearing tests and concurrent otolaryngologic evaluation. Symptoms of tinnitus, aural fullness, vertigo, or ear drainage also necessitate complete otolaryngologic evaluation.

Bibliography

Brown DK, Dort JC: Auditory neuropathy: when test results conflict, *J Otolaryngol* 30:46–51, 2001.
Griffiths TD: Central auditory pathologies, *Br Med Bull* 63:107–120, 2002.
Jerger J, Hayes D: The cross-check principle in pediatric audiometry, *Arc Otolaryngol* 102:614–620, 1996.
Johnson KC: Audiologic assessment of children with suspected hearing loss, *Otol Clin North Am* 35:711–732, 2002.
Lemkens N, Vermeire K, Brokx JP, et al: Interpretation of pure-tone thresholds in sensorineural hearing loss (SNHL): a review of measurement variability and age-specific references, *Acta Otorhinolaryngol Belg* 56:341–352, 2002.
Martin FN, Clack JG: *Introduction to Audiology*, ed 8, Needham Heights, MA, 2003, Allyn & Bacon.
Meurer J, Malloy M, Kolb M, et al: Newborn hearing testing at Wisconsin hospitals: a review of the need for universal screening, *WMJ* 99:43–46, 2000.
Murphy MR, Selesnick SH: Cost-effective diagnosis of acoustic neuromas: a philosophical, macroeconomic, and technological decision, *Otolaryngol Head Neck Surg* 127:253–259, 2002.
Pichora-Fuller MK, Souza PE: Effects of aging on auditory processing of speech, *Int J Audiol* 42(Suppl 2):2S11–2S16, 2003.
Rapin I, Gravel J: "Auditory neuropathy": physiologic and pathologic evidence calls for more diagnostic specificity, *Int J Pediatr Otorhinolaryngol* 67:707–728, 2003.
Rosenhall U: The influence of aging on noise-induced hearing loss, *Noise Health* 5:47–53, 2003.
Sininger YS: Audiologic assessment in infants, *Curr Opin Otolaryncol Head Neck Surg* 11:378–382, 2003.
Stewart MG: Outcomes and patient-based hearing status in conductive hearing loss, *Laryngoscope* 111(11 Pt 2):1–21, 2001.
Thornton AR, Raffin MJM: Speech-discrimination scores modeled as a binomial variable, *J Speech Hear Res* 21:507–518, 1978.
Vermeire K, Brokx JP, Lemkens N, et al: Speech recognition tests in sensorineural hearing loss, *Acta Otorhinolaryngol Belg* 57:169–175, 2003.
Watkin PM: Neonatal screening for hearing impairment, *Semin Neonatol* 6:501–509, 2001.
Zadeh MH, Selesnick SH: Evaluation of hearing impairment, *Comp Ther* 27:302–310, 2001.

CHAPTER 34

TINNITUS

Renee Banakis Hartl, MD, AuD and Ted H. Leem, MD, MS

KEY POINTS

1. Tinnitus is a relatively common disorder, with up to 15% of the population suffering from some degree of abnormal perception.
2. Most subjective tinnitus is hypothesized to result from changes in peripheral auditory function leading to central neural hyperexcitability and cortical reorganization.
3. Though most patients with tinnitus have hearing loss, up to 10% may show no changes in hearing sensitivity on standard audiometric evaluation.
4. Most therapy for subjective tinnitus focuses on integrating principles of sound masking, counseling, and/or psychotherapy.
5. The role of surgery for management of most tinnitus is limited.

Pearls

1. Pulsatile tinnitus may suggest a vascular malformation or neoplasm and indicate a need for radiologic evaluation.
2. MRI with gadolinium contrast is the imaging study of choice for evaluation of nonpulsatile tinnitus in order to evaluate for presence of a schwannoma of the vestibulocochlear nerve.
3. Palatal or stapedial myoclonus may cause a clicking tinnitus perception and can be associated with systemic disease, requiring additional evaluation.
4. High-dose salicylates are a known cause of reversible mild-to-moderate flat sensorineural hearing loss and tinnitus.

QUESTIONS

1. What is tinnitus?

   Tinnitus is an involuntary perception of sound that originates in the head and is not attributable to a perceivable external source. The word *tinnitus* is derived from the Latin *tinnire*, which means to ring. Tinnitus is often described as a "ringing" sound in the ear, but also includes descriptions such as buzzing, humming, roaring, hissing, and chirping. Tinnitus is a symptom and not a disease in itself.

2. What is the prevalence of tinnitus?

   It is generally accepted that about 10% to 15% of the population suffers from some degree of tinnitus, while 1% to 2% report that tinnitus has a severely negative impact on quality of life.

3. How can tinnitus be classified?

   Tinnitus has historically been classified as either objective (audible to an observer other than the patient) or subjective (perceptible by the patient alone). More useful classification includes description of tinnitus as either pulsatile or nonpulsatile, or categorization by location of injury or generation (external ear, middle ear, sensorineural, or central).

4. What are somatosounds?

   A more specific term for many forms of objective tinnitus, somatosounds are objective sounds that are created by the body and potentially audible to the examiner. Examples of somatosounds include perception of myoclonic contractions of the tensor tympani or pulsatile variations in blood flow in vessels near the ear.

5. What are the proposed mechanisms to explain subjective tinnitus?

   Both central and peripheral mechanisms have been proposed to explain the origin of tinnitus, but the exact cause remains unclear. Most tinnitus is associated with a cochlear abnormality, although not all patients with tinnitus have associated measurable changes in hearing. It has been proposed that sensory deprivation at the periphery leads to alterations in neural function at higher levels and persistence of these neural changes may contribute to the subjective perceptions of tinnitus. Tonotopic maps in the auditory cortex have been shown to reorganize in animal studies after sensory deprivation in a manner similar to somatosensory cortical organization changes after amputation, leading to the description of tinnitus as a "phantom limb" perception of the auditory cortex.

6. How is tinnitus evaluated?
No objective test is available to definitively verify tinnitus or identify its cause in most cases. An evaluation of tinnitus consists of a thorough case history, complete otologic exam, and an audiometric evaluation. Evaluation may also consist of administration of one of several validated questionnaires, such as the Tinnitus Handicap Inventory, the Tinnitus Handicap Questionnaire, or the Tinnitus Severity Index. Though these surveys provide little objective data, they can help to quantify the severity of impact on quality of life and may be used to track changes in tinnitus perception across various therapy modalities. Additional studies, such as imaging or vestibular evaluation, may be indicated depending on the initial presentation and differential diagnosis.

7. What is tinnitus matching and what is its value in assessment and treatment of subjective tinnitus?
Tinnitus matching is an audiometric evaluation that generally consists of pitch matching, loudness matching, and minimal suppression level (the amount of masking required to subjectively mask an individual's tinnitus). These more objective measures of tinnitus have little validity or clinical application, as tinnitus loudness, pitch, and maskability typically bear no relationship to the severity of the patient's experience or ability to benefit from treatment. Some treatment modalities, including individualized sound stimulation devices, may rely on pitch matching or minimum suppression levels to create customized listening programs targeted at masking an individual's tinnitus.

8. What signs or symptoms are suggestive of a vascular cause of tinnitus?
A pulsatile or throbbing quality that parallels the heartbeat should raise the index of suspicion. A reddish or blue mass behind the tympanic membrane may indicate a glomus tumor arising within the middle ear or a dehiscence of the jugular bulb or carotid artery. Arteriovenous malformations are uncommon but may occur between the occipital artery (passing medial to the mastoid process) and the transverse sinus. A venous hum may represent one of the more common causes of vascular tinnitus. It may signify impingement of the jugular vein by the second cervical vertebrae or suggest an underlying high-output cardiac condition, such as anemia, exercise, pregnancy, or thyrotoxicosis.

9. What is the imaging study of choice for nonpulsatile tinnitus?
MRI with gadolinium is the study of choice to exclude a vestibular schwannoma or other neoplasm of the cerebellopontine angle.

10. What is the imaging study of choice for pulsatile tinnitus?
Pulsatile tinnitus suggests a vascular neoplasm, vascular anomaly, or vascular malformation (although the cause may be as simple as transient otitis media). Glomus tumors are the most common type of vascular neoplasm. Most neoplasms and anomalies are best seen on bone windows of CT studies. Dural vascular malformations are often elusive on all cross-sectional imaging studies, and conventional angiography may be necessary to make this diagnosis. Flow-sensitive MR images show vascular loops compressing the eighth cranial nerve. Carotid dissections, aneurysms, atherosclerosis, and fibromuscular dysplasia can be identified on both MR/MR-angiographic studies and CT/CT-angiographic studies.
    Other causes such as otosclerosis and Paget's disease may be seen on CT scan. Idiopathic intracranial hypertension often shows characteristic findings of empty sella, thinning of the bony skull base, and prominent arachnoid pits. Multiple sclerosis is a rare cause of pulsatile tinnitus and is best seen on MR studies.

11. What causes of tinnitus are associated with pathology of the external ear canal?
Foreign bodies and cerumen accumulation often cause tinnitus. Hair, insects, and other small objects may come in contact with the tympanic membrane and motion may cause the perception of sound. The mandibular condyle is in close proximity with the external ear canal and disorder of the temporomandibular joint may result in a somatosound perception. Thorough case history and a careful examination are important to help rule out these causes, which often may be easily treated.

12. **What is palatal myoclonus?**
Palatal myoclonus is the regular, rhythmic contraction of the soft palate and pharyngeal musculature. The muscles involved are the tensor veli palatine, levator veli palatine, salpingopharyngeus, and superficial pharyngeal constrictor.

13. **How can palatal myoclonus be evaluated?**
The best way to detect palatal myoclonus is by using flexible nasopharyngoscopy in the awake patient to visualize the palate from a superior perch in the nasopharynx. Examining the palate from an oral cavity approach may lead to temporary extermination of the myoclonus while the mouth is stretched open. From a practical approach, both methods of examination should be used.

14. **What is stapedial myoclonus?**
The rhythmic contractions of the stapedius muscle of the middle ear are known to cause a clicking tinnitus. The tensor tympani may also demonstrate a similar middle ear myoclonus.

15. **How can stapedial myoclonus be evaluated?**
Myoclonus of the stapedius or tensor tympani musculature is best detected using audiometric immitance testing. Changes in middle ear impedance can be objectively measured in the absence of external stimuli and often correlated subjectively by the patient with the perception of clicking.

16. **What systemic diseases are associated with myoclonus?**
Multiple sclerosis, cerebrovascular accidents, intracranial neoplasms, trauma, syphilis, malaria, various psychogenic causes, and other degenerative processes.

17. **Describe the relationship between hearing loss and tinnitus.**
Most patients with tinnitus (about 85%) present with some degree of hearing loss, though not all patients with hearing loss develop tinnitus and all patients with tinnitus do not have abnormal hearing. About 10% of patients with tinnitus present with normal hearing.

18. **What objective changes in otologic function have been found in patients with tinnitus and clinically "normal" hearing?**
Recent studies have found that tinnitus patients with hearing thresholds within audiometrically normal limits demonstrate significantly smaller amplitudes of wave I of the ABR than individuals with similar thresholds that do not have tinnitus (Schaette, 2013). This suggests that possible early cochlear damage causing reduced neuronal input may be a contributing factor to the development of tinnitus, even in patients with clinically normal hearing.

19. **What is the relationship between noise exposure and tinnitus?**
With brief, isolated exposure to loud noise, most individuals experience temporary partial loss in hearing sensitivity and tinnitus that disappears within hours or days of the exposure. Repetitive excessive exposure to noise increases the risk of these changes becoming permanent.

20. **What is hyperacusis? What is the relationship between hyperacusis and tinnitus?**
Hyperacusis is decreased tolerance to sound stimuli of normally comfortable sound level and pitch. Individuals who suffer from hyperacusis often report that typically soft stimuli or sounds of a certain pitch are unbearable or painful. Some researchers believe that tinnitus and hyperacusis are two manifestations of the same alterations in auditory processing associated with decreased cochlear input and that almost all patients with hyperacusis eventually experience tinnitus.

21. **Which medications commonly cause tinnitus?**
Tinnitus is a known potential side effect of many medications (for a complete list, see Table 34-1). The medications more commonly associated with tinnitus as a side effect are salicylates and aminoglycosides.

22. **What are the effects of high-dose salicylates on tinnitus and hearing?**
High serum concentrations of salicylates and some nonsteroidal anti-inflammatory drugs (NSAIDs) cause a flat, bilateral hearing loss and tinnitus. The hearing loss is a mild to moderate sensorineural hearing loss of about 20 to 40 dB. Incidence rate of salicylate-induced ototoxicity is less than 1%. Salicylates act as competitive inhibitors of chloride at the anion binding site of prestin, the motor protein of the outer hair cell, resulting in reversible alteration in outer hair cell function. Both hearing loss and tinnitus are reversible within 24 to 72 hours of discontinuation of the offending medication.

Table 34-1. Common Medications That Can Cause Tinnitus

CLASS	EXAMPLES
ACE inhibitors	Enalapril, fosinopril (Monopril)
Anesthetics	Dyclonine, bupivacaine (Marcaine, Sensorcaine), lidocaine
Antibiotics	Aztreonam, ciprofloxacin, erythromycin estolate, erythromycin ethyl succinate/ sulfisoxazole (Pediazole), gentamicin (Garamycin), imipenem-cilastatin (Primaxin), sulfisoxazole, trimethoprimsulfamethoxazole, vancomycin
Antidepressants	Alprazolam (Xanax), amitriptyline (Elavil), desipramine, doxepin, fluoxetine (Prozac), imipramine, maprotiline (Ludiomil), nortriptyline (Pamelor)
Antihistamines	Aspirin-promethazine-pseudoephedrine (Phenergan), chlorpheniramine-phenylpropanolamine (Triaminic), clemastine (Tavist), pseudoephedrine-chlorpheniramine (Deconamine), pseudoephedrine-triprolidine (Actifed)
Antimalarials	Chloroquine, pyrimethamine-sulfadoxine (Fansidar)
Beta blockers	Betaxolol (Kerlone), carteolol (Cartrol), metoprolol (Lopressor), nadolol (Corgard), timolol (Timoptic)
Calcium channel	Diltiazem (Cardizem), nicardipine (Cardene), nifedipine blockers (Procardia)
Diuretics	Acetazolamide (Diamox), amiloride, ethacrynic acid
Narcotics	Dezocine (Dalgan), pentazocine (Talwin)
NSAIDs	Diclofenac (Voltaren), diflunisal (Dolobid), flurbiprofen (Ansaid), ibuprofen, indomethacin, meclofenamate (Meclomen), naproxen (Naprosyn), sulindac (Clinoril), tolmetin (Tolectin)
Sedatives/ Hypnotics/ Anxiolytics	Azatadine (Optimine), buspirone (BuSpar), chlorpheniramine phenylpropanolamine (Ornade)
Miscellaneous	Albuterol (Proventil), allopurinol, bismuth subsalicylate (Pepto-Bismol), carbamazepine (Tegretol), cyclobenzaprine (Flexeril), cyclosporine, diphenhydramine (Benadryl), flecainide, hydroxychloroquine (Plaquenil), iohexol (Omnipaque), isotretinoin (Accutane), lithium, methylergonovine (Methergine), nicotine polacrilex (Nicorette), prazosin, omeprazole (Prilosec), quinidine, recombinant hepatitis B vaccine (Recombivax), salicylates, sodium nitroprusside (Nipride), sulfasalazine (Azulfidine), tocainide

ACE = angiotensin-converting enzyme, NSAIDs = nonsteroidal anti-inflammatory drugs.

23. **What percentage of patients with acoustic neuromas have tinnitus as the presenting symptom?**
    Ten percent of patients with acoustic neuromas present with tinnitus; however, over 80% have tinnitus at some point during the course of the disease.

24. **How is auditory stimulation used in the treatment of tinnitus?**
    Various methods of treatment involve the use of auditory stimulation. Most early forms of treatment relied on tinnitus masking, or the use of external sound stimuli to cover up or mask the tinnitus. Environmental sounds generators, radios, televisions, fans, and custom devices worn like hearing aids with broadband masking generators have all been used with varying degrees of success. Hearing aids have also been shown to aid in tinnitus reduction when the pitch of the tinnitus is within the amplification range of the device. Individualized sound stimulation devices focus on providing an enriched acoustic environment to compensate for hearing loss with musical stimuli of customized frequency spectrum.

25. **What is tinnitus retraining therapy?**
Tinnitus retraining therapy (TRT) is a treatment modality composed of specific counseling strategies and sound therapy. The counseling aspect of TRT focuses on education regarding the neurophysiologic basis of tinnitus and decoupling of tinnitus perception from emotional, stress-based responses. Concurrent sound therapy attempts to reduce the strength of the tinnitus signal through gradual habituation. By reclassifying tinnitus and disengaging the emotionally driven responses, TRT seeks not to physiologically alter tinnitus but rather to decrease the negative impact on quality of life.

26. **What pharmacologic agents have been used as adjuvant therapy for tinnitus?**
No pharmacologic agent has been demonstrated to have any long-term reduction in tinnitus greater than that of placebo. Though the role of medication is limited in affecting an individual's perception of tinnitus, several drugs can be used to mediate the stress and anxiety that frequently accompany tinnitus. Tricyclic antidepressants and SSRIs have been used with moderate success in treating associated depression. Benzodiazepines are appropriate therapy to try in patients with severe stress from tinnitus, though they should be used with caution. Interestingly, IV lidocaine has been shown to decrease tinnitus, but its administration and side effects make this therapy impractical. For tinnitus caused by myoclonus, botulinum toxin has been used to temporarily paralyze the causative muscles.

27. **Describe the mechanism of action of lidocaine in tinnitus treatment.**
Lidocaine and several related anesthetics act as central nervous system depressants by inhibiting the influx of sodium and therefore reducing the number of action potentials. One theory to explain tinnitus pertains to the high basal firing rate of the normal auditory system and the loss of its natural inhibitors. Anesthetics are thought to augment or replace this natural inhibition process, holding tinnitus in check. At present, intravenous lidocaine is the only medication that can reliably stop tinnitus in many patients. However, it is impractical because of the short duration of action and intravenous administration.

28. **What is the role of complementary and alternative medicine in tinnitus treatment?**
No treatments available through complementary or alternative medicine have been shown to be effective at reducing tinnitus perception in randomized controlled trials. Meditation, acupuncture, controlled breathing, biofeedback, and hypnotherapy have not demonstrated reduction in tinnitus, but relaxation techniques are often beneficial in managing stress-related side effects of tinnitus. Relaxation techniques are often incorporated into cognitive behavioral therapy (CBT), which seeks to methodically identify and modify maladaptive behaviors associated with abnormal tinnitus perception.

29. **What is transcranial magnetic stimulation and how may it be beneficial in tinnitus treatment?**
Transcranial magnetic stimulation (TMS) relies upon electromagnetic induction to noninvasively generate low-level electric brain currents. It is proposed that these induced currents may inhibit the hyperexcited regions of the brain thought to be a source of subjective tinnitus perception. There is currently limited literature to support this treatment modality.

30. **What surgical treatments are available for tinnitus management?**
The role of surgery in the management of tinnitus is limited. Surgical management of pathologic conditions often associated with tinnitus, such as vascular malformations, otosclerosis, acoustic neuromas, and temporomandibular joint disorder, may improve subjective perceptions, but the majority of tinnitus sufferers do not have an identifiable pathology. Cochlear implantation in patients with bilateral profound hearing loss has been demonstrated to reduce or completely eliminate tinnitus in up to 86% of patients, though small percentages report a worsening or development of new tinnitus after surgery. For tinnitus related to myoclonus, placement of tympanostomy tubes is sometimes effective.

Bibliography

Andersson G, Vretblad P, Larsen HC, et al: Longitudinal follow-up of tinnitus complaints, *Arch Otolaryngol Head Neck Surg* 127:175–179, 2001.

Baguley D, McFerran D, Hall D: Tinnitus, *Lancet* 382:1600–1607, 2013.

Berry JA, Gold SL, Frederick EA, et al: Patient-based outcomes in patients with primary tinnitus undergoing tinnitus retraining therapy, *Arch Otolaryngol Head Neck Surg* 128:1153–1157, 2002.

Dauman R: Bouscau-Faure F: Assessment and amelioration of hyperacusis in tinnitus patients, *Acta Otolaryngol* 125(5):503–509, 2005.

Eggermont JJ, Roberts LE: The neuroscience of tinnitus, *Trends in Neuroscience* 27(11):676–682, 2004.

Folmer RL, Griest SE: Chronic tinnitus resulting from head or neck injuries, *Laryngoscope* 113:821–827, 2003.

Isaacson JE, Moyer MT, Schuler HG, et al: Clinical associations between tinnitus and chronic pain, *Otolaryngol Head Neck Surg* 128:706–710, 2003.

Jastreboff PJ: Phantome auditory perception (tinnitus): mechanisms of generation and perception, *Neurosci Res* 8:221–254, 1990.

Jastreboff PJ, Hazell JWP: *Tinnitus Retraining Therapy: Implementing the Neurophysiologic Model*, London, 2004, Cambridge University Press.

Langguth B, Kreuzer PM, Kleinjung T, et al: Tinnitus: causes and clinical management, *Lancet Neurol* 12:920–930, 2013.

Lockwood AH, Salvi RJ, Burkard RF: Tinnitus, *N Engl J Med* 347:904–910, 2002.

Nelson JJ, Chen K: The relationship of tinnitus, hyperacusis, and hearing loss, *Ear Nose Throat J* 83(7):472–476, 2004.

Schaette R: Tinnitus in men, mice (as well as other rodents), and machines, *Hear Res* 311:63–71, 2014. PMID: 24374091.

Tyler RS: *Tinnitus Treatment*, New York, 2006, Thieme.

Weissman JL, Hirsch BE: Imaging of tinnitus: a review, *Radiology* 216:342–349, 2000.

CHAPTER 35

EVALUATION OF THE VESTIBULAR SYSTEM AND VESTIBULAR DISORDERS

Carol A. Foster, MD

KEY POINTS

1. **Characteristics of Nystagmus in BPPV:** Nystagmus in BPPV is classically a torsional, upbeating positioning nystagmus triggered by the Dix-Hallpike test with the affected ear down. It has a paroxysmal quality, building to a peak and then disappearing over several more seconds. There is a latency of several seconds before it appears, and it fatigues with repeated Dix-Hallpike maneuvers.
2. **Vestibular Migraine:** There is a history of recurrent, severe, nauseating headaches or recurrent auras; vertigo spells vary in duration, from seconds or minutes up to days. It is common in people <50 years of age, and there is an increased risk of BPPV and Meniere's in this group.
3. **Ménière's Triad:** Hearing loss fluctuates, worsens during vertigo spells, and is associated with a sensation of fullness or pressure in the ear. Tinnitus fluctuates, can have a roaring quality, and is louder during vertigo spells. Vertigo is usually hours in duration, severe, and associated with vomiting.
4. **Characteristics of the Normal Caloric Response:** Cold water irrigation causes nystagmus beating away from the irrigated ear, whereas warm water irrigation causes nystagmus beating toward the irrigated ear. A useful mnemonic for nystagmus direction is **COWS** (**C**old **O**pposite, **W**arm **S**ame). The ear with the weakest response is the damaged ear.
5. **How to Test Each Inner Ear Sensor**
   a. Horizontal semicircular canal: Horizontal head impulse test, caloric examination, rotational chair tests
   b. Anterior semicircular canal: Vertical head impulse test, Dix-Hallpike test
   c. Posterior semicircular canal: Vertical head impulse test, Dix-Hallpike test
   d. Utricle: oVEMP
   e. Saccule: cVEMP

Pearls

1. Peripheral nystagmus becomes faster and more apparent when the patient gazes in the direction of the fast phase: a right-beating nystagmus worsens on right gaze, for example. This is called Alexander's Law.
2. You can often determine which ear is affected by horizontal or anterior canal BPPV by asking the patient if they previously had posterior canal BPPV treated, and on what side. Usually the same side will be affected. Alternatively, you can do treatment maneuvers for both sides.
3. Multisensory imbalance can be improved using walking aids. Trekking poles are helpful early in the disorder, but as the disease progresses, a rolling walker with handbrakes is the most effective treatment.
4. Patients with headaches and vertigo should be questioned about snoring. Sleep apnea is associated with morning headaches, worsens migraine, and can be associated with recurrent brief dizziness and progressive inner ear disorders such as Meniere's disease.
5. Peripheral vestibular losses of less than 50% are usually hard to detect by impulse testing. Caloric testing is better able to detect these mild to moderate lesions.

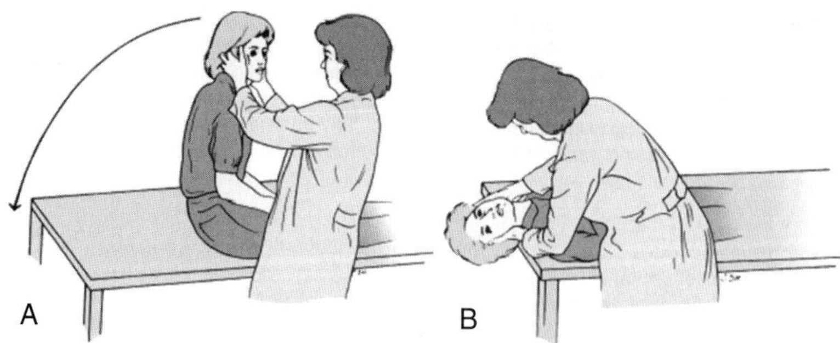

Figure 35-1. The Dix-Hallpike test. The Dix-Hallpike maneuver for the right ear. **A)** With the examiner on the seated patient's right side, the head is rotated 45 degrees toward the right shoulder. **B)** The patient is reclined rapidly into the supine position with the head turned toward the right. The position should be maintained for 15–30 seconds while the eyes are observed for nystagmus. *(Reprinted from Crane BW et al: Peripheral vestibular disorders. In Flint PW, et al: Cummings Otolaryngology: Head & Neck Surgery, 5 ed, Philadelphia, 2011, Mosby/Elsevier.)*

QUESTIONS

1. **When you evaluate a dizzy patient, what should your examination include?**
Careful observation for nystagmus and a check of the ears and hearing are always required. The neurologic examination should include an evaluation of cranial nerves and examination of cerebellar function by testing of coordination, gait, and balance. The neck should be evaluated for carotid artery bruits. Examination of the legs and feet for sensory lesions or range-of-motion restrictions is important. At the end of the exam, you should always perform a Dix-Hallpike maneuver (Figure 35-1) to rule out benign paroxysmal positional vertigo (BPPV), and head impulse testing to rule out vestibular loss.

2. **How do you properly examine a patient for nystagmus?**
Nystagmus has slow and quick components. The slow component is generated by the vestibular system and causes the eye to smoothly rotate. The fast phase represents a corrective response, a saccade that quickly returns the eyes to their original position. By convention, the direction of the nystagmus is named by its fast component, since to the observer the eyes appear to be "beating" in the direction of the saccades. You should evaluate for spontaneous nystagmus by viewing the patient's eyes with the eyes centered, then focused to the left and right. Direct the patient to focus the eyes upward, then downward. Note the direction of nystagmus for each eye position.

3. **How is the Dix-Hallpike maneuver performed?**
The Dix-Hallpike maneuver is a test for BPPV (Figure 35-1). The patient is seated on the examination table with the examiner on the side to be tested. Emphasize to the patient that the eyes should be kept open throughout the maneuver, so that you can observe nystagmus. To test the right ear, hold the patient's head turned 45 degrees to the right and then swiftly move the patient into the supine position until the head overhangs the table edge. Continue to support the patient's head throughout the test. After at least 30 seconds, assist the patient in reassuming the sitting position. The test is then repeated on the left. If the patient is elderly, frail, or has neck problems, the test can be done by lowering the head onto the table instead of allowing the head to overhang the edge of the table.

4. **What constitutes an abnormal Dix-Hallpike maneuver?**
Although this test has many implications, it is most valuable when used to diagnose posterior semicircular canal BPPV. A rotatory nystagmus and sensation of vertigo that begins several seconds after assuming the head-hanging position is characteristic of BPPV. The nystagmus fades after less than 1 minute, reverses direction upon sitting, and "fatigues" or decreases in intensity with repeated testing. For example, if the patient has a left pathologic ear, he or she will manifest a mixed vertical and rotatory nystagmus when positioned with the left ear down, and the upper poles of the eyes will appear to you as if they are beating toward the floor.

5. **Can BPPV affect the horizontal or anterior semicircular canals, too?**
Yes, horizontal canal BPPV causes a violent, purely horizontal paroxysm of nystagmus on Dix-Hallpike that can last for as long as a minute and often causes vomiting. Anterior canal BPPV causes a fine downbeating nystagmus that can be persistent for a few minutes on Dix-Hallpike testing. Repeating the Dix-Hallpike immediately after a BPPV treatment maneuver can cause particles to fall into the horizontal semicircular canal. Anterior canal BPPV is also more likely to appear in patients who have been recently treated with in-office or home maneuvers for posterior canal BPPV.

6. **Do other disorders cause nystagmus with the Dix-Hallpike maneuver?**
Other disorders of central or peripheral vestibular pathways may cause pathologic positional nystagmus. This kind of nystagmus usually does not fade away while the head remains in the hanging position, nor does it fatigue on repeated testing. It can appear when the patient is slowly brought to the supine position and does not require a quick movement like the Dix-Hallpike test to bring it out.

7. **What are the usual symptoms of BPPV?**
Typically, sudden episodes of vertigo are precipitated by specific head movements, usually in bed at night. For example, the patient may complain of vertigo precipitated by rolling over in bed, lying down into bed, or arising. These episodes are brief, lasting less than a minute. A change in hearing or tinnitus is not typical. Although BPPV becomes more frequent with age, it can occur in patients of any age group. This condition usually resolves spontaneously over a period of weeks to months. Failure to respond to treatment maneuvers is an indicator for formal vestibular testing.

8. **How is BPPV treated?**
This disorder usually disappears without treatment over several weeks, but the course can often be shortened dramatically by using therapeutic head maneuvers designed to rotate the particles out of the affected canal. The Epley maneuver, also called the canalith repositioning procedure, has proven very useful, with a success rate near 90%. Other liberatory maneuvers have also been described.

9. **A patient returns after a third episode of BPPV. Is there a home exercise for this condition?**
The half somersault maneuver has been shown to be a useful home exercise (Figure 35-2). The head is inverted in the somersault position, turned to face the elbow on the affected side, and then is raised first to back level and then fully upright, pausing for 30 seconds in each position. Patients who cannot perform the half somersault can use the Epley maneuver or the Semont maneuver at home but will usually require an assistant to help. It is best to wait 15 minutes between repetitions of maneuvers to avoid displacing newly removed particles back into the semicircular canals.

10. **You suspect that a patient's vestibular symptoms are due to migraine. On what grounds do you base your diagnosis?**
Migraine-associated dizziness is the most common cause of chronic dizziness in young adults. Although this disorder often has a benign course between attacks, it can cause serious debility. Migraine is believed to be genetic in origin, and is the most common cause of dizziness in children and young adults. Vertigo may occur as part of an aura, as part of the headache phase, or between the headaches, and it varies in duration from seconds to days. Typically the headaches are moderate to severe, last for hours, and are associated with nausea, photophobia, or phonophobia. Headaches may be accompanied by an aura, often consisting of visual illusions such as a scintillating scotoma, or they may occur without aura. There is an association between migraine and other more serious vertigo disorders, particularly Ménière's disease.

11. **How is migraine-associated dizziness treated?**
Migraine with vertigo can be treated with suppressants such as meclizine or promethazine if attacks are infrequent. However, prophylactic treatment is necessary if attacks are occurring more than once every few weeks. Tricyclic antidepressants such as amitriptyline are a good first-line choice; beta blockers, calcium channel blockers, topiramate, divalproex, and acetazolamide are also effective in some individuals. Medications should be tried for at least 1 month before another type is tried because the effect often builds over several weeks. Newer migraine treatments aimed at the headache phase, such as triptans, are generally not effective for migraine-associated vertigo spells.

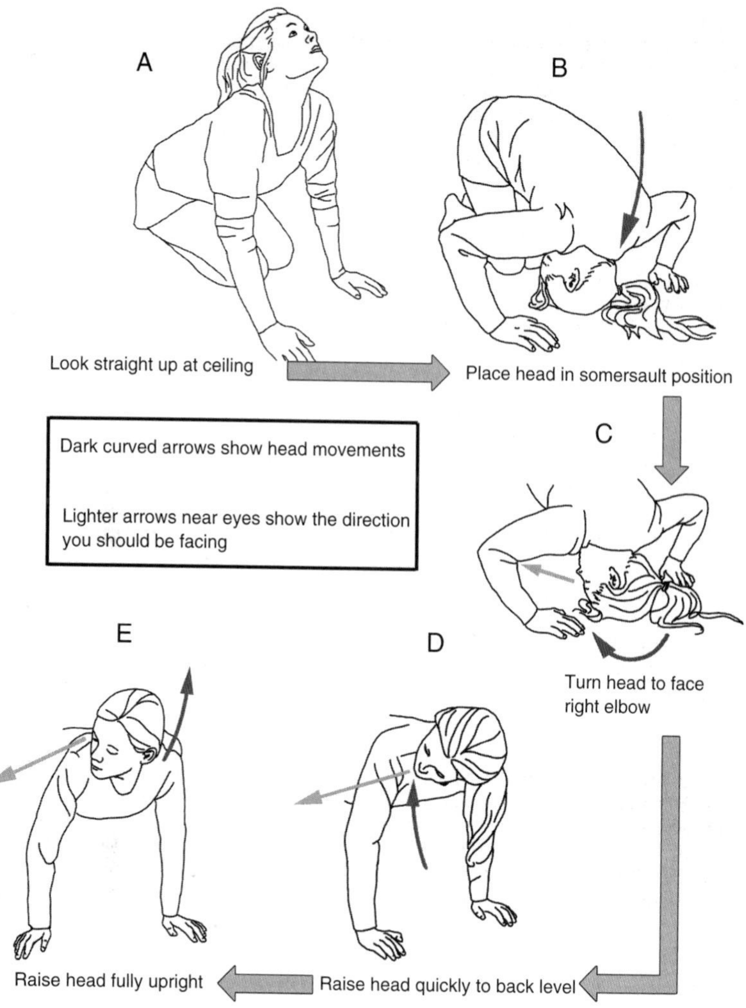

Figure 35-2. The Half Somersault maneuver. A) The head is rapidly tipped upward to face the ceiling. **B)** The head is then placed upside down on the floor. **C)** The head is rotated to face the elbow on the affected side and is maintained in this turned position (ex: R elbow for R posterior canal BPPV). **D)** The turned head is quickly lifted to back level. **E)** The turned head is then briskly raised to the fully upright position. Each position is held until the dizziness pauses or 30 seconds has elapsed. *(Reprinted from Foster CA, et al: Canal conversion and re-entry: a risk of Dix-Hallpike during canalith repositioning procedures, Otology & Neurotology 33:199–203, 2012.)*

12. Why do the elderly develop imbalance?

Normal balance depends on a normal vestibular system, normal vision and visual tracking, and normal sensation and proprioception in the lower extremities. Usually vision, visual tracking, and sensation in the feet become impaired with age. When coupled with any vestibular disorder, or with a gradual age-related decline in vestibular function, multisensory imbalance occurs. Affected people usually feel dizzy only when ambulating, and their dizziness is relieved when using a grocery store cart, for example.

13. **What is the typical course of viral infections of the eighth nerve?**
This acute unilateral vestibulopathy can be preceded by a nonspecific viral illness. Within hours to days, the patient experiences the sudden onset of vertigo. The vertigo reaches a peak rapidly and then gradually declines over a few days to weeks. Cochlear symptoms vary, ranging from normal hearing to a mild high-frequency hearing loss to sudden profound deafness in one ear. If there is no hearing loss, the disease is called *vestibular neuritis*. Total destruction of all auditory and vestibular function in one ear can occur with certain viruses, such as measles, mumps, or herpes zoster. After the severe symptoms have subsided, the patient may experience mild light-headedness with sudden movement that can persist for months. With time, however, the patient's vestibular system compensates, and the dizziness usually clears.

14. **How are viral inner ear infections treated?**
A brief course of steroids should be initiated within the first few days if possible. Vestibular suppressant medication, such as meclizine, diazepam, or promethazine, is used to control vomiting. Suppressants should be discontinued after a week because they interfere with the normal process of compensation to vestibular injuries. Patients who are still symptomatic at that time are good candidates for vestibular rehabilitation.

15. **Describe the head impulse test.**
This test of the vestibular system, also called the "head thrust test" (in awake patients) or the "doll's eye test" (in comatose patients) uses quick head rotation to demonstrate high-grade vestibular lesions in disorders such as vestibular neuritis. Awake patients should be asked to stare into your eyes during the test (Figure 35-3). Face the patient while holding the patient's head and then briskly turn the head to the right and to the left. Normally, the patient's gaze remains "locked" straight ahead on your eyes. The test is abnormal if the patient's gaze can be jerked away from yours by the quick head turn. In patients with peripheral vestibular loss, a series of "catch-up" or refixation saccades (Halmagyi's sign) may occur as the eyes attempt to regain focus on you. If the test results are abnormal with a right head turn, the patient has right vestibular injury; if abnormal to the left, the left ear is injured.

16. **What studies should be performed on patients with suspected inner ear disorders other than BPPV?**
Initially, an audiogram and a videonystagmogram (VNG) should be obtained. If these tests or the neurologic examination show an asymmetric or localizing finding, further studies are indicated. At this point, you should perform magnetic resonance imaging with gadolinium contrast to include the posterior fossa and internal auditory canals. If a congenital malformation of the temporal bone is suspected, an enhanced fine cut computed tomographic scan without contrast would be the most useful study. If the patient has long (more than 1 hour) spells of vertigo, laboratory studies may be beneficial, including a complete blood count, sedimentation rate, and antinuclear antibody testing. Tests to rule out HIV, syphilis, diabetes, clotting disorders, and lipid abnormalities may be useful if dictated by patient history.

17. **What is Ménière's disease?**
This is a set of symptoms associated with a chronically progressive, destructive disorder involving both the cochlea and labyrinth, resulting in permanent hearing loss and vestibular injury over time. It can affect one or both ears and follows a relapsing and remitting course. Spells typically last 30 minutes up to several hours. A number of disorders, such as autoimmune disease, human immunodeficiency virus infection, and syphilis can cause identical symptoms, so the term Ménière's disease is used only for cases in which the cause is unknown. The term is often used interchangeably with its pathologic description, *endolymphatic hydrops*. Patients with recurrent vertigo but without evidence of progressive hearing loss or permanent vestibular injury do not meet diagnostic criteria for this disorder.

18. **What history should I obtain in patients with Ménière's disease?**
Patients under the age of 50 should be asked about migraine headaches, since these are commonly associated with Ménière's disease in this age group. All patients should be questioned about snoring because there is an association with sleep apnea. Vascular risk factors such as a history of smoking, diabetes, vasculitis, MI, or stroke are also associated.

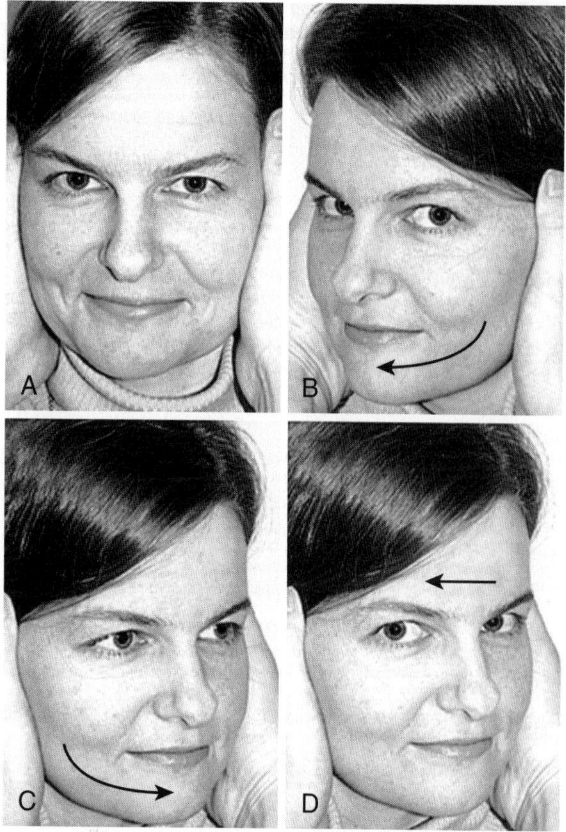

Figure 35-3. The Horizontal head impulse test. A) Starting position; **B)** when the head is turned rapidly toward the normal right ear, the eyes remained fixed on the examiner's; **C)** when the head is turned rapidly toward the abnormal left ear, the eyes move with the head and lose fixation with the examiner's; **D)** the eyes then return in a rightward refixation saccade to regain focus on the examiner's eyes. *(Reprinted from Hullar TE et al: Approach to the patient with dizziness. In Flint PW, et al: Cummings Otolaryngology: Head & Neck Surgery, 5 ed, Philadelphia, 2010, Mosby/Elsevier.)*

19. Describe the uses and limitations of caloric testing.
    Caloric tests reveal abnormalities by comparing the two ears to each other. Caloric tests examine only the function of the horizontal semicircular canals. Each ear is irrigated twice, using cold water and warm water, and the resulting nystagmus slow-phase velocities are measured. The symmetry of the paired responses is then calculated, giving two results, both expressed as a percentage: (1) canal paresis or unilateral weakness, describing the side and extent of a peripheral vestibular impairment; and (2) directional preponderance, suggesting an underlying tendency to nystagmus. If both ears have identical impairments, or if the impairments affect only the vertical canals or the otolith organs, a false negative test may result.

20. How can the otolith organs be tested?
    Vestibular evoked myogenic potential (VEMP) testing is able to assess the function of the otolith organs (Figure 35-3). Electrodes over the sternocleidomastoid muscles are able to detect electromyographic waveforms that result when the saccule is stimulated by loud sounds (cervical or cVEMP). Absence of the waveform on one side is a significant abnormality. However, the test is less reliable in patients over age 60, and in those with neck pain, stiffness or weakness. Delays in the

response can indicate a retrocochlear lesion on the affected side, and a lowered sound threshold for the response can be a sign of semicircular canal dehiscence. Electrodes positioned below the eyes can detect waveforms resulting from sound stimulation of the utricle (ocular or oVEMP).

21. What are the symptoms of superior semicircular canal dehiscence?
Patients typically report torsional vertigo that is triggered by loud sounds. Blowing the nose, sneezing or straining can set off spells. Some also report hearing internal bodily sounds, like their pulse or chewing, magnified in one ear. Others report a brief tinnitus brought on when the eyes move from side to side.

22. Are there tests to evaluate the function of the vertical semicircular canals?
Head impulse tests performed in the plane of the anterior or posterior semicircular canals can reveal refixation saccades if there is a loss of function in the tested canal. The head must be turned to one side and then tipped briskly upward or downward for these tests. You can sometimes see refixation saccades by looking at the eyes as you perform the test, but there are commercial systems that are better able to detect and record these high-acceleration responses.

BIBLIOGRAPHY

Dix MR, Hallpike CS: The pathology, symptomatology, and diagnosis of certain common disorders of the vestibular system, *Proc Royal Soc Med* 45:341–534, 1952.

Foster C, Zaccaro K, Strong D: Canal conversion and re-entry: a risk of Dix-Hallpike during canalith repositioning procedures, *Otol Neurotol* 33:199–203, 2012.

Foster C, Ponnappan A, Zaccaro K, et al: A comparison of two home exercises for benign positional vertigo: half somersault vs. Epley maneuver, *Audiol & Neurotol EXTRA* 2:16–23, 2012.

Halmagyi GM: Diagnosis and management of vertigo [see comment], *Clin Med* 5:159–165, 2005.

Halmagyi GM, Curthoys IS: A clinical sign of canal paresis, *Archives Neurol* 45:737–739, 1988.

Halmagyi GM, Weber KP, Aw ST, et al: Impulsive testing of semicircular canal function, *Prog Brain Res* 171:187–194, 2008.

Jacobson G, Shepherd N: *Balance Function Assessment and Management*, San Diego CA, 2008, Plural Publishing Inc.

Kerber KA, Baloh RW: The evaluation of a patient with dizziness, *Neurol: Clin Pract* 1:24–33, 2011.

Rosengren SM, Kingma H: New perspectives on vestibular evoked myogenic potentials, *Curr Opinion Neurol* 26:74–80, 2013.

Serra A, Leigh RJ: Diagnostic value of nystagmus: spontaneous and induced ocular oscillations, *J Neurol, Neurosurgery Psychiatry* 73:615–618, 2002.

HEARING AIDS AND IMPLANTABLE DEVICES

Allison Brower, AuD, MS

CHAPTER 36

KEY POINTS

1. A hearing aid consultation is recommended for any patient who exhibits hearing loss and complains of difficulty communicating.
2. The patient's type, configuration, and severity of hearing loss, their communication needs, and lifestyle all contribute to determination of the best individualized amplification option.
3. Indications for a bone-conduction hearing aid include: congenital malformations of the external and/or middle ear, chronically discharging ear, or single-sided deafness.
4. Cochlear implants have revolutionized the treatment of deafness, and criteria have expanded to include those individuals with significant residual hearing who do not receive adequate benefit from hearing aids.
5. Two ears are better than one—whether it is two hearing aids, a hearing aid and a cochlear implant or two cochlear implants.

Pearls

1. A conventional hearing aid consists of four main components: microphone, amplifier, receiver and battery.
2. Acoustic feedback occurs when amplified sound leaks out of the receiver back into the microphone.
3. There are several treatment options available for single-sided deafness, including CROS/BiCROS devices, bone conduction hearing aids worn on a headband, transcutaneous/percutaneous bone-anchored hearing aids, and bone conduction devices worn on the teeth.
4. MRI is contraindicated in patients with conventional CIs and fully implanted hearing aids because of the risk of device movement.
5. In cases of meningitis, the hearing aid trial can be bypassed and the child implanted under the age of 12 months due to the possibility of cochlear ossification.

QUESTIONS

1. **What are the major components of a digital hearing aid and how does each contribute to the function of the device?**
   In a very rough sense, the digital hearing aid has five major components: the microphone, the analog to digital converter, the microchip, the digital to analog converter, and the receiver. The microphone on the outside of the hearing aid picks up sound waves, and they are converted to an electrical signal. This signal is then passed through an analog/digital converter and sent to the microchip, which is essentially a tiny computer chip. The microchip filters the signal into bands and channels and manipulates the sound according to the user's hearing loss. The manipulated signal is converted back to an analog signal through the digital/analog converter. The analog signal is sent to the receiver where it is converted back to an acoustic signal that the patient hears.

2. **When should a patient be referred to audiology for a hearing aid consult?**
   A hearing aid consult should be recommended for those patients who exhibit hearing loss and report a disruption in communication with others. With improved hearing aid technology available today, hearing aids can enhance the quality of life for almost any patient with hearing loss, regardless of the type, severity or configuration.

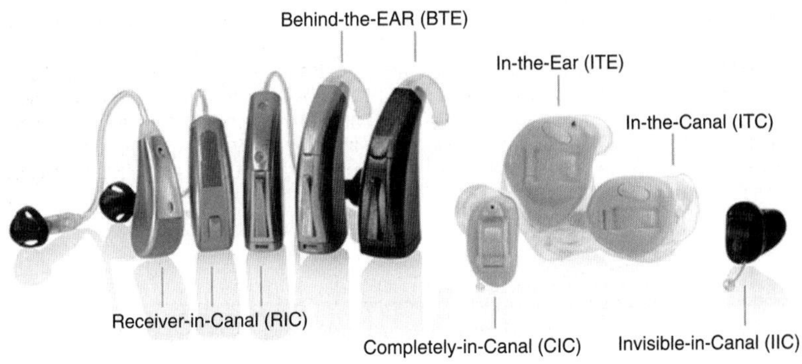

Figure 36-1. The different styles of hearing aids.

3. Name the most common styles of hearing aids (Figure 36-1).
   - Behind-the-ear (BTE) hearing aids
   - Receiver-in-the-canal (RIC) hearing aids
   - In-the-ear (ITE) hearing aids
   - In-the-canal (ITC) hearing aids
   - Completely-in-the-canal (CIC) hearing aids
   - Invisible-in-the-canal (IIC) hearing aids
   - Contralateral routing of sound (CROS) and bilateral CROS (BiCROS) hearing aids

4. What is acoustic feedback and what causes it?
   Acoustic feedback occurs when the acoustic signal leaks out from the receiver of the hearing aid and is picked up again by the microphone. This sound loop results in an unpleasant, high-pitched squealing sound. Feedback occurs most often in the instance of high-power hearing aids, ITE hearing aids, and hearing aids used in conjunction with a vented earmold or open-fit configuration. Feedback can also be an indication that the patient's earmolds are not inserted properly, are a poor fit, or the patient has outgrown the molds.

5. What is loudness recruitment and how is this phenomenon addressed in the hearing aid fitting?
   Loudness recruitment, or just "recruitment," refers to the abnormally rapid growth of loudness with increasing stimulus level, and is a common clinical symptom of sensorineural hearing loss. The theory of recruitment is that as the hair cells in the cochlea become damaged, normal adjacent hair cells are "recruited" to help hear the frequency of the damaged hair cell in addition to their own frequency. This increases the signal from the good hair cell and perceived loudness at the brain rapidly increases causing discomfort. One way to address recruitment in the hearing aid fitting is through the use of wide dynamic range compression (WDRC). WDRC improves the audibility of soft sounds and reduces discomfort of loud sounds by applying more gain to low-level inputs and less gain to high-level inputs.

6. What advancements in hearing aid technology have we seen in the last decade?
   Hearing aid technology is now close to completely digital. The most significant advancements lie in signal processing. Improvements are seen in the hearing aid's ability to make consistent changes to the directionality of the microphones, manipulation of the frequency, compression (non-linear amplification) and gain (amount of amplification applied to the input level), advanced digital noise reduction, digital speech enhancement, and acoustic feedback reduction. All of these features work together to improve the user's ability to understand speech in any environment. Binaurally integrated hearing systems use wireless connectivity to exchange information between the right and the left hearing aid and adjust the settings based on the user's listening environment. This technology significantly improves speech comprehension in the presence of background noise.

7. **How can an individual enhance hearing aid use in common and difficult listening situations?**
Wireless connectivity available in today's digital hearing aids allows for wireless communication between hearing aids and numerous forms of media devices. Individuals are now able to stream television, music, and phone calls wirelessly to their hearing aids through the use of an intermediary device between the hearing aids and the external source. This allows for a gateway to media connectivity and greater convenience in communication that was once not available to hearing aid users.

8. **What are indications for a bone conduction hearing aid?**
   - Congenital malformations of the external and/or middle ear (i.e., microtia/atresia)
   - Chronically discharging ear (i.e., chronic otitis media or mastoiditis)
   - Single-sided deafness
   - As an option for patients who cannot wear conventional hearing aids or are dissatisfied with outcomes

9. **What are the most common devices used to treat single-sided deafness (SSD)?**
A common treatment approach to SSD is the fitting of contralateral routing of sound (CROS) or bilateral CROS (BiCROS) amplification. Individuals who use a CROS system have normal or near-normal hearing in the better ear and no useable hearing in the poorer ear. A transmitting device with a microphone is placed on the poorer ear and a receiving instrument is placed on the better ear. Sound picked up by the transmitting device microphone is sent wirelessly to the receiving hearing instrument on the better ear. A BiCROS system is appropriate for those patients who exhibit some hearing loss in the better ear. In addition to the CROS, it has a second microphone located on the receiving hearing instrument that picks up and amplifies sound. Historically, patients using CROS or BiCROS systems have been dissatisfied with sound quality and cosmetic appearance, but advancements in hearing aid technology have improved CROS and BiCROS systems.

   A second common treatment option for SSD is bone conduction hearing aids. Bone conduction hearing aids use direct bone conduction to transmit sound vibrations directly to the inner ear through the skull. Bone conduction hearing aids can be worn on a softband, can be percutaneous or transcutaneous, and can even be worn on the teeth.

   Recent studies have evaluated the use of cochlear implants as treatment for SSD, although this is not an FDA-approved indication for CI.

10. **What are the challenges associated with percutaneous bone-anchored hearing aids and are nonsurgical bone conduction hearing aid options available?**
Postoperative complications associated with percutaneous bone-anchored hearing aids range anywhere from 8% to 59%. The two most common postoperative complications include infection or inflammation at the implant site, and failure of the device to osseointegrate. Longevity and health of the device are highly dependent on patient hygiene and at-home care of the implant. Even so, revision surgery is likely over the lifetime of the bone-anchored hearing implant. Other bone conduction hearing aid options include a transcutaneous bone-anchored hearing aid that is held in place via internal and external magnets. In addition, patients also have a nonsurgical bone conduction hearing aid option that transmits sound through the teeth. The device is composed of two parts: a custom-made in-the-mouth (ITM) device and a small BTE device that contains a microphone. Both parts are removable.

11. **What is an implantable hearing aid?**
An implantable hearing aid is designed for those individuals with mild to severe hearing loss who are unable to wear or do not wish to wear a conventional hearing aid. There is currently one FDA-approved fully implantable hearing device on the market. This device consists of three implantable components: the sound processor, a sensor, and a driver. Implantation of the device requires disruption of the ossicular chain, and the device then vibrates the ossicular chain directly.

12. **What are the challenges associated with implantable hearing aids?**
   - Capacity and recharging ability of batteries required to power the device
   - Adequate middle ear space necessary to house the device. Inadequate space can limit the amount of gain the device can provide, making it challenging to aid more severe degrees of hearing loss.

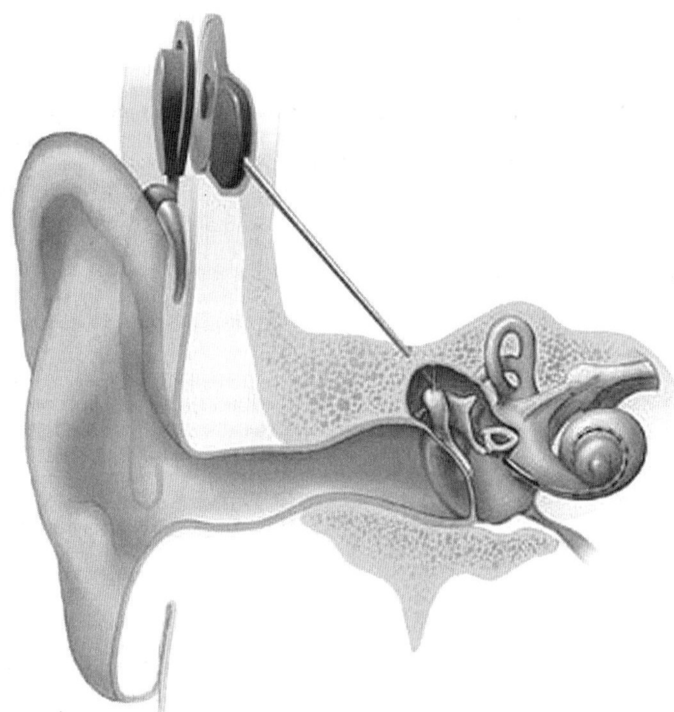

Figure 36-2. The cochlear implant system.

- Cost is significantly more than conventional hearing aids.
- Insurance coverage
- MRI contraindicated

13. **Describe a cochlear implant and how it works.**
A cochlear implant (CI) is a sophisticated, surgically implanted electronic device that is designed to produce useful hearing to a person with severe to profound sensorineural hearing loss by electrically stimulating the auditory nerve within the inner ear. It has become the standard treatment option for restoring hearing in those individuals with significant loss who no longer benefit from hearing aids. The device consists of internal and external components (Figure 36-2). The internal components consist of the receiver and the electrode array. The receiver is implanted just under the skin behind the ear, and the electrode array is inserted into the cochlea. The external components consist of a speech processor, microphone, and transmitting coil. The microphone picks up sound and sends the information to the speech processor, which digitally encodes the sound. The coded signals are then sent up the cable to the coil, which sends the information across the skin via FM radio frequency to the receiver implanted just under the skin. The receiver, via the electrode array, presents the information to the auditory nerve in the form of tiny electrical pulses, which then travel to the brain where they are perceived as sound.

14. **Describe how the electrical stimulation provided by a CI is perceived as sound to the patient.**
Specific characteristics of speech that are critical to word understanding are selectively coded by the speech processor. The coded signal is sent through the auditory nerve to the brain, where the code is interpreted into useful hearing sensations to enable speech understanding. The quality of the sound varies, but most recipients are able to understand speech without visual cues.

15. **What are the current FDA criteria for cochlear implant candidacy in the adult and pediatric populations?**
    - Adults (>18 years)
      - Bilateral moderate to profound hearing loss
      - Limited benefit from hearing aids as demonstrated by test scores of ≤50% sentence recognition in the ear to be implanted, and ≤60% in the contralateral ear or binaurally aided depending on insurance (≤40% in binaurally aided condition for Medicare)
      - All candidates should have realistic expectations regarding the cochlear implant process and outcomes, as well as exhibit a strong desire to be a part of the hearing world. A stable, quality support group available to the patient is strongly desired.
    - Children (2–17 years)
      - Bilateral severe to profound sensorineural hearing loss
      - Limited benefit from hearing aids as demonstrated by binaural amplification trial (at least 6 months) with word recognition scores of less than or equal to 30%
    - Infants (12–24 months)
      - Bilateral profound sensorineural hearing loss
      - No progress in auditory skill development with binaural hearing aids (at least 3 months trial except in cases of meningitis, where the hearing aid trial can be bypassed and implantation can be done under 12 months of age due to the possibility of cochlear ossification) and intervention.

    For children and infants, the placement of an educational plan and rehabilitation therapy that emphasizes development of auditory skills is imperative for successful outcomes with CI. High motivation and realistic expectations from family are strongly encouraged.

16. **What is the appropriate workup for an adult patient prior to receiving a CI?**
    - Assessment of unaided hearing thresholds
    - Audiological consult with a cochlear implant audiologist
    - Evaluation of aided thresholds and speech discrimination testing with appropriately fit, binaural hearing aids
    - Surgical consult with a cochlear implant surgeon
    - CT and/or MRI
    - Vestibular evaluation (VNG/VEMP)

17. **How does the workup differ for the pediatric CI candidate?**
    A team approach is highly recommended in cases of pediatric cochlear implant candidates. Team members should always include an ENT surgeon, pediatric audiologist, speech-language therapist, and the child's parents/family. Other recommended team members include: child psychologist or social worker, early intervention provider, and teacher(s) of the deaf. Upon completion of each member's evaluation, the team meets to discuss the patient and determine candidacy. A child's success with a cochlear implant is highly dependent on a supportive family and coordination and collaboration of all team members.

18. **Can individuals who have significant residual hearing receive a CI and is hearing preservation a possibility?**
    Historically, cochlear implants have been reserved as a method of treatment for those with severe to profound hearing loss. Advancements in implant technology have led to a notable expansion in cochlear implant candidacy criteria to now include those individuals with significant residual hearing. Cochlear implant manufacturers have designed specific electrode arrays with hearing preservation in mind. The use of these electrode arrays paired with a different surgical approach (round window insertion versus cochleostomy) has shown promising hearing preservation outcomes. The FDA recently approved use of the first hybrid cochlear implant device that combines electrical (CI) and acoustical (hearing aid) stimulation within one sound processor. The hybrid cochlear implant should be considered for those individuals with normal to near-normal low-frequency (<1000 Hz) hearing sloping to more severe thresholds in the high frequencies.

19. **What is bimodal stimulation and what are the binaural advantages one may experience?**
    Bimodal stimulation or bimodal hearing is the combined use of a cochlear implant (electrical input) in one ear, and a hearing aid (acoustic input) in the opposite ear. For cochlear implant patients

with some residual hearing in the nonimplanted ear, a conventional hearing aid should always be considered for the patient to achieve optimal hearing. Bimodal hearing has been shown to provide binaural advantages such as improved speech perception in the presence of background noise and improved sound localization. In addition, patients utilizing bimodal stimulation report overall improved and more natural sound quality, as well as improved speech perception.

20. **What are the major factors that have prognostic significance when predicting a patient's success with a cochlear implant?**
   - Pre- versus post-lingual deafness: Post-lingual hearing loss refers to the loss of hearing after the development of basic spoken language. Pre-lingual hearing loss occurs prior to the development of basic language skills. Post-lingually deafened patients will perform better with a CI than their pre-lingually deafened counterparts.
   - Length of deafness: The longer the individual has gone without hearing prior to receiving a cochlear implant, the poorer the outcome.
   - Amplification history: An ear that has been aided consistently and more recently will do better than an ear that has not been amplified in recent history.
   - Integrity of inner ear structures: Cochlear malformations present may require modification of conventional implantation and outcomes may be variable.
   - Motivation of the patient and family
   - Other existing medical conditions

21. **What cochlear malformations may be present and do they preclude cochlear implantation?**
   Minor anomalies such as cochlear dysplasia or malformation of the inner ear may include Mondini's malformation and enlarged vestibular aqueduct. Children presenting with abnormalities such as these may be implanted with relatively standard techniques and experience comparable outcomes to those with normal CTs. Major anomalies such as common cavity do not preclude cochlear implantation; however, surgical technique is more complicated and outcomes are less predictable.

22. **What is the difference between a cochlear implant and an auditory brainstem implant?**
   A cochlear implant works by stimulating fibers of the auditory nerve. In cases where the auditory nerve has been compromised during tumor removal, such as with neurofibromatosis type II (NF2) patients, a cochlear implant would not be appropriate. The auditory brainstem implant (ABI) was developed for patients in this situation. The ABI bypasses the cochlea and the auditory nerve and directly stimulates the brainstem. ABIs may also be indicated for those individuals with cochlear nerve deficiency and complete absence of a cochlear nerve. Outcomes are variable and hearing may be of limited quality.

23. **What are the advantages to a younger age of implantation?**
   Children who are born deaf or become deaf before spoken language is acquired have greater success developing age-appropriate language skills when they are implanted at a young age (before age 2 years). The FDA states that a child can receive a CI as young as one year of life. Earlier age of implantation allows these children to receive auditory information at a time when their brain is especially ready to learn language. Early placement of a CI can result in improved vocabulary outcomes, as well as improved speech perception and production outcomes.

CONTROVERSIES

24. **Cochlear implantation in the very young child (<12 months).**
   Current literature suggests that cochlear implantation before 1 year of age is both safe and efficacious. Insurance coverage may be a challenge as FDA criteria limit cochlear implantation to 12 months or older.

25. **CIs as treatment for single-sided deafness.**
   Recent studies have shown that cochlear implantation in those with single-sided deafness may improve sound localization and speech perception. Currently, SSD is not an approved indication for cochlear implantation, thus not covered by insurance. Further research is required to examine the benefits and likely challenges associated with cochlear implantation and SSD patients.

Bibliography

Adunka OF, Dillon MT, Adunka MC, et al: Cochleostomy versus round window insertions: influence on functional outcomes in electric-acoustic stimulation of the auditory system, *Otol Neurotol* 35(4):613–618, 2014.

Arnoldner C, Lin VY: Expanded selection criteria in adult cochlear implantation, *Cochlear Implants Int* 14(Suppl 4): S10–S13, 2013.

Azadarmaki R, Tubbs R, Chen DA, et al: MRI information for commonly used otologic implants: review and update, *Otolaryngol Head Neck Surg* 150(4):512–519, 2014.

Badrana K, Arya AK, Bunstone D, et al: Long-term complications of bone-anchored hearing aids: a 14-year experience, *J Laryngol Otol* 123(2):170–176, 2009.

Berrettini S, Passetti S, Giannarelli M, et al: Benefit from bimodal hearing in a group of prelingually deafened adult cochlear implant users, *Am J Otolaryngol* 31(5):332–338, 2010.

Birman CS, Elliott EJ, Gibson WP: Pediatric cochlear implants: additional disabilities prevalence, risk factors, and effect on language outcomes, *Otol Neurotol* 33(8):1347–1352, 2012.

Bovo R, Ciorba A, Martini A: Tinnitus and cochlear implants, *Auris Nasus Larynx* 38:14–20, 2011.

Clarós P, Pujol Mdel C: Active middle ear implants: Vibroplasty™ in children and adolescents with acquired or congenital middle ear disorders, *Acta Otolaryngol* 133(6):612–619, 2013.

Cosetti M, Roland JT Jr: Cochlear implantation in the very young child: issues unique to the under-1 population, *Trends Amplif* 14(1):46–57, 2010.

Doshi J, Sheehan P, McDermott AL: Bone anchored hearing aids in children: an update, *Int J Pediatr Otorhinolaryngol* 76(5):618–622, 2012.

Firszt JB, Holden LK, Reeder RM, et al: Auditory Abilities after Cochlear Implantation in Adults with Unilateral Deafness: A Pilot Study, *Otol Neurotol* 33(8):1339–1346, 2012.

Freeman SR, Stivaros SM, Ramsden RT, et al: The management of cochlear nerve deficiency, *Cochlear Implants Int* 14(Suppl 4):S27–S31, 2013.

Geers AE, Nicholas JG: Enduring advantages of early cochlear implantation for spoken language development, *J Speech Lang Hear Res* 56(2):643–655, 2013.

Gifford RH, Dorman MF, Skarzynski H, et al: Cochlear implantation with hearing preservation yields significant benefit for speech recognition in complex listening environments, *Ear Hear* 34(4):413–425, 2013.

Gurgel RK, Shelton C: The SoundBite hearing system: patient-assessed safety and benefit study, *Laryngoscope* 123(11): 2807–2812, 2013.

Hobson JC, Roper AJ, Andrew R, et al: Complications of bone-anchored hearing aid implantation, *J Laryngol Otol* 124(2): 132–136, 2010.

Kamal SM, Robinson AD, Diaz RC: Cochlear implantation in single-sided deafness for enhancement of sound localization and speech perception, *Curr Opin Otolaryngol Head Neck Surg* 20(5):393–397, 2012.

Kraus EM1, Shohet JA, Catalano PJ: Envoy Esteem Totally Implantable Hearing System: phase 2 trial, 1-year hearing results, *Otolaryngol Head Neck Surg* 145(1):100–109, 2011.

Morera C, Manrique M, Ramos A, et al: Advantages of binaural hearing provided through bimodal stimulation via a cochlear implant and a conventional hearing aid: a 6-month comparative study, *Acta Otolaryngol* 125(6):596–606, 2005.

Russell JL, Pine HS, Young DL: Pediatric cochlear implantation: expanding applications and outcomes, *Pediatr Clin North Am* 60(4):841–863, 2013.

Sheffield SW, Gifford RH: The benefits of bimodal hearing: effect of frequency region and acoustic bandwidth, *Audiol Neurootol* 19(3):151–163, 2014.

Siegert R, Kanderske J: A new semi-implantable transcutaneous bone conduction device: clinical, surgical, and audiologic outcomes in patients with congenital ear canal atresia, *Otol Neurotol* 34(5):927–934, 2013.

Syms MJ, Hernandez KE: Bone conduction hearing: device auditory capability to aid in device selection, *Otolaryngol Head Neck Surg* 150(5):866–871, 2014.

CHAPTER 37

INFECTIONS OF THE EAR

Melissa A. Scholes, MD

KEY POINTS

Essentials of Diagnosis of Otitis Media

- Moderate to severe bulging of the tympanic membrane or new otorrhea not associated with otitis externa
- Mild bulging of the tympanic membrane and less than 48 hours of otalgia or erythema of the tympanic membrane
- Middle ear effusion must be present as diagnosed by pneumatic otoscopy or tympanometry

Pearls

1. For a diagnosis of acute otitis externa, there must be a rapid onset (usually within 48 hours) of symptoms and signs of ear canal inflammation.
2. The most common bacterial pathogens contributing to acute otitis media are *Streptococcus pneumoniae* (35% to 40%), *Haemophilus influenza* (30% to 35%), and *Moraxella catarrhalis* (15% to 25%).
3. Amoxicillin remains the first-line therapy for acute otitis media because approximately 80% of bacterial isolates remain susceptible.
4. For a diagnosis of otitis media, a middle ear effusion must be present and confirmed by pneumatic otoscopy or tympanometry.
5. Pain is an important symptom of otitis externa and otitis media and needs to be treated appropriately.

QUESTIONS

1. What is otitis externa (OE)?

   Otitis externa is an infection of the skin of the external auditory canal (EAC), which can extend to surrounding structures such as the pinna, tragus, tympanic membrane, and regional lymph nodes.

2. What is the pathogenesis of OE?

   OE occurs when the protective mechanisms of the ear canal are disrupted. Cerumen, produced by glands in the cartilaginous ear canal, is bacteriostatic and also protects the ear canal by acting as a barrier to moisture. Cerumen is also slightly acidic, which aids in inhibiting infection. Cotton swabs can contribute to OE not only by removing the protective cerumen, but also by injuring the ear canal skin. If the skin of the ear canal is traumatized with a fingernail, ear plugs or foreign body, an infection may occur as well. Moist and humid environments also contribute to infections by weakening skin barriers. *Staphylococcus aureus* and *Pseudomonas aeruginosa* are the most common causative organisms.

3. What are the risk factors for acute otitis externa (AOE)? How do you prevent AOE?

   Water exposure is the most common culprit associated with AOE as seen in humid climates or from direct contact with water while bathing or swimming (so-called "swimmer's ear"). AOE can be prevented by reducing water exposure in the ear canal. Preventative measures include acidifying ear drops, removal of obstructing cerumen, drying the ear canal with a hair dryer (on a cool setting), ear plug use, and avoidance of direct ear canal trauma.

4. **What are the signs and symptoms of AOE?**
AOE usually presents as a rapid onset of intense ear pain. The pain is often out of proportion to exam and is exacerbated by palpation of the tragus and pinna. Signs of ear canal inflammation such as erythema, edema, and drainage must also be present. Ninety-eight percent of AOE is bacterial. Signs and symptoms include purulent ear drainage, otalgia (ear pain), plugged feeling in the affected ear, ear canal swelling, and debris in the ear canal. To be classified as acute the pain should be of less than 48 hours duration. Drainage from the ear canal may cause eczema of the outer ear.

5. **What is chronic otitis externa (COE)?**
Chronic otitis externa is defined as otorrhea with symptoms of otitis externa that are present for more than 6 weeks. The pain is often not as severe as acute OE. COE may occur after inadequate treatment of AOE.

6. **What is malignant otitis externa? What are other complications of OE?**
Malignant otitis externa is an infection of the skull base that can occur after acute or chronic OE. It is most often seen in elderly patients with diabetes and the immunocompromised. The infection can spread intracranially and cause cranial nerve deficits and is a life-threatening condition requiring intravenous antibiotic therapy and correction of the underlying immunocompromise. Other symptoms of malignant otitis media include a deep stabbing ear pain that is made worse with head motion, otorrhea, fever, loss of voice, dysphagia, and facial weakness. Less seriously, OE can spread and cause facial cellulitis. Chronic drainage from the ear canal can also cause irritation of the skin of the ear and neck.

7. **How do you treat OE?**
OE is best treated by debriding the ear of desquamated skin and cerumen, restoring the normal pH, topical antimicrobial therapy, and removal of causative agents. Fluoroquinolone drops are first-line therapy. If any systemic symptoms are present or the infection has spread outside the ear canal, systemic antibiotics that cover *S. aureus* are appropriate. If patients are predisposed to recurrent OE, 2 to 3 drops of a 1 : 1 solution of white vinegar and 70% ethyl alcohol can be instilled into the ear before and after swimming.

8. **What is bullous myringitis?**
Bullous myringitis is the formation of serous or hemorrhagic bullae on the tympanic membrane. It is associated with viral, *Streptococcus pneumoniae*, or staphylococcal infections. It is often very painful and may cause a conductive hearing loss. Supportive treatment is indicated including analgesics and anti-inflammatory medications. If signs of bacterial infection are present, then topical or oral antibiotics are appropriate.

9. **What is otitis media (OM)? What are the predisposing factors for OM?**
Otitis media is an infection of the middle ear space. It is common in younger children secondary to an immature immune system, eustachian tube dysfunction, and unfavorable anatomy. Other predisposing factors include colonization of the nasopharynx with otitis pathogens, upper respiratory infection, smoke exposure, bottle feeding, time of year, daycare attendance, and genetic susceptibility.

10. **What role does the eustachian tube play in otitis media?**
The eustachian tube (ET) runs from the anterior middle ear to the nasopharynx, and equalizes the pressure in the middle ear space. It is bony in its proximal portion and cartilaginous in its distal portion and is associated with four muscles: salpingopharyngeus, tensor veli palatini, tensor tympani, and levator veli palatine. The ET intermittently opens in response to different actions on these muscles including yawning, talking, and performing a Valsalva maneuver. The middle ear space is under constant negative pressure, and equalization by the ET prevents build-up of fluid. If the ET is dysfunctional for any reason, then fluid build-up occurs causing a middle ear effusion. Common causes for ET dysfunction include anatomic variants and viral infections with concomitant swelling. In children, the eustachian tube is flatter and less rigid, which can contribute to dysfunction (Figure 37-1). The fluid can then become infected from exposure to pathogens that are found in the nasopharynx.

11. **What are the most common bacterial pathogens found in OM? What are the most common organisms found in mastoiditis?**
Classically, the most common bacterial pathogens contributing to OM are *Streptococcus pneumoniae* (35% to 40%), *Haemophilus influenza* (30% to 35%), and *Moraxella catarrhalis* (15% to 25%).

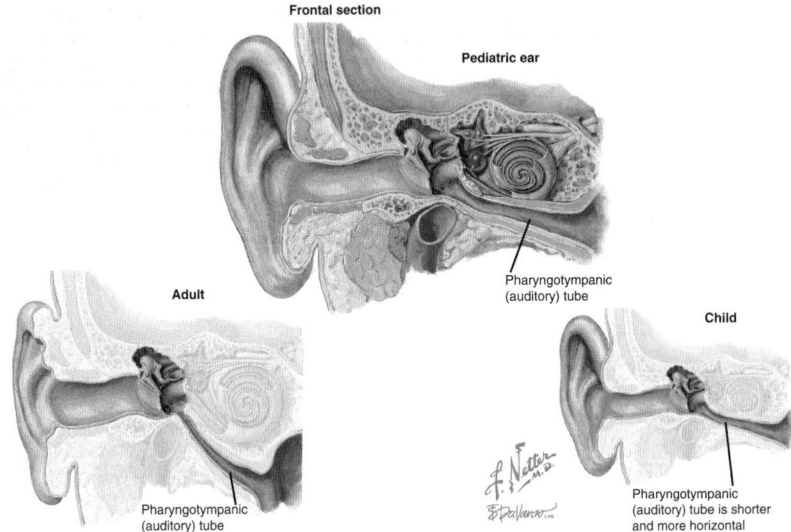

Figure 37-1. Eustachian tube anatomy. *(From Jong EC, Stevens DL: Netter's Infectious Diseases, 1e, Philadelphia, 2011, Saunders.)*

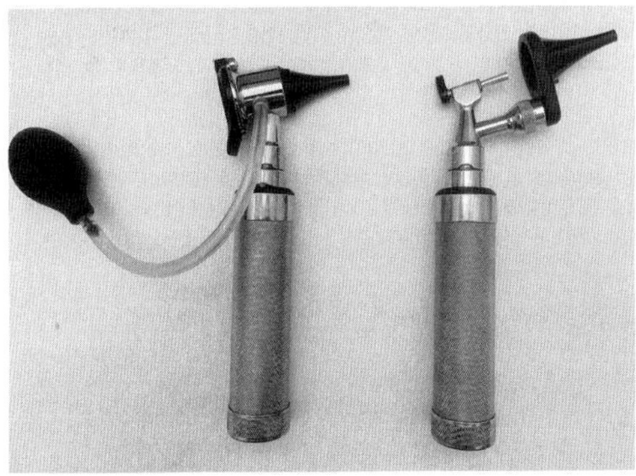

Figure 37-2. Closed and open head otoscopes.

Streptococcus pyogenes and *S. pneumoniae* are the most common pathogens found in mastoiditis. With the advent of the pneumococcal vaccine there has been a decrease in the number of infections from *S. pneumoniae* but an increase in infections from other bacteria such as *Staphylococcus aureus* and *H. influenzae*. There is a trend for an overall decrease in OM by about 6% to 7% since vaccinations were begun.

12. **What are biofilms and what is their role in otitis media?**
Biofilms are groups of microorganisms that reside in an extracellular matrix. The extracellular matrix is resistant to antibiotic penetration. Additionally, different bacteria in the biofilm can share host defense mechanisms and resistant genes. Biofilms have been found in the middle ear and nasopharynx of children with otitis media. It is thought that biofilms contribute to OM by shedding planktonic bacteria and inducing mucosal inflammation.

13. **What examination techniques are used in the diagnosis of otitis media?**
Any obstructing cerumen should be cleared from the ear canal to see the tympanic membrane. This can be done with an open operating otoscope (Figure 37-2) or under a microscope. Irrigation of the

ear canals should be used with caution in case there is an unrecognized tympanic membrane perforation. Water in the ear canal can also predispose to otitis externa. The tympanic membrane is examined for color, thickness, bulging, loss of landmarks, and presence of effusion. Loss of the light reflex is not specific for otitis media. Next, pneumatic otoscopy is performed with an insufflator bulb attached to a closed head otoscope. Gentle pressure is applied, which will cause a pressure change in the canal. If an effusion is present the ear drum will not move; in the absence of an effusion the ear drum will move. Only gentle pressure is needed. Too much pressure can cause pain. If pneumatic otoscopy cannot be performed, then tympanometry can be used to establish presence of an effusion.

14. **What tips for pneumotoscopy will help you perform an ear examination?**
    - Choose largest ear speculum to ensure a tight seal.
    - Insert the speculum into only the outer one third of the external canal to avoid pain from pressure on the bony canal.
    - Insert the speculum after compressing the bulb slightly, then release to check for movement. This helps avoid discomfort and can diagnose negative ear pressure.
    - Use only gentle pressure to minimally flutter the tympanic membrane.

15. **What antibiotics are used in the treatment of otitis media?**
    Amoxicillin remains the first-line therapy because approximately 80% of bacterial isolates remain susceptible. High dosages are used to help avoid resistance. Amoxicillin with clavulanic acid is used when the patient has failed clinically after 48 to 72 hours or has had amoxicillin in the last 30 days. In patients with penicillin sensitivity without severe reactions, cephalosporins are used. For children with IgE mediated allergic reactions, trimethoprim-sulfamethoxazole, clindamycin or a macrolide is used. Intramuscular ceftriaxone is usually reserved for failures of oral therapies (Tables 37-1 and 37-2).

16. **Are there other options besides antibiotics to treat OM?**
    Patients with minimal symptoms over 6 months of age can be observed for 48 to 72 hours. However, a plan should be in place if failure occurs, such as a "wait and see" prescription or an additional ear examination to ensure improvement.

17. **Is there any way to prevent OM?**
    The majority of episodes of otitis media occur in children because of anatomic issues as well as immaturity of the immune system. These factors cannot be changed. Avoidance of daycare centers, cigarette smoke, and bottle-propping can help. Breastfeeding has a protective effect by providing

Table 37-1. Treatment of Acute Otitis Media in an Era of Drug Resistance; Initial Immediate or Delayed Antibiotic Treatment

FIRST-LINE TREATMENT	ALTERNATIVE TREATMENT (IF PENICILLIN ALLERGIC)
1. Amoxicillin (80–90 mg/kg/day in two divided doses) • For children under age 2 yrs or children of all ages with severe symptoms, treat for 10 days • Age 2–6 yrs with mild-moderate symptoms, treat for 7 days • Over age 6 yrs with mild-moderate symptoms, treat for 5 days. or 2. Amoxicillin-clavulanate (90 mg/kg/day or amoxicillin, with 6.4 mg/kg/day of clavulanate in two divided doses) • For patients who have received amoxicillin in the previous 30 days or who have otitis-conjunctivitis syndrome.	1. Cefdinir (14 mg/kg/day in 1 or 2 doses) 2. Cefuroxime (30 mg/kg/day divided BID) 3. Cefpodoxime (10 mg/kg/day in 2 divided doses) 4. Ceftriaxone (50 mg IM or IV per day for 1 or 3 days) If unable to take oral medications 5. For children with severe penicillin allergies (IgE-mediated events): • Trimethoprim-sulfamethoxazole • Macrolide • Clindamycin (30–40 mg/kg/day, divided TID)

Table 37-2. Antibiotic Treatment after 48–72 Hours of Failure of Initial Antibiotic

RECOMMEND FIRST-LINE TREATMENT	ALTERNATIVE TREATMENT
1. Amoxicillin-clavulanate (90 mg/kg/day or amoxicillin, with 6.4 mg/kg/day of clavulanate in two divided doses) • For patients who have received amoxicillin in the previous 30 days or who have otitis-conjunctivitis syndrome or 2. Ceftriaxone (50 mg IM or IV per day for 3 days)	1. Ceftriaxone (50 mg IM or IV per day for 3 days) 2. Clindamycin (30–40 mg/kg/day, divided TID) with or without a third generation cephalosporin 3. Consider tympanocentesis • Consult specialist 4. Recurrence >4 weeks after initial episode: • A new pathogen is likely, so restart first-line therapy. • Be sure diagnosis is not OME, which may be observed for 3–6 months without treatment.

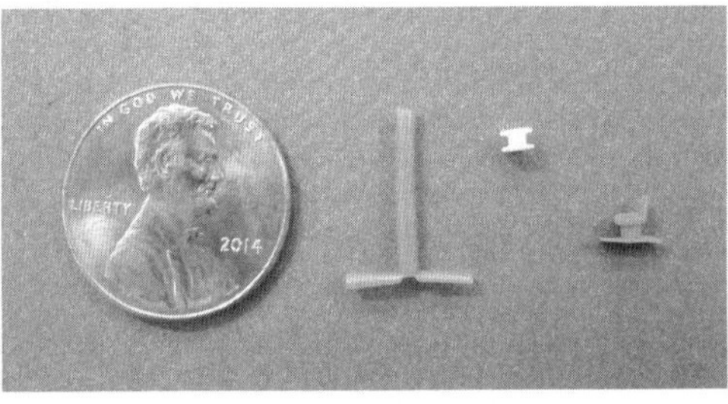

Figure 37-3. Different types of ear tubes.

maternal antibodies. Pacifier use may help to decrease episodes of AOM per one study. If a child has additional infections, such as pneumonia, an immune evaluation may be prudent. Antibiotic prophylaxis is not recommended because it contributes to resistance, can have side effects, and is not effective long term.

18. **What is otitis media with effusion (OME)?**
OME is the presence of an effusion in the middle ear without signs of acute inflammation. This can occur primarily from negative middle ear pressure from eustachian tube blockage as seen with adenoid hypertrophy, upper respiratory infection or from some other dysfunction. It can also be seen after an episode of acute otitis media after the inflammation has subsided. An effusion after AOM can be present for several weeks with 90% resolution by three months. OME must be differentiated from AOM because OME does not benefit from treatment with antibiotics.

19. **What is the medical treatment of OME?**
OME is not improved by administration of antibiotics, steroids, antihistamines or decongestants. Patient with an effusion lasting for more than 3 months should undergo testing of their hearing unless a child has risk factors for language delay, in which case they should be tested sooner. If a middle ear effusion is present for more than 3 months and there is a hearing loss, then tympanostomy tubes are often recommended.

20. **What are tympanostomy tubes? How do tympanostomy tubes help OME and AOM?**
Tympanostomy tube placement is the most common ambulatory surgery performed in the United States. The tubes are small cylinders usually with a flange or collar that sits in the tympanic membrane (Figure 37-3). The role of the tube is to drain fluid and equalize middle ear pressure. In children with acute otitis media, they prevent a build-up of middle ear fluid and subsequent inflammation and infection. In otitis media with effusion, they remove the effusion allowing for improvement in hearing. On average the tubes last for 6 months to a year. They are pushed out of the ear drum by the natural desquamation of the epithelial layer of the tympanic membrane.

Tympanostomy tubes are the main surgical treatment for recurrent otitis media and otitis media with effusion. There are specific surgical indications for each disease process.

21. Describe the surgical procedure of myringotomy and tympanostomy tube placement.
    Under microscopic vision the ear canal and tympanic membrane are visualized through a speculum. After evaluation of the ear drum and middle ear, a small incision is made in the anterior-inferior quadrant of the tympanic membrane to avoid the ossicles and chorda tympani. Any fluid is removed via suction and the ear tube is placed with gentle pressure.

22. What is chronic suppurative otitis media?
    Chronic suppurative otitis media is otorrhea from a perforated tympanic membrane. The perforation can occur from an acute otitis media or chronic middle ear effusion. Otorrhea can be the result of secretions entering the middle ear from the eustachian tube or from water exposure of the middle ear mucosa.

23. How is chronic suppurative otitis media treated?
    The first step is to clean the ear canal and secretions to evaluate the middle ear. You must rule out a cholesteatoma, which can also lead to chronic ear drainage. In the absence of cholesteatoma the ear is treated with topical antibiotic ear drops, usually ofloxacin. The patient is put on dry ear precautions to avoid any water exposure of the middle ear. If there are allergy issues or enlarged adenoids, these may need to be addressed to reduce secretions from the eustachian tube. A culture can be obtained to help direct antibiotic coverage in cases of recalcitrant drainage.

Bibliography

Bluestone CD, Stool SE, Alper CM, et al: *Pediatric Otolaryngology* (vol 1), ed 4, Philadelphia, 2002, Saunders.

Hay WW, Deterding RR, Levin MJ, et al: *Current Diagnosis and Treatment Pediatrics*, ed 22, New York, 2014, McGraw-Hill Medical.

Lieberthal AS, Carroll AE, Chonmaitree T, et al: The diagnosis and management of acute otitis media, *Pediatrics* 131(3):e964–e999, 2013.

Rosenfeld RM, Culpepper L, Doyle KJ, et al: Clinical practice guideline: otitis media with effusion, *Otolaryngol Head Neck Surg* 130:S95–S118, 2004.

Rosenfeld RM, Schwartz SR, Pynnonen MA, et al: Clinical practice guideline: tympanostomy tubes in children, *Otolaryngol Head Neck Surg* 149:S1S35, 2013.

CHAPTER 38

COMPLICATIONS OF OTITIS MEDIA

Jameson K. Mattingly, MD and Kenny H. Chan, MD

KEY POINTS

Pathophysiology of Complicated Otitis Media (OM)

1. Complications from OM can occur by different mechanisms.
2. Preformed pathways increase the risk of spread of infection from the middle ear and mastoid to adjacent areas.
3. The three main routes of spread of OM are hematogenous, direct extension, and propagation of thrombus.
4. The treatment of most complications will involve myringotomy and ventilation tube insertion, usually for persistent effusion or infection.
5. Complicated OM (COM) is associated with infections by bacteria with increased resistance including strains of *S. aureus, P. aeruginosa, K. pneumoniae,* and anaerobic bacteria.

Pearls

1. Most common pathogens associated with complications in AOM are *S. pneumonia, H. influenzae,* and *M. catarrhalis.*
2. Initial antibiotic regimens should be broad-spectrum, and the degree of CSF penetration should be considered.
3. Surgical intervention is warranted if there is no improvement on medical therapy, if complications develop, or with intracranial complications.

QUESTIONS

1. Describe the pathophysiology of complications related to acute otitis media (AOM).
   The pathophysiology of complicated otitis media (OM) largely depends on whether it arises in the setting of AOM or chronic suppurative otitis media (CSOM). AOM develops in previously healthy ears and is characterized by mucosal edema with exudation of fluid, bacterial proliferation, and the formation of byproducts of inflammation (pus). Infection then spreads contiguously into the mastoid. Given the lack of granulation tissue and bony erosion with AOM, infection spreads either hematogenously or through direct extension via preformed pathways.

2. Describe the pathophysiology of complications related to chronic suppurative otitis media (CSOM).
   CSOM is characterized by persistent mastoid and middle ear inflammation and infection. This can occur with or without cholesteatoma, tympanic membrane perforation, or persistent otorrhea through ventilation tubes. When infection and inflammation persist, mucosal edema blocks off the normal pathways for drainage and aeration between the mastoid and middle ear. Continued inflammation results in bony destruction and granulation tissue formation. Infection subsequently spreads through direct extension via bony erosion from cholesteatoma or osteitis, or possibly through preformed pathways (more commonly associated with AOM).

3. What are some examples of *preformed pathways*?
Examples of preformed pathways are congenital inner ear anomalies such as Mondini's malformation or an enlarged vestibular aqueduct, trauma from previous surgery, or prior temporal bone fractures. These pathways increase the risk of direct extension of infection in the middle ear and mastoid.

4. What are the three pathways that result in complicated OM?
The three main pathways that result in OM complications are hematogenous spread, direct extension though bony erosion or preformed pathways, and thrombophlebitis of local perforating (diploic) veins.

5. What is an example of *hematogenous* spread of infection with OM?
Meningitis is an example of hematogenous spread. Meningitis usually occurs as a result of AOM rather than CSOM, and classic symptoms include headache, nausea, nuchal rigidity, photophobia, altered mental status, and fever. Cerebrospinal fluid examination is critical, and many times computed tomography (CT) is performed to rule out other intracranial complications and mass lesions.

6. What are examples of *direct extension*?
Direct extension results in a variety of complications depending upon the area of spread. Complications such as postauricular abscess, Bezold's abscess, sigmoid sinus thrombosis, epidural abscess, and subdural empyema all result from direct extension (see Figure 38-1).

7. What is a Bezold's abscess?
A Bezold abscess is a complication of acute otomastoiditis where the infection erodes through the mastoid cortex medial to the attachment of sternocleidomastoid, at the attachment site of the posterior belly of the digastric muscle, and extends into the infratemporal fossa. Due to it being deep to the cervical fascia that envelops the sternocleidomastoid muscle and trapezius muscle, it is difficult to palpate.

8. What is the bacteriology of complicated OM?
Complicated otitis media characteristically has an increase in resistant organisms, and is often polymicrobial. Frequently cultured organisms include *P. aeruginosa, S. aureus* including methicillin resistant strains, *K. pneumoniae, P. acnes*, and *Bacteroides* species.

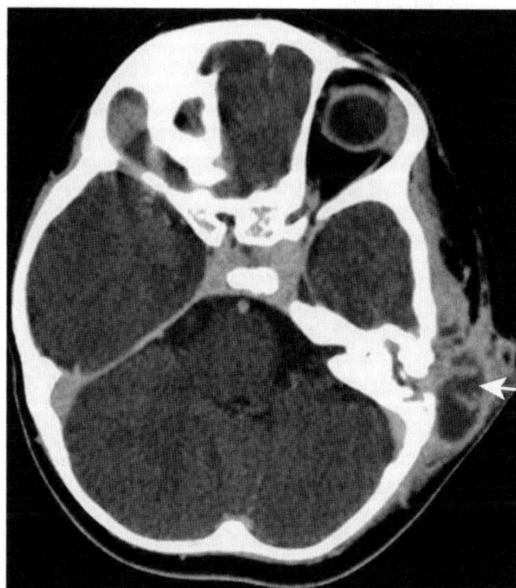

Figure 38-1. Axial CT scan with contrast demonstrating a postauricular abscess. *(From El-Kashlan H, Harker L, Shelton C, et al: Complications of Temporal Bone Infections. In Flint P, et al, editors:* Cummings Otolaryngology Head and Neck Surgery, *ed 5, Philadelphia, 2010, Mosby Elsevier, pp 1979–1998.)*

Table 38-1. Classification Schema for Complications of OM

EXTRACRANIAL/INTRATEMPORAL	INTRACRANIAL
Acute mastoiditis	Meningitis
Coalescent mastoiditis	Brain abscess
Chronic mastoiditis	Subdural empyema
Postauricular abscess	Epidural abscess
Bezold abscess	Lateral sinus thrombosis
Temporal abscess	Otitic hydrocephalus
Petrous apicitis	
Labyrinthe fistula	
Facial paralysis	
Acute suppurative labyrinthitis	
Encephalocele	
CSF leak	
Hearing loss (conductive and sensorineural)	

9. **What is the epidemiology of complications associated with OM?**
   The majority of complications associated with OM occur in children and young adults. Incidence varies among studies, but 60% to 80% of complications occur in the first two decades of life.

10. **What is the most common complication of OM?**
   The most common complication of OM is otitis media with effusion (OME). This entity is defined as middle ear effusion without signs of acute infection or inflammation, and may contribute to hearing loss.

11. **What is the classification schema for complications of OM?**
   Complications can be divided into intracranial or extracranial/intratemporal (Table 38-1).

12. **What are important presenting symptoms for complications of OM?**
   The signs and symptoms of OM and its associated complications can be quite broad, depending on the structures affected. Symptoms typically will begin with otalgia, irritability, and fever in AOM. CSOM may be initially more subtle, presenting with persistent purulent otorrhea. Patients may have postauricular pain, edema, otorrhea, and erythema with mastoid infection or abscess. Additionally, a patient's level of consciousness may be altered from intracranial complications. The time period of mental status change is variable based on the specific type of intracranial complication. The patient may exhibit papilledema, cranial nerve palsies, nuchal rigidity, or other neurologic findings.

13. **What is the role of imaging in the diagnosis of complicated OM?**
   A CT should be performed with contrast to assess for soft tissue and intracranial abscesses, inflammation, and flow voids in vessels. CT also allows evaluation of the osteology of the temporal bone specifically related to aeration of the middle ear and mastoid, bony dehiscence or erosions, and evaluation of cholesteatoma. However, it should be noted that imaging for OM is not needed unless there is worry about associated complications. Since the middle ear is connected to the mastoid air cell system, imaging of any acute OM likely will show mastoid opacification and thus may be interpreted as mastoiditis by the radiologist. Although CT offers excellent initial evaluation of suspected complications of OM and is much faster, MRI is more sensitive for diagnosis of intracranial complications. MRI detects subtle cerebral edema, dural enhancement, abscess, and vessel lumen patency more sensitively than CT. Both modalities are complementary to one another in diagnosis, management, and response to treatment. However, CT is a much quicker alternative than magnetic resonance imaging (MRI) in patients who are unstable or with altered mental status.

14. **What are important physical exam findings in complicated OM?**
A complete head and neck examination as well as a neurologic exam should be completed if there is any suspicion of complications of OM. The otologic exam may reveal signs of acute infection such as an erythematous, bulging, and opaque tympanic membrane, or may show perforation with purulent otorrhea, granulation tissue, or signs of a cholesteatoma. Postauricular or temporal abscesses may exhibit pain with palpation, erythema, and fluctuance. Vestibular symptoms may be present in certain cases with periods of imbalance, dysequilibirum, and vertigo.

Intracranial complications may present with papilledema, abducens nerve palsy, nuchal rigidity, positive Kernig or Brudzinski's signs, and altered mental status. Posterior superior sagging of the external auditory canal may be indicative of canal erosion from cholesteatoma. Facial nerve paralysis is not an uncommon finding, especially with bony dehiscence within the middle ear and resultant inflammation of the facial nerve. Petrous apicitis may present with abducens nerve palsy. It is therefore important to conduct a thorough cranial nerve examination.

15. **What are some eponyms that your attending might quiz you on?**
- *Queckenstedt's sign* is a test to determine whether cerebrospinal fluid (CSF) flow is obstructed in the subarachnoid space of the spinal canal by applying bilateral pressure on the internal jugular veins during lumbar puncture. No rise in pressure during this maneuver indicates obstruction of CSF flow as seen in meningitis or lateral sinus thrombophlebitis.
- *Gradenigo syndrome* is the triad of symptoms associated with petrous apicitis including retro-orbital pain, abducens nerve palsy, and otorrhea.
- *Bezold's abscess* is a cervical infection on the medial side of the mastoid deep to the digastric ridge that develops into an abscess.
- *Citelli abscess* is a cervical infection extending along the posterior belly of the digastric muscle that develops into an abscess.

16. **What is the general treatment for complications associated with AOM?**
Determining the status of the middle ear prior to infection is crucial in development of a treatment algorithm. Given that AOM develops in a previously normal ear without bony erosion and significant mucosal edema to block access to the mastoid, medical treatment with antibiotics is usually adequate to treat the otitis, and mastoidectomy is not needed. Sometimes myringotomy with or without tube placement is recommended. Treatments regarding specific complications vary and are discussed later in this chapter.

17. **What is the general treatment for complications associated with COM?**
As stated earlier, determining the status of the middle ear prior to infection is of the utmost importance. In CSOM, complications occur secondary to bony erosion, granulation tissue formation, or presence of cholesteatoma. In addition to bony erosion or cholesteatoma, infection can gain access to local structures through direct extension, and less frequently from a congenital anomaly. Infection may also propagate along vascular foramina from the mastoid to adjacent structures. Given the different pathophysiology of CSOM compared to AOM, the use of antibiotics and surgery are often complementary in management.

18. **What is the role of medical therapy in treating complications of OM?**
In almost all cases, intravenous (IV) antibiotics are the mainstay of therapy with initial broad-spectrum activity against aerobes and anaerobes. Until culture directed treatment can be obtained, initial regimens are meant to be broad and involve a combination of antibiotics such as vancomycin, a β-lactam antibiotic with a β-lactamase inhibitor (e.g., ampicillin-sulbactam), cephalosporins (e.g., ceftriaxone, cefepime, cefotaxime), and/or metronidazole. There may be significant institutional variability among antibiotics of choice depending on local patterns of resistance. Cerebrospinal fluid penetration should also be considered when intracranial complications are suspected. Treatment should be tailored once culture results are available.

19. **What is the role of anticoagulation with sigmoid sinus thrombosis due to OM?**
Sigmoid sinus thrombosis is an intracranial complication of OM. Mastoidectomy and antibiotics are well-established treatments with anticoagulation as a possible adjunct. Anticoagulation, though controversial, is thought to be beneficial in preventing clot extension and embolization, but current literature continues to be inconclusive regarding its use.

Table 38-2. General Treatment Strategies for Complications of OM Including Surgical Options

General Treatment Strategies for Complications of OM		
COMPLICATION	**MEDICAL TREATMENT**	**SURGICAL TREATMENT**
Acute mastoiditis	IV antibiotics	± Tympanocentesis, ± mastoidectomy
Coalescent mastoiditis	IV antibiotics	Mastoidectomy
Postauricular abscess	IV antibiotics	Incision and drainage, mastoidectomy
Bezold abscess	IV antibiotics	Incision and drainage, mastoidectomy
Temporal abscess	IV antibiotics	Incision and drainage, mastoidectomy
Petrous apicitis	IV antibiotics, ± steroids	± Mastoidectomy, ± petrous apex drainage
Labyrinthe fistula	± IV antibiotics	removal of cholesteatoma, ±fistula repair
Facial nerve paralysis	± IV antibiotics, ± steroids	± Tympanocentesis, ± facial nerve decompression, ± removal of cholesteatoma
Acute suppurative labyrinthitis	IV antibiotics, ± steroids	+± Mastoidectomy
Encephalocele, CSF leak	No antibiotics	Mastoid or middle fossa approach repair*
Meningitis	IV antibiotics, steroids	Tympanocentesis, ± mastoidectomy
Intraparenchymal brain abscess	IV antibiotics	± Incision and drainage*, mastoidectomy
Subdural empyema	IV antibiotics	Incision and drainage*, mastoidectomy
Epidural abscess	IV antibiotics	Incision and drainage, mastoidectomy
Sigmoid sinus thrombosis	IV antibiotics, ± anticoagulation, ± steroids	Mastoidectomy, ± clot removal, ± ligation of internal jugular vein
Otitic hydrocephalus	IV antibiotics, ± steroids, ± diuretics, ± anticoagulation	Mastoidectomy, ± clot removal, ± serial lumbar punctures

*Neurosurgical consultation.

20. **What is the role of surgical intervention?**
Table 38-2 depicts general treatment guidelines for complications of OM. Medical therapy without surgery may be warranted initially, especially in uncomplicated cases of acute mastoiditis. Surgery is usually recommended if there is failure to improve on medical therapy, development of complications, or presentation with intracranial complications. Surgery may range from myringotomy and tube insertion to mastoidectomy with intracranial decompression.

Special consideration must be given for complications associated with cholesteatoma because the removal of the cholesteatoma is required for adequate long-term treatment. IV antibiotics are usually warranted and neurosurgery consultation may be sought in both medical and surgical management of intracranial complications.

Bibliography

Casselbrant M, Mandel E: Acute otitis media and otitis media with effusion. In Flint P, et al, editors: *Cummings Otolaryngology Head and Neck Surgery*, ed 5, Philadelphia, 2010, Mosby Elsevier, pp 2761–2777.

Chole R, Sudhoff H: Chronic otitis media, mastoiditis, and petrositis. In Flint P, et al, editors: *Cummings Otolaryngology Head and Neck Surgery*, ed 5, Philadelphia, 2010, Mosby Elsevier, pp 1963–1978.

El-Kashlan H, Harker L, Shelton C, et al: Complications of temporal bone infections. In Flint P, et al, editors: *Cummings Otolaryngology Head and Neck Surgery*, ed 5, Philadelphia, 2010, Mosby Elsevier, pp 1979–1998.

Friedland DR, Pensak ML, Kveton JF: Cranial and intracranial complications of acute and chronic otitis media. In Snow J, Wackym P, editors: *Ballenger's Otorhinolaryngology Head and Neck Surgery*, ed 17, Ontario, 2009, BC Decker, pp 229–238.

Isaccson B, Mirabal C, Kutz W, et al: Pediatric otogenic intra-cranial abscesses, *Otolaryngol Head Neck Surg* 142: 434–437, 2010.

Osma U, Cureoglu S, Hosgoglu S: The complications of chronic otitis media: report of 93 cases, *J Laryngol Otol* 114:97–100, 2000.

Psarommatis IM, Voudouris C, Douros K, et al: Algorithmic management of pediatric acute mastoiditis, *Intl J Pediatr Otorhinolaryngol* 76(6):791–796, 2012.

Singh B, Maharaj TJ: Radical mastoidectomy: its place in otitic intracranial complications, *J Laryngol Otol* 107: 1113–1118, 1993.

Sitton MS, Chun R: Pediatric otogenic lateral sinus thrombosis: role of anti-coagulation and surgery, *Intl J Pediatr Otorhinolaryngol* 76:428–432, 2012.

Yorgancilar E, Yildrum M, Gun R, et al: Complications of chronic suppurative otitis media: a retrospective review, *Eur Arch Otorhinolaryngol* 270:69–76, 2013.

CHAPTER 39

TYMPANOMASTOIDECTOMY AND OSSICULAR CHAIN RECONSTRUCTION

Brianne Barnett Roby, MD and Patricia J. Yoon, MD

KEY POINTS

1. Key landmarks for a mastoidectomy are the tegmen, sigmoid sinus, lateral semicircular canal, incus, and posterior canal wall.
2. A mastoidectomy is the surgical removal of the mastoid air cells. It is indicated for certain types of infection, cholesteatoma, and approaches to other landmarks in the temporal bone.
3. Different types of mastoidectomies are performed based on the extent of the ear disease, and include a canal wall up mastoidectomy and canal wall down mastoidectomy.
4. Ossicular chain reconstruction is performed when there is a disruption between any of the ossicles.

Pearls

1. A canal wall down mastoidectomy is indicated when there is a semicircular canal fistula or posterior canal wall damage due to cholesteatoma, a sclerotic mastoid prevents adequate visualization with a wall up mastoidectomy, or the patient is unable to follow up or undergo additional surgeries for proper monitoring of recurrent cholesteatoma.
2. A second look procedure is indicated in a canal wall up mastoidectomy for cholesteatoma and is performed 6 to 12 months after initial surgery to look for recurrence of cholesteatoma.
3. The facial recess is bordered anteriorly by the chorda tympani, posteriorly by the facial nerve, and superiorly by the incus buttress.
4. A PORP is indicated when stapes suprastructure is present, whereas a TORP is indicated when the stapes suprastructure is not present.

QUESTIONS

1. **What is a mastoidectomy? What is a tympanomastoidectomy?**
The mastoid is a portion of the temporal bone that houses air cells connected to the middle ear space. A mastoidectomy is a surgical procedure in which mastoid bone and air cells are removed. A tympanomastoidectomy is a tympanoplasty plus mastoidectomy. This procedure is commonly used to address chronic ear disease in the mastoid bone as well as a tympanic membrane that is perforated, severely retracted, or involved with cholesteatoma.

2. **What are the main types of mastoidectomy?**
There are a number of different types of mastoidectomy surgery, broadly grouped into canal wall up (CWU) and canal wall down (CWD) procedures.
In a canal wall up (CWU) mastoidectomy, the mastoid air cells are removed, leaving the posterior external auditory canal wall intact. The borders of a complete mastoidectomy are the tegmen superiorly, the sigmoid sinus posteriorly, and the posterior canal wall anteriorly.
A canal wall down (CWD) mastoidectomy is one in which the mastoid air cells are removed along with the posterior wall of the external auditory canal. This creates a mastoid cavity or "bowl." With this procedure, a meatoplasty is also usually performed, which widens the opening of the outer

ear canal in order to improve visualization and access to the mastoid bowl. A canal wall down mastoidectomy effectively "exteriorizes" the mastoid.

In a modified radical mastoidectomy the canal wall is taken down and the epitympanum, mastoid antrum, and external auditory canal are converted into a common cavity. The middle ear space, tympanic membrane, and ossicles are preserved. This procedure is sometimes called the Bondy modified radical mastoidectomy.

In a radical mastoidectomy, a CWD mastoidectomy is performed and the tympanic membrane and ossicles, except for the stapes, are also permanently removed. These structures are not reconstructed.

3. **What are the indications for a mastoidectomy?**
The most common indication for a mastoidectomy is chronic disease such as cholesteatoma or mastoiditis. A mastoidectomy is also indicated for some complications of acute otitis media, such as acute mastoiditis or a subperiosteal abscess.

A mastoidectomy is a key portion of the approach for cochlear implantation or facial nerve decompression. A mastoidectomy may be performed as part of a transmastoid approach for excision of temporal bone tumors, such as vestibular schwannoma, glomus tumor, or meningioma. In unusual cases, a mastoidectomy may be required for repair of a cerebrospinal fluid leak.

4. **What are the important landmarks in mastoidectomy surgery? (Figure 39-1)**
The superior border of a mastoidectomy is the tegmen, which is the thin bone layer separating the middle cranial fossa from the ear. The posterior border is the sigmoid sinus. The anterior border is the posterior wall of the external auditory canal. The deep (medial) border is the lateral semicircular canal and incus, which are found in the aditus ad antrum, the connection between the mastoid cavity and the middle ear space. Another key landmark is the facial nerve.

5. **When is a canal wall down procedure indicated?**
A canal wall down procedure is indicated in the following situations:
- Cholesteatoma involving the sinus tympani area, not accessible transcanal or through the facial recess
- Semicircular canal fistula with adherent cholesteatoma matrix
- The posterior canal wall is extensively damaged by disease

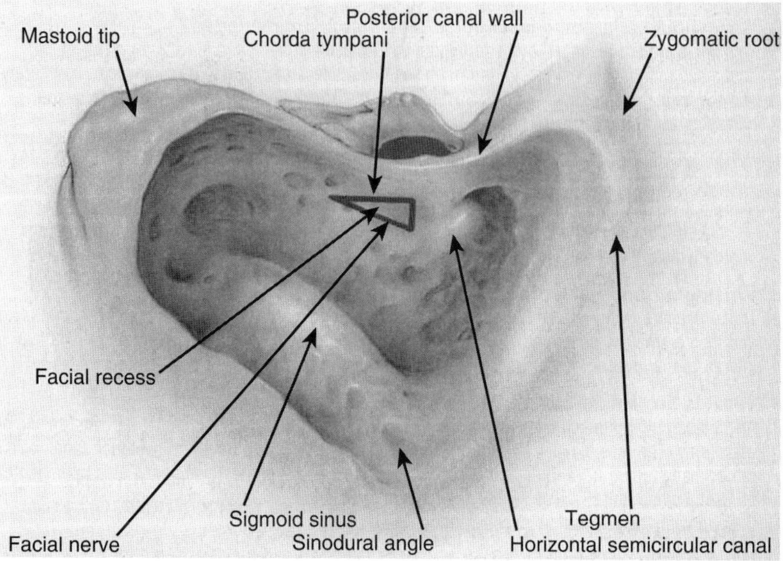

Figure 39-1. Landmarks in mastoidectomy surgery. *(From Nelson RA: Temporal Bone Surgical Dissection Manual from the House Ear Institute, Los Angeles, ed 3. Antonio De la Cruz and Jose N Fayad. Figure 10.)*

- The mastoid is contracted and sclerotic, preventing adequate visualization and access via a CWU approach
- Unresectable cholesteatoma matrix on the dura or posterior cranial fossa
- Attic or mastoid cholesteatoma in a patient unable to maintain follow-up or unable to safely tolerate further surgery

6. **What are the disadvantages of a CWD mastoidectomy?**
The mastoid bowl often fills with cerumen and requires periodic debridement to prevent infection. Although not necessarily unsightly, the meatoplasty is often visible. Hearing outcomes may be slightly diminished due to the change in the acoustic properties of the ear canal. Water restrictions are recommended due to risk of mastoid bowl infection.

7. **What are the disadvantages of a canal wall up (CWU) procedure?**
There is a higher chance of recurrent or residual cholesteatoma, as exposure of the attic, antrum, and facial recess is more limited if the canal wall is left intact. Patients that have had a CWU procedure are more likely to require a "second look" procedure in the operating room whereas patients undergoing a CWD mastoidectomy can often be monitored in the clinic.

8. **What is a second look procedure?**
For patients who have had cholesteatoma removed using the CWU technique, a second look surgery may be performed several months later (typically 6 to 12 months) to determine whether there is recurrent or residual disease that was not visible at the time of the previous surgery and could not be detected on office examination.
The procedure is performed several months later to allow time for any microscopic residual disease to grow large enough to be visualized. However, one should not wait too long, as residual or recurrent cholesteatoma may grow large enough to cause damage to ear structures.

9. **What is a facial recess approach? What are the borders of the facial recess?**
The facial recess is an area within the mastoid that frequently contains air cells and is a pathway to the middle ear space. The facial recess is bordered anteriorly by the chorda tympani, posteriorly by the facial nerve, and superiorly by the incus buttress. The facial recess air cells are at the same level as the tip of the short process of the incus. The facial recess may be opened up to help eradicate cholesteatoma, and is also used in cochlear implantation to allow introduction of the electrode through the middle ear space into the round window.

10. **How should a lateral semicircular canal fistula be managed?**
This is most often managed by performing a CWD mastoidectomy and leaving a portion of squamous matrix over the fistula. In rare cases, the cholesteatoma may be removed in its entirety and the fistula patched with a graft. Suctioning of the area should be avoided to preserve the endolymph within the canal.

11. **What are the potential complications of a mastoidectomy?**
Major complications include facial nerve injury, sensorineural hearing loss, cerebrospinal fluid leak, and dural venous sinus injury.
Minor complications include temporary change in taste sensation from manipulation of the chorda tympani, vertigo, and tympanic membrane perforation.

12. **What is a Bondy atticotomy?**
This procedure involves a limited approach to an attic cholesteatoma. An endaural incision is used and then a small atticoantrostomy is performed. The bone overlying the attic is then taken down to inferior to the level of the disease. The pars tensa and the ossicular chain are left intact.

13. **What is an "inside-out" mastoidectomy?**
An "inside-out" approach usually begins endaurally by raising a tympanomeatal flap and drilling an atticotomy. The mastoid air cells are drilled starting from the atticotomy and posterior canal wall, rather than starting from the mastoid cortex as with a traditional mastoidectomy. This approach can be useful when there is a very low-lying tegmen or anteriorly placed sigmoid sinus which can limit the approach for a typical atticoantrostomy.

14. **What are the indications for an ossicular chain reconstruction?**
The ossicular chain is composed of the three bones of the middle ear: the malleus, incus, and stapes (Figure 39-2). Ossicular chain reconstruction is performed when conductive hearing loss is

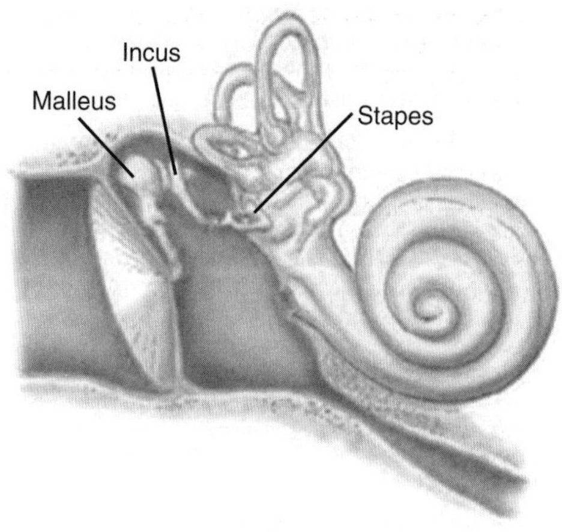

Figure 39-2. Ossicular chain. *(Modified from Dorland's Illustrated Medical Dictionary, 32 ed. Philadelphia, Saunders 2011.)*

due to a disruption or abnormality of these bones. The disruption may be due to trauma, congenital abnormalities, chronic ear disease, cholesteatoma, or surgery. Osteoclastic properties of cholesteatoma often erode the ossicular chain. Ossicular chain reconstruction is undertaken when the ear is felt to be free of disease, which is often not until a second look or subsequent procedure.

15. What are contraindications for an ossicular chain reconstruction?
Acute otitis media at time of reconstruction is an absolute contraindication. Relative contraindications include persistent middle ear disease such as cholesteatoma, dehiscent facial nerve overlying the oval window, or an only hearing ear.

16. What are some of the different prostheses that may be used in ossicular chain reconstruction and their specific indications?
Two broad categories exist: Partial ossicular chain prostheses (PORPs) and total ossicular chain prostheses (TORPs). A PORP is used when the stapes suprastructure is present where the PORP can sit on the stapes head and then connect the tympanic membrane. A TORP sits on the stapes footplate and extends to contact the tympanic membrane. A cartilage graft is placed on the head of the prosthesis to help prevent extrusion through the tympanic membrane.
TORPs and PORPs are made of different materials, commonly titanium and hydroxyapatite-polyethylene.
Bone cement is useful in certain situations, such as reconstructing the long process of the incus and in stabilizing prostheses.

17. What is an incus interposition graft?
An incus interposition graft can be used when there are abnormalities of either the incudomalleal joint or the incudostapedial joint, but with normal malleus and stapes. The incus is removed and sculpted with a groove to accommodate the malleus and a cup to hold the stapes capitulum. The carved incus is then placed back between the malleus and stapes, making sure it makes proper contact with both.

18. What are the expected outcomes for ossicular reconstruction surgery?
It is important to set realistic expectations for patients undergoing ossicular reconstruction. Results are quantified based on the postoperative air–bone gap achieved and are stratified as follows: excellent (<10 dB), good (11 to 20 dB), fair (21 to 30 dB). Success is dependent on multiple factors, including absence or presence of a mobile stapes superstructure, eustachian tube function and middle ear status, and presence or absence of the canal wall. Hearing outcomes are generally more successful with PORPs than with TORPs.

19. **What are potential complications of ossicular reconstruction surgery?**
Complications include perilymphatic fistula resulting in sensorineural hearing loss and vertigo, extrusion or displacement of the prosthesis, tympanic membrane perforation, facial nerve injury, and change in taste sensation.

20. **What is endoscopic ear surgery and what are its advantages?**
Traditional ear surgery is performed under a microscope and the field of view via a transcanal approach is limited by the narrowest portion of the ear canal. A mastoidectomy is therefore often required even when the mastoid is free of disease in order to gain visualization and access to the attic, facial recess, and hypotympanum. In recent years, the use of rigid surgical endoscopes for cholesteatoma surgery has increased in popularity. Both 0-degree and angled rigid endoscopes through the ear canal allow for a wider field of view within the middle ear and allow visualization of areas that cannot be seen using the microscope. With the use of endoscopes and specially designed endoscopic ear surgery instruments, surgery for cholesteatoma and other middle ear problems is now possible in many cases through much smaller postauricular or even transcanal incisions with significantly improved visualization.

Bibliography

Ayache S, Tramier B, Strunski V: Otoendoscopy in cholesteatoma surgery of the middle ear. What benefits can be expected?, *Otol Neurotol* 29(8):1085–1090, 2008.

Brackmann DE, Shelton C, Arriaga MA, editors: *Otologic Surgery*, ed 3, Philadelphia, 2010, Elsevier.

Coker NJ, Jenkins HA, editors: *Atlas of Otologic Surgery*, Philadelphia, 2001, WB Saunders Company.

Hathiram BT, Khattar VS, editors: Chap 15. *Atlas of Operative Otorhinolaryngology and Head and Neck Surgery*, Philadelphia, PA, 2013, Jaypee Medical Publishers, pp 112–123.

Johnson J, Rosen C, editors: *Bailey's Head and Neck Surgery: Otolaryngology*, ed 5, Baltimore, 2013, Lippincott Williams and Wilkens, pp 2447–2486.

Lalwani A, editor: Chap 44. *Current Diagnosis and Treatment in Otolaryngology Head and Neck Surgery*, ed 3, New York, 2012, McGraw Hill Medical.

Lalwani AK, Grundfast KM, editors: *Pediatric Otology and Neurotology*, Philadelphia, 1998, Lippincott Raven Publishers.

Myers EN, editor: Chap 114 and 115. *Operative Otolaryngology*, Philadelphia, 2008, Saunders Publishing, pp 1167–1176.

CHAPTER 40

OTOSCLEROSIS

Jameson K. Mattingly, MD and Herman Jenkins, MD

KEY POINTS

1. Otosclerosis involves the otic capsule
2. Originates from altered bony metabolism with ongoing resorption and deposition of disorganized bone
3. Results in fixation of the ossicular chain producing conductive hearing loss
4. Can also rarely involve the cochlea resulting in "cochlear otosclerosis"
5. Possible contributing factors include measles infection, autoimmunity, multiple endocrine abnormalities, and low fluoride consumption

Pearls

1. The most common presentation of otosclerosis is progressive conductive hearing loss, although it can rarely present with sensorineural hearing loss.
2. Although not required for diagnosis, many patients will have a positive family history.
3. Medical therapies, including sodium fluoride and bisphosphonates, are controversial in their clinical effectiveness.

QUESTIONS

1. **Define otosclerosis.**
   Otosclerosis is derived from the Greek word "hardening of the ear." In a broad sense it is defined as altered bony metabolism in the otic capsule with ongoing resorption and deposition of bone. This process results in fixation of the ossicular chain and resultant conductive hearing loss (CHL).

2. **Describe the epidemiology of otosclerosis.**
   Otosclerosis most commonly occurs in Caucasians in the second to fifth decades of life, with a female to male preponderance of 2:1. Bilateral disease occurs in 80% of patients, and approximately 20% to 30% develop sensorineural hearing loss (SNHL).

3. **What is the pathophysiology of otosclerosis?**
   Otosclerosis is a localized remodeling process of bone occurring in and around the otic capsule. In the normal state, endochondral calcification is usually complete in the otic capsule at one year of age with little remodeling thereafter. The disease process of otosclerosis is the result of abnormal prolonged remodeling of bone in and around the otic capsule by osteoblasts and osteoclasts. This process results in poorly organized bone that becomes metabolically active, well-vascularized bone (spongiotic), and/or densely mineralized (sclerotic) bone (Figure 40-1). The end result in classic otosclerosis is fixation of the stapes footplate, usually beginning anteriorly with posterior progression to complete footplate involvement.

4. **What are the initial symptoms of otosclerosis?**
   The characteristic presentation of otosclerosis is adult-onset progressive unilateral or bilateral conductive hearing loss. Although less likely, otosclerosis can present with SNHL due to "cochlear otosclerosis." Some patients report improved hearing in noisy environments, referred to as "paracusis of Willis." The second most common complaint is tinnitus. Vestibular symptoms are rarely reported.

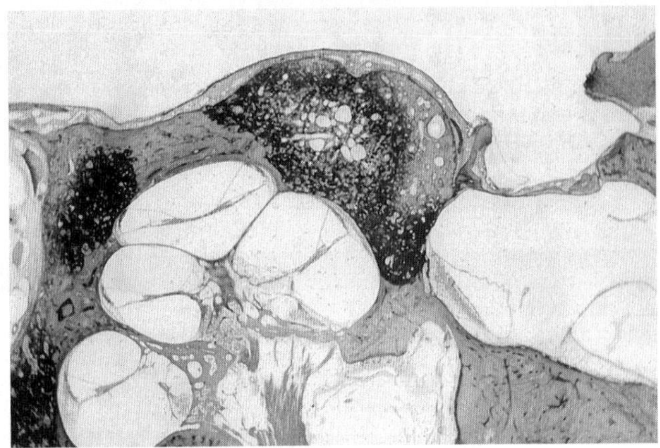

Figure 40-1. Multiple otosclerotic lesions around the cochlea and anterior to the stapes footplate. *(Adapted from Flint PW, Haughey BH, Lund VJ, et al, editors: Cummings Otolaryngology: Head & Neck Surgery, ed 5, Philadelphia, 2010, Mosby.)*

5. **Does genetics play a role in the development of otosclerosis?**
   Studies of families with otosclerosis have supported an autosomal dominant pattern of inheritance with incomplete penetrance. Within these groups multiple genes have been implicated, although there is significant heterogeneity of the genetic pattern. Although genetic factors likely influence the development of otosclerosis, approximately half of all cases arise without a positive family history.

6. **What other factors may be causative in the development of otosclerosis?**
   Although literature supporting various etiologies is limited, persistent measles infection, autoimmunity, multiple endocrine factors, and low fluoride consumption have been implicated in the development of otosclerosis.

7. **What is the Schwartze sign?**
   Schwartze sign is a reddish hue seen though the tympanic membrane reflecting the increased vascularity of the bone over the promontory. Although this may be seen early in the disease process, this finding is not present in all cases.

8. **What physical exam findings are expected in patients with otosclerosis?**
   Physical exam findings of patients with otosclerosis are limited. Most present with a normal external auditory canal and tympanic membrane with an occasional Schwartze sign. Rinne and Weber tuning fork exams will typically reveal bone conduction to be greater than air conduction, and lateralization to the affected side, respectively, although these findings are not specific for otosclerosis.

9. **What are the expected audiogram findings of otosclerosis?**
   Audiometric studies typically show a CHL that is worse at low frequencies. The Carhart notch is characteristic of otosclerosis showing an apparent SNHL at 2000 Hz.

10. **What is a Carhart notch?**
    A Carhart notch (Figure 40-2) is a decrease in bone thresholds on an audiogram at 2000 Hz which can be seen in otosclerosis and other pathologies affecting the middle ear. It is thought to be caused by inertia of the ossicular chain. It is not sensitive or specific for otosclerosis.

11. **What role does acoustic immitance testing play in diagnosis of otosclerosis?**
    Tympanometry will typically show an A_s configuration reflecting normal middle ear pressure, but decreased amplitude indicative of some degree of ossicular chain fixation. The stapedial reflex may be present in early portions of the disease process, but may show abnormalities including biphasic reflexes. Reflexes become absent with progression of the disease to stapes fixation.

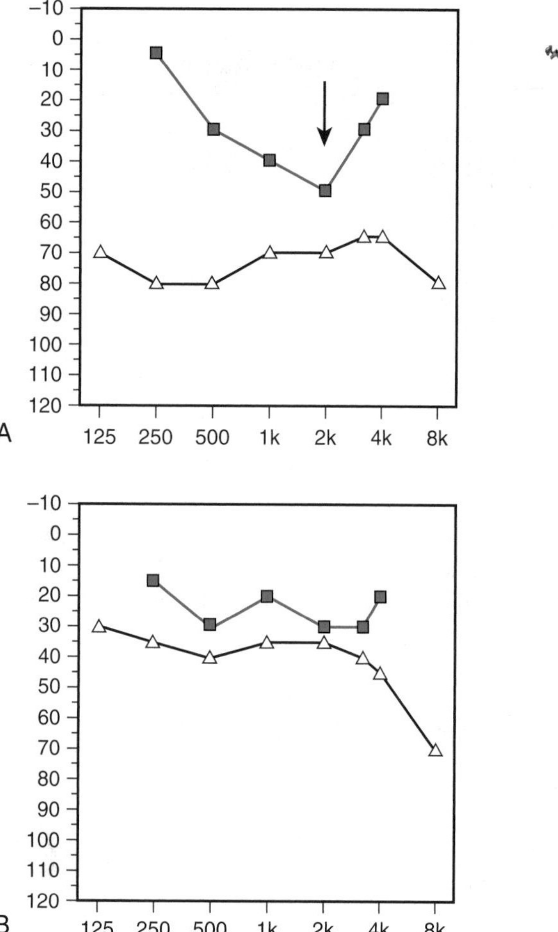

Figure 40-2. Pure-tone audiogram (PTA; **A,** preoperative PTA, **B,** postoperative PTA). There is preoperative conductive hearing loss as shown by a characteristic Carhart notch *(black arrow),* which implies bone conduction impairment at 2 kHz. After the ossicular chain was reconstructed using a total ossicular replacement prosthesis (TORP), postoperative audiometric evaluations done at a 6-month follow-up visit demonstrated closure of the air–bone gap and disappearance of the Carhart notch. *(From Kim KW, Jun H-S, Im GJ, et al: Isolated otosclerosis of the incus in a Korean woman, Auris Nasus Larynx 38(5): 654–656, 2011.)*

12. Does imaging play a role in otosclerosis?
    Imaging modalities in otosclerosis such as computed tomography (CT) and magnetic resonance imaging (MRI) are not routinely needed. However, recent studies have suggested high resolution CT, along with physical and audiometric data, to be highly sensitive in diagnosing otosclerosis. In addition to assisting in diagnosis, CT may also provide information helpful for surgical planning and prevention of complications.

13. Does medical treatment play a roie in otosclerosis?
    Current medical therapy is aimed at decreasing bone remodeling, specifically targeting osteoclastic activity. Much of this theory has been based on success with treatment of osteoporosis. Possible medical therapies include bisphosphonates and sodium fluoride. Given the success of surgical

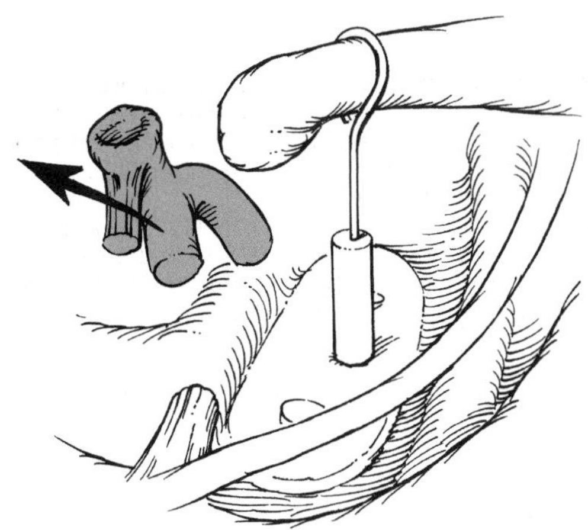

Figure 40-3. Stapes prosthesis from the incus into the stapedotomy fenestra after removal of the stapes suprastructure. *(Adapted from Flint PW, Haughey BH, Lund VJ, et al, editors: Cummings Otolaryngology: Head & Neck Surgery, ed 5, Philadelphia, 2010, Mosby.)*

treatment and unknown efficacy, no medical therapies are consistently recommended. Hearing aids offer a successful nonsurgical alternative for correction of hearing loss associated with otosclerosis.

14. **Describe the surgical treatment of otosclerosis.**
There are currently multiple techniques in use for correction of otosclerosis. Regardless of variations in technique, current literature reports successful outcomes in greater than 90% of patients measured by closure of their preoperative air–bone gap.
In general, the goal of surgery is to allow transmission of sound from the tympanic membrane through the ossicular chain to the oval window while bypassing the fixed stapes footplate. This process typically involves some variation of removal of the arch of the stapes, fenestration or partial removal of the stapes footplate, and insertion of a prosthesis connecting the incus to the oval window (Figure 40-3). In cases of incus necrosis, a prosthesis connecting the malleus to the oval window can be used.

15. **Are there any special considerations in patients with bilateral otosclerosis?**
Bilateral otosclerosis occurs in approximately 70% of cases. When electing to operate on a patient with bilateral disease, the poorer hearing ear is generally operated on first, and followed by, if successful, the contralateral ear 6 months later.

16. **What are the risks associated with stapes surgery?**
Risks that should be considered during informed consent include SNHL (including deafness), vertigo, facial nerve injury, loss or change of taste, continued conductive hearing loss, prosthesis extrusion or displacement, and tympanic membrane perforation.

17. **Discuss the important points regarding revision stapes surgery.**
Despite the success of stapes surgery, need for revision is not uncommon. Common reasons for revision surgery include CHL, vertigo, SNHL, and distortion of sound. Prior to undergoing revision stapes surgery other factors for these symptoms should be thoroughly explored. CT of the temporal bones is warranted to evaluate the middle ear, the indwelling prosthesis, and to rule out other causes of CHL such as superior semicircular canal dehiscence. Revision surgery is associated with decreased success and increased risk of SNHL (including deafness) in comparison to primary surgery.

18. **What lasers are best suited for stapedotomy?**
Multiple lasers have been used for stapedotomy, including argon, potassium titanyl phosphate (KTP), erbium yttrium aluminum garnet (Er-YAG), and CO_2 lasers. These lasers have various characteristics that make them appealing. Although the literature is limited regarding lasers best suited for stapedotomy, the CO_2 laser has been most commonly used and prior studies have favored this device due to potentially better closure of air–bone gaps.

19. What should be done if a persistent stapedial artery or overriding facial nerve is encountered intraoperatively?

Persistent stapedial arteries and an overriding facial nerve are anatomic variants that can be encountered during stapes surgery. The surgery can generally proceed if these are encountered, but additional precautions should be taken. An overriding facial nerve can usually be retracted gently to allow access to the stapes footplate for creating the fenestra. Persistent stapedial arteries historically were approached with caution due to the risk of hemorrhage and ischemia to neural structures if damaged. The latter concern is mostly theoretical as no cases have been reported. Hence, coagulation or ligation of the artery can be performed if needed. However, if surgery cannot proceed safely, the procedure should be terminated to prevent undue risk to the patient. The patient can then be referred for alternative treatments such as hearing amplification.

Bibliography

Altmann F, Glasgold A, Macduff JP: The incidence of otosclerosis as related to race and sex, *Ann Otol Rhinol Laryngol* 76:377–392, 1967.

Chole RA, McKenna M: Pathophysiology of otosclerosis, *Otol Neurotol* 22:249–257, 2001.

Glasscock M III, Storper I, Haynes D, et al: Twenty-five years of experience with stapedectomy, *Laryngoscope* 105: 899–904, 1995.

House J, Cunningham C: Otosclerosis. In Flint P, et al, editors: *Cummings Otolaryngology Head and Neck Surgery*, ed 5, Philadelphia, 2010, Mosby Elsevier, pp 2028–2035.

Jenkins H, McKenna M: Otosclerosis. In Snow J, Wackym P, editors: *Ballenger's Otorhinolaryngology Head and Neck Surgery*, ed 17, Ontario, 2009, BC Decker, pp 247–251.

Kursten R, Schneider B, Zrunek M: Long-term results after stapedectomy versus stapedotomy, *Am J Otol* 15(6):804–806, 1994.

Lagleyre S, Sorrentino T, Calmels MN, et al: Reliability of high-resolution CT scan in diagnosis of otosclerosis, *Otol Neurotol* 30(8):1152–1159, 2009.

Schrauwen I, Van Camp G: The etiology of otosclerosis: a combination of genes and environment, *Laryngoscope* 120:1195–1202, 2010.

Shea J: Forty years of stapes surgery, *Am J Otol* 19:52–55, 1998.

Ziya Ozuer M, Olgun L, Gultekin G: Revision stapes surgery, *Otolaryngol Head Neck Surg* 146(1):109–113, 2011.

CHAPTER 41

CHOLESTEATOMA

Jameson K. Mattingly, MD and Kenny H. Chan, MD

KEY POINTS

Surgical Management of Cholesteatoma

1. Multiple techniques exist for removal of cholesteatomas.
2. Canal wall up procedures maintain a physiologic ear canal, but have increased risk of residual and recurrent disease.
3. Canal wall down procedures provide superior visualization of disease during surgery, but may require periodic cleaning and createdifficulty with hearing aids, and possible water restriction.
4. Ossiculoplasty may be needed to improve hearing if ossicles are damaged.
5. Otoendoscopy may improve visualization of cholesteatoma in certain areas.

Pearls

1. Cholesteatomas are usually classified into congenital, primary acquired, and secondary acquired types.
2. Cholesteatomas characteristically become infected and/or erode bone resulting in a variety of complications.
3. CT is the most commonly used imaging modality to evaluate cholesteatomas.
4. Surgery is the definitive treatment with the primary goal of complete eradication of disease, followed by preservation hearing, and the overall improvement of ear hygiene.
5. Second-stage operations are commonly performed to evaluate for residual and recurrent disease.

QUESTIONS

Pathophysiology, Etiology, and Classification

1. What is a cholesteatoma?
   Cholesteatomas are epidermal inclusion cysts of the temporal bone composed of squamous epithelium and associated debris. These masses enlarge over time and become destructive, commonly with surrounding inflammation and granulation tissue.
   The word *cholesteatoma* was first used to describe its light color and gross resemblance to cholesterol crystals under microscopy. This observation turned out to be incorrect—there is no cholesterol or fat in cholesteatomas.

2. What are the different types of cholesteatoma?
   The three main types are congenital, primary acquired, and secondary acquired (Table 41-1).

3. Briefly describe the different pathways of formation.
   Congenital cholesteatomas are thought to originate from keratinizing squamous epithelium of the middle ear cleft. Although the etiology remains unknown, multiple theories exist to describe the origin of the squamous epithelium. These theories include epidermoid cell rests within the middle ear (most favored theory), squamous metaplasia, epithelial migration through tympanic membrane (TM) microperforations, and deposition of desquamated epithelial cells from amniotic fluid.
   Primary acquired cholesteatomas usually arise in the setting of retraction of the TM, usually as a result of otitis media and chronic eustachian tube dysfunction. Although usually arising from the pars flaccida, they can more rarely develop in the pars tensa. Secondary acquired cholesteatomas, alternatively, arise in the setting of TM perforations with epithelial migration. Multiple theories exist

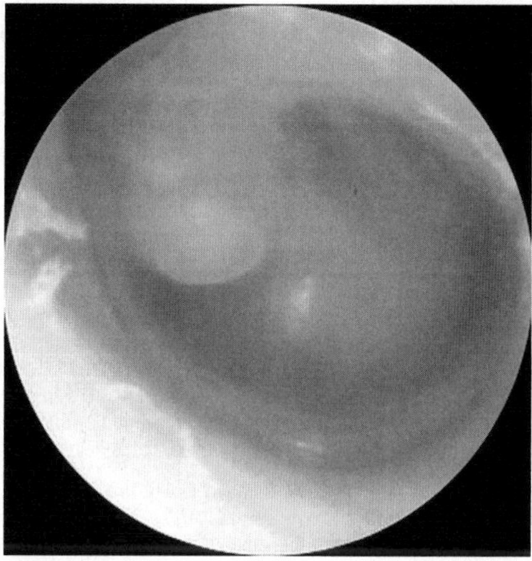

Figure 41-1. Congenital cholesteatoma behind an intact tympanic membrane. *(From Flint PW, Haughey BH, Lund VJ, et al, editors: Cummings Otolaryngology: Head & Neck Surgery, ed 5, Philadelphia, 2010, Mosby.)*

Table 41-1. Various Types of Cholesteatomas and Their Associated Origin

TYPE	ORIGIN
Congenital	Keratinizing epithelium in middle ear cleft with an intact TM
Primary acquired	Occurs in the setting of TM retraction
Secondary acquired	Occurs in the setting of TM perforation

to explain the pathogenesis of acquired cholesteatomas including: TM invagination, migration of epithelium though TM perforations, basal cell hyperplasia, squamous metaplasia, and implantation.

4. **What is the invagination theory?**
Invagination is the most accepted theory of primary acquired cholesteatomas. TM retraction results from negative middle ear pressure due to eustachian tube dysfunction, poor pneumatization of the mastoid, inflammation, and/or TM atrophy. Progressive retraction forms a pocket resulting in disrupted normal epithelial migration and drainage of keratin debris. As this process progresses, a cholesteatoma forms.

5. **Why treat cholesteatoma?**
Cholesteatomas have a propensity to become recurrently infected and erode bone. Once infected, eradication of an infection may be very difficult, and can result in a variety of intracranial and extracranial complications associated with chronic otitis media. The bacterial flora associated with cholesteatomas are also different from those in acute otitis media. Infections associated with cholesteatomas are frequently polymicrobial with an increase in anaerobes and antibiotic-resistant bacteria.
Bone erosion can affect various structures in the temporal bone that can result in hearing loss, vestibular dysfunction, facial nerve injury, and intracranial complications. Bone erosion is thought to be due to the influx of inflammatory mediators due to chronic inflammation and infection that results in an imbalance of bone remodeling favoring resorption.

6. **How does a congenital cholesteatoma present?**
Congenital cholesteatomas usually present as white or yellow masses in the *anterior superior* quadrant of the middle ear (Figure 41-1). Unlike acquired cholesteatomas, congenital cholesteatomas usually arise in the setting of an intact TM with an absence of otorrhea. Many times

they are asymptomatic, and other symptoms vary depending on the extent of the disease. Presenting symptoms include slowly progressive conductive hearing loss (CHL), vertigo, facial nerve paralysis, or intracranial infection.

7. **How do acquired cholesteatomas present?**
Acquired cholesteatomas usually present as *posterior superior* retraction pockets seen at the margin of the TM with surrounding keratin debris. Acquired cholesteatomas may or may not have TM perforations with persistent foul-smelling otorrhea and granulation tissue. Presenting symptoms, as in congenital cholesteatoma, vary depending on the extent of the disease and can include many of the same features mentioned in the prior paragraph.

Preoperative Assessment

8. **What is the role of imaging in the preoperative assessment?**
Computed tomography (CT) is frequently used to augment physical examination in those suspected of having a cholesteatoma. Although not required for uncomplicated cases, CT provides valuable information regarding extent of disease, involved structures, and relevant anatomy that assists in preoperative planning. CT may also prove to be very helpful in revision cases. Magnetic resonance imaging (MRI) is less commonly used, but is helpful in evaluating intracranial complications.

9. **What is the one CT finding commonly seen in acquired cholesteatoma that your attending likely will ask about?**
Blunting or erosion of the scutum is a common finding on CT in those with cholesteatoma. The scutum is a bony prominence in the lateral portion of the middle ear and superior portion of the external auditory canal.

10. **What is significant about finding cholesteatoma around the oval and round windows or eroding into the lateral semicircular canal?**
Cholesteatoma around the round window poses an increased risk of sensorineural hearing loss (SNHL) and suppurative labyrinthitis. In addition to the increased risk of suppurative labyrinthitis and SNHL, erosion into the lateral semicircular canal or disease around the oval window can rarely result in a perilymphatic fistula.

11. **What are the risks you would discuss with the patient or the family in obtaining surgical consent for cholesteatoma surgery?**
See Table 41-2.

12. **Are audiograms useful in the treatment and management of cholesteatoma?**
Preoperative audiograms are indicated to assess baseline hearing, and for long-term follow-up after surgical removal. There are also medical-legal implications in the event of an operative complication.

Surgical Management

13. **What are the standard surgical approaches?**
There are various surgical approaches, including tympanotomy for disease contained in the mesotympanum, atticotomy, cortical mastoidectomy, canal wall up or down mastoidectomy, and modified-radical and radical mastoidectomy. Regardless of the type of surgery performed, the goal

Table 41-2. Risks of Surgery During Cholesteatoma Removal

Incomplete removal of disease	Need for second-stage surgery
Hearing loss, including deafness	Facial nerve injury
Vertigo	CSF leak
Encephalocele	Change/alteration in taste
Bleeding	Infection

is for complete removal of disease, preservation of hearing, prevention of residual or recurrent disease, and improvement of ear hygiene. The specific surgical approach is mainly determined by extent of disease as well as surgeon comfort level. Facial nerve monitoring should also be considered, especially during revision surgery or cases with extensive disease. Facial nerve monitoring has been shown to improve identification of dehiscences, and although small, decreases rates of nerve injury, particularly in cases involving a facial recess approach.

Atticotomy is mainly used when disease is limited lateral to the malleus and incus as well as in the "attic." Cortical mastoidectomy with or without facial recess is used with cholesteatoma extending medially to the ossicles and into the mastoid through the antrum.

The decision of canal wall up or down procedure is largely based on the ability to perform complete removal of cholesteatoma. Canal wall down procedures have been shown to provide improved postoperative physical exam, and superior intraoperative visualization of disease, specifically in difficult to view areas of the middle ear. Canal wall up procedures, alternatively, allow for preserved anatomy, and an improved ability for reconstruction resulting in a more physiologic middle ear with decreased aural care, improved ability to use hearing aids, and no water restrictions.

14. **Why are surgeons reluctant to perform a canal wall down mastoidectomy, especially in young children?**
Although canal wall down mastoidectomy procedures provide superior visualization during and after cholesteatoma removal, they often result in difficulty reconstructing the middle ear and subsequent problems with the mastoid cavity. These include the need for life-long canal cleaning with increased risk of persistent otorrhea. It may also result in long-term water restrictions, vertigo induced by temperature changes with air or water exposure, and impaired use of hearing aids.

15. **Why is a second-stage procedure required?**
Planned second-stage procedures are performed due to increased rates of recurrence, especially in the pediatric population, and for evaluation of residual disease. Recurrent cholesteatomas are thought to be due to underlying chronic disease, such as eustachian tube dysfunction, creating a new retraction pocket for cholesteatoma formation. Residual disease is common with extensive cholesteatomas where disease was left inadvertently or intentionally due to involvement of critical structures.

Although common, the timing and decision to perform a second-stage procedure is not well established, and mainly depends on surgeon experience. It should also be noted that certain factors such as location of disease correlate with a higher risk of recurrence. Once the middle ear is deemed safe and free of cholesteatoma, an ossiculoplasty may be performed during a second look surgery.

16. **What is the timing for the second-stage procedure?**
The timing of a second-stage procedure is debated, but is typically performed 9 to 12 months after the original procedure in adults and 6 to 9 months after the original procedure in children.

17. **Describe other techniques used in cholesteatoma surgery.**
The use of otoendoscopy has increased in recent years to allow better visualization of areas known to have a high incidence of residual disease. Endoscopy allows structures out of the linear view of a microscope to be viewed, and may offer a less invasive approach in second-stage procedures.

Mastoid cavity obliteration is sometimes considered to prevent future retraction pocket formation and recurrent cholesteatoma. This procedure involves a canal wall down mastoidectomy followed by a posterior wall reconstruction. The middle ear and mastoid are separated from one another, and the mastoid is filled with an inert material. This technique allows the superior visualization and removal of cholesteatoma associated with a canal wall down technique, but decreased complications such as the need for frequent cleaning, difficulty with hearing aids, and water restriction.

18. **What's new in cholesteatoma follow-up?**
Although second-stage procedures are commonly used for evaluation for recurrent and residual cholesteatoma, new imaging sequences may be acceptable alternatives and prevent needless surgery. MRI has the advantage over CT in differentiating soft tissues and fluid in the middle ear and mastoid. Specifically, non–echo-planar-based diffusion-weighted MRI has been shown to have a high reliability in detecting cholesteatoma recurrence.

Bibliography

Adams M, El-Kashlan H: Tympanoplasty and ossiculoplasty. In Flint P, et al, editors: *Cummings Otolaryngology Head and Neck Surgery*, ed 5, Philadelphia, 2010, Mosby Elsevier, pp 1999–2008.

Badr-el-Dine M: Value of ear endoscopy in cholesteatoma surgery, *Otol Neurotol* 23(5):631–635, 2002.

Chole R, Nason R: Chronic otitis media and cholesteatoma. In Snow J, Wackym P, editors: *Ballenger's Otorhinolaryngology Head and Neck Surgery*, ed 17, Ontario, 2009, BC Decker, pp 218–227.

Chole R, Sudhoff H: Chronic otitis media, mastoiditis, and petrositis. In Flint P, et al, editors: *Cummings Otolaryngology Head and Neck Surgery*, ed 5, Philadelphia, 2010, Mosby Elsevier, pp 1963–1978.

Hulka G, McElveen JT: A randomized, blinded study of canal wall up versus canal wall down mastoidectomy determining the differences in viewing middle ear anatomy and pathology, *Am J Otol* 19:574–578, 1998.

Li P, Linos E, Gurgel R, et al: Evaluating the utility of non-echo-planar diffusion-weighted imaging in the pre-operative evaluation of cholesteatoma: a meta-analysis, *Laryngoscope* 123(5):1247–1250, 2013.

Mutlu C, Khashaba A, Saleh E, et al: Surgical treatment of cholesteatoma in children, *Otolaryngol Head Neck Surg* 113(1):56–60, 1995.

Noss R, Lalwani A, Yingling C: Facial nerve monitoring in middle ear and mastoid surgery, *Laryngoscope* 111:831–836, 2001.

Schraff S, Strasnick B: Pediatric cholesteatoma: a retrospective review, *Int J Pediatr Otorhinolaryngol* 70(3):385–393, 2006.

Vercruysse J, De Foer B, Somers T, et al: Mastoid and epitympanic bony obliteration in pediatric cholesteatoma, *Otol Neurotol* 29:953–960, 2008.

CHAPTER 42

FACIAL NERVE

Scott Mann, MD and Stephen P. Cass, MD

KEY POINTS

1. The facial nerve is complex and more than a just a motor nerve. In addition to motor fibers, the facial nerve carries visceral motor, general sensory, and special sensory fibers to the following structures:
   - Parasympathetic input to the lacrimal, submandibular, and sublingual glands
   - Taste from the tongue (special sensory)
   - Sensation from auricular skin (general sensory)
   - Sympathetic input to the middle meningeal artery
2. The facial nerve is anatomically divided into three segments:
   - Intracranial (pontine, cerebellar-pontine angle, and internal auditory canal); 23 to 24 mm in length
   - Intratemporal (the fallopian canal); 20 to 30 mm in length
   - Extratemporal (from the stylomastoid foramen to the muscles of facial expression, posterior belly of digastric, stylohyoid and postauricular muscles); 15 to 20 mm
3. The extratemporal facial nerve trunk can be found as it exits the temporal bone via the stylomastoid foramen in several ways:
   - Finding the tragal pointer
   - Following the digastric muscle
   - Finding the tympanomastoid fissure
   - Following a peripheral branch proximally
   - Drilling out the mastoid
4. While Bell's palsy is the most common cause of facial nerve paralysis, not all facial palsies are Bell's palsy. For facial nerve paralysis, think neoplasm rather than Bell's palsy if any of the following are present:
   - Slow, progressive onset
   - Other cranial nerve involvement
   - Palpable mass in the parotid gland or a mass visible in the middle ear
   - Adult with unilateral middle ear effusion
5. Treatment of Bell's palsy includes:
   - Oral steroids within 72 hours of symptom onset.
   - Oral antivirals should not be used alone for Bell's palsy (no proven benefit) but are an option in combination with oral steroids.
   - Imaging is not required if a patient has a history and physical exam consistent with Bell's palsy.
   - Education on eye care and the importance of physician follow-up until recovery occurs.

Pearls

1. A common mnemonic for the five major motor branches to the facial muscles is: **T**o **Z**anzibar **B**y **M**otor **C**ar (Figure 42-1).
2. Passive upper eyelid closure can occur by relaxation of the levator palpebrae muscle (innervated by the oculomotor nerve), so upper eyelid motion is not always indicative of an intact facial nerve.
3. The labyrinthine segment of the facial nerve is the narrowest portion of the fallopian canal, making it the area most susceptible to entrapment neuropathy during nerve swelling.
4. The geniculate ganglion lies at the junction of the labyrinthine and tympanic segments of the facial nerve. The geniculate ganglion contains special sensory ganglion cells serving taste. The first branch of the facial nerve (greater superificial petrosal nerve containing parasympathetic fibers to the lacrimal gland) exits the anterior margin of the geniculate ganglion.
5. The marginal mandibular and temporal branches of the facial nerve are the branches most at risk during parotidectomy, rhytidectomy, and repair of mandibular fracture.

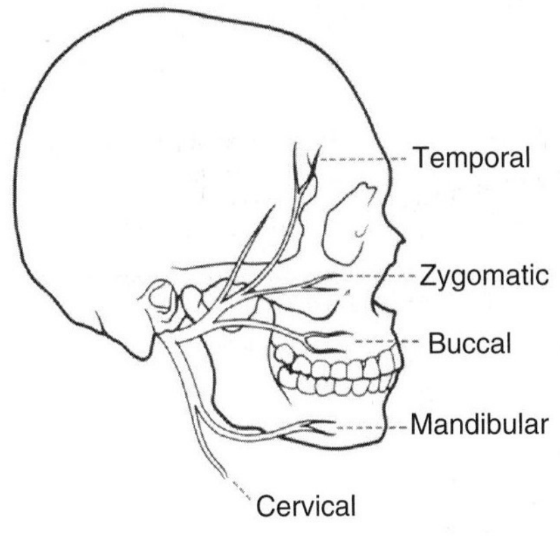

Figure 42-1. The five major motor branches to the facial muscles. *(From May M, Schaitkin B: The Facial Nerve, May's 2 ed, New York, 2000, Thieme.)*

Examination Pearls

1. Since the facial nerve is the nerve of the second branchial arch, it innervates all muscles derived from it. It is this association that makes remembering the muscles easier.
2. Any adult who has a unilateral otitis media with effusion associated with a facial paralysis needs to be evaluated for more than just Bell's palsy. Think about occult neoplasm.
3. The facial nerve is capable of regeneration. The extent of recovery is most dependent on the degree of initial injury (neuropraxia versus neurotmesis) with the single most important clinical factor being whether the nerve slowly lost function over days or lost it immediately at the time of the trauma.

QUESTIONS

1. **What types of nerve fibers are carried by the facial nerve?**
   The facial nerve carries both motor and sensory nerve fibers (Figure 42-2). These include:
   - Special visceral efferent: Motor innervation of the muscles of facial expression, stylohyoid, stapedius, platysma, and posterior belly of the digastric muscle
   - General visceral efferent: Parasympathetic innervation of the lacrimal, submandibular, sublingual, minor salivary, mucosal glands of the nose, and palate
   - Special sensory afferent: Taste from the anterior two thirds of the tongue, palate, and tonsillar fossa
   - Somatic sensory afferent: Sensation from the external ear canal and skin of the concha portion of the auricle
   - General visceral afferent sensory: Sensation from the nasal mucosa, palate, and pharynx

2. **What branchial arch is associated with the facial nerve during development?**
   Second branchial arch. All muscles innervated by the facial nerve are second arch derivatives, as well as the stapes suprastructure, styloid process, stylohyoid ligament, and the lesser cornu of the hyoid.

3. **Name the three anatomic segments of the fallopian canal, their course, and their length (Figure 42-3).**
   - Labyrinthine segment: From fundus of IAC (meatal foramen) to the geniculate ganglion; 3 to 5 mm. The labyrinthine segment represents the narrowest portion of the fallopian canal at 1 mm.
   - Tympanic segment: From geniculate ganglion to pyramidal process; 8 to 11 mm. Begins at the second genu (the first genu is intrapontine). The bony covering of the facial nerve is often dehiscent in this segment. This is the most common site of iatrogenic injury during ear surgery
   - Mastoid segment: From pyramidal process to stylomastoid foramen; 10 to 14 mm

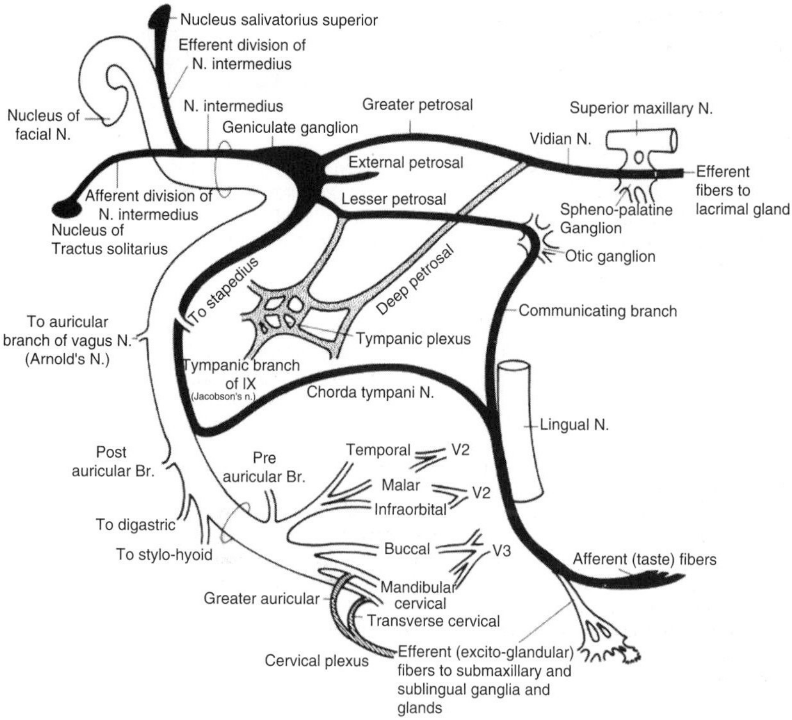

Nucleus salivatorius superior
Efferent division of N. intermedius
N. intermedius
Greater petrosal
Superior maxillary N.
Nucleus of facial N.
Geniculate ganglion
Vidian N.
External petrosal
Efferent fibers to lacrimal gland
Afferent division of N. intermedius
Nucleus of Tractus solitarius
Lesser petrosal
Spheno-palatine Ganglion
Otic ganglion
To stapedius
Deep petrosal
Communicating branch
To auricular branch of vagus N. (Arnold's N.)
Tympanic plexus
Tympanic branch of IX
(Jacobson's n.)
Chorda tympani N.
Lingual N.
Post auricular Br.
Pre auricular Br.
Temporal
V2
Malar
V2
Infraorbital
To digastric
To stylo-hyoid
Buccal
V3
Afferent (taste) fibers
Greater auricular
Mandibular cervical
Transverse cervical
Cervical plexus
Efferent (excito-glandular) fibers to submaxillary and sublingual ganglia and glands

Figure 42-2. Diagram of the facial nerve. *(From May M, Schaitkin B: The Facial Nerve, May's 2 ed, New York, 2000, Thieme.)*

CPA (15.8 mm)
IAC (8–10 mm)
LAB (3–5 mm)
Tymp. (11 mm)
Mast. (13 mm)
SMF

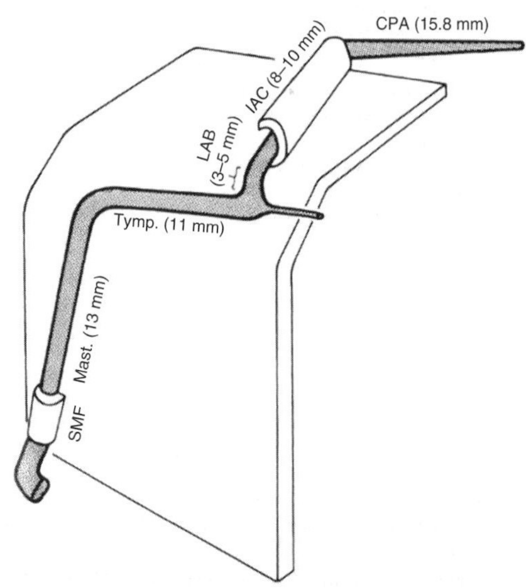

Figure 42-3. Anatomic segments of the fallopian canal. *(From May M, Schaitkin B: The Facial Nerve, May's 2 ed, New York, 2000, Thieme.)*

4. **What is the nervus intermedius?**
The nervus intermedius is a division of the facial nerve that carries its nonbranchial motor components. It is anatomically adjacent to but separate from the main trunk of the facial nerve as it exits the brainstem and then fuses with the facial nerve within the internal auditory canal. The chorda tympani is the terminal extension of the nervus intermedius.

5. **What is the chorda tympani?**
The chorda tympani carries parasympathetic innervation to both the submandibular and sublingual glands and special sensory afferents from the anterior two thirds of the tongue. It branches off from the mastoid segment of the facial nerve and traverses the middle ear before exiting the tympanic cavity through the petrotympanic fissure to join the lingual branch of the trigeminal nerve. Stretching or cutting of this nerve during middle ear surgery produces transient taste alteration.

6. **What is the pes anserinis?**
The pes anserinus ("goose's foot") is the first major branching of the extratemporal facial nerve after it leaves the stylomastoid foramen. This branching usually splits the nerve into upper and lower divisions. More distally the branching is variable but normally forms five major branches (see Figure 42-1):
   - **T**emporal: frontalis, corrugator supercilii, procerus, and upper orbicularis oculi
   - **Z**ygomatic: lower orbicularis oculi
   - **B**uccal: zygomaticus major and minor, levator anguli oris, buccinator, and upper orbicularis oris
   - **M**arginal mandibular: lower orbicularis oris, depressor anguli oris, depressor labii inferioris, and mentalis
   - **C**ervical: platysma

7. **During parotid surgery, what are the landmarks for identifying the facial nerve?**
There are a number of methods to find the main trunk:
   - Identify the tragal pointer, which is a triangular extension of the tragal cartilage. The main trunk of CN VII typically lies 10 mm inferior and 10 mm deep to this landmark.
   - Follow the posterior belly of the digastric muscle to the styloid process. The stylomastoid foramen lies deep to this structure and is where the nerve exits the temporal bone. Typically it is 25 mm deep to the skin's surface. NOTE: In children under the age of 2 the mastoid is not well developed, and the facial nerve lies much closer to the surface of the skin than would otherwise be expected.
   - Find the tympanomastoid fissure. The nerve can be found 6 to 8 mm inferior to the end of the fissure.
   - Identify a peripheral branch (e.g., marginal mandibular) and follow it proximally.
   - Perform a mastoidectomy to find the mastoid portion of the nerve and follow it out of the stylomastoid foramen.

8. **What are the three types of nerve injury?**
   - **Neuropraxia** results when a lesion stops the axoplasm flow within an axon, blocking electrical conduction. Examples would include traumatic swelling or pharmacologic blockade. The nerve is viable and returns to normal function when the blockade is corrected. Electrophysiologic testing reveals normal function, except that the electromyogram fails to show voluntary motor action potentials because they are not conducted across the blockade.
   - **Axonotmesis** is a state of Wallerian degeneration distal to the lesion with preservation of the motor axon endoneural sheaths. Examples would include mild crush or stretch injuries. Electrically, the nerve shows rapid and complete degeneration, with loss of voluntary motor units. Regeneration to the motor end plates will occur, as long as the endoneural tubules are intact.
   - **Neurotmesis** is characterized by both Wallerian degeneration and loss of endoneural tubules. Electrophysiologic studies yield evidence of complete nerve degeneration. Regeneration is dependent on many factors, including the integrity of the endoneurium, perineurium, and epineurium and the extent of ischemia and scarring around the lesion.

9. **What is synkinesis?**
If a facial nerve lesion results in Wallerian degeneration, subsequent axon regeneration may result in "cross-wiring" in which voluntary movement of one facial muscle group induces involuntary movement of another. For example, after recovering from a facial palsy a patient may have squinting whenever he or she smiles. Although this is usually thought to occur from aberrant routing of

Table 42-1. House-Brackmann Facial Nerve Grading System

GRADE	GROSS CHARACTERISTICS	MOTION CHARACTERISTICS
I. Normal	Normal facial appearance in all areas	Normal facial function in all areas
II. Mild Dysfunction	Slight weakness noticeable only on close inspection. Normal symmetry and tone at rest	Forehead: moderate to good function Eye: complete closure with minimal effort Mouth: slight asymmetry
III. Moderate Dysfunction	Obvious but not disfiguring asymmetry. Normal symmetry and tone at rest	Forehead: slight to moderate movement Eye: complete closure with effort Mouth: slightly weak with maximum effort
IV. Moderately Severe	Obvious weakness with possible dysfunction	Forehead: none Eye: incomplete closure Mouth: asymmetric with maximum effort
V. Severe Dysfunction	Only minimally perceptible motion. Asymmetry at rest	Forehead: none Eye: incomplete closure Mouth: slight movement
VI. Total Paralysis	No movement and obvious asymmetry at rest	No movement at any level

regenerating axons, it is also proposed to be the result of ephaptic transmission (abnormal connections between axons) and postsynaptic hyperexcitability.

10. **What is the House-Brackmann Facial Nerve Grading System?**
This grading system is used to classify the degree of function of the facial nerve following its recovery after injury (Table 42-1).

11. **What is Bell's palsy?**
Bell's palsy is the most commonly diagnosed cause of facial paralysis. The etiology is thought to be a viral neuropathy caused by the herpes simplex virus. Most importantly, it is a diagnosis of exclusion with the following minimum diagnostic criteria:
    - Paralysis or paresis of all facial muscle groups on one side of the face
    - Sudden onset
    - Absence of signs of central nervous system (CNS) disease, ear disease, or a parotid mass

    It often follows a viral prodrome with a typical 3- to 5-day duration and a peak in symptoms at 48 hours. The patient may have a widened palpebral fissure, diminished taste, difficulty chewing, hyperesthesia in one or more branches of the fifth cranial nerve, facial pain, and hyperacusis. In 14% of patients with Bell's palsy, family history will be positive. Some 12% of patients may have recurrent facial paralysis, either ipsilateral or contralateral.

    HSV has been shown to be present within the geniculate ganglion of affected individuals, in contrast to the normal population in which this is rare. It has been proposed that reactivation of this virus in the geniculate ganglion causes swelling and subsequent paralysis. Bell's palsy accounts for roughly 70% of acute facial palsies. However, it is important to remember that this is a diagnosis of exclusion.

12. **List the common etiology categories of facial paralysis.**
    - Congenital: Möbius syndrome, congenital unilateral lower lip paralysis, Melkersson-Rosenthal syndrome, dystrophic myotonia
    - Traumatic: Temporal bone fractures, intrauterine compression, birth trauma/forceps delivery, facial contusions or lacerations, penetrating wounds to face or ear, iatrogenic injury (parotid/ear/cranial surgery, embolization for epistaxis, mandibular block anesthesia)

- Infection: Bell's palsy, herpes zoster oticus, otitis media with effusion, acute mastoiditis, malignant otitis externa, tuberculosis, Lyme disease, acquired immunodeficiency syndrome, mononucleosis, influenza, encephalitis, malaria, syphilis, botulism
- Idiopathic: Recurrent facial palsy
- Neoplasia: Cholesteatoma, carcinoma, acoustic neuroma, meningioma, facial neuroma, glomus jugulare or tympanicum, leukemia, hemangioblastoma, osteopetrosis, histiocytosis, rhabdomyosarcoma
- Metabolic/systemic: Diabetes, hyperthyroidism, pregnancy, autoimmune disorders, sarcoidosis, hypertension
- Neurologic: Guillain-Barré syndrome, multiple sclerosis, Millard-Gubler syndrome

13. **What elements of the history and physical examination are important in evaluating a facial paralysis?**
With a good history, the wide differential diagnosis listed above can be narrowed significantly. Identifying factors for systemic and/or infectious causes is mandatory. Any palsy with slow progression or without improvement after 3 months should be considered a neoplasm until proven otherwise. Additional signs of possible tumor involvement include facial twitching, other cranial nerve involvement, hearing loss, recurrent episodes of facial paralysis, a mass behind the tympanic membrane or in the parotid gland, unilateral eustachian tube dysfunction, skin lesions suggesting skin cancer, and/or prolonged ear pain.
Bell's palsy and herpes zoster oticus may also have associated numbness in the middle and lower face, otalgia, hyperacusis, decreased tearing, or altered taste sensation.

14. **How can you distinguish whether the lesion causing facial paralysis is peripheral or central?**
A unilateral central lesion (supranuclear) will spare the upper face, since these muscles receive both crossed and uncrossed fibers. Lesions of the peripheral system involve both the upper and the lower face. A central lesion is also suggested by the lack of emotional facial movement as well as decreased lacrimation, taste, and salivation on the ipsilateral side. Cortical lesions are also frequently associated with tongue or hand dysfunction.

15. **Which radiologic studies should be part of the diagnostic workup for a patient with a facial paralysis?**
Routine radiologic tests are not indicated for the assessment of every patient presenting with a facial nerve paralysis. The need for such studies is based on both the clinical history and the course of the paralysis (i.e., if a neoplasm is suspected). If radiologic imaging is deemed necessary, high-resolution computed tomography (CT) or magnetic resonance imaging (MRI) are the studies of choice. MRI scans are superior to CT in imaging the nerve at the cerebellopontine angle and internal auditory canal. Gadolinium-enhanced MRI is the test of choice for facial nerve paralysis secondary to inflammatory, neoplastic, and other nontraumatic etiologies. CT, on the other hand, is preferred for the evaluation of traumatic seventh nerve paralysis and other etiologies involving the temporal bone such as cholesteatoma.

16. **What is Schirmer's test?**
Schirmer's test is a method to assess parasympathetic innervation to the lacrimal gland via the greater superficial petrosal nerve. The procedure entails placing small filter paper strips in the conjunctival fornix of each eye and measuring lacrimation by comparing the length of paper moistened by tear flow over a 5-minute period. An abnormal Schirmer's test occurs with <15 mm lacrimation or a 25% reduction as compared to the contralateral eye.

17. **Describe the electrophysiologic tests that are important in evaluating a patient with a facial paralysis?**
    - **Nerve Excitability Test (NET):** In this study, a 1/sec^2 wave pulse, which is 1 msec in duration, is applied over both the affected and the unaffected facial nerves. Thresholds for minimal facial muscle response are recorded and compared. A 3- to 4-mA or greater difference is considered significant, suggesting denervation. This test is not accurate during the first 72 hours after onset of paralysis, since it takes 3 days for Wallerian degeneration to occur.
    - **Maximal Stimulation Test (MST):** A variation of the NET, the MST stimulates the ipsilateral and contralateral facial muscles at a level sufficient to depolarize all motor axons underlying the stimulator. Therefore, it utilizes maximal as opposed to minimal stimulation to evaluate muscular

response. The results of the test are recorded as a subjective account of the difference in facial muscle movement between the normal and involved sides. Generally, it is thought that the MST becomes abnormal before the NET and is therefore a better prognostic indicator. However, the MST is limited by its lack of objectivity.

- **Electroneuronography (ENoG):** ENoG measures and compares the amplitudes of the muscle summation potentials that are elicited when a supramaximal level of current is applied over the main trunk of the facial nerve on the affected and unaffected sides. The peak-to-peak amplitude is directly proportional to the number of intact motor axons, thus providing a gauge to assess neuronal degeneration. For example, an evoked summation potential of 5% to 10% indicates 90% degeneration. This test is commonly used to predict who may benefit from a surgical facial nerve decompression. Just like the MST, it is only accurate after Wallerian degeneration has occurred so it must be performed more than 72 hours after onset of symptoms. To accurately predict which patients may benefit from surgical decompression, ENoG must be performed within 2 weeks of the onset of symptoms.
- **Electromyography (EMG):** EMG is complementary in the evaluation of acute facial paralysis, helping to eliminate false positive results obtained by NET, MST, and ENoG. The EMG determines the activity of the muscle rather than the activity of the nerve. This test can (1) provide information regarding intact motor units in the acute phase and (2) confirm the integrity of intact axons in the recovery phase, detecting reinnervation potentials 6 to 12 weeks before the return of facial muscle function is clinically evident. However, unlike NET, MST, and ENoG, an EMG cannot assess the degree of degeneration or prognosis for recovery.
- **Audiometry:** Audiometry should be performed to evaluate for conductive and sensorineural hearing losses. Conductive hearing losses are most consistent with middle ear tumors, cholesteatomas, and other middle ear processes involving the tympanic segment of the facial nerve. Sensorineural hearing losses may indicate neoplastic conditions such as acoustic neuroma, meningioma, and facial nerve neuromas, which affect the nerve in the cerebellopontine angle or internal auditory canal.

18. What is the most important complication following the onset of facial paralysis?

Exposure keratitis in the eye of the affected side can lead to vision loss. It is caused by (1) paralysis with inability to close the eyelid completely, (2) diminished tearing, and (3) loss of corneal sensitivity if there is coexistent trigeminal nerve dysfunction. Evidence for corneal irritation includes redness, itching, foreign-body sensation, and visual blurring. Avoidance of this complication involves using artificial tears 4 to 5 times/day. While sleeping, ophthalmic lubricant should be instilled along with taping the eyelid shut. The eye should be protected from wind, foreign bodies, and drying with glasses and/or moisture chambers. Surgical placement of a gold weight within the eyelid can facilitate full closure in complete paralysis. An ophthalmology consult should be obtained for these patients.

19. What are crocodile tears?

Injuries to the facial nerve may be associated with aberrant nerve regeneration. Fibers that normally innervate the salivary glands may regenerate to innervate the lacrimal gland. This leads to "crying" when the patient eats (gustatory tearing). Similarly, these fibers can regenerate to innervate sweat glands in the skin, leading to gustatory sweating (Frey's syndrome).

20. How do you treat facial nerve paralysis medically?

- If infectious processes are involved, appropriate treatment with antimicrobial and/or antiviral agents, in addition to eradication of the infectious nidus (i.e., mastoidectomy/ myringotomy) should be instituted.
- A course of oral steroids, if initiated within the first 72 hours after onset of symptoms, may improve recovery via decreased inflammation.
- Electrophysiologic assessment of the extent of nerve damage provides valuable information, particularly in cases in which surgical decompression may be a treatment option.
- Prophylactic eye care to protect against exposure keratitis should be initiated in all patients with a facial nerve paralysis.
- For Bell's palsy, specifically, the current recommendation for treatment is (1) oral steroids to begin within 72 hours of onset of symptoms, (2) optional oral acyclovir in addition to steroids if started within 72 hours of onset of symptoms, and (3) eye care.

Table 42-2. Surgical Strategies as Determined by Etiology

CLINICAL SCENARIO	SURGICAL INTERVENTION
Facial paralysis due to trauma	Nerve decompression, anastomosis
Paralysis secondary to acute OM	Myringotomy
Nerve paralysis due to chronic OM	Decompression, mastoidectomy
Iatrogenic injury to facial nerve	Decompression, anastomosis
Complete idiopathic paralysis	Decompression

21. **When is surgical treatment indicated?**
Surgical intervention may take multiple forms depending on the etiology of the facial nerve lesion. Bony decompression of the facial nerve may improve recovery in certain cases where total paralysis is present with evidence of rapid severe nerve degeneration. Serial studies with ENoG have shown that when the number of motor fibers falls to less than 10% of normal (tested prior to day 14 post-onset), the recovery rate of normal function is substantially decreased. It is therefore at this level that surgical exploration/decompression is most likely to be considered. In Bell's palsy, swelling in the labyrinthine segment causes an entrapment neuropathy, which is decompressed via a middle fossa craniotomy.

Table 42-2 is a list of possible surgical strategies by etiology.

22. **If the nerve is cut during surgery, can it be fixed?**
Yes. Several techniques may be employed for repairing a transected or partially transected nerve. A common clinical rule of thumb is that if greater than 50% of the nerve is transected, it should be repaired.

Direct anastomosis involves repair of the perineurium with exact end-to-end approximation. An 8-0 monofilament suture is used to approximate the nerve ends together without tension at the anastomosis. Grafting can also be utilized if there is loss of a segment of the nerve; great auricular or sural nerves can be used for interposition grafts. Jump grafts from other cranial nerves (such as CN XII) have also been used successfully to reanimate the facial muscles in cases in which the proximal facial nerve is not present. Cross nerve grafts connected to the contralateral facial nerve can also be used.

23. **What is the association between facial nerve paralysis and otitis media? Mastoiditis? Cholesteatoma?**
In otitis media (OM), facial palsy can present as a complication of acute suppurative OM, OM with effusion, and chronic OM. The palsy results from an inflammatory reaction or bacterial toxins within the bony fallopian canal. In both mastoiditis and cholesteatoma, compression of the nerve and inflammatory response can result in facial nerve palsy.

The mainstay of treatment, particularly if the palsy is a complication of OM, is to eradicate the infection with a combination of aggressive antibiotic therapy and surgical drainage via myringotomy or tympanomastoid surgery. Facial palsy secondary to coalescent mastoiditis can be managed surgically with myringotomy followed by a mastoidectomy. The presence of cholesteatoma requires surgical management.

24. **Describe the most common traumatic injuries to the facial nerve.**
Traumatic injuries to the facial nerve generally fall within two categories, penetrating wounds and temporal bone fractures.

Penetrating wounds of the cheek, face, or parotid gland may lacerate the facial nerve trunk or one of its branches. Nerve injuries such as these can often be repaired with direct anastomosis. Generally, the results of facial nerve repairs are good; however, repairs of the main trunk usually result in synkinesis during the regenerative process.

Temporal bone fractures involve the facial nerve via laceration or contusion injury within the bony fallopian canal. Eighty to ninety percent of temporal bone fractures are longitudinal (parallel to the petrous bone) and will have an associated facial nerve injury only 20% of the time. In contrast, transverse temporal bone fractures (perpendicular to the petrous bone) account for only 15% of cases but have an associated facial nerve injury about 50% of the time. A facial paralysis that occurs immediately following nonpenetrating head trauma is suggestive of laceration or impingement of the nerve within the bony fallopian canal. In these instances, surgical exploration with decompression or repair may be required. If, however, the paralysis develops in a delayed fashion, medical management with steroids and electrophysiologic monitoring to map the course of recovery are indicated.

25. **What are the most common facial nerve tumors?**
The two most common facial nerve tumors are facial schwannomas (facial neuromas) and geniculate ganglion hemangiomas. Facial schwannomas arise from the myelin-producing Schwann cells. Hemangiomas of the geniculate ganglion arise from the vascular plexus surrounding the ganglion. These tumors are often observed initially but many will require treatment due to growth and/or progressive facial nerve paralysis.

26. **What are herpes zoster oticus and Ramsay Hunt syndrome?**
Herpes zoster oticus is characterized by intense ear pain and vesicles on the external auditory canal and concha. It is caused by reactivation of the dormant herpes zoster (chickenpox) virus within the afferent sensory neurons of the facial nerve. If this progresses to involve the efferent motor axons of the facial nerve, a facial palsy can result. When both a facial palsy and painful vesicles are present, it is referred to as Ramsay Hunt syndrome. Hearing loss and vertigo may also occur. Treatment includes narcotic analgesics for pain relief, oral corticosteroids to decrease inflammation, and acyclovir to inhibit viral DNA replication. Topical antibiotic drops may also be used if there is concern for secondary bacterial otitis externa. Additionally, the facial paresis may affect eyelid closure and place the orbit at risk for dryness and excoriation and possible permanent damage.

Bibliography

Baugh RF, et al: Clinical practice guideline: Bell's palsy, *Otolaryngol Head Neck Surg* 149(3 Suppl):S1–S27, 2013.

Carrasco VN, Zdanski CJ, Logan TC, et al: Facial nerve paralysis. In Lee KJ, et al, editors: *Essential Otolaryngology Head and Neck Surgery*, ed 8, Stamford, CT, 2003, Appleton & Lange, pp 169–191.

Chang CY, Cass SP: Management of facial nerve injury due to temporal bone trauma, *Am J Otol* 20:96–114, 1999.

De Diego JI, Prim MP, De Sarria MJ, et al: Idiopathic facial paralysis: a randomized, prospective, and controlled study using single-dose prednisone versus acyclovir three times daily, *Laryngoscope* 108(4 Pt I):573–575, 1998.

Dulguerov P, Marchal F, Wang D, et al: Review of objective topographic facial nerve evaluation methods, *Am J Otol* 20:672–678, 1999.

Gidley PW, Gantz BJ, Rubinstein JT: Facial nerve grafts: from cerebellopontine angle and beyond, *Am J Otol* 20:781–788, 1999.

Jackson CG, von Doersten PG: The facial nerve. Current trends in diagnosis, treatment, and rehabilitation, *Med Clin North Am* 83:179–195, x, 1999.

Marenda SA, Olsson JE: The evaluation of facial paralysis, *Otolaryngol Clin North Am* 30:669–682, 1997.

Ramsey MJ, DerSimonian R, Holtel MR, et al: Corticosteroid treatment for idiopathic facial nerve paralysis: a meta-analysis, *Laryngoscope* 110(3 Pt 1):335–341, 2000.

Ruckenstein MJ: Evaluating facial paralysis. Expensive diagnostic tests are often unnecessary, *Postgrad Med* 103:187–188, 191–192, 1998.

CHAPTER 43

SURGERY FOR VERTIGO

Scott Mann, MD and Stephen P. Cass, MD

KEY POINTS

1. Most forms of vertigo are not managed surgically. Most patients with vertigo can attain significant improvement with conservative nonsurgical measures.
2. Ménière's disease is a clinical diagnosis based on these features:
   - Definitive vertigo lasting 20 minutes or longer
   - More than one episode of vertigo
   - Hearing loss
   - Tinnitus or aural fullness
3. Surgical treatment options for medical failure in Ménière's disease include:
   - Intratympanic steroid perfusion
   - Endolymphatic sac surgery
   - Intratympanic gentamicin ablation
   - Surgical labyrinthectomy
   - Vestibular nerve section
4. There is no surgical procedure that improves hearing in Ménière's disease.
5. BPPV arises from free-floating posterior canal endolymph particles.
   - Most cases can be treated by particle repositioning (Epley maneuver).
   - Recurrent BPPV is common
   - For intractable or recurrent typical BPPV, posterior semicircular canal occlusion is a safe and effective procedure.

Pearls

1. Vestibular compensation is a central nervous system process that is critical for improvement of the vestibulo-ocular reflex and gait stability after loss of peripheral vestibular (labyrinthine) function. Vestibular specific physical therapy can help expedite this process.
2. BPPV commonly follows an episode of vestibular neuritis. In this situation vestibular physical therapy (in addition to canalith repositioning) is often helpful to promote full recovery.
3. Superior semicircular canal dehiscence can mimic other otologic diseases because it can present with conductive hearing loss similar to otosclerosis, ear fullness, and autophony similar to a patulous eustachian tube, and vertigo similar to Ménière's disease.
4. The key finding that distinguishes conductive hearing loss due to SSCD from that caused caused by otosclerosis is an intact ipsilateral stapedial reflex.

QUESTIONS

1. **What is the general role of surgery in the treatment of vertigo?**
   Most forms of vertigo are not managed surgically. Management of patients with vertigo and balance disorders demands diagnostic acumen, clinical judgment, and both medical and surgical skills. The most important step in treating vertigo is correctly diagnosing the cause. Only then can appropriate treatment recommendations be made. Though surgery is an option for some causes of vertigo, often it is not the first treatment offered. Many patients with a condition amenable to surgical treatment can attain significant improvement with conservative measures alone. However, when patients are carefully selected surgical intervention can be highly successful.

2. **What are the most common vertigo conditions with surgical options?**
   - Meniere's disease
   - BPPV
   - Superior semicircular canal dehiscence

3. **What are some alternatives to surgery in patients with vertigo?**
   As stated, the most important step in treating vertigo is identifying the correct cause. The appropriate nonsurgical treatment is dictated by an accurate diagnosis. Some common forms of conservative management include:
   - Vestibular rehabilitation therapy
   - Pharmacologic therapy (diuretics, migraine medications, vestibular suppressants)
   - Dietary changes
   - Canalith repositioning maneuvers

4. **Which patients should be considered for surgical intervention?**
   As a general rule, surgery should only be considered for the treatment of vertigo if a patient meets the following three criteria:
   - Vertigo caused by unilateral peripheral vestibular dysfunction, with absolute certainty of which side is affected
   - Vertigo must be disabling.
   - No signs or symptoms of central vestibular system dysfunction that could impair postoperative vestibular compensation

5. **How does American Academy of Otolaryngology-Head and Neck Surgery (AAO-HNS) advise reporting of vertigo control in Ménière's Disease?**
   18 to 24 months following treatment, divide the number of episodes per 6 months by the number of episodes in the 6 months prior to treatment.
   - Grade A: Complete control (0%)
   - Grade B: Substantial control (1% to 40%)
   - Grade C: Partial control (41% to 80%)
   - Grade D: No Control (81% to 120%)
   - Grade E: Worse (>120%)
   - Grade F: Secondary treatment required due to disabling vertigo

6. **What are the surgical options for the treatment of Ménière's disease?**
   Procedures to control vertigo in Ménière's disease can be divided into ablative and nonablative procedures. Ablative procedures include gentamicin middle ear injections, labyrinthectomy, and vestibular nerve section. The most common nonablative procedures are endolymphatic shunt surgery and intratympanic steroid perfusion. The ablative procedures have greater vertigo control rates than the nonablative procedures but require vestibular compensation to limit post-treatment disequilibrium

7. **What are the possible types of endolymphatic shunt surgery?**
   - Shunting: Placement of synthetic shunt to drain endolymph
   - Drainage: Incision of the sac to allow endolymph drainage
   - Decompression: To improve sac function of endolymph absorption

8. **Describe the Sham Surgery Trial by Thomsen et al, 1981.**
   - Double-blinded placebo-control study
   - Compared cortical mastoidectomy without decompression versus endolymphatic shunt
   - Conclusion: "We are therefore of the opinion that the impact of surgery on the symptoms of Ménière's disease is completely nonspecific and unrelated to the actual shunt procedure."

9. **What is a vestibular nerve section?**
   A vestibular nerve section is a procedure in which the vestibular division of the eighth cranial nerve is selectively divided to remove vestibular function from the affected side (Figure 43-1). The approaches that can be used to perform vestibular nerve section include:
   - Middle fossa
   - Retrolabyrinthine
   - Retrosigmoid
   - Translabyrinthine (See Chapter 44)

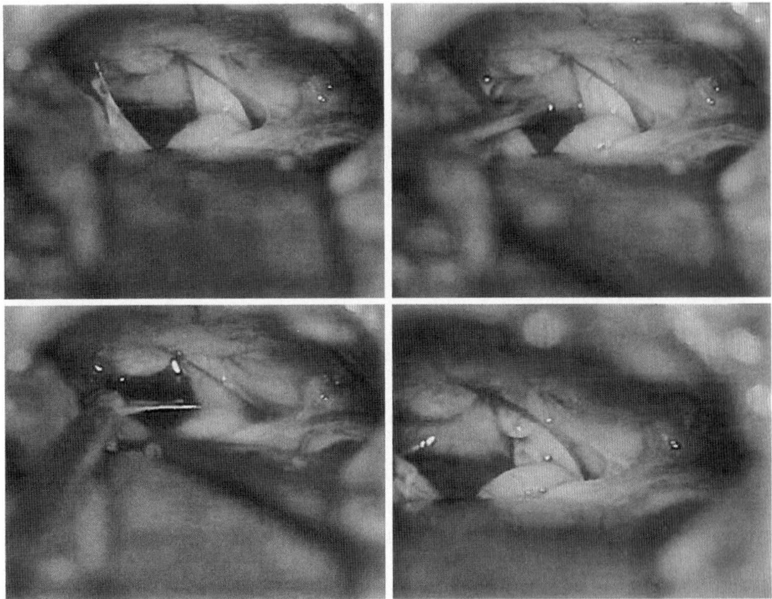

Figure 43-1. Vestibular nerve sectioning (retrosigmoid approach).

10. What are the potential complications of vestibular nerve section?
    - Facial paralysis
    - Hearing loss
    - CSF leak
    - Persistent disequilibrium

11. What is the most reliable treatment for vertigo due to Ménière's disease?
    Labyrinthectomy is the most reliable surgical treatment, but hearing is sacrificed. In this procedure, all of the vestibular neuroepithelium can be removed. This effectively ends all aberrant information produced by the diseased ear, but hearing function cannot be preserved.

12. What is benign paroxysmal positional vertigo (BPPV) and when is the treatment surgical?
    BPPV is a condition in which free-floating otolith particles within semicircular canals activate the canal ampulla and cause vertigo during head movements. These particles can often be repositioned with maneuvers such as the Epley maneuver. Recurrence is common but maneuvers can be repeated as often as needed. However, if the symptoms are intractable or recurrences are frequent, surgery can be considered. The surgical options available include:
    - Posterior semicircular canal occlusion: This procedure plugs the posterior semicircular canal, preventing free-floating particles from activating the canal ampulla (Figure 43-2).
    - Vestibular neurectomy: This procedure eliminates all vestibular function from the affected ear and is rarely used for BPPV.
    - Singular neurectomy: This procedure removes the innervation to the posterior canal ampulla. It was the first surgical procedure for BPPV but is technically difficult and carries a significant risk of hearing loss.

13. What is Tullio's phenomenon?
    - Sound-induced dizziness, vertigo, or nystagmus
    - First described by Tullio in 1928. He demonstrated that fenestration of the bony labyrinth renders it sound sensitive.
    - Can also happen in syphilis or Lyme disease

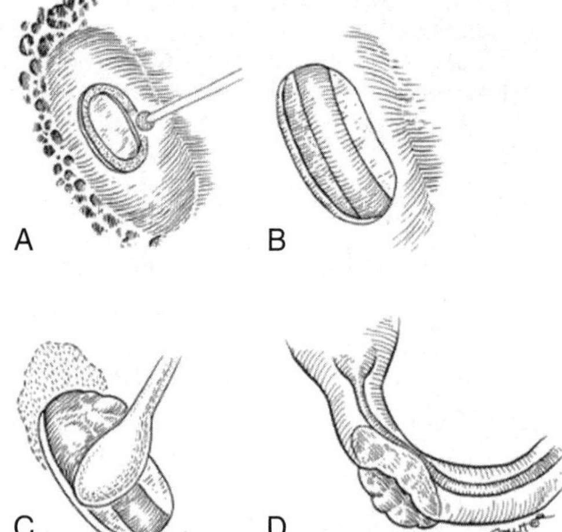

Figure 43-2. A–D, Technique for plugging semicircular canal. *(From Myers E: Operative Otolaryngology Head and Neck Surgery, Vol II. Philadelphia, 1997, Saunders, Figure 117-44.)*

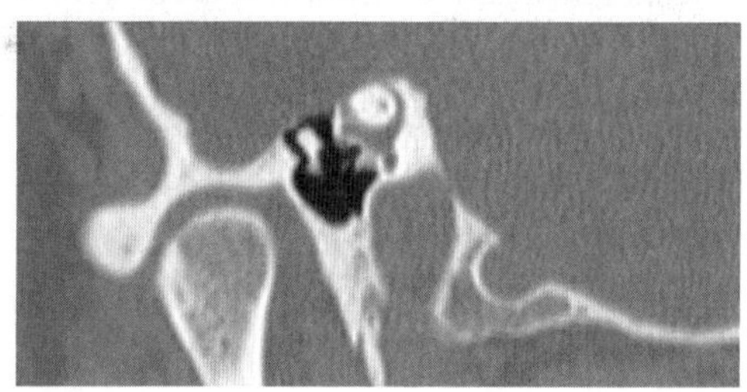

Figure 43-3. CT scan showing superior semicircular canal dehiscence (oblique sagittal view).

14. What is semicircular canal dehiscence?
    Semicircular canal dehiscence is a thinning or complete absence of the temporal bone overlying the superior semicircular canal (Figure 43-3).

15. What are the characteristic clinical symptoms of superior semicircular canal dehiscence (SSCD)?
    - Sound, pressure, or vibration induced vertigo
    - Hearing loss: usually a low-frequency conductive loss with better than 0-dB bone conduction threshold
    - Autophony (voice seems unusually loud) and a "blocked ear" feeling

16. What testing is used to confirm a diagnosis of superior semicircular canal dehiscence?
    - Vestibular evoked myogenic potentials (VEMP) demonstrate abnormally low thresholds.
    - High-resolution CT scan of the temporal bone reveals dehiscence of the bony covering that separates the superior canal from the dura mater (see Figure 43-2).

17. What causes SSCD?
    The cause is not clearly understood and may be multifactorial. In the developmental hypothesis the cause is thought to be due to incomplete ossification of the semicircular canals. SSCD is also noted when chronic increased intracranial pressure is present and can be found in association with temporal-mastoid encephalocele.

18. What are the treatment options for SSCD?
    - Educate the patient on the condition.
    - PE tubes can be helpful to reduce pressure-induced vertigo.
    - Ear plugs can be helpful to reduce exposure to loud sounds.
    - Surgery to plug or resurface the affected semicircular canal when the patient fails other measures or has intractable symptoms.

19. What surgical techniques are used in SSCD?
    - Middle fossa craniotomy to expose the superior semicircular canal is the gold standard approach. The dehiscence is then resurfaced.
    - Transmastoid approaches can also be used to plug the semicircular canal or cap the dehiscence with cartilage.

Bibliography

Agarwal SK, Parnes LS: Transmastoid superior semicircular canal occlusion, *Otol Neurotol* 29:363–367, 2008.

Bhattacharyya N, Baugh R, Orvidas L, et al: Clinical practice guideline: benign paroxysmal vertigo, *Otolaryngol Head Neck Surg* 139:S47–S81, 2008.

Cass SP: Surgery for vertigo. In Myers E, editor: *Operative Otolaryngology Head and Neck Surgery* (vol II), Philadelphia, PA, 1997, Elsevier, pp 1396–1432.

Kemink JL, Telian SA, Graham MD, et al: Transmastoid labyrinthectomy: reliable surgical management of vertigo, *Otolaryngol Head Neck Surg* 101:5–10, 1989.

Minor LB, et al: Superior canal dehiscence syndrome, *Am J Otol* 21:9–19, 2000.

Parnes LS, McClure JA: Posterior semicircular canal occlusion for patients with intractable benign paroxysmal positional vertigo, *Ann Otol Rhinol Laryngol* 99:330, 1990.

Thomsen J, et al: Placebo effect in surgery for Meniere's disease, *Arch Oto* 107:271–277, 1981.

Zhou G, Gopen Q, Poe DS: Clinical and diagnostic characterization of canal dehiscence syndrome: a great otologic mimicker, *Otol Neurotol* 28:920–926, 2007.

NEUROTOLOGY

J. Eric Lupo, MD, MS and John C. Goddard, MD

CHAPTER 44

KEY POINTS

1. Unilateral sensorineural hearing loss, tinnitus, and disequilibrium are the hallmark presenting symptoms of a cerebellopontine angle (CPA) mass.
2. Magnetic resonance imaging (MRI) of the internal auditory canals (IACs) with gadolinium is the gold standard for diagnosis of acoustic neuroma (AN) and other lesions of the CPA.
3. Several surgical approaches are available for excision of a CPA lesion. The particular approach chosen should be influenced by the location and size of the lesion, age of the patient, and the presence of serviceable hearing.
4. Observation, surgery, and radiotherapy are acceptable treatment modalities for AN and paragangliomas.
5. The best treatment for AN or paragangliomas should be individualized after discussion of treatment options and consideration of overall health status, age, and tumor characteristics.

Pearls

1. Understanding the anatomy of the cerebellopontine angle (CPA) is key to diagnosis and management of pathology occurring in this location. Know the classic CT and MR characteristics of tumors in this area.
2. Know the staging system and surgical options for temporal bone SCC.
3. The Hitzelberger sign is numbness of the medial, posterior, or superior external auditory canal caused by an acoustic neuroma compressing CN VII.

QUESTIONS

1. **Describe the anatomy of the cerebellopontine angle (CPA).**
The CPA is a complex three-dimensional CSF-filled space in the posterior fossa of the cranial cavity (Figure 44-1). The clivus and petrous portion of the temporal bone delineate the anterolateral boundary. The posterior boundary includes the ventral surface of the brainstem and cerebellum. Medially lies the pons and medulla of the brainstem. The superior boundary includes the cerebellum and middle cerebellar peduncle. The inferior limit is the cerebellar tonsil. The CPA is the region through which cranial nerves VII and VIII travel laterally and superiorly from the brainstem to the internal auditory canal (IAC). The trigeminal nerve is located superiorly in the CPA and travels anteriorly from the pons to Meckle's cave. Cranial nerves IX, X, and XI are located inferiorly.

2. **If you are positioned at the CPA looking laterally into the IAC, what is the relationship between the facial, cochlear and vestibular nerves?**
The facial nerve lies anterior and superior, with the cochlear division of the eighth cranial nerve lying anterior and inferior. The superior vestibular nerve lies posterior and superior, while the inferior vestibular nerve occupies the posterior and inferior position. Bill's bar is a vertical crest of bone separating the facial nerve and superior vestibular nerve at the lateral end of the IAC. The transverse crest separates the superior and inferior portions of the lateral IAC. The spatial relationships of the facial-vestibulocochlear nerve complex change during their transit through the IAC, as the facial nerve originates anterior to the vestibulocochlear nerve complex at the brainstem and occupies an anterosuperior position in the fundus of the IAC.

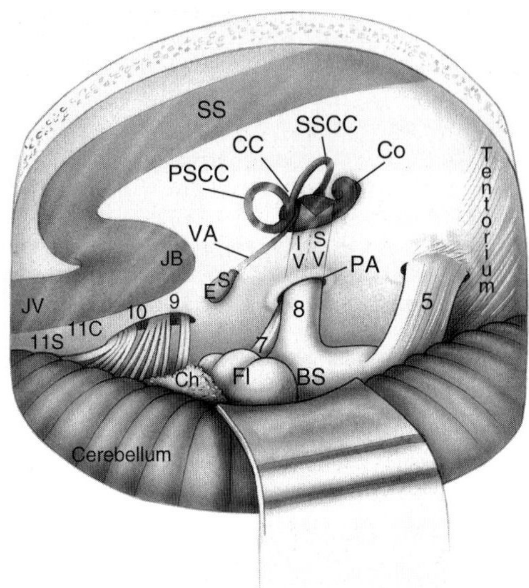

Figure 44-1. Retrosigmoid craniotomy (left side) illustrating the surgical anatomy of the posterior fossa exposure. The venous sinuses and inner ear structures have been made visible to help clarify their relationships to intracranial structures. BS, brainstem; CC, common crus; Ch, choroid plexus; Co, cochlea; ES, endolymphatic sac; Fl, flocculus; IV, inferior vestibular nerve; JB, jugular bulb; JV, jugular vein; PA, porus acusticus; PSCC, posterior semicircular canal; SS, sigmoid sinus; SSCC, superior semicircular canal; SV, superior vestibular nerve; VA, vestibular aqueduct. Cranial nerves: 5, trigeminal; 7, facial; 8, cochleovestibular; 9, glossopharyngeal; 10, vagus; 11C, accessory (cranial portion); 11S, accessory (spinal portion). *(From Jackler RK, Brackmann DE (eds.): Surgical Neurotology: An Overview. Neurotology, 2 ed. Philadelphia: Elsevier Mosby, 2005, p. 686.)*

3. **What are the vascular relationships within the CPA?**
   There are three major arterial branches of the vertebrobasilar system that traverse the CPA. From inferior to superior arise the posterior inferior cerebellar artery (PICA), the anterior inferior cerebellar artery (AICA), and the superior cerebellar artery (SCA). Disruption of the PICA leads to the lateral medullary syndrome (Wallenberg's syndrome) consisting of dysphagia, dysarthria, vocal cord paralysis, vertigo, facial paralysis, ataxia, ipsilateral Horner's syndrome, and hemisensory disturbance. The AICA follows a tortuous path with a loop lying laterally in the CPA in close association with the facial and cochleovestibular nerve roots. Disruption of the AICA leads to symptoms based on location of injury with hemiplegia and cranial nerve dysfunction from medial injury and ataxia from more lateral injury. The *internal auditory artery*, the blood supply to the labyrinth, is a branch of the AICA. The superior cerebellar artery is located superiorly within the CPA.

4. **What is the differential diagnosis for a CPA mass?**
   - Vestibular schwannoma/Acoustic neuroma (60% to 90%)
   - Meningioma (3% to 7%)
   - Epidermoid (2% to 4%)
   - Other cranial nerve schwannomas (V, VII, IX, X, XI) (1% to 4%)
   - Arachnoid cysts (1% to 2%)
   - Rare: Metastasis, hemangioma, lipoma, chordoma, chondrosarcoma, dermoid, neuroepithelial tumors, endolymphatic sac tumors, ependymoma, glioma, astrocytoma, medulloblastoma, choroid plexus papilloma, aneurysm, arteriovenous malformation

5. **What is an acoustic neuroma (AN)?**
   Also known as a vestibular schwannoma, an AN is a benign tumor arising from the Schwann cells of the eighth cranial nerve. These tumors tend to arise lateral to the obersteiner-redlich zone (transition

zone of central/peripheral myelin) and may affect either the superior or inferior vestibular nerve (inferior > superior). With continued tumor growth, the tumor extends medially to the CPA and may lead to marked brainstem compression. The incidence of sporadic AN is 10 per 1,000,000.

6. **Are ANs associated with inherited syndromes?**
ANs are associated with the autosomal dominant syndromes of neurofibromatosis (NF) types 1 and 2. NF1 (von Recklinghausen's disease) is associated with intracranial and extracranial neuromas; however, fewer than 5% of patients develop AN. In contrast, NF2 is associated with bilateral AN in over 90% of patients. The presence of bilateral ANs is diagnostic of NF2. NF1 is related to a gene defect on chromosome 17, whereas NF2 may be caused by various types of NF2 gene mutations at locus 22q12.2.

7. **What is the natural history of AN?**
Acoustic neuromas typically grow at a rate of 1 to 2 mm/year, but occasionally the growth rate may be as rapid as 2 cm/year or greater. Conversely, the AN may not exhibit future growth after diagnosis. As the tumor grows, extension medially into the CPA is common and encroachment on the brainstem, cerebellum, and/or adjacent cranial nerves may occur. A large CPA component may also cause obstructive hydrocephalus due to fourth ventricle compression. Although usually slow-growing, if left untreated, these tumors are lethal due to brainstem compression or intracranial hypertension.

8. **What are the presenting signs and symptoms of an AN?**
Presenting signs and symptoms of AN often depend on the size of the AN, which may be small (<1.5 cm), medium (1.5 to 2.5 cm), large (2.5 to 4 cm) or giant (>4 cm). Small, intracanilicular (within the IAC) tumors present with symptoms associated with dysfunction of CN VIII such as hearing loss, tinnitus, or vertigo. As the tumor grows, hearing loss may worsen and disequilibrium may develop. With brainstem compression, facial hypesthesia ensues due to fifth cranial nerve involvement. Severe brainstem compression leads to symptoms of acute or chronic hydrocephalus such as headache, nausea/vomiting, and mental status changes. The most common symptom of AN is hearing loss (95%), while tinnitus is prominent in 56% to 63% and disequilibrium in 46% to 61%. There is substantial variability in the presenting symptoms of AN. For instance, sudden sensorineural hearing loss secondary to AN has been seen in up to 1% of patients. Facial weakness is a rare finding associated with larger tumors. *Hitzelberger's sign*, numbness on the posterior aspect of the concha caused by interruption of sensory fibers of the facial nerve by a mass such as AN, was assessed historically before the era of modern radiographic diagnosis.

9. **How is AN typically diagnosed?**
As patients typically present for evaluation of a unilateral hearing loss, audiometry is often the initial diagnostic test. Unilateral pure-tone sensorineural hearing loss with disproportionate loss of speech discrimination is suggestive of a retrocochlear lesion. Acoustic reflex testing is useful, as 88% of patients with AN have absent reflexes or abnormal reflex decay. Auditory brainstem response (ABR) testing may also be quite useful, detecting 95% of tumors. A delay in the latency of wave V of 0.2 msec or greater is considered abnormal. The false negative rate of ABR is 18% to 30%, especially for small intracanalicular lesions. In the setting of a negative ABR with strong suspicion for AN, a stacked ABR technique improves detection of small AN. Magnetic resonance imaging (MRI) with gadolinium enhancement, however, is the gold standard for diagnosing AN. ANs are isointense to brain on T1 images and mildly hyperintense on T2 with fairly avid enhancement following gadolinium contrast administration.

10. **How are ANs treated?**
There are three main treatment modalities for AN. The decision on which modality to choose depends on many different factors. Observation with repeated imaging is an option for patients with AN, particularly elderly patients with small tumors. As the tumor enlarges there may be progression of cranial nerve dysfunction with eventual brainstem compression. Morbidity from treatment increases with increasing size of AN. Given the potential of late complications caused by tumor growth, younger patients with AN require treatment. Effective modalities include surgical excision or radiotherapy. Surgery may or may not entail a hearing preservation approach; this decision is based on the amount of residual hearing present and the location and size of the tumor. Radiation therapy may be preferentially used for those who cannot tolerate a surgical procedure or who have a limited life expectancy. Stereotactic radiosurgery is the most commonly utilized form of radiotherapy, although external beam therapy is also performed.

11. **Is surgery or radiotherapy preferable for the treatment of AN?**
Treatment for a given AN depends on many factors, including the tumor size, location, age of the patient, residual hearing, vestibular symptoms, and preference of the patient. Understanding the risks and benefits of each modality is critical for patient counseling. Rates of cranial nerve palsies are low with each modality and are influenced by the extent of surgery (gross total resection vs. near-total or sub-total resection) and radiation dose (less with marginal doses of 13 Gy) along with surgeon and treatment center experience. The rate of recurrence of surgically excised AN ranges from 1% to 20% depending on extent of resection. The rates of regrowth after radiosurgery have been reported at 5% to 15%. Radiation offers the advantage of earlier return to normal activity. Variation in protocols for radiation therapy and the paucity of long-term follow-up, however, make it difficult to interpret the data for patient counseling on long-term results.

12. **What are the results of AN treated with radiotherapy?**
There are different protocols utilized to treat AN including stereotactic radiosurgery (SRS), where radiation is delivered in a single fraction, or stereotactic radiotherapy (SRT), where radiation is delivered in fractions. Two common systems for delivering radiation in treatment for AN are the Gamma Knife system, a cobalt-60 system, and the CyberKnife system, a linear-accelerator based system. Current radiation doses are on the order of 1200 to 1300 rad, which results in a decreased incidence of cranial nerve palsies compared to higher doses used previously. Reports of progression-free survival and rates of tumor control are comparable between protocols and between systems. Rates of 10-year progression-free survival for AN range from 92% to 98% with overall rates of tumor control 93% to 99%. Complications associated with radiation include trigeminal neuropathies (0% to 27% for SRS), facial nerve palsy/paresis (0% to 23%), and hearing loss which appears to worsen over long-term follow-up. Radiation-induced carcinogenesis is a rare potential late complication of radiation for acoustic neuromas.

13. **What are the primary surgical approaches for ANs? List advantages and disadvantages of each.**
See Table 44-1.

14. **What are additional lateral skull base approaches to the CPA and their primary indication?**
   - **Retrolabyrinthine:** Posterior craniotomy between the sigmoid sinus and otic capsule providing limited exposure of the posterior fossa used for vestibular neurectomy.
   - **Transcochlear:** Anterosigmoid posterior fossa craniotomy providing an enhanced view of the anterior aspect of the CPA extending the translabyrinthine craniotomy. Meningiomas medial to the IAC, chordomas, chondrosarcomas, as well as residual/recurrent AN may be approached in this manner.
   - **Infratemporal fossa:** Approach used to access tumors of the temporal bone extending inferior to the jugular foramen near the petrous internal carotid artery (ICA) or tumors of the deep lobe of the parotid gland with temporal bone involvement.

15. **What is a meningioma?**
Meningiomas are benign tumors thought to arise from arachnoidal cap cells associated with the arachnoid villi in the CPA. Meningiomas account for 20% of intracranial neoplasms and are the second most common lesion of the CPA. These lesions are generally sporadic. Like AN, they may be seen with greater incidence in NF2. Although these lesions are benign, 5% may become malignant. Presentation of a meningioma depends on location and involvement of nearby structures. Meningiomas in the CPA present similarly to ANs with hearing loss, tinnitus, and imbalance. Classic imaging characteristics include enhancement on a postcontrast MRI with a characteristic dural tail and hyperostosis observed on CT. For growing or symptomatic meningiomas, surgical resection is warranted. SRS or SRT for small lesions (<3 cm) or for postsurgical residual disease may provide tumor growth control.

16. **What postoperative complications may follow excision of a CPA tumor?**
Cerebrospinal fluid (CSF) leaks occur in approximately 10% to 15% of postoperative patients. These typically present as fluid collections beneath the postauricular skin for transmastoid approaches and supra-auricular skin for middle fossa surgery. CSF leaks may also present as clear otorrhea or rhinorrhea. Reapplication of a pressure dressing and bed rest is often sufficient for these to resolve. Lumbar drainage may be required in some while additional fat obliteration of the mastoid may be

Table 44-1. Advantages and Disadvantages of Surgical Approaches to the Cerebellopontine Angle

APPROACH	INDICATIONS	ADVANTAGES	DISADVANTAGES
Translabryinthine	• ANs larger than 2.0 cm (hearing preservation unlikely) • Small ANs without serviceable hearing • Approach for facial nerve decompression and vestibular neurectomy in the presence of poor hearing • Exposure for other CPA tumors with poor hearing	• Versatile, wide, more anterior exposure • Reduced incidence of headache • Highest rate of preserved facial nerve function depending on tumor size (98.5% anatomic, 75% HB I-IV) • Facial nerve identified laterally at fundus • May repair facial nerve during surgery • No cerebellar retraction • Low recurrence rate	• Total hearing loss • Short-term vertigo if poor preop compensation • CSF leak 4% to 14% • Requires a fat graft
Retrosigmoid	• ANs with servicable hearing and minimal involvement of the IAC (not extending to the lateral portion of the IAC) • Meningiomas with limited IAC involvement	• Versatile wide exposure • Hearing preservation possible • Facial nerve preservation possible	• Fundus not visualized • Comparatively more cerebellar retraction • Postoperative headache (up to 65%) • Limited visualization of ventral brainstem • CSF leak (risk slightly higher than translabyrinthine)
Middle Fossa	• Small intracanalicular ANs with <1.0cm CPA extension • Superiorly based meningiomas of the IAC/petrous bone	• Durable hearing preservation possible (65%) • Excellent preservation of facial nerve function (91% to 95%)	• Not recommended for patients >65y because dura is fragile and adherent • Must work around facial nerve to remove tumor • CSF leak (equivalent to translabyinthine)

necessary for resolution. *Meningitis* is an uncommon sequela but should be considered after any surgery that exposes the subarachnoid space. Typical signs and symptoms of altered mental status, headache, meningismus, and fever are noted. Aggressive culture-directed antibiotic therapy after lumbar puncture is mandatory. *Facial nerve dysfunction* may be present after AN excision. The majority of these injuries are due to manipulation of the nerve during tumor excision rather than nerve interruption. If the nerve is severed, it should be immediately repaired either with an end-to-end approximation or with a suitable transposition graft. If the nerve does not recover function, various facial reanimation procedures exist. Other less common complications include stroke, cerebral edema, air embolus, cerebellar ataxia, and death (<1%).

17. **What is the differential diagnosis of a petrous apex lesion?**
    - Inflammatory: cholesterol granuloma, cholesteatoma, mucocele
    - Infectious: petrous apicitis, osteomyelitis
    - Neoplastic: schwannoma, meningioma, paraganglioma, chordoma, sarcoma, nasopharyngeal carcinoma, metastatic lesions (renal cell, lung, breast, prostate)
    - Anatomic variants: asymmetric pneumatization (up to 35%)
    - Vascular: carotid artery aneurysm

18. **What is a cholesterol granuloma? How can it be distinguished from other petrous apex lesions, and how is it treated?**
    A cholesterol granuloma is a reactive lesion that occurs after hemorrhage into petrous apex air cells. On CT, a punched-out bony lesion is present with an isodense mass that exhibits rim enhancement with intravenous contrast. The lesion is hyperintense on both T1 and T2 weighted MRI images, whereas cholesteatomas and mucoceles are hypointense on T1 and hyperintense on T2. Symptomatic cholesterol granulomas are treated with procedures to drain the lesion to other aerated portions of the skull. Depending on anatomic location of the cholesterol granuloma, the lesion may be drained through a transsphenoidal approach if located medially within the temporal bone or through an infralabyrinthine or infracochlear approach to the petrous apex.

19. **What is jugular foramen syndrome? What lesions are typically responsible?**
    The jugular foramen syndrome, also termed Vernet's syndrome, is paresis or paralysis of the cranial nerves that exit this canal: IX, X, and XI. The hypoglossal nerve exits through the hypoglossal canal and is thus usually unaffected. The most common lesions of the jugular foramen include paragangliomas, schwannomas, meningiomas, metastatic lesions, and jugular vein thrombosis.

20. **What is a paraganglioma? How does it present?**
    A paraganglioma (a.k.a. glomus tumor) is a benign tumor that arises from the paraganglionic cell rests of the adventitia of the jugular bulb (glomus jugulare) or on the promontory of the cochlea associated with the tympanic plexus of CN IX and X (glomus tympanicum). As such, a glomus jugulare tumor typically arises near the jugular foramen and may extend into the middle ear or inferiorly into the neck. The glomus tympanicum arises within the middle ear and grows to fill the middle ear cleft. Patients with these tumors present with pulsatile tinnitus, conductive hearing loss, aural fullness, and—when extending extracranially or into the jugular foramen—cranial neuropathies. A purplish-red mass is often visible via otoscopy and application of positive pressure causes the tumor to blanch (Brown's sign); a bruit may often be auscultated.

21. **What is the blood supply of jugular paragangliomas?**
    Jugular paraganiomas are supplied by the ascending pharyngeal artery while glomus tympanicum lesions are supplied by the inferior tympanic artery, a terminal branch of the ascending pharyngeal artery.

22. **How are paragangliomas associated with the temporal bone staged?**
    The Fisch staging system is often used to classify temporal bone paragangliomas based on their extension into adjacent structures and their intracranial extension (Table 44-2).

23. **How are paragangliomas treated?**
    Paragangliomas can be excised surgically. The location and extent of the disease dictates the surgical approach necessary for removal, ranging from transtympanic approaches for small glomus tympanicum lesions to more involved infratemporal fossa approaches for type C lesions. Lesions with intracranial extension require combined transcranial and transtemporal approaches. Radiotherapy is also used to treat these lesions, either with external radiotherapy or stereotactic

Table 44-2. Fisch Staging System for Paragangliomas of the Temporal Bone

CLASSIFICATION	ANATOMIC EXTENT
A	Tumor limited to the middle ear cleft involving the promontory (glomus tympanicum)
B	Tumor limited to the tympanomastoid area but not involving the jugular bulb
C	Tumor originates in the jugular bulb and erodes the bone surrounding the jugular bulb
C1	May erode carotid foramen but does not invade carotid
C2	May involve the vertical carotid canal
C3	Tumor invasion of the horizontal portion of the carotid canal
De1/2	Intracranial extension but extradural <2 cm (De1) or >2 cm (De2)
Di1/2	Intracranial and intradural extension <2 cm (Di1) or >2 cm (Di2)
Di3	Unresectable intracranial extension

Table 44-3. University of Pittsburgh Staging System

T STAGE	ANATOMIC EXTENT	MANAGEMENT
T1	Limited to EAC with bony erosion	Lateral temporal bone resection (LTBR)
T2	Limited EAC bony erosion or limited (<0.5 cm)	LTBR
T3	Eroding bony EAC (full-thickness) with limited involvement, or involving middle ear or mastoid	LTBR or sub-total temporal bone
T4	Eroding cochlea, petrous apex, medial wall of carotid, jugular foramen	Sub-total or total temporal bone resection

radiosurgery. For jugular foramen tumors with extension to the middle ear leading to conductive hearing loss, a multimodal approach may be employed with surgical excision of the middle ear component and radiation of the skull base component.

24. **What are the neurovascular relationships at the jugular foramen?**
The jugular foramen is divided into a vascular compartment, the pars vascularis, which receives the sigmoid sinus and transitions to the jugular bulb before continuing as the internal jugular vein. The more anterior, smaller component, the pars nervosa, transmits CN IX, X, and XI and the inferior petrosal sinus. The two compartments are separated by a fibrous or bony septation. CN IX is the more anterior of the three nerves as they enter the neck (anterior to ICA). CN XI is most posterior (anterior to IJV). CN X lies medial to CN IX and XI and extends between the ICA and IJV.

25. **What is the most common malignancy of the external auditory canal (EAC)?**
Squamous cell carcinoma is the most common malignancy of the EAC, followed by basal cell carcinoma and adenoid cystic carcinoma. Squamous cell carcinoma is commonly misdiagnosed as chronic otitis externa and is frequently associated with otorrhea and pain. Conductive hearing loss may be present with early lesions, whereas sensorineural hearing loss or vertigo suggests extensive disease with labyrinthine invasion. Facial nerve paresis is an ominous sign in squamous cell carcinoma of the temporal bone.

26. **How is squamous cell carcinoma of the EAC staged and treated? What are the outcomes?**
The University of Pittsburgh staging system for EAC tumors is the most widely accepted system (Table 44-3). Two-year survival rates by stage are as follows: T1, 100%; T2, 80%; T3, 50%; and T4, 15%.

Bibliography

Hasegawa T, Kida Y, Kato T, et al: Long-term safety and efficacy of stereotactic radiosurgery for vestibular schwannomas: evaluation of 440 patients more than 10 yrs after treatment with gamma knife surgery, *J Neurosurg* 118:557–565, 2013.

Moody SA, Hirsch BE, Myers EN: Squamous cell carcinoma of the external auditory canal: an evaluation of a staging system, *Am J Otol* 21:582–588, 2000.

Muckle RP, De la Cruz A, Lo WM: Petrous apex lesion, *Am J Otol* 19:219–225, 1998.

Schwartz MS, Kari E, Strickland BM, et al: Evaluation of increased use of partial resection of large vestibular schwannomas: Facial nerve outcomes and recurrence/regrowth rates, *Otol Neurotol* 34(8):1456–1464, 2013.

Sheehan JP, Tanaka S, Link MJ, et al: Gamma Knife surgery for the management of glomus tumors: a multicenter study, *J Neurosurg* 117(2):246–254, 2012.

Wang AC, Chinn SB, Than KD, et al: Durability of hearing preservation after microsurgical treatment of vestibular schwannoma using the middle cranial fossa approach, *J Neurosurg* 119:131–138, 2013.

CHAPTER 45

TEMPORAL BONE TRAUMA

Vincent Eusterman, MD, DDS

KEY POINTS

1. The temporal bone is made up of five components (squamous, tympanic, petrous, mastoid, styloid) and fractures generally follow natural lines of weakness at the sutures, canals, and foramina.
2. Temporal bone injuries primarily affect hearing, balance, and the facial nerve and each require separate evaluation.
3. The petrous bone is extremely solid and protects the auditory and vestibular organs within the otic capsule in temporal bone trauma.
4. CT scan classification of temporal bone fractures often does not correlate with the signs and symptoms of the fracture; the physical examination still offers the most clinical relevance.
5. Persistent CSF drainage after conservative therapy requires surgical intervention to prevent meningitis.

Pearls

1. Periorbital and mastoid ecchymoses following basal skull fractures are known as "raccoon eyes" and "Battle's sign," respectively.
2. CSF leak is common in temporal bone fractures and usually stops within 7 days.
3. The most common site of injury to the facial nerve is in the perigeniculate region.
4. The most common hearing loss associated with temporal bone trauma is conductive hearing loss.

QUESTIONS

1. What are the common causes of temporal bone trauma and how frequent is this injury?

Temporal bone trauma can be classified as blunt or penetrating. Blunt trauma is most commonly the result of motor vehicle accidents (31%), followed by assaults, falls, and motorcycle accidents. Penetrating trauma is almost exclusively due to gunshot wounds. Temporal bone trauma is most common in the second through fourth decades of life and most often in males. In head trauma of sufficient magnitude to fracture the skull, 14% to 22% of these patients sustain a temporal bone fracture. When fractures occur, 90% are associated with intracranial injuries and 9% are associated with cervical spine injuries. Sixty percent are open fractures, draining bloody otorrhea or CSF fluid, and 8% to 29% occur bilaterally.

2. What important structures course through the temporal bone that may be subject to injury during temporal bone trauma?

The temporal bone is extremely complex; it houses ossicles, cochlear and vestibular organs, the vestibulocochlear nerve (IIX), the facial nerve (VII), the carotid artery, and the jugular vein. Other nerves passing near or through the temporal bone are the abducens nerve (VI), glossopharyngeal nerve (IX), vagus nerve (X), and spinal accessory nerve (XI), which can also be injured during temporal bone fractures. The multiple foramina and canals in the skull base weaken the bone and are responsible for the patterns seen in temporal bone fractures.

3. The temporal bone has several parts; what are they?

The *squamous portion* is a flat plate that is the lateral wall of the middle cranial fossa housing the middle meningeal artery; it includes the zygomatic arch and glenoid fossa. The *tympanic portion* is a horseshoe-shaped incomplete ring of bone that makes up most of the external auditory canal.

Medially it forms the tympanic sulcus which holds the tympanic membranes annular ligament. The *styloid process* projects inferiorly from the vaginal process of the temporal bone. It lies anterior to CN VII and lateral to the carotid artery. The *petrous portion* is the pyramid-shaped medial portion of the temporal bone that separates the middle and posterior cranial fossa. It is extremely solid and protects the auditory and vestibular organs within the otic capsule. The internal auditory canal is located medially on the posterior surface. The inferior surface contains the carotid canal and the jugular foramen. The posterior part of the petrous bone contains the *mastoid*, which is filled with air cells and lined with mucous membrane.

4. **What are the important elements of the initial history of a patient with temporal bone trauma in an emergency?**
   The initial history should include the mechanism of injury, time of onset of symptoms, presence or absence of hearing loss, vertigo, and facial weakness. In facial nerve trauma, the prognosis and approach to treatment depend partially on whether the onset of paralysis was immediate of delayed. Often, patients with severe head trauma that results in temporal bone fractures are unconscious. In these cases, the history must be obtained from family, paramedics, and emergency department personnel.

5. **How are temporal bone fractures classified?**
   Temporal bone fractures are classically described as either longitudinal or transverse; however, most fractures are actually in an *oblique* or *mixed pattern* (Figure 45-1). They can also be described as *otic capsule-sparing* or *disrupting* to emphasize the functional sequelae of the fracture, and other authors have described them according to the portion of the temporal bone involved (squamous, tympanic, mastoid, and petrous).

6. **Describe "longitudinal temporal bone fractures" and their significance.**
   Traditionally longitudinal fractures are most common, accounting for 80% of temporal bone fractures. They are otic capsule sparing in 95% and are caused by blunt trauma to the temporoparietal region. They extend from the squamous part of the temporal bone, down the external auditory canal (EAC), through the middle ear (disrupting the ossicular chain), parallel to the long axis of the petrous pyramid to the foramen lacerum. Up to 30% of the time they can extend to the opposite temporal bone and become bilateral. These fractures have a 20% incidence of facial nerve injury and often produce conductive hearing loss (CHL) rather than sensorineural hearing loss (SNHL). Tympanic membrane rupture and ear canal lacerations are common and can be associated with cerebrospinal fluid (CSF) otorrhea.

7. **Describe "transverse temporal bone fractures" and their significance.**
   Transverse fractures are associated with high morbidity and fortunately are less common, representing 20% of temporal bone fractures. The injury usually results from severe blunt trauma to the occiput or frontal region. The fracture often begins at the foramen magnum and crosses the long

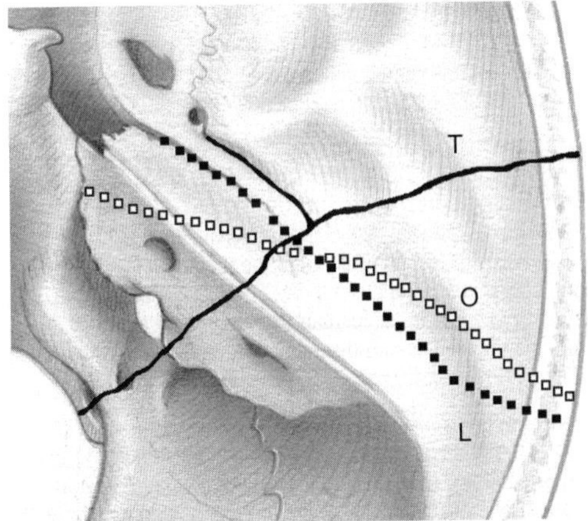

Figure 45-1. Temporal bone fractures, longitudinal (L), transverse (T), and oblique (O).

axis of the petrous pyramid at right angles and can have a higher incidence of otic capsule disruption. They have a 50% facial nerve injury rate, severe SNHL or mixed (CHL + SNHL) hearing loss, with intense vertigo. Because the tympanic membrane is usually intact, CSF leakage into the middle ear usually presents as CSF rhinorrhea via the eustachian tube.

8. **What physical findings should you look for when evaluating someone with suspected temporal bone fracture?**
   - *Facial nerve weakness* may be sudden or delayed in onset; documentation is important because sudden loss of function may require urgent intervention.
   - *Hearing loss* may be conductive, sensorineural or both; hearing can be tested in the awake patient with a 512-Hz tuning fork and deferred in the unconscious patient.
   - *Nystagmus* results from vestibular injury or perilymphatic fistula. Sudden severe vertigo with SNHL is associated with otic capsule disruption.
   - *Tympanic membrane and external auditory canal lacerations* are often seen with longitudinal fractures.
   - *Hemotympanum* is blood within the middle ear space.
   - *CSF otorrhea* occurs through a lacerated ear drum most often with longitudinal fractures.
   - *CSF rhinorrhea* occurs through the eustachian tube with an intact TM, which is commonly seen in transverse fractures.
   - *Battle's sign* is postauricular ecchymosis arising from bleeding from the mastoid emissary vein.
   - *Raccoon eyes* is periorbital ecchymosis arising from middle and anterior cranial fossa fractures from meningeal tears that cause venous sinus bleeding into the orbit.

9. **What complications are associated with temporal bone fracture?**
   - *Facial nerve injury* is common and may be temporary or permanent.
   - *CSF leak* is common and generally improves within 7 days.
   - *Hearing loss* is common and may be conductive, sensorineural or both.
   - *Vertigo* is common and may be mild to very severe and constant or positional.
   - *Vascular injuries* are uncommon except in severe blunt or penetrating trauma where angiography for carotid, vertebral, and middle meningeal artery injury may be required.
   - *Facial hypesthesia or hypoesthesia* is uncommon and due to injury to the trigeminal nerve on the surface of the petrous bone in Meckel's cave.
   - *Diplopia* is uncommon and due to abducens nerve injury as it courses through Dorello's canal.
   - *Cholesteatoma* may be a late finding from displaced canal skin or tympanic membrane skin into the middle ear or mastoid spaces.

10. **Describe the difference between penetrating and blunt temporal bone trauma.**
    Although less frequent, penetrating trauma of the temporal bone is most often from gunshot injury and more severe. It is more destructive than blunt injury with intracranial complications to the temporal lobe, cranial nerves, and the carotid artery. The facial nerve is commonly injured in its vertical or extratemporal segments. The destructive nature is associated with missile velocity. High-velocity missiles penetrate the bone and cause temporary cavity formation and secondary missile formation from dislodged bone fragments. Angiography of the carotid and vertebral arteries should be done. Injuries of these vessels are often treated at the time of angiography.

11. **What are the best imaging studies for temporal bone fracture?**
    Patients with severe head trauma often have a computed tomography (CT) scan of the head to assess for intracranial hemorrhage. Additional imaging of the temporal bone with axial and coronal thin-section high-resolution CT scanning with bone algorithms is indicated in the presence of facial paralysis, CSF leakage, EAC fracture and canal disruption, vascular injury, and conductive hearing loss. Preoperative assessment with a CT scan for patients with significant conductive hearing loss may be necessary for information to guide surgical exploration and ossicular reconstruction. Carotid angiography, MRA, or CTA may be indicated for patients with transient or persistent neurologic deficits. Conventional radiographs no longer play a role in the evaluation of patients with suspected temporal bone fracture.

12. **What physical findings on initial examination of a temporal bone fracture might require early surgical intervention by the otolaryngologist?**
    Facial nerve injury, CSF leak, hearing loss, and vertigo on initial examination may warrant early surgical intervention. The finding of most importance to the otolaryngologist is immediate onset of

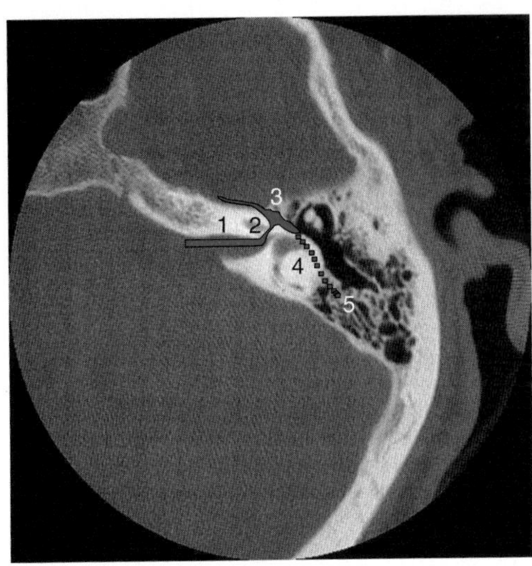

Figure 45-2. CT image of the facial nerve through the left temporal bone, segments include from proximal to distal; 1) meatal segment, 2) labyrinthine segment, 3) perigeniculate area, 4) "horizontal" or tympanic segment, and descending to the stylohyoid foramen as the 5) "vertical" or mastoid segment.

facial nerve paralysis. Patients with immediate onset of paralysis likely represent an injury that would result in a poor outcome; these patients may require facial nerve exploration, decompression, nerve repair, or nerve grafting. A fine cut (1 mm) CT scan of the temporal bone that suggests bony impingement or transection can be helpful in deciding to explore and repair the nerve.

13. **What are the most likely sites of facial nerve injury in temporal bone fractures?**
The site of facial nerve injury is in the *perigeniculate region* in most patients, possibly from tethering by the GSPN. Damage can also occur in the "horizontal" or tympanic segment and in the labyrinthine segment by direct injury or nerve edema (Figure 45-2). Chang and Cass reviewed surgical findings of four types of facial nerve pathology after temporal bone trauma. The authors' review of 67 longitudinal fractures from three studies revealed that 76% of fractures had bony impingement or intraneural hematoma, and 15% had transection. The remainder had no visible pathology except neural edema. In contrast, of 11 transverse fractures reviewed, 92% were transected, and 8% had bony impingement.

14. **How is an injured facial nerve evaluated in an obtunded or unconscious patient?**
Facial nerve evaluation begins after stabilization of serious and life-threatening injuries. Facial nerve examination by gross facial function in the unconscious patient can be elicited as a grimace in response to painful stimuli. Patients with immediate onset of paralysis can be tested with the *Hilger nerve stimulator,* using NET (minimal nerve excitability testing) and MST (maximum stimulation test) between days 3 and 7 post injury. If no loss of stimulability occurs the patient is observed. If the nerve loses stimulability within 1 week of the injury, facial nerve exploration is considered. *Electroneuronography (ENoG)* uses bipolar stimulating and recording electrodes. Evoked compound muscle action potential (CAP) is measured and the diminution in amplitude is indicative of percentage of degenerated nerve fibers. If ENoG demonstrates more than 90% degeneration of the CAP at 6 days and more than 95% in 14 days, recovery is unlikely and surgical exploration or decompression of the facial nerve may be indicated. Traditional *electromyography (EMG)* performed by monopolar intramuscular recording electrodes shows voluntary activity (innervated muscle) and fibrillation potentials (denervated muscle). EMG is most useful 2 to 3 weeks after paralysis and offers little additional information in the acute setting for a decision to operate.

15. **What are the surgical approaches to facial nerve decompression?**
Facial nerve injuries involving the otic capsule with loss of hearing are explored by a *translabyrinthine* approach. For otic capsule sparing fractures and intact hearing two approaches are used. In patients with well-aerated mastoid air cells or with ossicular discontinuity, a *transmastoid/*

supralabyrinthine approach is used. In patients with poorly aerated mastoid cells or when a severed facial nerve is encountered in the supralabyrinthine approach, a combined *transmastoid/middle cranial fossa* technique is used.

16. **What causes CSF otorrhea and rhinorrhea and what are the dangers?**
CSF leaks occur in 17% of temporal bone fractures and represent a serious risk of meningitis. Fractures in the floor of the middle cranial fossa drain into the middle ear (epitympanum and antrum) and mastoid air cells. *CSF otorrhea* results when the tympanic membrane is perforated and *CSF rhinorrhea* results when the tympanic membrane is intact and CSF exits through the eustachian tube into the nose. CSF fistulas of 7 days or less have a 5% to 10% incidence of meningitis, and those for more than 7 days have a 50% to 90% incidence of meningitis. Otic capsule fractures have a higher risk of delayed meningitis due to the inability of enchondral bone to remodel and heal.

17. **How is persistent CSF fistula treated?**
CSF fistulas generally close within 7 to 10 days with bed rest, head elevation, and avoiding activities that increase intracranial pressure. Antibiotics are not routinely prescribed in cases with CSF leakage, for fear of masking early infection and development of drug resistance. Patients should be questioned frequently about meningeal symptoms of headaches with nuchal rigidity and photophobia. A lumbar puncture should be performed if meningitis is suspected, before beginning antibiotic therapy. If spontaneous resolution does not occur, lumbar drainage is attempted for 72 hours and surgical exploration can be considered. Otic capsule disrupting fractures with profound sensorineural hearing loss are treated with mastoidectomy and middle ear obliteration. In this procedure, the middle ear contents are removed, temporalis fascia is used to cover the fracture line, the middle ear is obliterated with an abdominal fat graft, and the eustachian tube and EAC are closed. Otic capsule sparing fracture treatment depends on the location of the fracture and accessibility. Most are closed through a mastoidectomy and facial recess approach. Those associated with brain herniation or areas difficult to reach are treated by middle fossa craniotomy.

18. **What are the types of vertigo that occur following temporal bone trauma?**
There are five types of posttraumatic vertigo. The most common form of posttraumatic vertigo is *concussive injury* to the membranous labyrinth. These patients have a positional vertigo with a normal VNG, requiring only symptomatic treatment. Otic capsule disrupting temporal bone fractures produce a *severe ablative vertigo* with intensity that will decrease after 7 to 10 days and then decrease steadily over the following 1 to 2 months, leaving an unsteady feeling that lasts 3 to 6 months until compensation occurs. Intense nystagmus (third degree) is present initially, with the fast component beating away from the fracture site. This nystagmus progressively diminishes in intensity and then disappears over time. *Posttraumatic benign positional vertigo* is usually delayed on onset and is treated by the Epley maneuver. *Posttraumatic vertigo and fluctuating SNHL* may indicate a perilymphatic fistula which is initially treated with conservative measures and can require surgical closure. Last, *posttraumatic endolymphatic hydrops* may develop much later and presents as fluctuating hearing loss, tinnitus, and aural fullness with vertigo. Treatment is similar to that of Ménière's disease.

19. **What kinds of hearing loss are seen with temporal bone trauma? How are they treated?**
Conductive hearing loss (CHL) is the most common type of hearing loss associated with temporal bone trauma. It is usually temporary and caused by blood in the middle ear, edema or tympanic membrane perforation. It may be persistent if the injury results in failure of the perforation to heal or an ossicular discontinuity. The incus is most prone to fracture and joint separation due to its minimal stabilizing elements. The malleus and stapes are stabilized by multiple ligaments, tendons, and the tympanic membrane. Surgical exploration of the middle ear with CHL is usually done 3 to 6 months after injury as 75% of these patients return to normal. Those with persistent tympanic membrane perforation or ossicular discontinuity will require tympanoplasty and ossicular chain reconstruction. *Sensorineural hearing loss (SNHL)* is less common and results from an otic capsule disruption injury. It may also occur from a perilymphatic fistula, noise injury, concussion injury, or direct injury to the central auditory system. Longitudinal fractures commonly produce a CHL with high tone SNHL from inner ear concussion. Transverse fractures commonly produce a severe SNHL or mixed (SNHL and CHL) loss.

CONTROVERSIES

20. **Should a paralyzed facial nerve be explored after temporal bone fracture?**
Recommendations for surgery are based on three poor prognostic factors for spontaneous improvement: (1) immediate onset of paralysis, (2) amount of worsening on ENoG testing, and (3) evidence of nerve transection or bony impingement by CT scan.

Pros: Patients with immediate onset of complete facial paralysis following temporal bone trauma have a relatively poor prognosis. This is often due to transection of the facial nerve and the time of injury. Extensive data from nonrandomized studies in the treatment of Bell's palsy support the use of ENoG in the prognosis of an intact facial nerve that meets criteria for degeneration. Data on its use to guide treatment of traumatic facial paralysis are only emerging and confined to case series which suggest a favorable prognosis in patients with degeneration to less than 90% of normal within 6 days or less than 95% of normal within 14 days after injury (Figure 45-3).

Cons: Approximately 50% of patients with immediate-onset, complete paralysis recover normal or near-normal facial function. Surgical indications for posttraumatic intratemporal facial paralysis are poorly defined and randomized controlled studies of surgical versus nonsurgical treatments do not exist. Most recommendations for exploration of the facial nerve are based on personal opinion and data from case series to identify poor prognostic factors and the population most likely to benefit from surgery. The use of ENoG criteria for temporal bone trauma surgery is limited, as it has been more studied in Bell's palsy. More than 90% of individuals without poor prognostic factors listed above are likely to recover near-normal facial function (House-Brackmann grade 1 or 2) (Table 45-1) with conservative treatment.

21. **Should patients with CSF leak due to temporal bone fracture receive antibiotics?**
The incidence of meningitis in patients with CSF leaks ranges from 2% to 88%, with the most significant factor being the duration of leakage. The incidence of meningitis in temporal bone fractures without CSF fistula is low and antibiotic prophylaxis has no role in these cases. The use of

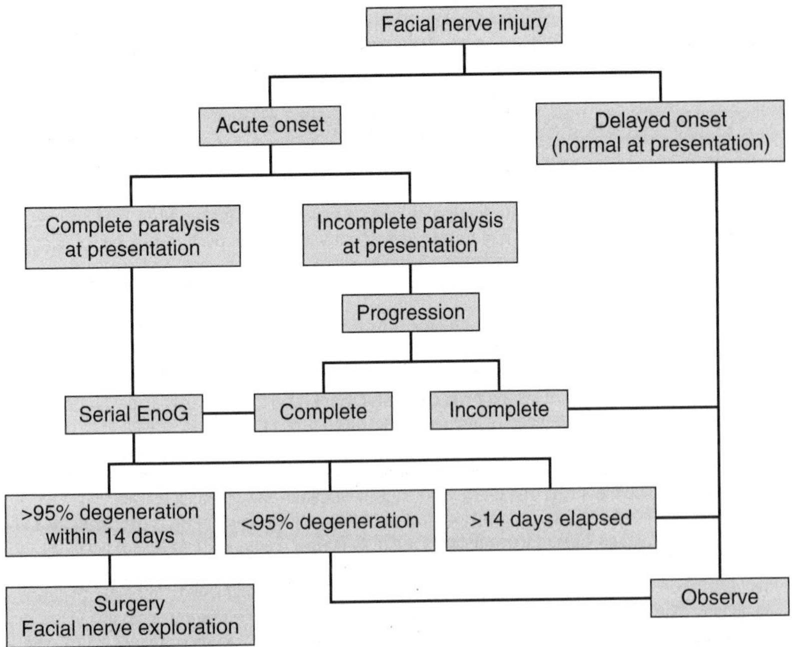

Figure 45-3. Proposed algorithm for the management of traumatic injury to the facial nerve. *(From Massa N. Intratemporal bone trauma, http://emedicine.medscape.com/article/846226-overview.)*

Table 45-1. House-Brackmann Classification of Facial Nerve Function

GRADE	DESCRIPTION	CHARACTERISTICS
I	Normal	Normal facial function in all areas
II	Slight Dysfunction	Slight weakness noticeable on close inspection; may have very slight synkinesis
III	Moderate Dysfunction	Obvious, but not disfiguring, difference between two sides; noticeable, but not severe, synkinesis, contracture, or hemifacial spasm; complete closure with effort
IV	Moderate Severe Dysfunction	Obvious weakness or disfiguring asymmetry; normal symmetry and tone; incomplete eye closure
V	Severe Dysfunction	Only barely perceptible motion; asymmetry at rest
VI	Total Paralysis	No movement

(From House JW, Brackmann DE: Facial nerve grading system. Otolaryngol Head Neck Surg 93:146–147, 1985.)

antibiotic prophylaxis in temporal bone fractures with CSF leak is controversial because its use has not been shown to be beneficial in small studies, and appears only minimally significant in meta-analysis.

Bibliography

Alvi A, Bereliani A: Acute intracranial complications of temporal bone trauma, *Otolaryngol Head Neck Surg* 119:609–613, 1998.

Brodie HA: Prophylactic antibiotics for posttraumatic cerebrospinal fluid fistulae. A meta-analysis, *Arch Otolaryngol Head Neck Surg* 123:749–752, 1997.

Brodie HA: Management of temporal bone trauma. In Flint W, Haughey BH, Lund VJ, et al, editors: *Cumming's Otolaryngology: Head and Neck Surgery*, ed 5, Philadelphia, 2010, Mosby Elsevier, pp 2036–2047.

Brodie HA, Thompson TC: Management of complications from 820 temporal bone fractures, *Am J Otol* 18:188–197, 1997.

Chang CY, Cass SP: Management of facial nerve injury due to temporal bone trauma, *Am J Otol* 20:96–114, 1999.

Dahiya R, Keller JD, Litofsky NS, et al: Temporal bone fractures: otic capsule sparing versus otic capsule violating clinical and radiographic considerations, *J Trauma* 47:1079–1083, 1999.

DiBiase P, Arriaga MA: Post-traumatic hydrops, *Otolaryngol Clin North Am* 30:1117–1122, 1997.

Fisch U: Surgery for Bell's palsy, *Arch Otolaryngol* 107:1–11, 1981.

Gantz B, Rubinstein JT, Gidley P, et al: Surgical management of Bell's palsy, *Laryngoscope* 109:1177–1188, 1999.

Ghorayeb BY, Yeakley JW: Temporal bone fractures: longitudinal or oblique? The case for oblique temporal bone fractures, *Laryngoscope* 102:129–134, 1992.

Johnson F, Semaan MT, Megerian CA: Temporal bone fracture: evaluation and management in the modern era, *Otolaryngol Clin North Am* 41:597–618, 2008.

Kang HM, Kim MG, Boo SH, et al: Comparison of the clinical relevance of traditional and new classification systems of temporal bone fracture, *Eur Arch Otorhinolaryngol* 269:1893–1899, 2012.

Leech PI, Paterson A: Conservative and operative management of cerebrospinal fluid leakage after closed head injury, *Lancet* 1:1013–1115, 1973.

MacGee EE, Cauthen JC, Brackett CE: Meningitis following acute traumatic cerebrospinal fluid fistula, *J Neurosurg* 33:312–316, 1970.

Massa N: Intratemporal bone trauma. Available at http://emedicine.medscape.com/article/846226-overview.

Morgan WE, Coker NJ, Jenkins HA: Histopathology of temporal bone fractures: implications for cochlear implantation, *Laryngoscope* 104:426–432, 1994.

Patel A, Groppo E: Management of temporal bone trauma, *Craniomaxillofac Trauma Reconstr* 3:105–113, 2010.

Rafferty MA, McConn-Walsh R, Walsh M: A comparison of temporal bone fractures classification systems, *Clin Otolaryngol* 31:287–291, 2006.

Resnick DK, Subach BR, Marion DW: The significance of carotid canal involvement in basilar cranial fracture, *Neurosurgery* 40:1177–1181, 1997.

Ulrich K: Verletzungen des Gehorlorgans bel Schadelbasisfrakturen (Ein Histologisch und Klinissche Studie), *Acta Otolaryngol Suppl* 6:1–150, 1926.

V

Pediatric Otolaryngology

PEDIATRIC ENT ANATOMY AND EMBRYOLOGY WITH RADIOLOGY CORRELATES

CHAPTER 46

Stephen S. Newton, MD and David M. Mirsky, MD

QUESTIONS

1. **What is the foramen of Huschke?**
   The foramen tympanicum, also known as the foramen of Huschke, is an anatomic variation in the tympanic portion of the temporal bone. When present, it is located at the anteroinferior aspect of the external auditory canal (EAC), posteromedial to the temporomandibular joint (TMJ). In most children, the foramen tympanicum gradually becomes smaller and completely closes before the age of 5 years, but it occasionally persists. Because no neural or vascular structures pass through this defect, it is not a true foramen. Persistence of the foramen tympanicum may also predispose the person to the spread of infection or tumor from the EAC to the infratemporal fossa, and vice versa.

2. **How does the size and shape of the external auditory canal differ between children and adults?**
   In adults, the EAC has a near sigmoid shape with the cartilaginous portion angling posteriorly and superiorly and the bony portion angling anterior inferiorly. Pulling the helix posterosuperiorly straightens the EAC and allows for better visualization of the tympanic membrane. In the infant the EAC is nearly straight. It then elongates and changes shape up till about age 9 when it is nearly adult size.

3. **What is a dimeric tympanic membrane?**
   The tympanic membrane is made up of three layers: an inner membranous layer, a middle fibrous layer that gives rigidity to the membrane, and an outer squamous layer. If a tympanic membrane perforation does not heal with the fibrous layer incorporated, then that newly healed portion has only the two layers (dimeric) and results in a thin, floppy segment. This thinned segment is more easily retracted into the middle ear and can affect conduction of sound to the ossicles.

4. **Why are the tympanic membrane and ossicles required for normal hearing?**
   Sound as it is presented to us travels through air, while our hearing organs within the inner ear are bathed in fluid. If we attempt to transmit sound from air to fluid there is a 99.9% loss in energy, which is known as an impedance mismatch. The impedance mismatch is overcome by a series of mechanical advantages including a tympanic membrane that is 21 times the size of the stapes footplate, and ossicles that create a lever force of 1.3×. Together these overcome the mismatch in impedance and allow for near full transmission of all sound energy into the inner ear.

5. **What are the innervations of the tensor tympani and stapedius muscles?**
   The tensor tympani is derived from the first pharyngeal arch and thus is innervated by a branch of the fifth cranial nerve. The stapedius muscle is derived from the second arch and thus is innervated by a branch from the seventh cranial nerve. The dampening effects of these two muscles can result in a reduced sound transmission of 15 dB.

6. **Why is the stapes shaped like a stirrup?**
   The stapedial artery is transiently present in fetal development connecting the future external carotid arterial system with the internal carotid system. This vessel goes through the middle ear and the primordial stapes creating the structure of the stapes known as the obturator foramen. A persistent stapedial artery (Figure 46-1) is very rare and may be associated with pulsatile tinnitus, conductive hearing loss, and an absent ipsilateral foramen spinosum.

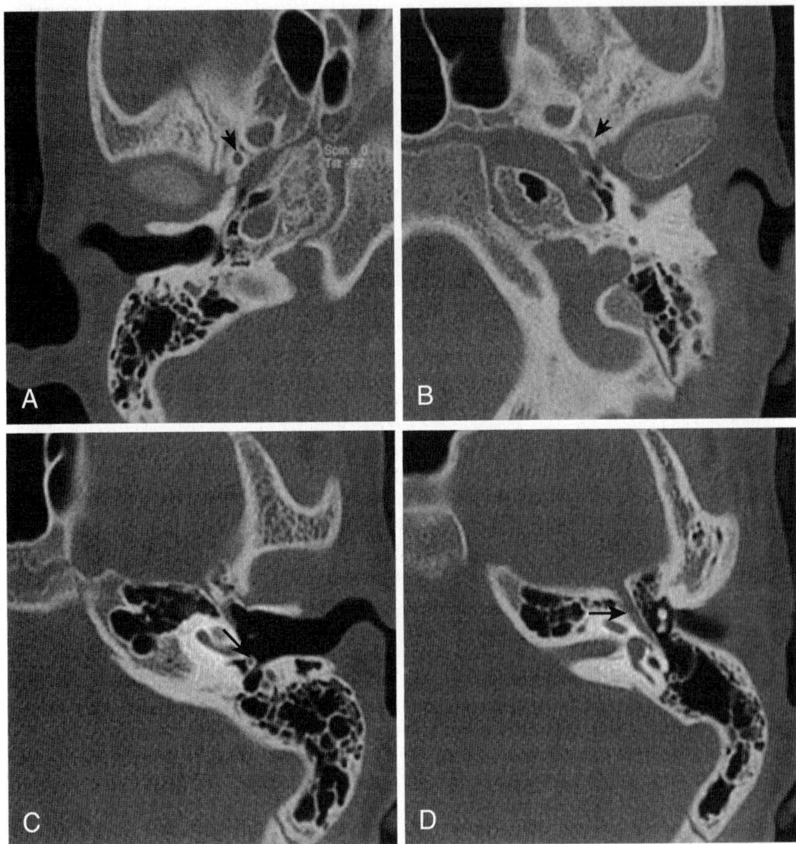

Figure 46-1. Persistent stapedial artery. Axial CT images reveal **(A)** a normal foramen spinosum on the right *(arrowhead)* and **(B)** an absent foramen spinosum on the left *(arrowhead)*. Images acquired more cephalad through the left ear illustrate the course of the persistent stapedial artery **(C)** ascending in a small canal on the surface of the posterior cochlear promontory *(arrow)*, and **(D)** resulting in an enlarged anterior tympanic segment of the facial nerve canal (arrow).

7. What are the two most common congenital abnormalities of the ossicles?
   The two most common ossicular abnormalities are a congenitally fixed stapes and incudostapedial discontinuity. Isolated abnormalities of the stapes are more likely to be unilateral while congenital abnormalities of the other ossicles are more likely to be bilateral.

8. What are the nerves that run through the middle ear?
   Jacobson's nerve is a branch of CN IX and runs across the tympanic promontory innervating the middle ear mucosa and eustachian tube and providing parasympathetic innervation to the parotid gland. Arnold's nerve is a branch of the vagus nerve that gives sensory innervation to the external auditory canal. This nerve is sometimes stimulated when cleaning the ear and can make a patient cough. The chorda tympani nerve branches from the descending portion of the facial nerve (Figure 46-2) and runs medial to the malleus before exiting the middle ear through the petrotympanic fissure. Finally, the facial nerve may be dehiscent superior to the oval window or may be positioned within the middle ear in congenitally malformed ears.

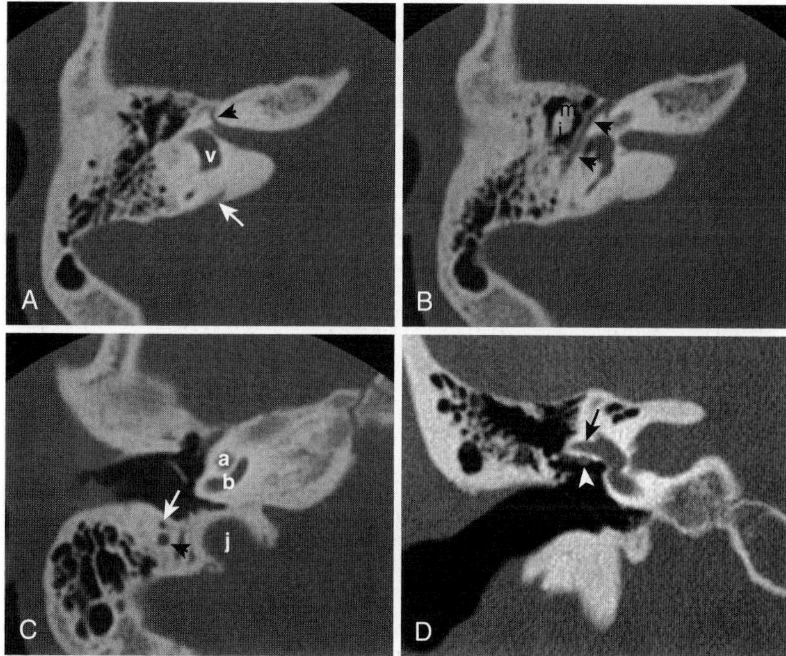

Figure 46-2. Facial nerve. Axial CT images demonstrate the course of the facial nerve *(black arrowheads)*, including **(A)** the labyrinthine segment, **(B)** the tympanic segment, and **(C)** the mastoid segment. Coronal reformat CT image **(D)** illustrates the course of the tympanic segment *(white arrowhead)* passing under the lateral semicircular canal (arrow). Relevant anatomy includes **(A)** the vestibule (v) and vestibular aqueduct *(white arrow)*, **(B)** the interrelationship between the head of the malleus (m) and body of incus (i) in the epitympanum, and **(C)** the apical and basal turns of the cochlea (a & b), the jugular bulb (j), and the chorda tympani *(white arrow)*.

9. **What are the named segments of the facial nerve that run through the temporal bone and which is the narrowest?**
The *internal auditory canal segment* of the facial nerve is 7 to 8 mm in length and runs superior to the cochlear nerve (think of the mnemonic "7up/Coke down"). The *labyrinthine segment* extends from the internal auditory canal to the geniculate ganglia; this is the narrowest segment and most prone to damage secondary to trauma and/or swelling. The *tympanic segment* runs from the geniculate ganglion to the second genu, running in the medial wall of the tympanic cavity over the round window and below the bulge of the lateral semicircular canal. The final segment is the *mastoid* or *vertical segment* (Figure 46-2).

10. **What is the cochleariform process and what is its relationship to the facial nerve?**
The cochleariform process is a curved ridge of bone that houses the tendon of the tensor tympani muscle. This ridge of bone is also a good landmark denoting the anterior position of the tympanic portion of the facial nerve.

11. **What are the boundaries of the sinus tympani?**
The borders of the sinus tympani are formed by the ponticulus superiorly and subiculum inferiorly. This space is difficult to visualize during surgery without the use of a mirror or angled endoscope. Clinically this area is important during surgery for cholesteatoma, as the cholesteatoma may have grown into the sinus and can be difficult to extract.

12. **What is the promontory of the middle ear?**
This bulge on the medial surface of the middle ear represents the prominence of the basal turn of the cochlea.

13. **What are some commonly described developmental abnormalities of the cochlea and when does developmental arrest occur?**
    - Cochleovestibular Aplasia, formerly known as a Michel deformity (arrest third week): Complete absence of cochlear and vestibular structures (Figure 46-3)
    - Cochlear Aplasia (arrest late third week): Absent cochlea; normal, dilated or hypoplastic vestibule and semicircular canals
    - Common Cavity (arrest fourth week): Cochlea and vestibule form a common space (Figure 46-4)
    - Incomplete Partition Type I (arrest fifth week): Cystically enlarged cochlea without internal architecture; dilated vestibule, mostly enlarged internal auditory canal
    - Cochlear hypoplasia (arrest sixth week): Distinctly recognizable separation of cochlear and vestibular structures; small cochlear bud
    - Incomplete Partition Type II, formerly known as a Mondini deformity (arrest seventh week): Cochlea with 1½ turns, cystically dilated middle and apical turn (cystic apex), slightly dilated vestibule (Figure 46-5)

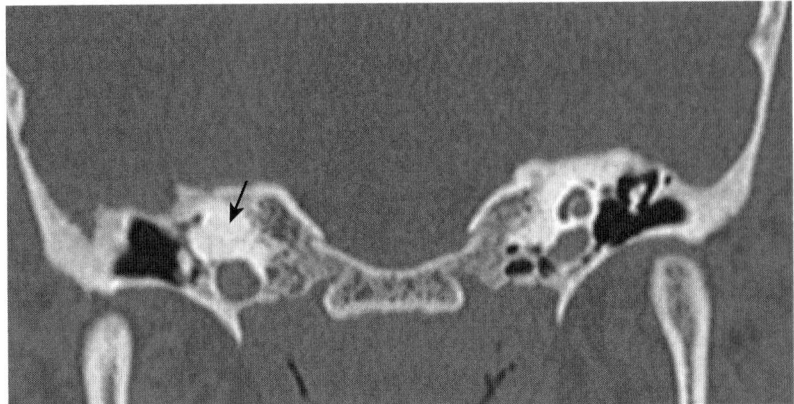

Figure 46-3. Complete labyrinthine aplasia. Coronal reformat CT image shows complete absence of all inner ear structures on the right *(arrow)* representing arrested otic placode development prior to the third week of gestation.

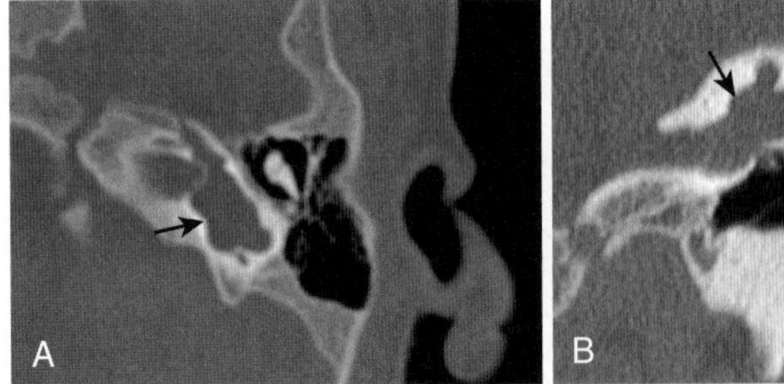

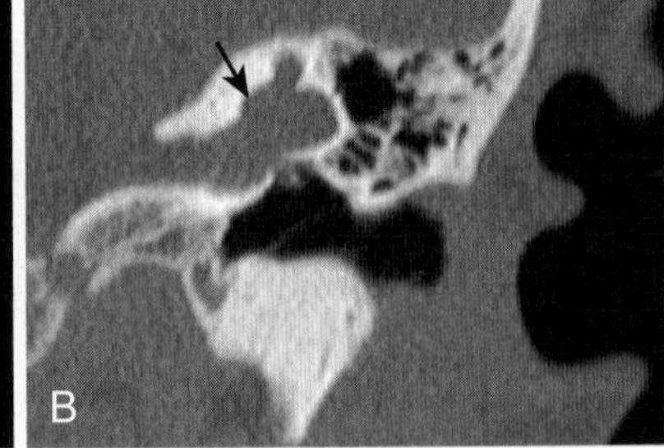

Figure 46-4. Common cavity malformation. (A) Axial and **(B)** coronal reformat CT images demonstrate a featureless common cavity representing a rudimentary cochlea, vestibule, and semicircular canals *(arrows)*. In this anomaly, otic placode development is arrested in the fourth gestational week, following differentiation into the otocyst.

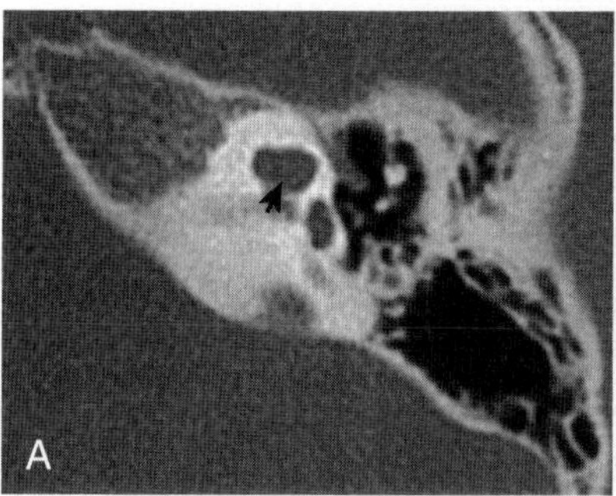

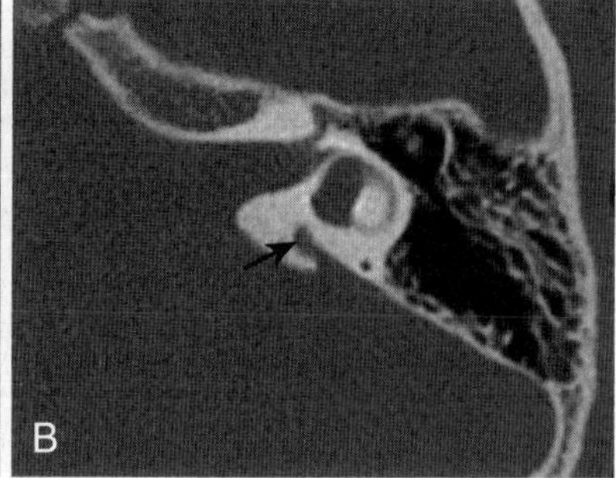

Figure 46-5. Cochlear incomplete partition type II. (A) Axial CT image reveals deficiency of the interscalar septum between the middle and apical turns (arrowhead) in this patient with a **(B)** large vestibular aqueduct *(arrow)*.

14. Of the above developmental deformities which are the most common?
Incomplete partition type II followed by a common cavity

15. What is the most common finding on a CT scan of a profoundly deaf child?
The most common finding is a radiographically normal inner ear. It is presumed that the malformation is limited to the membranous labyrinth, which cannot be seen by our imaging modalities and represents 90% of children with profound hearing loss.

16. Why are children more prone to nasoseptal hematomas?
The cartilage of children is more pliable and less likely to fracture. As the cartilage bends or buckles this can create a shearing force that results in separation between the perichondrium and the cartilage and bleeding within this space.

17. What paranasal sinuses are present at birth? Describe the development of the paranasal sinuses.
    - **Ethmoid:** The anterior and posterior ethmoid sinuses are the most developed sinuses and are present at birth.
    - **Maxillary:** The maxillary sinuses are present at birth but are only millimeters in size. The maxillary sinuses then undergo a biphasic growth pattern with rapid development in the first three years and then again between ages 7 to 12.
    - **Frontal:** The frontal sinuses are generally not present at birth and develop as extensions of ethmoid air cells anteriorly and superiorly into the frontal bone. At 2 years of age this development starts in the vertical phase of growth with near adult size achieved by the early teen years. Approximately 5% of people do not develop a unilateral frontal sinus and another 5% never develop any frontal sinuses.
    - **Sphenoid:** Pneumatization of the sphenoid bone does not start to occur until 3 to 4 years of age and reaches adult size by 12 to 15 years of age.

18. What are the developmental spaces of the nasal frontal region that are possible paths for dermoid, encephalocele, and nasal gliomas?
During development, dural projections extend through the anterior neuropore (primitive frontonasal region) and approximate with the subcutaneous region. This includes the *fonticulus frontalis* (a transient fontanelle between the inferior frontal bone and nasal bone), the *foramen cecum*, and the prenasal space. When these spaces close, failure of involution can result in nasal dermoids, encephaloceles, and nasal gliomas.

19. How does ossification and normal development of the nasofrontal region affect imaging characteristics and choice of imaging for congenital nasal frontal masses?
In the first 6 to 8 months of life the nasal frontal process, nasal bones, and ethmoid bones are unossified with CT attenuation similar to brain and nasal cartilage. With normal nasal secretions this

can give the false impression of a bony dehiscence in this region with possible connection to the frontal nasal mass. In addition, the frontal process, nasal bones, and crista galli lack fat in the first 8 months of life, resulting in similar intensity to brain on T1-weighted images. Because of this variability, MR imaging is the modality of choice for assessing the nasofrontal region in young children.

20. What muscles form the paratubal support for the eustachian tube?
The tensor veli palatini, tensor tympani, levator veli palatini, and salpingopharyngeus. The tensor veli palatini is the primary dilator of the eustachian tube, which allows for equalization for pressure between the nasopharynx and the middle ear space with contraction.

21. How does the eustachian tube vary between infants and adults?
Besides being significantly smaller, the infant eustachian tube is either in a horizontal direction or 10 degrees from horizontal while the adult eustachian tube is at a 45-degree angle. It is believed that this angle in infants affects the function of the tensor veli palatini.

22. What are the divisions of the pharynx and their boundaries?
The pharynx is divided into the nasopharynx, oropharynx, and hypopharynx.
- Nasopharynx: Superior to the soft palate, posterior to the choanae, with the skull base as the superior extent
- Oropharynx: Superior border is the soft palate, inferior boundary is the base of tongue (level of the hyoid), and the anterior borders are the palatoglossal arch and circumvallate papillae
- Hypopharynx: Level of the epiglottis down to the level of the inferior border of the cricoid cartilage

23. Why are neonates considered obligate nasal breathers?
In neonates the larynx is elevated with the epiglottis in apposition to the soft palate. This allows the infant to drink and breathe simultaneously, but this also means that infants have difficulty breathing through their mouths (Figure 46-6).

24. What is the anatomy of the tonsillar fossae?
The palatine tonsils are surrounded by the tonsillar fossa that is made up of the palatoglossus muscle (anterior tonsillar pillar) anteriorly and the palatopharyngeus muscle (posterior tonsillar pillar) posteriorly.

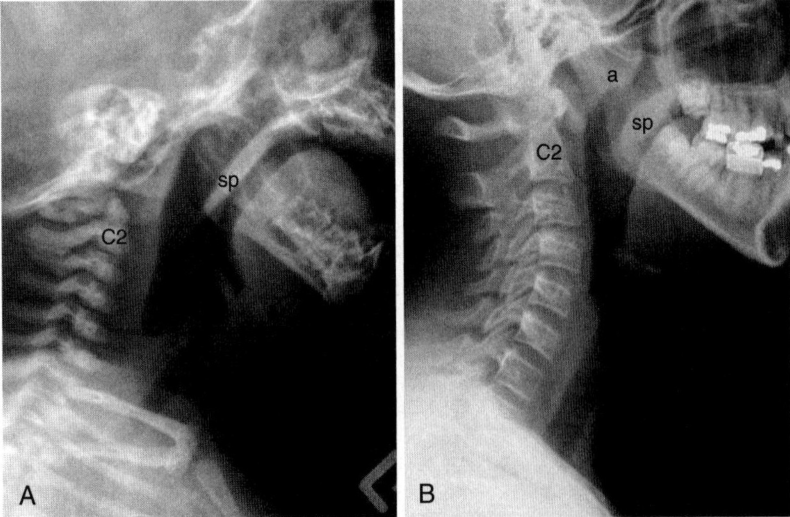

Figure 46-6. Normal airway. Lateral radiographs in **(A)** a 13-day-old and **(B)** a 14-year-old illustrate normal airway anatomy. a: adenoids; sp: soft palate; e: epiglottis; ae: aryepiglottic folds; h: hyoid; C2: odontoid process.

25. **What is the blood supply to the palatine tonsils?**
Five arteries primarily provide the blood supply: dorsal lingual artery, ascending palatine artery (facial artery), tonsillar branch of the facial artery, ascending pharyngeal artery (external carotid), and the lesser palatine artery (descending palatine artery). The venous drainage is via the peritonsilar plexus into the lingual and pharyngeal veins, and then to the internal jugular vein. While not supplying the palatine tonsils, the internal carotid artery is approximately 2.5 cm posterolateral to the tonsils.

26. **What is Waldeyer's ring?**
Heinrich von Waldeyer was an anatomist who described the lymphoid tissue in the posterior nasopharynx and oropharynx. The ring named in his honor is composed of the lingual tonsils, pharyngeal tonsils (adenoids), and palatine tonsils. This ring of the immune system samples pathogens that enter the upper aerodigestive pathway, and is involved in the synthesis of humoral immunoglobulins and production of lymphocytes.

27. **What is a bifid uvula and what is its potential significance?**
A bifid uvula is an abnormality in closure of the most posterior aspect of the soft palate resulting in a uvula with a forked tip. This may signify a possible submucosal cleft, where the mucosa of the secondary palate is normal but the underlying muscular sling may be incomplete with irregular attachments. This may result in abnormal motion of the palate and poor closure of the velopharynx, leading to speech and swallowing difficulties secondary to velopharyngeal insufficiency.

28. **Which pharyngeal arches develop into the larynx and how does this affect its innervation?**
The larynx develops from the fourth and sixth pharyngeal arches. The fourth arch is associated with the superior laryngeal nerve and the sixth arch is associated with the recurrent laryngeal nerve.

29. **What is the narrowest part of the larynx in children and adults?**
The narrowest part of the infant larynx is the cricoid cartilage. This is in contrast to the narrowest part of the adult larynx, which is the rima glottis or glottic opening. Because the narrowest part of the airway in young children is a rigid cartilaginous ring, an endotracheal tube that is too large may cause ischemic injury to the surrounding mucosa and result in scarring and eventual subglottic stenosis.

30. **Why does the recurrent laryngeal nerve wrap around the aortic arch on the left and subclavian artery on the right?**
The sixth arch, which is important in laryngeal development, is also important in the development of the aortic arch and subclavian artery. As portions of the sixth arch descend to form these great vessels it carries the recurrent laryngeal nerve with it. A nonrecurrent laryngeal nerve on the right is a rare entity associated with an aberrant right subclavian artery (abnormal development of the sixth arch) (Figure 46-7).

31. **What are the external laryngeal and internal laryngeal nerves?**
Both are branches of the superior laryngeal nerve. The external laryngeal nerve innervates the cricothyroid muscle and the inferior constrictor muscles of the pharynx. The internal laryngeal nerve only receives afferents (sensation) from the supraglottic larynx and has no motor function.

32. **How do congenital airway and esophageal obstruction affect amniotic fluid levels during pregnancy?**
Abnormalities or compression of the upper airway or esophagus can decrease or prevent the infant's ability to swallow amniotic fluid, resulting in polyhydramnios.

33. **What is CHAOS?**
CHAOS stands for congenital high airway obstruction syndrome. It is a failure of the airway to recannulate during embryological development of the larynx (laryngeal atresia) (Figure 46-8) or upper trachea. If this is not identified prenatally the survival rate is very low because the patient is unable to be ventilated unless there is a corresponding tracheoesophageal fistula.

34. **Describe the normal shape of tracheal rings and how they are different from the cricoid cartilage.**
The cricoid cartilage is a complete cartilaginous ring whereas the tracheal rings are incomplete with a membranous wall that is shared with the esophagus. This C-shaped tracheal ring allows for the

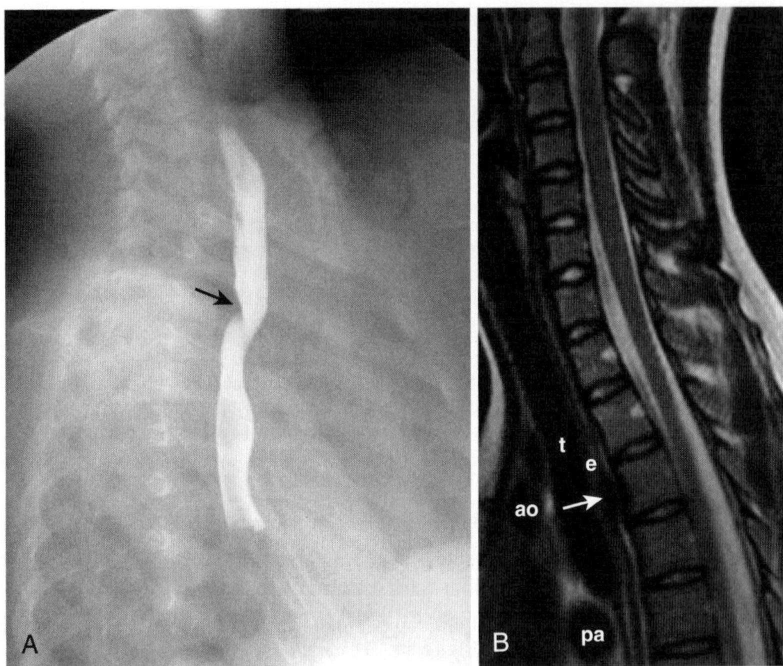

Figure 46-7. Aberrant subclavian artery. A, Oblique image from an esophagram shows an extrinsic posterior indentation on the esophagus *(black arrow)*. **B,** Sagittal T2-weighted image of the cervical spine, in a different patient, reveals an aberrant right subclavian artery *(white arrow)* coursing posterior to the trachea (t) and esophagus (e). (pa: pulmonary artery, ao: aorta).

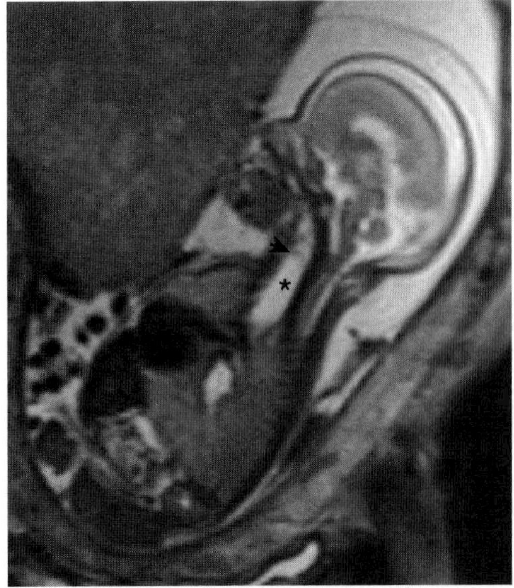

Figure 46-8. Laryngeal atresia. Sagittal HASTE image from a fetal MRI reveals a high airway obstruction, at the level of the larynx (arrowhead), with distension of the distal trachea (asterisk) secondary to failure of the airway to recannulate during embryogenesis.

needed rigidity to maintaining the airway throughout respiration but also allows for larger boluses of food to pass through the esophagus.

35. **What is the blood supply to the trachea?**
    There are lateral pedicles that run the length of the trachea and esophagus that supply blood to the trachea. These pedicles obtain their blood supply from the inferior thyroid, subclavian, supreme intercostal, internal thoracic, innominate, and superior and middle bronchial arteries.

36. **What is Killian's triangle?**
    Also known as Killian's dehiscence, this is a weakened area of the pharyngeal wall located between the inferior constrictor and the cricopharyngeus muscle. Excessive pressure within the lower pharynx and impaired relaxation/spasm of the cricopharyngeus during swallowing can lead to a diverticulum of this region called a Zenker's diverticulum.

Bibliography

Ahmad SM, Soliman A: Congenital anomalies of the larynx, *Otolaryngol Clin N AM* 40:177, 2007.

Hedulund G: Congenital frontonasal masses: developmental anatomy, malformations, and MR imaging, *Pediatr Radiol* 36:647, 2006.

Jackler RK: Congenital malformations of the inner ear. In Cummings CS, et al, editors: *Otolaryngology—Head and Neck Surgery*, ed 2, Chicago, 1993, Mosby-Yearbook, 152: 9.

Lacout A, Marscot-Dupuch K, Smoker WR, et al: Foramen tympanicum, or foramen of Huschke: pathologic cases and anatomic CT study, *AJNR* 26(6):1317, 2005.

Park HY, Han DH, Lee JB, et al: Congenital stapes anomalies with normal eardrum, *Clin Exp Otolaryngol* 2(1):33, 2009.

Poje CP, Rechtweg JS: Structure and function of the temporal bone. In Wetmore RF, Munts HR, McGill TJ, editors: *Pediatric Otolaryngology Principles and Practice Pathways*, ed 2, New York, 2012, Thieme, chapter 8.

Salassa JR, Pearson BW, Payne WS: Gross and microscopical blood supply of the trachea, *Ann Thorac Surg* 24(2):100, 1977.

Sennaroglu L, Saatci I: A new classification for cochleovestibular malformations, *Laryngoscope* 112:2230, 2002.

Sibergleit R, Quint DJ, Mehta BA, et al: The persistent stapedial artery, *AJNR* 21:572, 2000.

Spaeth J, Krugelstein U, Schlondorff G: The paransal sinuses in CT-imaging: development from birth to age 25, *Int J Pediatr Otorhinolaryngol* 39(1):25, 1997.

CHAPTER 47

THE ACUTE PEDIATRIC AIRWAY

Leah J. Hauser, MD and Tendy Chiang, MD

KEY POINTS

1. The assessment of the acute pediatric airway patient includes general appearance (degree of distress), vital signs, skin color, and level of consciousness.
2. Stridor is not a diagnosis but rather a symptom or physical sign of turbulent airflow. Localization of the site of turbulence can be guided by the phase(s) of respiration in which stridor is present.
3. In general, a rapid onset of airway compromise requires immediate attention, whereas chronic mild stridor without distress can be managed in an outpatient setting.
4. Croup is a common viral infection in children. Most cases can be managed conservatively on an outpatient basis; atypical or recurrent episodes requiring prolonged medical management require further evaluation.
5. Always ask about the possibility of foreign body aspiration when evaluating a pediatric patient with acute airway obstruction.

Pearls

1. The pediatric airway is significantly smaller than the adult airway; inflammation and narrowing of the airway can be far more clinically significant in an infant than a similar degree of edema in an adult.
2. Multilevel airway obstruction should be considered in children with syndromes.
3. Bilateral choanal atresia classically presents with respiratory distress and cyanosis at birth that is relieved with crying.
4. Respiratory distress with inspiratory or biphasic stridor in the setting of a strong cry raises suspicion for bilateral true vocal cord paralysis.
5. Epiglottitis can frequently be managed nonoperatively with medical management. Younger patients are more likely to require operative intervention.
6. Urgent intervention is necessary for suspicion of button battery ingestion.

QUESTIONS

1. **How does an infant's airway differ anatomically from an adult's?**
   An infant larynx is one third the size of an adult larynx. The subglottis is the narrowest segment of the pediatric airway compared to the glottis in an adult. The average diameter of a term infant subglottis is about 3.5 mm compared to 10 to 14 mm for an adult.
   The neonatal larynx is initially located at vertebral level C2-3, allowing for the supraglottic structures to interdigitate with the soft palate. This protects and optimizes the airway for infant feeding (suck-swallow-breathe pattern). The larynx descends throughout development to level C7 by adulthood.

2. **What unique physiological and mechanical properties of the pediatric airway increase the risk of respiratory compromise in infants versus adults?**
   In smaller airways, minimal swelling can produce a significant narrowing of the airway. This is because of Poisuelle's law, which states that resistance is inversely proportional to the radius to the fourth power. As such, 1 mm of obstruction in the infant subglottis (4 mm) leads to a 16-fold increase in resistance and a 75% decrease in airway cross-section compared to the same

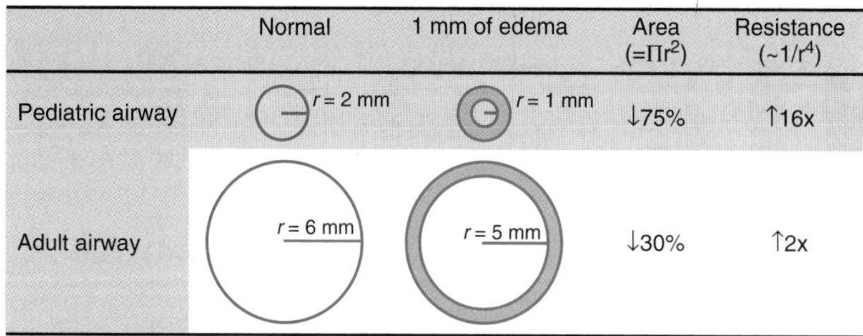

Figure 47-1. Impact of minimal swelling on the pediatric versus adult airway. According to Poiseuille's law, resistance is inversely proportional to the radius to the fourth power. A minimal amount of edema in the pediatric airway will have a more significant impact on airway diameter and resistance compared to the same amount of edema in an adult. *(Adapted from Albert D, Boardman S, Soma M: Evaluation and management of the stridulous child. In Flint PW, Haughey BH, Lund VJ, et al, editors: Cummings Otolaryngology: Head & Neck Surgery, ed 5, Philadelphia, 2010, Mosby, pp 2896–2911.)*

obstruction in an adult airway (12 mm), which only causes a 30% decrease in cross-sectional area and a 2-fold increase in resistance (Figure 47-1). Additionally, quicker oxygen desaturations occurs in children due to a greater chest wall compliance allowing easier collapse, a higher oxygen consumption at baseline, and a smaller lung capacity.

3. What is stridor? What is stertor?

Stridor is a respiratory noise produced by turbulent airflow in the airway. It is not a diagnosis or disease but rather a symptom that indicates narrowing or obstruction of the upper airway. It is a harsh, high-pitched noise that can resemble a squeak or a whistle. *Stertor* resembles snoring and indicates pharyngeal obstruction.

4. Identify the three types of stridor.

Inspiratory stridor reflects airflow impairment above or at the level of the vocal cords. It is generally high pitched when occurring at the vocal cords and may be low pitched (stertor) when obstruction is above the vocal cords (pharynx or supraglottic larynx).

Expiratory stridor is classically caused by obstruction in the distal trachea or bronchi. It gives rise to a more prolonged, sonorous sound and a prolongation of the expiratory phase of respiration.

Biphasic stridor has both an inspiratory and expiratory component and is suggestive of a fixed lesion. This typically suggests a narrowing of the subglottic region, though fixed narrowing in other locations can also result in this sound.

5. What are the signs of impending respiratory failure?

- Biphasic stridor or quiet breathing after prolonged stridor and increased work of breathing
- Suprasternal and/or subcostal retractions
- Abdominal breathing/accessory muscle use
- Nasal flaring
- Diaphoresis
- Mental status changes
- Neck hyperextension or a "tripod" position (sitting leaning forward with chin up, mouth open, and bracing hands on the bed)
- Tachypnea, tachycardia
- Given compensatory mechanisms (tachypnea, tachycardia), oxygen desaturation is a late and ominous sign that frequently indicates impending decompensation
- Pallor and cyanosis can accompany hypoxia

6. What is the differential diagnosis of respiratory distress that presents immediately at birth?

Airway obstruction that is present at birth is characteristic of a fixed anatomical narrowing of the airway. This can be due to obstruction at the level of the nose, oral cavity/oropharynx, hypopharynx, larynx, and trachea (Table 47-1).

Table 47-1. Differential Diagnosis of Neonatal Airway Obstruction by Anatomic Site

SITE OF OBSTRUCTION	DIFFERENTIAL
Nose	Rhinitis, piriform aperture stenosis, nasolacrimal duct cyst, nasal mass, choanal atresia, encephalocele or meningocele, midface hypoplasia (Crouzon's, Down syndrome, etc.)
Oral Cavity/Oropharynx	Micrognathia (Pierre Robin, Treacher-Collins, etc.), macroglossia (Down syndrome), lingual thyroid, masses, cysts
Larynx	Laryngomalacia, vocal fold paralysis, subglottic stenosis, laryngeal web, laryngeal atresia, cysts or masses
Trachea	Tracheomalacia/bronchomalacia, tracheal stenosis or atresia, extrinsic/vascular compression (vascular ring, double aortic arch, pulmonary artery sling, etc), complete tracheal rings

Albert D, Boardman S, Soma M: Evaluation and management of the stridulous child. In Flint PW, Haughey BH, Lund VJ, et al, editors: Cummings Otolaryngology: Head & Neck Surgery, ed 5, Philadelphia, 2010, Mosby, Table 205-1.

7. **What are the possible causes of neonatal nasal obstruction?**
   The differential diagnosis includes rhinitis, piriform aperture stenosis, nasolacrimal duct cysts, midline nasal masses, and choanal atresia. Because neonates are obligate nasal breathers until 4 to 6 months of age, the classic presentation of respiratory distress from neonatal nasal obstruction results in difficulty breathing/cyanosis that is relieved with crying.

8. **What is choanal atresia?**
   Choanal atresia is a failure of the posterior nasal cavity to communicate with the nasopharynx, postulated to represent the failure of the nasobuccal membrane to rupture. Two thirds of cases are unilateral and usually present later in life with chronic rhinorrhea and congestion. Bilateral atresia usually presents in the neonatal period with cyanotic events during feeding that are relieved with crying. Fifty percent to 75% of patients will have an associated congenital anomaly.
   Diagnosis is made by failure to pass catheters through the nose and confirmed with flexible endoscopy and CT scan. Treatment is surgical resection of the atretic plate to create patent choanae.

9. **Name a common genetic syndrome with which choanal atresia is associated.**
   Choanal atresia is a component of the CHARGE syndrome:
   - C = Coloboma
   - H = Heart anomalies
   - A = Atresia of the choanae
   - R = Retardation of growth and development
   - G = Genitourinary disorders (hypoplasia for males)
   - E = Ear anomalies and/or hearing loss

10. **What is Robin sequence? What are other causes of obstruction at the same level?**
    Robin sequence (RS) describes a triad of micrognathia, glossoptosis, and airway obstruction. Glossoptosis and retrognathia result in obstruction at the level of the base of tongue and oropharynx. Micrognathia and glossoptosis can prevent fusion of palatal shelves at the midline, resulting in a U-shaped cleft palate.
    RS can occur in isolation or with a syndrome (Treacher Collins, Stickler, velocardiofacial syndrome, and many others). Presence of a syndrome with mandibular hypoplasia should raise suspicion for multilevel obstruction.

11. **Discuss the evaluation and management of children with Robin sequence.**
    In addition to a complete history and physical, flexible fiber-optic/rigid laryngoscopy, bronchoscopy, sleep endoscopy, and polysomnogram are commonly used to characterize the degree of obstruction.

Many cases of RS can be managed with supplemental oxygen, prone positioning, placement of a nasopharyngeal trumpet, and/or continuous positive airway pressure (CPAP). Failure to thrive, obstructive sleep apnea, and respiratory failure require escalation of management.

Definitive surgical management options include tongue-lip adhesion, mandibular distraction, and tracheostomy.

12. **Name four congenital laryngeal anomalies that cause respiratory distress. What is the most common congenital laryngeal anomaly?**
    - Laryngomalacia (most common)
      - Collapse of the supraglottic larynx resulting in inspiratory stridor
      - May result from aryepiglottic fold shortening, redundant supraglottic tissue, and/or hypotonia
    - Vocal fold paralysis
    - Congenital subglottic stenosis
    - Congenital laryngeal web

13. **What is the cause of bilateral vocal fold paralysis (BVCP)?**
    Bilateral vocal cord paralysis is most commonly idiopathic (46%). Other causes include Arnold Chiari malformation, cerebral palsy, hydrocephalus, spina bifida, birth trauma or hypoxia. Workup consists of an MRI of the brain to evaluate for intracranial abnormalities, genetic consultation to evaluate for chromosomal abnormalities, and laryngoscopy with palpation of the cricoarytenoid joint to delineate BVCP from joint fixation.

14. **How does bilateral vocal fold paralysis present and how is it managed?**
    Patients typically present at birth with respiratory distress and inspiratory or biphasic stridor. Flexible fiber-optic laryngoscopy should be performed to evaluate supraglottic architecture and cord mobility. The mainstay of treatment is tracheotomy; most cases of idiopathic BVCP demonstrate recovery of function in time, and decannulation is often possible.

15. **How do infections of the different divisions of the larynx differ in presentation? Which pathogens are most commonly associated with each?**
    See Table 47-2.

16. **What radiographic findings are classically found in supraglottitis, croup and bacterial tracheitis?**
    (Figure 47-2).
    - Supraglottitis: "Thumb sign" on lateral neck x-ray
      - Thickening and rounding of the epiglottis with loss of the normal air space of the vallecula
    - Croup: "Steeple sign" on AP neck x-ray
      - Narrowing at the level of the subglottis

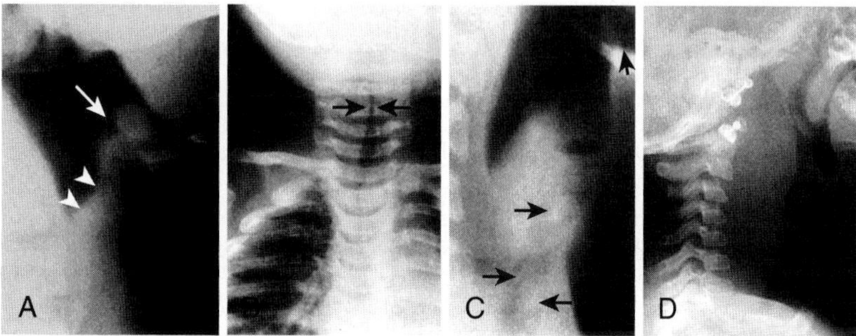

Figure 47-2. Imaging characteristics of pediatric airway infections. **A,** Supraglottitis. Rounded epiglottis *(white arrow)*, thickened aryepiglottic folds *(white arrowheads)*, and distention of the hypopharyngeal space. **B,** Croup. Narrowed subglottis *(black arrows)*, showing a "steeple sign." **C,** Bacterial tracheitis. Tracheal lumen obscured by sloughed mucosa *(black arrows)*. Note normal epiglottis *(black arrowhead)*. **D,** Retropharyngeal abscess. Widened retropharyngeal soft tissues compared to the vertebral bodies. *(Adapted from Duncan NO: Infections of the airway in children. In Flint PW, Haughey BH, Lund VJ, et al, editors: Cummings Otolaryngology: Head & Neck Surgery, ed 5, Philadelphia, 2010, Mosby, pp 2803–2811, Figures 197-8, 197-3, 197-10, and 197-13.)*

Table 47-2. Clinical Characteristics of Airway Infections by Location

	SUPRAGLOTTITIS	LARYNGITIS	CROUP	TRACHEITIS
Age	2–7 yrs	Any	6 mo–3 yrs	6 mo–8 yrs
Onset	Rapid*	Slow	Slow	Rapid
Prodrome	None or mild URI*	URI	URI	URI*
Fever	High*	No	None or low grade*	High*
Hoarseness	No, but voice muffled and speech limited due to severe pain*	Yes*	Yes	Yes
Stridor	Usually none. Inspiratory stridor is a late finding indicating severe infection/obstruction	Absent	Inspiratory initially, may progress to biphasic in severe cases	Biphasic
Cough	None	Variable	Barky*	Barky
Odynophagia/ Drooling	Yes*	No	No	No
Toxic Appearance	Yes	No	No	Yes*
Pathogen	*Haemophilus influenza*, type B Group A B-hemolytic *Streptococci*	Multiple viruses	Parainfluenza virus Respiratory syncytial virus (RSV)	*Staphylococcus aureus* *Moraxella catarrhalis*

*indicates classic feature.
Adapted from Duncan NO: Infections of the airway in children. In Flint PW, Haughey BH, Lund VJ, et al, editors: Cummings Otolaryngology: Head & Neck Surgery, ed 5, Philadelphia, 2010, Mosby, Table 197-1.

- Bacterial tracheitis: "Pseudomembranes" on lateral neck x-ray
  - Ratty or irregular tracheal borders indicative of thick, purulent secretions or sloughing mucosa

17. **What is another name for supraglottitis? Describe the change in incidence in the last several decades.**
Epiglottitis is another name for supraglottitis, but this is somewhat inaccurate because this clinical entity typically involves the entire supraglottis. Most cases of supraglottitis were due to hemophilus influenza type b (HIB), the incidence of which has dropped dramatically since implementation of the HIB vaccine in 1988.

18. **Discuss the presentation and management of supraglottitis.**
Patients with supraglottitis most commonly present with odynophagia (pain with swallowing), dysphagia (difficulty swallowing), voice change (muffled voice, hoarseness), and difficulty tolerating secretions. Stridor and respiratory distress are less common signs, but suggest an impending surgical emergency. The "tripod" positioning of the patient is associated with respiratory distress.
Management consists of close airway surveillance with possible operative intervention to establish an airway. Parents are counseled that intervention spans a wide spectrum from direct laryngoscopy or fiber-optic endotracheal intubation to placement of a tracheotomy; however, in most cases, this is not necessary. Airway intervention is more common in younger patients, with a mean of 4 years of age (almost two thirds are 2 years old or younger). Anxiety-provoking maneuvers should be avoided when handling a patient with a tenuous airway; all instrumentation and interventions should be performed in the operative suite.

If operative intervention is necessary, direct laryngoscopy should be performed after the airway is secured to obtain swab cultures from the epiglottis and evaluate for an abscess at the lingual surface of the epiglottis. Intravenous antibiotics should be started and a 10- to 14-day course should be completed. Extubation can generally be accomplished within 48 hours when supraglottic edema improves and an air leak is present around the endotracheal tube.

19. **How is croup managed?**
Croup is very common; 3% to 5% of all children have one episode in their lifetime. Most cases can be managed conservatively with supportive care only. For more significant symptoms, corticosteroids have been shown to decrease hospitalization rate and severity of disease. Generally one dose of dexamethasone is sufficient and nebulized racemic epinephrine can also be used to decrease airway edema. Between 85% and 99% of patients can be managed as outpatients. Hospitalized patients should be treated with repeated doses of intravenous dexamethasone and racemic epinephrine until symptoms resolve. Only 1% to 5% of patients require intubation for severe airway obstruction.
Direct laryngoscopy should be considered in very young children or those with recurrent or severe croup to rule out underlying airway pathology (i.e., subglottic stenosis, hemangioma, subglottic cyst, etc).

20. **How is bacterial tracheitis managed?**
Though severity of symptoms is usually not as dramatic as in acute epiglottitis, airway obstruction is not infrequent with bacterial tracheitis and management includes rigid bronchoscopy with debridement of secretions. About 60% to 80% require intubation and repeated endoscopies can be performed for recurrent plugging and crusting. Extubation can be achieved after fevers resolve, secretions diminish, and an air leak is present around the endotracheal tube. Intravenous antibiotics are directed toward *Staphylococcus aureus* for a 10- to 14-day course.

21. **Describe how pharyngeal infections can lead to airway obstruction.**
Peritonsillar, parapharyngeal, and retropharyngeal abscesses can all present with airway obstruction and require surgical drainage for management. Peritonsillar abscesses present with a "hot potato" voice and stertor, as the level of obstruction is at the oropharynx. Airway symptoms are usually milder than with parapharyngeal and retropharyngeal abscesses. Parapharyngeal and retropharyngeal abscesses present with fevers, sore throat, dysphagia, and decreased neck mobility and should be considered in the differential diagnosis of croup and bacterial tracheitis. Airway obstruction is more likely and severe with retropharyngeal abscesses. Management of the airway should be carefully planned in patients with large abscesses. Care should be taken with sedation because endotracheal intubation can be challenging or even impossible and the airway can be lost. Tracheostomy may have to be considered. See Figure 47-2, panel D.

22. **When evaluating a pediatric patient with acute airway obstruction, what should always be included in the history of present illness?**
Always ask if there is concern for or possibility of foreign body (FB) aspiration. About half of aspiration events are not witnessed. If the foreign body does not immediately cause airway obstruction, symptoms can be more subtle and mimic other airway infections, asthma, or pneumonia. A high index of suspicion should be maintained for FB aspiration and history regarding possible aspiration events should always be included when working up children with airway symptoms.

23. **What are risk factors for foreign body aspiration?**
FB aspiration is most common in toddlers between 1 and 3 years of age. This is because they are more likely to explore their environment with their mouths, they have poor coordination of swallowing, they lack posterior dentition necessary for chewing food properly, they lack an appreciation of what is edible, and they are likely to be playing while eating. Other risk factors include male gender and developmental delay or neurologic impairment.

24. **Which items have the highest risk for aspiration?**
Toddlers are most likely aspirate or ingest incompletely chewed food, most commonly nuts, seeds, and beans. Other common objects include small plastic or metal toys or pieces. Coins are the most common esophageal foreign bodies.

25. What are the symptoms of foreign body aspiration?

Symptoms vary depending on the location of the foreign body and how long it has been present.

- Larynx: FB in the larynx can cause an airway emergency requiring emergent intervention. Patients can present with obstruction, cough, and hoarseness. Delay in diagnosis can allow edema to progress and cause a partial obstruction to become a complete obstruction.
- Trachea: Symptoms include stridor, wheezing, dyspnea, and coughing. Hoarseness is absent in comparison to laryngeal FB.
- Bronchi: This is the most common location for airway FB to lodge (80% to 90%). The classic triad of cough, wheeze, and decreased unilateral breath sounds may not always be present, but nearly all patients will have at least one of these symptoms.
- Esophagus: Dysphagia, odynophagia, drooling, and vomiting are common symptoms of esophageal foreign bodies. Esophageal FB are more common than airway FB. Common sites of esophageal FB are at the cricopharyngeus and at the level where the esophagus crosses the aortic arch.

26. What is the x-ray of choice in diagnosis for airway foreign bodies?

Inspiratory and expiratory chest films. As the lodged FB can cause air to enter but not escape, air trapping or hyperinflation can be appreciated on x-ray and exaggerated by the expiratory phase. Other changes seen on plain films include atelectasis and pneumonia. Radiopaque objects and those in the bronchi are more likely to be detected on x-ray. A negative film should not rule out FB aspiration, as between 25% and 50% of patients can have completely normal radiographs.

27. What is the management of foreign body aspiration? Which situations require urgent intervention?

Management includes direct laryngoscopy and bronchoscopy for evaluation and endoscopic removal of the foreign body. Intubation and treatment with steroids are considered for those patients with severe obstruction, mucosal damage, or significant airway edema. Bronchial foreign bodies can result in postobstructive pneumonia distal to the point of obstruction. Always consider evaluation of the esophagus when a child presents with airway obstruction or a positive history and has a normal bronchoscopy because esophageal foreign bodies can cause effacement of the airway. Coins in the esophagus have a high rate of passage through the GI tract and watchful waiting can be considered in older children and those in the distal esophagus when there are no signs of airway compromise.

Urgent intervention is necessary for acute or potential airway obstruction, concern for esophageal injury, or suspicion of disc battery ingestion.

28. Discuss button battery ingestion and describe the differences in management compared with ingested coins.

A button battery can be mistaken for a coin, but will often have a characteristic "double halo" or "double ring" sign on AP view or may have a step off on lateral view.

The incidence of button battery ingestion has remained relatively stable (about 10 to 12 per million per year), but there has been a dramatic rise in complications and fatalities over the past 10 years as more household objects utilize batteries and battery size has increased. Though hearing aid batteries are the most commonly ingested battery, they are smaller, pass more easily, and pose less of a risk of serious injury to the aerodigestive tract.

Urgent intervention is indicated because button batteries can begin to cause mucosal damage due to caustic injury within 1 hour and esophageal perforation can occur within 6 hours. Twelve percent of young children who ingest batteries greater than 20 mm in diameter will experience a major complication, such as perforation, tracheoesophageal fistula, major vessel injury, esophageal stricture, vocal cord paralysis, or cervical spine injury.

Bibliography

Acevedo JL, Lander L, Choi S, et al: Airway management in pediatric epiglottitis: a national perspective, *Otolaryngol Head Neck Surg* 140:548–551, 2009.

Albert D, Boardman S, Soma M: Evaluation and management of the stridulous child. In Flint PW, Haughey BH, Lund VJ, et al, editors: *Cummings Otolaryngology: Head & Neck Surgery*, ed 5, Philadelphia, 2010, Mosby, pp 2896–2911.

Daniel SJ: The upper airway: Congenital malformations, *Ped Respiratory Rev* 7S:S260–S263, 2006.

DeRowe A, Massick D, Beste DJ: Clinical characteristics of aero-digestive foreign bodies in neurologically impaired children, *Int J Pediatr Otorhinolaryngol* 62(3):243–248, 2002.

Duncan NO: Infections of the airway in children. In Flint PW, Haughey BH, Lund VJ, et al, editors: *Cummings Otolaryngology: Head & Neck Surgery*, ed 5, Philadelphia, 2010, Mosby, pp 2803–2811.

Holinger LD, Poznanovic SA: Foreign bodies of the airway and esophagus. In Flint PW, Haughey BH, Lund VJ, et al, editors: *Cummings Otolaryngology: Head & Neck Surgery*, ed 5, Philadelphia, 2010, Mosby, pp 2935–2943.
Jatana KR, Litovitz T, Reilly JS, et al: Pediatric button battery injuries: 2013 task force update, *Int J Pediatr Otorhinolaryngol* 77:1392–1399, 2013.
Kuo M, Rothera M: Emergency management of the paediatric airway. In Graham JM, Scadding GK, Bull PD, editors: *Pediatric ENT*, Heidelberg, 2007, Springer, pp 183–188.
Messner AH: Congenital disorders of the larynx. In Flint PW, Haughey BH, Lund VJ, et al, editors: *Cummings Otolaryngology: Head & Neck Surgery*, ed 5, Philadelphia, 2010, Mosby, pp 2866–2875.
Nisa L, Holtz F, Sandu K: Paralyzed neonatal larynx in adduction. Case series, systematic review, and analysis, *Int J Pediatr Otorhinolaryngol* 77:13–183, 2013.
Pasagolu I, Dogan R, Demircin A, et al: Bronchoscopic removal of foreign bodies in children: retrospective analysis of 822 cases, *Thorac Cardiovasc Surg* 39:95–98, 1991.
Sidell DR, Kim IA, Coker TR, et al: Food choking hazards in children, *Int J Pediatr Otorhinolaryngol* 77:1940–1946, 2013.
Stroud RH, Friedman NR: An update on inflammatory disorders of the pediatric airway: epiglottitis, croup, and tracheitis, *Am J Otolaryngol* 22:268–275, 2001.

CHAPTER 48

CHRONIC PEDIATRIC AIRWAY DISEASES

Brook K. McConnell, MD and Jeremy D. Prager, MD

KEY POINTS

1. In the evaluation of pediatric airway disorders, flexible fiber-optic laryngoscopy is the best initial imaging modality in the stabilized patient. Based on initial fiber-optic examination, additional exam under anesthesia including direct laryngoscopy and bronchoscopy may be indicated.
2. Laryngomalacia and unilateral vocal cord paralysis are the first and second most common causes of stridor in the infant. History, physical, and flexible laryngoscopy while awake allow diagnosis of these more common conditions. Additional plain films of the neck and fluoroscopic studies will help the provider evaluate for less common lesions.
3. Since the advent of softer material endotracheal tubes for prolonged intubation, subglottic stenosis has become less common in premature infants. Choose the smallest endotracheal tube that provides adequate ventilation and limit the total duration of time the patient is intubated to minimize the risk of subglottic stenosis. Endoscopic and open surgical techniques remain the mainstay of treatment for subglottic stenosis.
4. Children who present with symptoms such as choking with oral intake, chronic cough, recurrent pneumonia, and chronic lung disease consistent with aspiration should undergo evaluation for anatomic disorders of the upper aerodigestive tract.
5. Current management of RRP is based on repeat endoscopic excision of airway lesions using various modalities emphasizing removal of disease while preserving function.
6. Pediatric aspiration is most commonly evaluated using modified barium swallow studies and/or fiber-optic endoscopic evaluation of swallowing. Choice of modality can be tailored to the individual patient and each one can be used to facilitate selection of a safe diet for patients.

Pearls

1. Laryngomalacia is the most common cause of stridor in the infant. In most cases, it resolves by age 2 years without surgical intervention. Unilateral vocal cord paralysis in the pediatric population is most commonly iatrogenic in etiology and represents the second most common cause of stridor.
2. The most common cause of subglottic stenosis is iatrogenic scarring related to endotracheal intubation.
3. In the setting of chronic aspiration, pediatric otolaryngologists must maintain a high index of suspicion for laryngeal cleft.
4. Infantile hemangiomas are the most common tumors of infancy. The majority are found within the head and neck.
5. HPV vaccination has the potential to significantly decrease the transmission of recurrent respiratory papillomatosis. Vaccines for RRP must address viral subtypes 6 and 11.

QUESTIONS

LARYNGOMALACIA

1. **List the three most common congenital disorders of the larynx.**
In order of most to least common: laryngomalacia, vocal cord paralysis, subglottic stenosis.

2. **What is stridor?**
Stridor is an audible breath sound due to turbulent airflow from airway narrowing.

3. **What is the most common cause of stridor in the neonate and infant?**
Laryngomalacia.

4. **Describe the characteristics of laryngomalacia.**
There are several theories regarding the etiology of laryngomalacia, including anatomic changes resulting in short folds of tissue between the epiglottis and arytenoids as well as neuromuscular control of the supraglottis. Inspiratory stridor occurs with collapse of the supraglottic tissue on inspiration. Affected infants typically present with intermittent inspiratory stridor within the first two weeks of life. Stridor is usually worse with feeding, while supine, or while agitated. The child may need to take breaks while feeding to breathe. The majority of cases are self-limited, with resolution of symptoms by age 18 months. However, approximately 10% of patients will experience significant upper airway obstruction resulting in feeding difficulties, failure to thrive, pectus excavatum, apneic episodes, cyanosis, and hypoxia. These patients warrant consideration for surgical intervention.
Patients may have associated gastroesophageal reflux disease (GERD). This condition may contribute to airway edema, further compromising the airway. Acid suppression may improve mild cases of laryngomalacia and is often instituted empirically.
Diagnosis is made with awake flexible fiber-optic laryngoscopy, which allows for rapid diagnosis without need for anesthesia.

SUBGLOTTIC STENOSIS

5. **What is the typical size of the pediatric airway?**
Airway size is determined based on the narrowest portion of the airway. In the pediatric population, this site is the subglottis at the level of the cricoid cartilage. In a term infant, the subglottic lumen measures 4.5 to 5.5 mm.

6. **How is an endotracheal tube size chosen?**
Endotracheal and tracheostomy tube sizes are based on the inner diameter of the tube. For example a 4.0 endotracheal or tracheostomy tube correlates to an inner diameter of 4 mm. The smallest tube that provides adequate ventilation should be chosen. Several size-predictive formulas exist and are based on parameters such as age, height, weight, and/or finger width. One commonly used formula is based on the age of the patient: inner diameter = 4 + age/4. This formula is more accurate for older children.

7. **Describe the characteristics of subglottic stenosis.**
Subglottic stenosis (SGS) is narrowing of the subglottis and can be either congenital or acquired. Congenital SGS occurs in the absence of a history of endotracheal intubation or other causes of acquired stenosis. Causes of congenital SGS include an elliptical cricoid, congenital narrowing (as in Down syndrome), and trapped first tracheal ring.
Acquired stenosis is more common than congenital SGS. Endotracheal intubation is the most common acquired cause. Duration of intubation and endotracheal tube size are the two most important factors in the development of stenosis. Stenosis occurs as a result of pressure necrosis and subsequent scar formation. Prevention of subglottic stenosis via selection of the proper endotracheal tube and a short duration of intubation is ideal. Other causes include neck trauma, laryngeal procedures, caustic ingestions, radiotherapy, and tracheal infection. Diagnosis is made at the time of direct laryngoscopy and bronchoscopy.

8. **Describe the most commonly used grading system for subglottic stenosis.**
The Myer-Cotton classification system is the most widely used system for grading the degree and severity of subglottic stenosis (Figure 48-1).

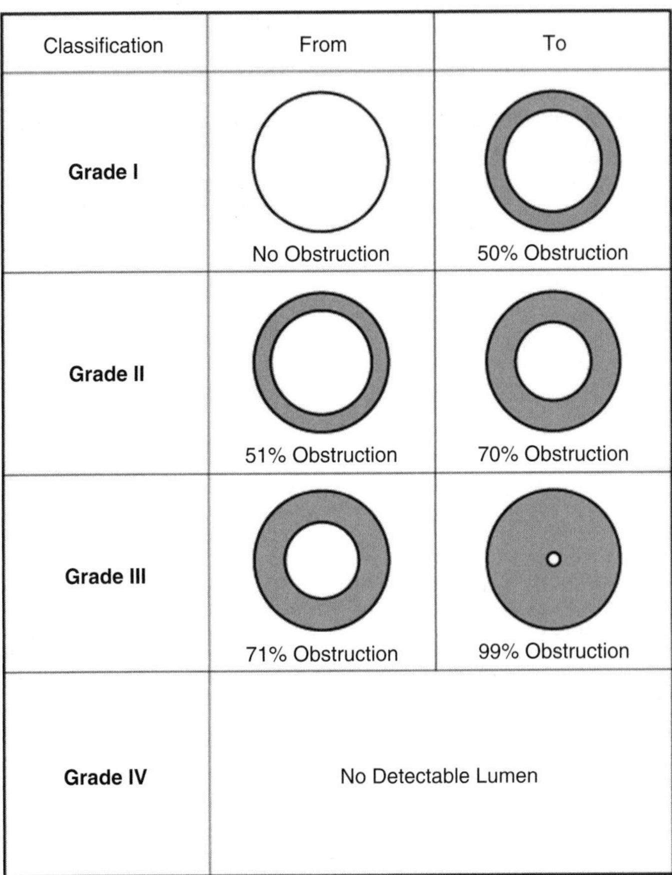

Figure 48-1. The Myer-Cotton Classification System. *(Used with permission. Myer CM III, O'Connor DM, Cotton RT: Proposed grading system for subglottic stenosis based on endotracheal tube size, Ann Otol Rhinol Laryngol 103:319, 1994.)*

9. **How is subglottic stenosis treated?**
Surgical methods of managing subglottic stenosis include endoscopic and open transcervical techniques. Choice of method depends on many patient factors including degree of stenosis, comorbid conditions, and age of the lesion. Thin weblike lesions that are identified early, when the scar is immature, may be amenable to endoscopic procedures including scar lysis by balloon dilation. More mature, thicker lesions with greater superior-inferior dimension may require augmentation or resection procedures. Augmentation procedures involve placing cartilage grafts into the airway to make the lumen bigger. Resection procedures involve removing the affected segment and anastomosing the airway.

LARYNGEAL CLEFT

10. **What is the underlying embryologic defect that leads to the development of a laryngeal cleft?**
The tracheoesophageal septum forms from two opposing ridges in the midline of the primordial aerodigestive tract into what will eventually become the larynx/trachea and the esophagus. The septum forms in a caudal to cranial direction. Laryngeal clefts are a result of incomplete

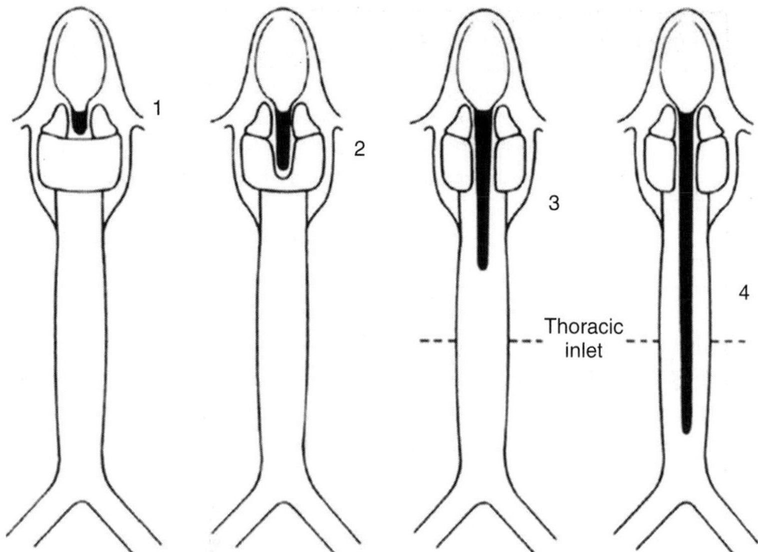

Figure 48-2. Benjamin-Inglis Classification System. Type 1: The cleft is isolated to the supraglottic interarytenoid region located above or at the level of the vocal cords. Type 2: The cleft extends into the upper portion of the cricoid but not through the inferior border. Type 3: The cleft extends through the inferior border of the cricoid cartilage, can variably extend into the cervical trachea. Type 4: The cleft extends into the thoracic trachea and may extend to the carina. *(From Chien W, Ashland J, Haver K, Hardy SC, et al: Type 1 laryngeal cleft: establishing a functional diagnostic and management algorithm,* Int J Pediatr Otorhinolaryngol *70(12):2073–2079, 2006.)*

development and fusion of the tracheoesophageal septum resulting in an abnormal communication between the airway and the hypopharynx/esophagus.

11. **Describe the most commonly used classification system for laryngeal clefts.**
The Benjamin-Inglis system is the most commonly used classification system (Figure 48-2).

12. **Discuss the typical presentation of laryngeal clefts.**
The presentation of this anomaly depends on the severity of the defect. For type I and certain type II laryngeal clefts, symptoms may be subtle and include hoarse voice, mild stridor, chronic cough, lingering upper respiratory infections, and recurrent pneumonia. Because the presentation may be subtle, a high index of suspicion is needed to make the diagnosis. More severe types of laryngeal clefts present at birth with respiratory distress and aspiration with po intake.

13. **Which syndromes are associated with laryngeal cleft?**
See Table 48-1.

Unilateral Vocal Cord Paralysis

14. **What is the most common cause of unilateral vocal cord paralysis?**
Iatrogenic complications are the leading cause of unilateral vocal fold paralysis with patent ductus arteriosus (PDA) ligation resulting in left vocal cord paralysis being the most frequent cause. The incidence of iatrogenic vocal cord paralysis has increased as the number of pediatric cardiothoracic procedures has increased. Other surgical procedures that can lead to unilateral vocal fold paralysis include repair of tracheoesophageal fistulas and esophageal atresia repair. Birth trauma may also result in vocal cord paralysis.

Unilateral vocal cord paralysis also may be congenital in origin. Arnold Chiari malformations can lead to vocal cord paralysis but are classically thought to cause bilateral rather than unilateral paralysis. Other less commonly encountered causes of unilateral paralysis include neoplasms of the central nervous system, neck, or mediastinum causing recurrent laryngeal nerve dysfunction.

Table 48-1. Syndromes Associated with Laryngeal Cleft

Opitz-Frias	Characterized by craniofacial anomalies such as cleft lip and palate, genitourinary abnormalities, and midline airway malformations such as laryngeal cleft
Pallister Hall Syndrome	Congenital hypothalamic hamartoblastoma, hypopituitarism, polydactyly, imperforate anus, cardiac abnormalities, and renal malformations
VACTERL Association	**V**ertebral anomalies, **A**nal atresia, **C**ardiac anomalies, **T**racheoesophageal fistula, **E**ar malformation, **R**enal anomalies, **L**imb anomalies
CHARGE Syndrome	**C**oloboma, **H**eart disease, choanal **A**tresia, growth and mental **R**etardation, **G**enital anomalies, **E**ar anomalies

15. **Describe the clinical course of unilateral vocal cord paralysis.**
Unilateral vocal cord paralysis presents with stridor, a weak cry, and feeding difficulty with possible aspiration. This condition is the second most common cause of stridor in the infant. The diagnosis is made with an awake, flexible fiber-optic laryngoscopy. Further workup may be needed in patients in whom an underlying cause is not apparent (idiopathic). Imaging the course of the recurrent laryngeal nerve from skull base to mediastinum may be performed to identify potential etiologies. Patients with difficulty feeding may benefit from evaluation for aspiration via modified barium swallow or fiber-optic endoscopic evaluation of swallowing.
Seventy percent of idiopathic causes of unilateral vocal cord paralysis are expected to resolve spontaneously, most within 6 months of age. Cases of iatrogenic paralysis are less likely to resolve, with 35% of patients noted to recover function at 16-month follow-up. For those patients who are severely symptomatic, vocal cord medialization may improve speech and swallow function at the cost of increasing airway narrowing at the glottis and stridor.

Airway Hemangioma

16. **What is an infantile hemangioma?**
Infantile hemangiomas are benign vascular neoplasms that develop during infancy as a result of disordered angiogenesis. These lesions may occur throughout the body but are most commonly found within the head and neck, including the airway. Symptoms and signs are dependent on the location and natural history of the hemangioma. These are the most common tumors of infancy.

17. **What signs and symptoms could indicate the presence of an airway hemangioma?**
Infantile hemangiomas of the airway present in early infancy during the rapid proliferative phase with symptoms of progressive airway compromise. Patients may present with biphasic stridor or a chronic cough which may be misdiagnosed as croup. Failure to respond to standard treatment should lead to consultation with ENT. A particularly high degree of suspicion is warranted in the stridulous child with cutaneous hemangiomas of the lower face. Up to 50% of patients with cutaneous hemangiomas within a beard distribution will have a synchronous airway lesion. Diagnosis of an airway hemangioma is made on fiber-optic laryngoscopy and/or direct laryngoscopy in the operating room. Plain films of the neck may reveal an asymmetric narrowing of the subglottis as well.

18. **What is the standard treatment of a subglottic infantile hemangioma?**
While many infantile hemangiomas do not require treatment, those in the airway and in particular those in the subglottis warrant therapy. Medical therapy includes oral systemic steroids and propranolol. Steroids aim to stop angiogenesis and decrease surrounding inflammation and swelling. Systemic steroid treatment, however, is only effective in the proliferative phase. Multiple studies have documented rapid regression of hemangiomas with the use of propranolol. The exact mechanism to explain the effect of propranolol on hemangiomas has not been identified.
Surgical therapy is an option for those patients who are not adequately treated with medical therapy alone. Endoscopic treatment includes laser treatment and steroid injection into the lesion. In addition, the lesion may be excised via open transcervical approach. Finally, tracheostomy may be needed in certain patients in order to bypass the site of obstruction in the subglottis until spontaneous involution occurs.

Tracheomalacia

19. What is tracheomalacia?

Tracheomalacia is softness/collapsibility of the trachea. It is diagnosed during rigid or flexible bronchoscopy when there is greater than 50% loss of airway diameter during coughing. Lateral chest x-rays during inspiratory and expiratory phases may also demonstrate collapsibility of the tracheal airway. Tracheomalacia presents as expiratory stridor (sometimes biphasic), barky cough, and prolonged or recurrent pulmonary infections. This condition may be classified as extrinsic or intrinsic.

Intrinsic tracheomalacia occurs if the tracheal cartilage is weak or absent. The majority of children with intrinsic tracheomalacia outgrow the condition during the first few years of life. Management for these children includes the potential need for early intervention for pulmonary illnesses, inhaled steroids for airway edema, and the understanding that the barky cough is not necessarily croup. A condition commonly associated with intrinsic tracheomalacia is tracheoesophageal fistula.

Extrinsic tracheomalacia implies that a structure outside of the airway is compressing the tracheal cartilage. This is most commonly related to cardiac and vascular anomalies (i.e., vascular rings which may encircle the airway). A barium esophagram may suggest a vascular ring encircling the airway. Rigid bronchoscopy and CT or MRI are also diagnostic of vascular ring.

Papilloma

20. What is recurrent respiratory papillomatosis?

Recurrent respiratory papillomatosis (RRP) is a neoplasm of the airway that is caused by human papilloma virus (HPV). It is the most common benign neoplasm of the pediatric larynx, leading to symptoms of dysphonia and stridor. This disease does occur in adults and tends to be less aggressive.

21. What are the most common types of HPV that lead to RRP?

HPV types 6 and 11 are the most common HPV types that lead to RRP. Specific viral types are associated with disease severity. For example, HPV 11 subtype has been associated with more airway obstruction, tracheal disease, pulmonary disease, and need for tracheostomy.

22. How is RRP transmitted?

Vertical transmission via contact through an infected birth canal is the proposed method of disease transmission from mother to child. It has been suggested that newly acquired genital lesions are more likely to shed viral particles, which is thought to account for the higher incidence of disease in patients born to young mothers of low socioeconomic status. However, the overall risk of contracting RRP from a mother with active genital condylomata at the time of birth is generally low (1 in 231 to 400). Cesarean section is then likely of limited use to prevent vertical transmission, especially given the risks and significant costs associated with the procedure. The American Academy of Pediatrics and the American College of Obstetricians and Gynecologists do not currently recommend cesarean section to solely protect the neonate from HPV infection.

23. List the risks factors for the development of RRP.

- First born child
- Teenage mother
- Vaginal delivery (it should be noted that several cases exhibit in utero transmission)

24. How is RRP treated?

There is no single treatment modality that has been shown to eradicate RRP once and for all. The current mainstay of therapy is surgical reduction of disease burden (to debulk as much disease as possible while maintaining normal morphology and anatomy). Methods include cold steel excision with or without powered instrumentation (e.g., microdebrider) versus laser excision (carbon dioxide, potassium titanium phosphate (KTP)).

Adjuvant medical treatments also exist, though none have demonstrated efficacy in double blind, randomized controlled trials. The most well-known adjuvant therapy is topical injection of the antiviral medication cidofovir. There are multiple statements from the RRP Task Force regarding counseling on and potential use of cidofovir as an option.

Table 48-2. Four Phases of Swallowing

Oral preparatory phase	Bolus formation
Oral propulsive phase	Transport of bolus to the pharynx
Pharyngeal phase	Transport of the food bolus from the pharynx into the esophagus. During this phase, the nasopharynx is closed, breathing stops, the vocal cords adduct, the larynx rises, and the base of tongue and pharyngeal muscles propel the bolus to the esophagus.
Esophageal phase	Peristaltic contraction of the esophagus moves the bolus from the upper esophageal sphincter, into the body of the esophagus, through the lower esophageal sphincter, and into the stomach.

25. **How is RRP prevented?**
HPV vaccination is likely the most important mode of prevention. There are currently multiple vaccines in development and one commercially available FDA-approved vaccine. Gardasil is a quadrivalent HPV vaccine which addresses HPV subtypes 6, 11, 16, and 18.

Aspiration

26. **Define aspiration. How does it differ from penetration?**
Aspiration occurs when a material passes from the upper airway below the true vocal cords. Alternatively, penetration occurs when a material passes into the larynx but not past the true vocal cords. Penetration deep into the larynx is a risk factor for aspiration.

27. **List the four phases of swallowing.**
See Table 48-2.

28. **How do abnormalities of the phases of swallowing contribute to aspiration?**
Any abnormality, whether anatomic or functional, of any phase of swallowing can contribute to swallowing dysfunction and ultimately result in aspiration. Dysfunction can be broken down into the affected phase of swallowing. For example, vocal cord paralysis can result in abnormal glottic closure during the pharyngeal phase of swallowing and possible aspiration. Neurologic disorders, on the other hand, can result in muscular weakness and dysfunction of any phase of swallowing.

29. **What are anatomic abnormalities that may predispose a pediatric patient to aspiration?**
Cleft palate, tracheoesophageal fistula, laryngeal cleft, macroglossia, and micrognathia are all examples of anatomic abnormalities of the head and neck that can lead to dysfunctional swallow and aspiration.

It is important to note that neurologic conditions, hypotonia, and certain syndromes (e.g., Down syndrome) are highly associated with aspiration during oral intake. Providers should keep this in mind when caring for these select patient populations.

30. **Discuss the workup of suspected pediatric aspiration.**
Evaluation for aspiration includes obtaining a history consistent with aspiration (coughing and choking with feeds, recurrent pneumonia, wheezing, respiratory distress, etc.) as well as supportive radiographic or endoscopic testing. Modified barium swallow studies (MBS) are used to evaluate the oral cavity, pharynx, and upper esophagus during swallowing. During MBS, different consistencies of barium preparations are given to the patient during fluoroscopy of the upper aerodigestive tract. Penetration and aspiration with different consistencies may be noted and recommendations regarding safe oral intake can be made.

Flexible or fiber-optic endoscopic evaluation of swallowing (FEES) is an additional method of evaluating the airway during oral intake. FEES relies on the direct visualization of swallow via a nasopharyngeal fiber-optic examination. During the examination, the patient is asked to swallow foods of varying consistency. MBS and FEES each have their strengths and weaknesses as tools for the evaluation of aspiration. Patients may undergo both exams in order to gain the greatest amount of information regarding their disease process.

BIBLIOGRAPHY

Benjamin B, Inglis A: Minor congenital laryngeal clefts: diagnosis and classification, *Ann Otol Rhinol Laryngol* 98:417, 1989.

Cole F: Pediatric formulas for the anesthesiologist, *Am J Dis Child* 94:672, 1957.

Derkay CS, Wiatrak B: Recurrent respiratory papillomatosis: a review, *Laryngoscope* 118:1236–1247, 2008.

Derkay C: Cidofovir for recurrent respiratory papillomatosis (RRP): a re-assessment of risks, *Int J Pediatr Otorhinolaryngol* 69:1465, 2005.

Fried M: *The Larynx*, ed 2, St. Louis, 1996, Mosby, pp 15–24.

Jacobs IN, Finkel RS: Laryngeal electromyography in the management of vocal cord mobility problems in children, *Laryngoscope* 112:1243, 2002.

King BR, Baker MD, Braitman LE, et al: Endotracheal tube selection in children: a comparison of four methods, *Ann Emerg Med* 22:530, 1993.

King EF, Blumin JH: Vocal cord paralysis in children, *Curr Opin Otolaryngol Head Neck Surg* 17:483–487, 2009.

Kosko JR, Derkay CS: Role of cesarean section in prevention of recurrent respiratory papillomatosis—is there one?, *Int J Pediatr Otorhinolaryngol* 35:31, 1996.

Myer CM III, O'Connor DM, Cotton RT: Proposed grading system for subglottic stenosis based on endotracheal tube sizes, *Ann Otol Rhinol Laryngol* 103:319, 1994.

Olney DR, Greinwald JH Jr, Smith RJ, et al: Laryngomalacia and its treatment, *Laryngoscope* 109:1999, 1770.

Orlow SJ, Isakoff MS, Blei F: Increased risk of symptomatic hemangiomas of the airway in association with cutaneous hemangiomas in a "beard" distribution, *J Pediatr* 131:643, 1997.

Peridis S, Pilgrim G, Athanasopoulos I, et al: A meta-analysis on the effectiveness of propranolol for the treatment of infantile airway hemangiomas, *Int J Pediatr Otorhinolaryngol* 75:455, 2011.

Truong MT, Messner AH, Kerschner JE, et al: Pediatric vocal fold paralysis after cardiac surgery: rate of recovery and sequelae, *Otolaryngol Head Neck Surg* 137:780–784, 2007.

Wiatrak BJ, Wiatrak DW, Broker TR, et al: Recurrent respiratory papillomatosis: a longitudinal study comparing severity associated with human papilloma viral types 6 and 11 and other risk factors in a large pediatric population, *Laryngoscope* 114:1, 2004.

CHAPTER 49

PEDIATRIC ADENOTONSILLAR DISEASE, SLEEP DISORDERED BREATHING AND OBSTRUCTIVE SLEEP APNEA

Norman R. Friedman, MD and Patricia J. Yoon, MD

KEY POINTS

1. There are no studies to date that demonstrate significant alterations in the immune system following an adenotonsillectomy.
2. Penicillin is the initial drug of choice for culture-positive streptococcal infections. Resistance to penicillin or first-generation cephalosporins has not been reported.
3. SDB is not a benign condition. It has been associated with social, behavioral, and neurocognitive problems, including decreased quality of life, growth impairment, and cardiovascular complications. Recent studies also suggest that SDB is associated with systemic inflammation.
4. Obstructive sleep apnea requires a PSG to make the diagnosis. Sleep disordered breathing is a clinical diagnosis.
5. The AAO/HNS guidelines strongly recommend against the routine administration of antibiotics postoperatively.
6. Ibuprofen is no longer contraindicated as a pain option following an adenotonsillectomy.
7. Tylenol with codeine is contraindicated due to an FDA black box warning. Both codeine and hydrocodone are metabolized to a more active compound. For hydrocodone, the analgesic activity is attributed to hydromorphone not hydrocodone.
8. Post-tonsillectomy bleeding can be a life-threatening complication and should be evaluated by an otolaryngologist.

Pearls

1. The classic rash associated with scarlet fever appears on the neck and face and then spreads and looks like a sunburn with tiny bumps. The rash will blanch when one presses on it.
2. If mononucleosis is suspected, amoxicillin should be avoided because it may cause a salmon-colored rash.
3. The most common indication for a tonsillectomy is SDB, followed by recurrent tonsillitis.
4. A submucous cleft palate is associated with a higher incidence of postadenoidectomy VPI.

QUESTIONS

ANATOMY AND FUNCTION

1. What is Waldeyer's ring?
   Waldeyer's ring is the lymphoid tissue surrounding the entrance to the aerodigestive tract. The structures composing this ring are the faucial (palatine) tonsils, pharyngeal tonsils (adenoid), and the lingual tonsil located at the base of the tongue.
2. Where are the adenoid and tonsils located?
   The adenoid is located midline along the posterior aspect of the nasopharynx at the level of the posterior chonae and extend laterally to the eustachian tube orifices. The palatine tonsils lie in a

fossa along the lateral walls of the oropharynx, between the anterior and posterior pillars. They extend superiorly from the soft palate down inferiorly to the tongue base. Here, they can appear to blend into the lingual tonsils. The palatine tonsils, in contrast to the lingual tonsils and adenoid, have a distinct capsule.

3. **Describe the blood supply to the palatine tonsils.**
The tonsils are supplied by several branches of the external carotid artery, including the tonsillar and ascending palatine branches of the facial artery, the ascending pharyngeal artery, the dorsal lingual branch of the lingual artery, and the palatine branch of the internal maxillary artery. The tonsillar branch of the facial artery provides the main blood supply.

4. **How is tonsillar hypertrophy graded?**
Tonsil size is graded as 1 to 4 according to the percentage projection from the anterior tonsillar pillar toward the midline. A 1 tonsil projects 0% to 25% from the anterior tonsillar pillar toward the midline; 2 projects 25% to 50%; 3 projects 50% to 75%; and 4 projects 75% to 100%. Tonsils graded 4 are sometimes referred to as "kissing" tonsils because they touch in the midline. The presence of enlarged tonsils does not necessarily mean that there will be disrupted breathing. Obstructive sleep apnea (OSA) arises as a combination of anatomic and neuromuscular factors.

5. **What is the function of the tonsils and adenoid?**
The tonsils and adenoid are predominantly B-cell lymphoid structures that probably play a role in secretory immunity. They are appropriately positioned for exposure to inhaled and ingested antigens, which can induce immunoglobulin and lymphokine production. Hyperplasia is thought to result from B-cell proliferation during exposure to high doses of antigen. It is generally accepted that removal of tonsils and adenoid does not produce a clinically significant immunologic deficiency. Tonsils and adenoid are immunologically most active between the ages of 4 and 10 years, and tend to involute after puberty. There are no studies to date that demonstrate significant alterations in the immune system following an adenotonsillectomy.

6. **What are tonsilloliths?**
Tonsillar concretions, or tonsilloliths, are whitish, cheesy, malodorous, foul-tasting lumps that can form in the tonsillar crypts. They arise from bacterial growth and retained debris, and although they are often asymptomatic, tonsilloliths can cause problems with halitosis, foreign body sensation, and otalgia. Conservative management includes gargling and expression and removal of tonsilloliths by the patient, performed with cotton swabs or a dental water jet device.

INFECTIONS

7. **How does bacterial tonsillitis present?**
Sudden onset of throat pain, odynophagia, enlarged erythematous tonsils with exudate, halitosis, fever, malaise, and tender cervical nodes are classic symptoms and signs of acute tonsillitis. The classic rash associated with scarlet fever appears on the neck and face and then spreads and looks like a sunburn with tiny bumps. The rash will blanch when one presses on it. Viral pharyngitis tends to be milder in presentation and usually without exudates. There may be an associated cold, cough, conjunctivitis, diarrhea, and rash. EBV is a notable exception.

8. **Name the most common infectious etiologic agents involved in adenotonsillar disease.**
Group A β–hemolytic streptococcus (GABHS) is the most common cause of acute tonsillitis and can be associated with such serious sequelae as rheumatic fever and poststreptococcal glomerulonephritis. Numerous other organisms, however, are commonly associated with adenotonsillar disease, including non-GABHS bacteria, and beta-lactamase–producing organisms such as *Bacteroides* species, nontypable *Haemophilus* species, *Staphylococcus aureus*, and *Moraxella catarrhalis*. Common viral pathogens include adenovirus, coxsackievirus, parainfluenza, enteroviruses, Epstein-Barr virus (EBV), herpes simplex virus, and respiratory syncytial virus.

9. **Describe the otolaryngologic manifestations of mononucleosis.**
Mononucleosis is caused by EBV and often produces an exudative tonsillitis that may appear indistinguishable from bacterial infections. Signs and symptoms of mononucleosis include high fever, malaise, generalized lymphadenopathy, enlarged tonsils with yellow-gray exudates, odynophagia, dysphagia, palatal petechiae, and hepatosplenomegaly. Useful lab results include

lymphocytosis and the presence of atypical lymphocytes, as well as a positive Monospot and heterophil antibody titers. If mononucleosis is suspected, amoxicillin should be avoided because it may cause a salmon-colored rash.

10. **How should adenotonsillar infection be treated?**
It can be difficult to distinguish viral from bacterial tonsillitis/pharyngitis. Most viral infections are self-limited and require only supportive care. If a bacterial infection is suspected, a rapid streptococcus detection test should be performed. If the test results are negative but suspicion for streptococcal tonsillitis is high, a throat culture should be performed. Penicillin is the initial drug of choice for culture-positive streptococcal infections. Resistance to penicillin or first-generation cephalosporins has not been reported. Tetracyclines, sulfonamides, and quinolones should not be used for treating GAS infections. If a child is a suspected strep carrier, the most effective treatment is clindamycin for 10 days.

11. **What is a peritonsillar abscess? How does it present?**
A peritonsillar abscess is a collection of pus in the potential space that surrounds the tonsil, between the tonsillar capsule and the superior constrictor muscle of the lateral pharyngeal wall. This process develops when infection penetrates the tonsillar capsule and enters the peritonsillar space. Over half of patients who present with peritonsillar abscess have a history of prior tonsillitis. Symptoms include throat pain, fever, dysphagia, a "hot potato" or muffled voice, trismus, and drooling. Examination reveals infected, swollen tonsils. The peritonsillar area is inflamed and swollen, usually unilaterally, with a bulge in the soft palate superior to the tonsil and displacement of the uvula toward the contralateral side.

12. **How is a peritonsillar abscess managed?**
Needle aspiration with recovery of pus can be diagnostic and therapeutic and has been shown to be effective over 90% of the time. This procedure can usually be performed in the office or emergency department. After drainage, an antibiotic with strong gram-positive and anerobic coverage, such as clindamycin, is recommended. Tonsillectomy is recommended if a patient has had more than one peritonsillar abscess. It is performed after complete resolution of the infection. In selected cases, a quinsy tonsillectomy (tonsillectomy in the presence of abscess) is indicated, such as when drainage fails to adequately treat the abscess, or sometimes in children, who often require a general anesthetic for drainage anyway.

Sleep Disordered Breathing

13. **How is obstructive sleep apnea (OSA) different from sleep disordered breathing (SDB)?**
OSA is a diagnosis that requires an abnormal polysomnogram. SDB is a clinical diagnosis with the following features: snoring with associated gasping, labored breathing, and daytime symptoms that may include hyperactivity, inattention, poor concentration, and excessive sleepiness (Box 49-1).

Box 49-1. Clinical Features of SDB

I. Nighttime symptoms:
   1. Habitual snoring
   2. Gasping, pauses, labored breathing
   3. Other symptoms that may be related to SDB include night terrors, sleep walking, and secondary enuresis

II. Daytime symptoms:
   1. Feeling unrefreshed after sleep
   2. Attention deficit
   3. Hyperactivity
   4. Emotional lability
   5. Temperamental behavior
   6. Poor weight gain
   7. Daytime fatigue
   8. Other symptoms that are suggestive of disruptive breathing patterns include daytime mouth breathing or dysphagia.

Box 49-2. Standard Components of a PSG Report

Sleep efficiency: Total sleep time divided by total recording time. This indicates how well the child slept.

Sleep architecture: Another indication of how well the child slept. An elevated amount of Stage 1 sleep suggests a disrupted sleep pattern. The amount of REM sleep is important because REM sleep is associated with muscle atonia. In the absence of REM sleep, one may underestimate the severity of obstruction.

Oxygen distribution and nadir: The oxygen distribution gives an indication of the gas exchange. The nadir is important because it helps determine if a child should be admitted for observation following a tonsillectomy.

End tidal CO_2 distribution: Some children may not have may obstructive events, but rather prolonged periods of partial obstructive hypoventilation that can only be detected by an elevated end tidal CO_2.

Obstructive index: Total number of obstructive respiratory events (obstructive apneas, obstructive hypopneas, and mixed apneas).

Central index: Total number of central apneas and central hypopneas.

Other Elements

Video: Comments on the appearance of the child during sleep. Some children may not have an elevated obstructive index, but may look pitiful with retractions, loud snoring, and paradoxical respirations (where the chest and abdomen, instead of rising up and down together, looks like a see-saw).

Morning-after questionnaire: To insure the parent feels that the sleep patterns were typical during the study.

14. What are the indications for requesting a polysomnogram?
According to the 2011 AAO/HNS guidelines one should obtain a preoperative polysomnogram prior to an adenotonsillectomy in the following circumstances: obesity, Down syndrome, craniofacial abnormalities, neuromuscular disorders, sickle cell disease, mucopolysaccharidoses, or if history and physical examination are discordant.

15. What does one assess during a sleep study?
The information contained in a sleep study allows one to evaluate sleep quality, degree of obstruction, and gas exchange (Box 49-2).

16. What are the criteria to diagnose OSA?
Most clinicians agree and recent research suggests that an obstructive apnea/hypopnea index greater than 5 events an hour is clinically relevant.

17. What is the P crit?
The P crit is a measure of airway collapsibility. The P crit of an airway will determine whether a patient has complete airway obstruction, partial obstruction, or no obstruction. A more negative P crit is indicative of an airway that is less prone to collapse (stiffer airway).

18. Does nasal patency matter?
Yes. A more patent nasal passage allows one to move air more easily into the upper airway. With a more patent nasal airway, the higher volume of air entering the pharynx will distend the upper airway and make it less likely to collapse.

19. Does an adenotonsillectomy cure OSA?
Adenotonsillectomy is not universally curative for OSA. Studies often have differing criteria for success of resolution of OSA after surgery. A large 2010 multicenter retrospective review of treatment outcomes for OSA after adenotonsillectomy gives somes clues to success. In order of influence, the following factors were associated with less improvement: age >7 years, elevated BMI, presence of asthma, and more severe OSA preoperatively (AHI >10 events/hour).

20. What are nonsurgical treatment options for residual OSA?
    - One study in children with mild residual OSA (AHI >1 but <5 events/hour) who were treated with anti-inflammatory therapy consisting of oral montelukast and intranasal nasal steroid for 12 weeks had normalization of their AHI.
    - Noninvasive ventilation is a nonsurgical treatment for OSA. Positive pressure is applied via a nasal mask to splint open the upper airway. Effectiveness is determined by how compliant the child is.
    - For children who have malocclusion and a contracted maxilla, rapid maxillary expansion has resulted in a dramatic improvement.

21. **What diagnostic tests are available to help identify the anatomic site of obstruction of a child with OSA?**
A cine MRI or drug induced sleep endoscopy will facilitate identification of sites of anatomic obstruction. Additional surgical interventions after adenotonsillectomy include an inferior turbinate reduction, lingual tonsillectomy, posterior tongue base reduction, and supraglottoplasty.

ADENOTONSILLECTOMY

22. **What are the indications for performing an adenotonsillectomy?**
The most common indication is SDB, followed by recurrent tonsillitis. Other less common indications include dypshagia due to large tonsils and suspected malignancy. AAO-HNS guidelines recommend surgical intervention for recurrent tonsillitis under the following circumstances: 7 infections in a 12-month period, 5 infections per year for 2 consecutive years, or 3 infections per year for 3 consecutive years.

23. **What are the clinical criteria for a throat infection to be counted as an acute tonsillitis to meet the AAO/HNS criteria for an adenotonsillectomy?**
See Box 49-3.

24. **List the contraindications for tonsillectomy and adenoidectomy.**
    1. Bleeding disorders
    2. Anemia
    3. Poor anesthetic risk due to uncontrolled medical illness
    4. Acute infection

25. **How are tonsils removed?**
The tonsil is dissected along the plane between the tonsillar capsule and the superior constrictor muscle. Tonsillectomy can be performed using either a "cold" or "hot" technique, and the merits of one over the other are much debated. In "cold" dissection, a superior mucosal incision is created with a knife, and then blunt dissection separates the tonsil from the tonsillar bed. The tonsil is then amputated at its inferior aspect, often using a snare. The "hot" technique employs electrocautery to cut and coagulate simultaneously. Some studies suggest that "cold" dissection may lead to less postoperative pain; however, there may be less intraoperative blood loss with electrocautery. Other devices have also been introduced for tonsillectomy, including lasers and ultrasonic and radiofrequency devices. Proponents cite advantages such as less postoperative pain; however, these advantages remain to be proven.

26. **Are any special precautions required in performing tonsillectomy and adenoidectomy on children with Down syndrome?**
About 12% of patients with Down syndrome have atlantoaxial instability. Cervical spine manipulations should be undertaken with the greatest of care when positioning these patients for surgery because neck extension may cause spinal cord compression. One also should be aware that these children have smaller airways so should initially be intubated with a tube that is smaller than their age-appropriate size.

27. **In patients with long-standing adenotonsillar obstruction, what pulmonary problem can occur after adenotonsillectomy?**
Pulmonary edema. The long-term obstruction by adenotonsillar tissue produces a state of increased positive end-expiratory pressure (PEEP). With removal of the obstructing tissue, the excess PEEP is suddenly relieved and fluid moves into the interstitial and alveolar spaces, resulting in pulmonary

Box 49-3. Clinical Criteria for an Acute Tonsil Infection

Presence of a sore throat & at least one of the following:
1. Cervical lymphadenopathy (lymph nodes tender or 2 cm)
2. Tonsillar exudates
3. Positive group A β-hemolytic streptococcus culture
4. Fever greater than 38.3° C

Table 49-1. Complications of Tonsillectomy and Adenoidectomy

I. Acute	Airway obstruction due to edema Postobstructive pulmonary edema
II. Subacute	Postoperative hemorrhage Dehydration and weight loss
III. Delayed	Velopharyngeal insufficiency Nasopharyngeal stenosis

edema with decreased blood oxygen saturation. This can occur intraoperatively or a few hours later. Treatment involves diuresis for mild cases, or intubation with reestablishment of increased PEEP in severe cases.

28. **List possible complications of tonsillectomy and adenoidectomy.**
See Table 49-1.

29. **What are the criteria to admit a child postoperatively after T&A for overnight monitoring?**
- Younger than 3 years of age with a diagnosis of SDB
- Abnormal polysomnogram with either an obstructive apnea/hypopnea index of ≥10 events per hour, or an oxygen saturation nadir <80%
- A child who has complications following the surgery, which may include hypoxemia, obstruction or poor oral intake. Social factors may also play a role, especially if there is not a reliable mode of transportation to return to the hospital or the family lives far from the hospital.
- Although the AAO/HNS clinical practice guideline advocates for preoperative polysomnogram for children with certain comorbidities, if a sleep study was not performed one should strongly consider hospital observation since one would not know the severity of the obstruction. It is also reasonable to have a low threshold to observe a child with complex heart disease.

30. **Should one administer perioperative antibiotics?**
The AAO/HNS guidelines strongly recommend against the routine administration of antibiotics postoperatively. There is no evidence that antibiotics aid recovery and there is the risk of adverse reactions, including rash, upset stomach, allergy, and inducing bacterial resistance.

31. **What should be given for post-tonsillectomy pain?**
Tylenol with codeine is contraindicated due to an FDA black box warning. Both codeine and hydrocodone are metabolized to a more active compound. For hydrocodone, the analgesic activity is attributed to hydromorphone not hydrocodone. Since the conversion to hydromorphone occurs via the CYP2D6 pathway (the same pathway codeine uses when converting to morphine) the concern for variability in response between ultra-rapid and poor metabolizers exists—oversedation in ultra-rapid metabolizers and minimal pain relief in poor metabolizers. The presence of ultra-rapid metabolizers is highest in the Ethiopian African population (29%) and lowest in Northern Europeans (1% to 2%).

NSAID use has been controversial but since 2011 has become more acceptable. A Cochrane review demonstrated NSAID safety with the exception of ketorolac. Particularly in the immediate postoperative period, NSAIDs may theoretically induce some platelet dysfunction. One study in adults demonstrated that reversible inhibition of platelets lasted for 6 to 8 hours after administration of 400 mg of ibuprofen. It may be prudent to wait for at least 8 hours prior to ibuprofen administration after an adenotonsillectomy to allow for clot maturation. Besides medications, families need to be educated on what to expect following surgery, and to encourage good hydration, which will lessen pain.

32. **What does the postoperative management of adenotonsillectomy involve?**
Expect significant pain and fatigue for about 1 week, and often longer in teenagers and adults. Children should plan to take 7 to 10 days off from school, and strenuous activity should be avoided for 2 weeks. Pain control is important to promote oral intake of liquids and to prevent dehydration. Diet may be advanced as tolerated; many recommend a soft diet.

Throat and/or ear pain (referred pain), halitosis, and low-grade fevers are normal after surgery. No further bleeding should occur. If fresh blood is seen, it should be brought to the attention of the otolaryngologist immediately. There may be some blood-tinged saliva around postoperative day 5 to 7, when the "scab" falls off the surgical site. If this does not stop within several minutes, or if it should worsen, medical attention should be sought.

33. What is the incidence of postoperative tonsillectomy bleeding?
The rate of primary hemorrhage (occurring within 24 hours of surgery) ranges from 0.2% to 2.2%. The rate of secondary hemorrhage (occurring more than 24 hours after surgery) has been quoted as anywhere from 0.1% to 3%.

34. How is postoperative bleeding managed?
A patient presenting to the emergency department with a post-tonsillectomy bleed should be examined by an otolaryngologist. The tonsillar fossae should be carefully examined, looking for active bleeding sites or evidence of a clot. If active bleeding is encountered, it should be controlled with cautery and/or suture ligation. If no abnormality is seen and only minimal bleeding is reported, then observation is reasonable. If a clot is present without active bleeding, the patient should be admitted for overnight observation, ready for surgery in case bleeding should reoccur. Depending on the history, a hematocrit and coagulation profile may be drawn. The threshold for admission and intervention should be lower in smaller children who have a lower blood volume to begin with.

ADENOID

35. What problems are caused by the adenoid?
Adenoid can become acutely and chronically infected. Symptoms may be difficult to differentiate from bacterial or viral upper respiratory infections and are often mislabeled as "sinusitis." Adenoiditis commonly presents as fever, purulent rhinorrhea, nasal obstruction, and otalgia. Postnasal drip, congestion, chronic cough, and halitosis can occur during chronic infections.

Adenoid hypertrophy can cause nasal obstruction, contribute to obstructive sleep apnea, and result in hyponasal speech. Chronic hypertrophy and mouth breathing can also cause alterations in craniofacial growth. "Adenoid facies" is characterized by an open mouth, facial elongation, a high arched palate, an open anterior bite with protrusion of the upper incisors, and flattened midface. It is also believed that adenoid play a role in patients with recurrent otitis media or effusions by mechanically obstructing the eustachian tubes and by providing a bacterial nidus for infection.

36. How is the adenoid evaluated?
In patients with suspected adenoid hypertrophy, breathing and speech should be assessed. Words that emphasize nasal emission such as "mommy" can be useful in demonstrating hyponasality. The nose should be examined for other causes of obstruction such as enlarged turbinates. The adenoid cannot be seen by looking in the mouth or the anterior nose, but it is generally assumed that children with significant obstructive symptoms who require tonsillectomy will have enlarged adenoid as well. The adenoid is visualized at the time of surgery and removed accordingly. Lateral neck radiography and fiber-optic endoscopy can be used to assess the adenoid if there is diagnostic uncertainty.

37. What nonsurgical therapies are available for adenoiditis or adenoid hypertrophy?
    1. Antibiotics are used to treat infectious adenoiditis.
    2. Nasal steroid sprays can improve adenoidal hypertrophy.

38. List the indications for adenoidectomy.
    1. Recurrent acute or chronic adenoiditis
    2. Nasal obstruction with chronic mouth breathing
    3. Hyponasal speech
    4. Craniofacial growth abnormalities
    5. Obstructive sleep apnea
    6. Recurrent otitis media or persistent effusion in patients who have undergone prior tympanostomy tube placement (adenoidectomy usually performed in conjunction with a subsequent tube placement procedure)

39. **How is the adenoid removed?**
Adenoidectomy is performed transorally, and the nasopharynx is visualized using a laryngeal mirror. Tissue can be removed by the following methods:
   1. Curetting is the traditional method for adenoidectomy. The curette is positioned high in the nasopharynx against the septal vomer and then swept inferiorly, thereby cutting out the adenoid tissue. Hemostasis is achieved by packing followed by suction cautery.
   2. Suction cautery can be used to fulgurate the adenoid tissue. This method is associated with less intraoperative blood loss and is ideal for smaller adenoid, although it can be used routinely as well.
   3. The microdebrider can be used to shave away adenoid tissue. Care must be taken to avoid injury to surrounding structures with powered instrumentation.

40. **Why can velopharyngeal insufficiency (VPI) occur after adenoidectomy?**
VPI occurs when there is incomplete closure of the soft palate against the posterior pharyngeal wall during speech and swallowing. VPI results in hypernasal speech and nasopharyngeal regurgitation. In children, adenoid tissue significantly adds to the bulk of the posterior pharyngeal wall. An adenoidectomy reduces this bulk and can lead to incomplete closure. Most cases are temporary, but persistent or severe cases may require speech therapy and/or surgical treatment.
The incidence of VPI after adenoidectomy ranges from 1/1500 to 1/10,000 in healthy patients. The incidence is much higher in patients with palatal disorders.

41. **Why should one always inspect and palpate the palate prior to adenoidectomy?**
A submucous cleft palate is associated with a higher incidence of postadenoidectomy VPI. Signs of a submucous cleft include a bifid uvula, zona pellucida, and notching of the posterior hard palate. In the presence of these findings, a superior pole adenoidectomy is recommended. This procedure removes obstructing tissue from the choanal area but preserves bulk in the posterior pharyngeal wall.

Bibliography

Baugh RF, Archer SM, Mitchell RB, et al: American Academy of Otolaryngology-Head and Neck Surgery Foundation: clinical practice guideline: tonsillectomy in children, *Otolaryngol Head Neck Surg* 144(1 Suppl):S1–S30, 2011. doi: 10.1177/0194599810389949. PMID: 21493257.

Bhattacharjee R, Kheirandish-Gozal L, Spruyt K, et al: Adenotonsillectomy outcomes in treatment of obstructive sleep apnea in children: a multicenter retrospective study, *Am J Respir Crit Care Med* 182(5):676–683, 2010.

Casselbrant ML: What is wrong in chronic adenoiditis/tonsillitis anatomical considerations, *Int J Pediatr Otorhinolaryngol* 49:S133–S135, 1999.

Friedman M, LoSavio P, Ibrahim H, et al: Radiofrequency tonsil reduction: safety, morbidity, and efficacy, *Laryngoscope* 113:882–887, 2003.

Goldsmith AJ, Rosenfeld RM: Tonsillectomy, adenoidectomy, and UPPP. In *surgical Atlas of Pediatric Otolaryngology*, Hamilton, Ontario, 2002, BC Decker, pp 380–405.

Goldstein NA, Armfield DR, Kingsley LA, et al: Postoperative complications after tonsillectomy and adenoidectomy in children with Down syndrome, *Arch Otolaryngol Head Neck Surg* 124:171–176, 1998.

Hong Y, Gengo M, Rainka M, et al: Population pharmacodynamic modeling of aspirin- and ibuprofen-induced inhibition of platelet aggregation in healthy subjects, *Clin Pharmacokinet* 47(20):129–137, 2008.

Hultcrantz E, Linder A, Markstrom A: Tonsillectomy or tonsillotomy? A randomized study comparing postoperative pain and long-term effects, *Int J Pediatr Otorhinolaryngol* 51:171–176, 1999.

Jones KL: Chromosomal abnormality syndromes: Down syndrome. In *Smith's Recognizable Patterns of Human Malformation*, ed 5, Philadelphia, 1997, Saunders, pp 8–10.

Kheirandish L, Goldbart AD, Gozal D: Intranasal steroids and oral leukotriene modifier therapy in residual sleep-disordered breathing after tonsillectomy and adenoidectomy in children, *Pediatrics* 117(1):e61–e66, 2006. PubMed PMID: 16396849.

Koltai PJ, Solares CA, Koempel JA, et al: Intracapsular tonsillar reduction (partial tonsillectomy): reviving a historical procedure for obstructive sleep disordered breathing in children, *Otolaryngol Head Neck Surg* 129:532–538, 2003.

Marcus CL, Brooks LJ, Draper KA, et al: American Academy of Pediatrics: Diagnosis and management of childhood obstructive sleep apnea syndrome, *Pediatrics* 130(3):e714–e755, 2012. doi: 10.1542/peds.2012-1672. [Epub 2012 Aug 27]; [Review]. PMID: 22926176.

Marcus CL, Brooks LJ, Draper KA, et al: American Academy of Pediatrics: Diagnosis and management of childhood obstructive sleep apnea syndrome, *Pediatrics* 130(3):576–584, 2012. doi: 10.1542/peds.2012-1671. [Epub 2012 Aug 27]; PMID: 22926173.

Marcus CL, Moore RH, Rosen CL, et al: Childhood Adenotonsillectomy Trial (CHAT). A randomized trial of adenotonsillectomy for childhood sleep apnea, *N Engl J Med* 368(25):2366–2376, 2013. doi: 10.1056/NEJMoa1215881. [Epub 2013 May 21]; PubMed PMID: 23692173. PubMed Central PMCID: PMC3756808.

Nicklaus PJ, Herzon FS, Steinle EW: Short-stay outpatient tonsillectomy, *Arch Otolaryngol Head Neck Surg* 121: 521–524, 1995.

Nunez DA, Provan J, Crawford M: Postoperative tonsillectomy pain in pediatric patients: Electrocautery (hot) versus cold dissection and snare tonsillectomy: a randomized trial, *Arch Otolaryngol Head Neck Surg* 126:837–841, 2000.

Paradise JL: Tonsillectomy and adenoidectomy. In Bluestone CD, Stool SE, Alper CM, et al, editors: *Pediatric Otolaryngology*, ed 4, Philadelphia, 2002, W.B. Saunders, pp 1210–1222.

Randall DA, Hoffer ME: Complications of tonsillectomy and adenoidectomy, *Otolaryngol Head Neck Surg* 118:61–68, 1998.

Richardson MA: Sore throat, tonsillitis, and adenoiditis, *Med Clin North Am* 83:75–83, 1999.

Roland PS, Rosenfeld RM, Brooks LJ, et al: American Academy of Otolaryngology—Head and Neck Surgery Foundation: Clinical practice guideline: polysomnography for sleep-disordered breathing prior to tonsillectomy in children, *Otolaryngol Head Neck Surg* 145(1 Suppl):S1–S15, 2011. [Epub 2011 Jun 15]; PMID: 21676944.

Tan HL, Gozal D, Kheirandish-Gozal L: Obstructive sleep apnea in children: a critical update, *Nat Sci Sleep* 5:109–123, 2013. eCollection 2013. Review. PubMed PMID: 24109201. PubMed Central PMCID: PMC3792928.

Wiatrak BJ, Woolley AL: Pharyngitis and adenotonsillar disease. In Cummings CW, Fredrickson JM, Harker LA, et al, editors: *Otolaryngology Head & Neck Surgery*, vol 5, ed 3, St. Louis, 1998, Mosby, pp 188–215.

CONGENITAL MALFORMATIONS OF THE HEAD AND NECK

CHAPTER 50

Craig Quattlebaum, MD and Sven-Olrik Streubel, MD, MBA

KEY POINTS

1. A hemangioma is typically absent at birth and undergoes proliferation before reaching the involution stage.
2. Lymphatic malformations are not true tumors but grow commensurately with the patient and can rapidly expand with infection, bleeding, or trauma.
3. Sistrunk procedure involves removal of the anterior portion of the hyoid and results in decreased recurrence rates for TDCs.
4. Laryngomalacia will usually resolve by 1 year of age. Surgical treatment with supraglottoplasty is reserved for cases of significant breathing or feeding problems.
5. Infants are obligate nasal breathers and the presence of bilateral choanal atresia is a life-threatening anomaly at birth.

Pearls

1. A "beard"distribution of hemangioma in a stridulous child should raise suspicion for subglottic hemangioma.
2. Branchial cleft anomalies track deep to the structures of their own arch and superficial to the structures of the subsequent arch.
3. Always evaluate for normal thyroid prior to removing thyroglossal duct cyst.
4. Pseudotumor of infancy (SCM tumor) responds to conservative treatment by 1 year of age in 80%.
5. The differential for midline nasal mass includes glioma, dermoid, and encephalocele. Imaging should always be obtained prior to excision for diagnosis and to rule out intracranial extension.

QUESTIONS

1. **What is the differential for a congenital neck mass?**
   See Table 50-1.

2. **What is a thyroglossal duct cyst (TDC) and how does it form?**
   TDCs are the most common congenital neck mass in the pediatric population. At 3 weeks of gestation, the thyroid gland forms from a diverticulum at the oral tongue (the foramen cecum). As development continues this diverticulum descends to fuse with components of the fourth and fifth branchial pouch, anterior to or through the hyoid, and to the thyroid's final location in the neck. At 5 to 8 weeks, the tract formed by this descent obliterates leaving the foramen cecum proximally and the pyramidal lobe of the thyroid distally. Incomplete obliteration results in a TDC anywhere along this tract. Because of its origin, a TDC generally elevates with extrusion of the tongue.

3. **What must be considered before surgical treatment and what is the treatment of choice?**
   Preoperative evaluation for TDC should include preoperative thyroid ultrasound to rule out an ectopic thyroid gland. Failure to do so could mean removing the patient's only functioning thyroid tissue along with the cyst.

Table 50-1. Differential Diagnosis of Congenital Neck Mass

SITE	CHARACTERISTICS
Midline	
Thyroglossal duct cyst	Elevates with swallowing
Dermoid cyst	Usually submental, moves with skin
Teratoma	Firm, CT with calcification, rare in neck
Plunging ranula	Midline, cystic, extends to floor of mouth
Lateral	
Branchial cleft cyst	Deep to anterior border of SCM, fluctuant
Lymphangioma	Soft, compressible, transilluminate, CT/MRI
External laryngocoele	Air-filled, protrude through thyrohyoid membrane, hoarseness, cough, CT helpful
SCM tumor	Firm, painless, discrete, fusiform mass
Extensive	
Lymphangioma	Thin-walled, multiloculated cysts
Hemangioma	Red/bluish soft mass, size increases with cry

CT, Computed tomography; SCM, sternocleidomastoid; MRI, magnetic resonance imaging.
Adapted from Wetmore R, Potsic W: Differential diagnosis of neck masses. In Cummings CW, Frederickson JM, Harker LA, et al, editors: Otolaryngology Head and Neck Surgery, ed 3, St. Louis: Mosby, 1998, p. 248–261.

Historically, recurrence of a TDC was very high (38% to 70%). The Sistrunk procedure includes excision of the cyst, the tract connecting it to the foramen cecum, and the central portion of the hyoid bone resulting in a recurrence rate of 2.6% to 5%. It is also notable that rarely (less than 1%), TDCs can harbor malignancy. This is usually well differentiated thyroid carcinoma. Complete removal with Sistrunk offers an excellent cure rate.

4. **Two additional midline masses are teratomas and dermoid cysts. How do these differ?**
Teratomas are composed of all three germ layers and are larger and typically more symptomatic than dermoid cysts. They are often diagnosed by prenatal ultrasound and 30% are associated with hydramnios secondary to esophageal obstruction. Dermoid cysts are composed of only ectoderm and mesoderm and form from entrapped epithelium along the lines of embryonic fusion (midline). They will enlarge over time as they fill with sebaceous material and have characteristic "cheesy" contents upon excision.

5. **What are the types of branchial anomalies (BA) and how do they form?**
An understanding of the embryology is crucial to the identification and management of BAs. At 4 weeks gestation there are 4 pairs of branchial arches and 2 rudimentary arches. These are externally lined with ectoderm and internally lined with endoderm, with mesoderm between. The arches are separated by pouches internally and clefts externally. These clefts and pouches are gradually replaced with mesenchyme forming well-defined anatomic stuctures. When the clefts and pouches persist, BAs are formed. There are three types:
    1. Cyst: remnant with no internal or external opening. Lined with squamous epithelium.
    2. Sinus: remnant with an external opening, often draining to the skin. Often lined with ciliated columnar epithelium.
    3. Fistula: remant with internal (aerodigestive tract) and external opening (skin). Also lined with ciliated columnar epithelium.

6. **Discuss the types of BAs in relation to their developmental origin. Where would you expect them to track?**
BAs follow a predictable course, as each branchial arch has an associated artery, cranial nerve, muscles (innervated by the cranial nerve of that arch), and skeletal/cartilagenous structure. The course of a BA is deep to the structures derived from its own arch and superficial to the structures of the subsequent arches (Table 50-2). First branchial cleft cysts are rare (1% of BA) and present as a cyst, sinus, or fistulae between the external auditory canal and the submandibular area. Type 1

Table 50-2. Courses of Branchial Anomilies

PHARYNGEAL ARCH	ARCH ARTERY	CRANIAL NERVE	SKELETAL ELEMENTS	MUSCLES
1	Terminal branch of maxillary artery	Maxillary and mandibular division of trigeminal (V)	Incus, malleus, Mackel's cartilage, upper portion of auricle, maxilla, zygomatic, squamous portion of temporal bone, mandible	Muscles of mastication (temporalis, masseter, and pterygoids), mylohyoid, anterior belly of digastric, tensor tympani, tensor veli palatini
2	Stapedius artery (embryologic) and corticotympanic artery (adult)	Facial nerve (VII)	Stapes, styloid process, stylohyoid ligament, lesser horns and upper rim of hyoid, lower portion of auricle	Muscles of facial expression (orbicularis oculi, orbicularis oris, fronto-occipitalis, buccinator), posterior belly of digastric, stylohyoid, stapedius
3	Common carotid artery, most of internal carotid	Glossopharyngeal (IX)	Lower rim and greater horn of hyoid	Stylopharyngeus
4	Left: Arch of aorta; Right: Right subclavian artery; Original sprouts of pulmonary arteries	Superior laryngeal branch of vagus (X)	Laryngeal cartilages (Derived from the 4th arch cartilage, originate from lateral plate mesoderm)	Constrictors of pharynx, cricothyroid, levator veli palatini
6	Ductus arteriosus; roots of definitive pulmonary arteries	Recurrent laryngeal branch of vagus (X)	Laryngeal cartilages (derived from the 6th-arch cartilage; originate from lateral plate mesoderm)	Intrinsic muscles of larynx

first BAs track lateral to the facial nerve and are duplications of the external auditory canal while Type 2 first BAs are typically medial to the nerve. Both can terminate at the EAC or middle ear. The main differentiation is that Type 1 first BAs do not contain mesoderm while type 2 BAs do. They usually require parotidectomy and facial nerve dissection for excision. Second branchial cleft anomalies are most common (95%) and are found along the anterior border of the SCM. They track between the internal and external carotid arteries and terminate at the tonsillar fossa. Third and fourth branchial anomalies are rare and present lower along the anterior border of the SCM and terminate in the ipsilateral piriform sinus. Because of the embryology, the tract of a fourth BA on the right loops under the subclavian, while on the left will travel to the mediastinum and under the aortic arch before leading to the piriform.

7. What is a pseudotumor of infancy?
This refers to a firm rounded mass within the sternocleidomastoid (SCM) muscle. Also called SCM tumor of infancy or fibromatosis coli, it presents usually 2 to 3 weeks after birth. The mass is characterized histologically by dense fibrous tissue and the absence of striated muscle. Implicated in the etiology is birth trauma, ischemia of muscle, or intrauterine positioning. Conservative treatment and physical therapy results in resolution by 1 year of age in greater than 80% of cases.

8. What is the differential for a midline nasal mass?
   - **Nasal dermoid:** Most common of the three. Nasal dermoids present as a noncompressible mass over the nasal dorsum, anywhere from the glabella to the columella. There is usually an assocated midline pit with hair at the opening. Treatment is surgical excision.
   - **Glioma:** Likely forms when a cranial suture closes, isolating a portion of brain tissue from the cranial cavity. They can sometimes have a fibrous stalk that maintains a connection to the CNS but by definition they do not contain herniated dura.
   - **Encephalocele:** A herniation of meninges and brain matter through a bony skull base defect. The mass will illuminate and will enlarge with straining or crying (Furstenberg's sign). All midline masses should be imaged prior to operative planning (MRI and CT may be complementary).

9. What is choanal atresia (CA)?
At 1 in 8000 live births, CA is the most common congenital nasal anomaly. It is more commonly unilateral, right-sided, and affects females more than males. The choana is the posterior nasal aperture by which air flows from the nasal cavity into the nasopharynx. It can be bony or membranous with most recent data citing membranous as more common. Because infants are obligate nasal breathers, bilateral CA (usually associated with a syndrome or association such as CHARGE, Crouzon, or Treacher-Collins) is life-threatening. Atresia is suspected when a 5–6 French catheter cannot be passed into the nasopharynx at birth.

10. What is the most common cause of stridor in infants? What are the classic findings on exam?
Laryngomalacia accounts for 60% to 75% of all congenital laryngeal anomalies. The associated stridor is caused by the airflow dynamics of the supraglottic tissues (epiglottis, aryepiglottic folds, arytenoids) upon inspiration. Typically infants have few to no symptoms at birth but gradually develop high-pitched inspiratory stridor in the first weeks of life that usually resolves by 1 year of age. In cases where laryngomalacia causes significant breathing or feeding problems it is treated with supraglottoplasty. Because of its dynamic nature, laryngomalacia must be diagnosed with endoscopic visualization while the infant is awake and breathing. An omega-shaped epiglottis and foreshortened aryepiglottic folds are the classic finding. Laryngomalacia is usually associated with significant laryngoesophageal reflux making acid supression first line in nonsurgical therapy.

11. How common is congenital vocal fold immobility?
Congenital immobility of one or both vocal cords is the second most common congenital laryngeal disorder. Unilateral immobility may manifest as a weak or breathy cry, poor feeding, or aspiration. Bilateral immobility, while thankfully less common, can be life-threatening and results in biphasic stridor at birth. Etiology is often idiopathic but can include birth trauma, hydrocephalus, spina bifida, cerebral palsy, and Arnold-Chiari malformation.

12. What are the two most common malformations of the subglottis?
Congenital subglottic stenosis (SGS) is defined as a diameter of <4 mm in the newborn (3 in the premature infant) and can be considered congenital only prior to any attempt at intubation. The stenosis can be membranous (more common, less severe) or cartilagenous. SGS will typically

present in the first few months of life with biphasic or inspiratory stridor and recurrent/persistent croup. Depending on the severity of stenosis, treatment can include watchful waiting with medical management of episodic croup, anterior cricoid split, or tracheostomy.

A hemangioma of the subglottic area classically presents in the third or fourth week of life with inspiratory or biphasic stridor, harsh cough, abnormal cry, and failure to thrive. Approximately 50% of infants with subglottic hemangioma have additional cutaneous hemangiomas. Spontaneous regression of these lesions often occurs by 5 years of age. When the lesion is obstructing the airway, treatment options include beta blockers, cryotherapy, sclerotherapy, systemic or intralesional steroid, open surgical resection, tracheostomy, and laser ablation.

13. What is a laryngotracheal cleft?

Laryngeal and laryngotracheal clefts are uncommon posterior clefts of varying severity caused by incomplete development of the tracheoesophageal septum. Presentation includes a hoarse cry, cyanosis, coughing, choking, stridor, aspiration, and recurrent pneumonia depending on the length of the cleft.

They are classified into 4 types based on the distal extent of the cleft:

Type 1 is an interarytenoid cleft with absence of the interarytenoid muscle (above the level of the vocal cords)
Type 2 extends into the upper cricoid
Type 3 involves the entire cricoid with or without extension into the cervical trachea
Type 4 cleft extends into the thoracic trachea

14. Name the five types of tracheoesophageal anomalies and discuss their presentation and diagnosis.

- Esophageal atresia with distal tracheoesophageal fistula (≈85%)
- Isolated esophageal atresia without fistula (≈8%)
- Tracheoesophageal fistula without atresia or H-type (≈5%)
- Esophageal atresia with proximal tracheoesophageal fistula (≈1%)
- Esophageal atresia with proximal and distal tracheoesophageal fistula (≈0.5% to 1%)

When atresia is present, there are copius oral secretions with episodes of coughing and respiratory distress with feeds in the first few days of life. Symptoms depend on the severity of atresia. A nasogastric tube cannot be passed. The H-type fistula can present later with chronic feeding difficulties and recurrent respiratory distress and/or pneumonia. Diagnosis can be made with a barium esophagram and/or endoscopy.

15. What are the two classifications of tracheal malformations? What causes them?

Intrinsic malformations are caused by improper development of the trachea. Examples of intrinsic malformations include tracheal agenesis (not compatible with life), congenital tracheal stenosis (often with complete tracheal rings), and tracheomalacia.

Extrinsic causes of tracheomalacia are secondary to compression of the airway from the structures that surround it. Causes include vascular compression (e.g., innominate artery, double aortic arch, right aortic arch with persistent ductus or ligamentum arteriosum), masses in the neck and mediastinum, and thyromegaly.

16. What are the most common external auricular deformities?

Lop ear is the most frequent, and treatment involves molding the fold of the superior crus in the early neonatal period. Stahl's ear is the result of an abnormal fold in the scapha and responds to pressing out of this area. Protruding ear is third most common, and the percentage increases during growth. Correction is achieved by affixing the posterior helical rim to the posterior retroauricular region with surgical tape. More recently, surgeons have also used dental wax to mold the ear in addition to taping.

17. How are microtia deformities described?

Microtia is hypoplasia of the external ear. It can be associated with or without atresia of the external auditory canal (EAC). It may be present as an isolated deformity or may be associated with other anomalies (e.g., Treacher Collins, Goldenhar's syndrome). There is no universal classification scheme, but type I includes a normal auricle or one with deformities that are mild and will not require the use of additional skin or cartilage for reconstruction. Type II deformities are those where some structures of a normal auricle are recognizable and reconstruction will require additional skin and/or cartilage. Type III are those with no recognizable landmarks of the auricle or canal. These will require large amounts or cartilage and skin for reconstruction.

18. **How are most type III microtias managed?**
Current therapy for microtia is multistage (2 to 4 stages) reconstructive surgery using an autologous rib graft for the framework. Stage I consists of cartilage implantation. Stage II is done 2 to 3 months after and is transfer of the lobule. Stage III involves elevation of the cartilage graft and postauricular skin grafting, and stage IV reconstructs the tragus. Initial workup should always include audiologic evaluation, and placement of a bone anchored hearing device before 1 year of age should be considered in cases of bilateral hearing loss. While the optimal timing of repair is controversial, the usual age is between 6 and 8 years.

19. **Explain the anomalies of the first branchial groove.**
The first branchial groove gives rise to the EAC. Anomalies are divided into aplasia, atresia, stenosis, and duplication of the EAC. Aplasia occurs when the first branchial groove does not develop. The groove usually persists as a tract. Atresia anomalies occur when the EAC is present but the lumen fails to develop, leaving a core of bone, fibrous tissue, or both. Stenosis occurs when the lumen is narrowed, which occurs in varying degrees of severity. Duplication occurs when the EAC develops normally, but the tract persists from the canal to the skin of the neck.

20. **How do cup ear deformities and prominent ear deformities differ?**
A cup ear deformity is a congenital malformation of the auricle in which the upper and middle portions are abnormal and the lower portion is normal. The upper portion is bent forward and downward. The middle portion is generally large and at a 90-degree angle from the skull. It can be present in various degrees of severity. In a prominent ear deformity, the child has protruding ears. Measured from the mastoid to the ear, this produces an angle of 40 degrees or a distance of 20 mm. Both cup ear and prominent ear deformities can be improved with reconstructive surgery.

21. **How do hemangiomas and vascular malformations differ?**
Hemangiomas are rarely present at birth and undergo a rapid postnatal proliferation phase followed by slow involution. They are the most common neonatal tumor (10% incidence) and demonstrate increased capillary tubule formation in vitro. A vascular malformation (VM) is always present at birth and is not a tumor as there is no cellular hyperplasia or cellular proliferation. VMs are a product of abnormal morphogenesis of vascular channels. They do not proliferate or involute but can grow larger with hypertrophy of existing cells or filling of cystic spaces with trauma, infection, and hormonal changes. They are classified as either low flow (capillary malformations, venous malformations, lymphatic malformations, or combined types) or high flow (arterial malformations and arteriovenous malformations).

22. **What syndromes or findings are associated with vascular malformations and hemangiomas?**
In Sturge-Weber, a facial capillary malformation (port wine stain) in the region of CN V1 is a classic finding and should raise suspicion for a vascular malformation of the leptomeninges on that side.
Klippel Trenaunay syndrome describes a cutaneous capillary malformation with an underlying venous/lymphatic malformation and is associated with skeletal overgrowth of a limb.
Though not a named syndrome, a beard distribution of cutaneous hemangiomas should raise suspicion for subglottic hemangioma.

Bibliography

Acierno S, Waldhausen J: Congenital cervical cysts, sinuses and fistulae, *Otolaryngol Clin N Am* 40:161–176, 2007.

Ahmad S, Soliman A: Congenital anomalies of the larynx, *Otolaryngol Clin N Am* 40:177–191, 2007.

Chandra R, Gerber M, Holinger L: Histologic insight into the pathogenesis of severe laryngomalacia, *Int J Pediatr Otorhinolaryngol* 61:31–38, 2001.

Matsuo K, Hayashi R, Kiyono M, et al: Nonsurgical correction of congenital auricular deformities, *Clin Plast Surg* 17:383–395, 1990.

Muriaki C, Quatela V: Reconstruction surgery of the ear. In Cummings CW, Frederickson JM, Harker LA, et al, editors: *Otolaryngology Head and Neck Surgery*, ed 3, St. Louis, 1998, Mosby, pp 439–460.

Radowski D, Arnold J, Healy GB, et al: Thyroglossal duct remnants: Preoperative evaluation and management, *Arch Otolaryngol Head Neck Surg* 117:1378, 1991.

Sandu K, Monnier P: Congenital tracheal anomalies, *Otolaryngol Clin N Am* 40:193–217, 2007.

Toynton SC: Aryepiglottoplasty for laryngomalacia: 100 consecutive cases, *J Laryngol Otol* 115:35–38, 2001.

CHAPTER 51

CLEFT LIP AND PALATE

Gregory C. Allen, MD, FACS, FAAP

KEY POINTS

1. The etiology of cleft lip and palate is multifactorial, including both syndromic and nonsyndromic causes.
2. Embryologically, clefts of the lip and primary palate are due to failure of fusion between the medial nasal prominence and the maxillary prominence, the lateral nasal prominence, or both.
3. The Millard, or rotation, advancement is the most common technique for repair of the unilateral cleft lip.
4. VPI is hypernasality during speech or reflux of saliva or food into the nasopharynx during swallowing. VPI occurs when the nasopharynx and oropharynx are not successfully separated by complete palatal closure during certain speech sounds or during swallowing.

Pearls

1. A higher frequency of cleft lip and palate occurs in Native Americans, those of Asian descent, and those of Latin American descent (1 : 400). The lowest frequency is reported in African Americans (1 : 1500 to 2000). Cleft palate alone is fairly consistent among ethnic groups at 1 : 2000. There is a male predominance in cleft lip and palate, and a female predominance in cleft palate alone.
2. Cleft lip and palate most commonly occur together (50%). Cleft palate alone occurs in 35%, and cleft lip alone in 15%. Left unilateral cleft lip and palate is the most common.
3. Know the classic characteristics of cleft nose deformity.

QUESTIONS

1. **Who cares for children with cleft lip and palate?**
It is generally agreed that a multidisciplinary team best treats children with cleft lip and palate. This team is usually composed of a diverse group of clinicians, including otolaryngologists, plastic surgeons, pediatric dentists, orthodontists, occupational therapists, pediatricians, speech therapists, audiologists, social workers, geneticists, psychologists, and feeding specialists/nutritionists. Each team member provides expertise in an area needed in the treatment of children who are born with a cleft.

2. **Are there guidelines regarding the care of children with cleft lip and/or palate?**
A report about children with special needs issued in 1987 by the Surgeon General of the United States stressed that the care of children with clefts should be comprehensive, coordinated, culturally sensitive, specific to the needs of the individual, and readily accessible. The Maternal and Child Health Bureau recognized that children with clefts and/or other craniofacial anomalies have special needs and in 1991 provided funding to the American Cleft Palate-Craniofacial Association (ACPA) to develop standards for their health care. As part of these parameters of care, it has been recommended that treatment of cleft and craniofacial conditions occur in a team setting. In 1993, the ACPA released Parameters for Evaluation and Treatment of Patients with Cleft Lip/Palate or Other Craniofacial Anomalies. These parameters have been revised several times, most recently in 2009, and serve as a basis for teams to achieve and maintain accreditation.

3. **Summarize the guidelines for the cleft palate team.**
   - The team should consist of an operating surgeon, orthodontist, speech-language pathologist, and at least one additional specialist from otolaryngology, audiology, pediatrics, genetics, social work, psychology, and general pediatric or prosthetic dentistry, who meet face to face at least six times per year to evaluate and develop treatment plans for the team's patients.

- The team should evaluate at least 50 patients per year.
- The team should have at least one surgeon who operates on at least 10 primary cleft lips and/or palates per year.
- The team should coordinate treatment and ensure that a primary care physician evaluates each patient.
- The team should ensure that its members attend periodic continuing education programs about cleft lip and palate.
- Figure 51-1 demonstrates example times/ages when specific concerns are most often addressed.

4. **Describe the difference in frequency of clefting in regard to race and gender.**
The overall reported frequency of children being born with a cleft lip and/or palate is approximately 1:700. A higher frequency of cleft lip and palate occurs in Native Americans, those of Asian descent, and those of Latin American descent (1:400). The lowest frequency is reported in African Americans (1:1500 to 2000). Cleft palate alone is fairly consistent among ethnic groups at 1:2000. There is a male predominance in cleft lip and palate, and a female predominance in cleft palate alone.

5. **What are some of the causes of cleft lip/palate?**
Clefts can be generally classified as syndromic or nonsyndromic. Single gene transmissions, chromosomal aberrations, teratogenic effects, or environmental exposures can cause syndromic clefting. Over 400 syndromes are associated with cleft lip/palate. Nonsyndromic clefts have a non-Mendelian inheritance pattern. There is not a clear understanding of the factors involved in the occurrence of cleft lip/palate. Concordance rates in monozygotic and dizygotic twins are 40% to 60% and 5%, respectively. These findings indicate a major genetic component, but environmental factors are also implicated. Recurrence rates for cleft lip/palate and isolated cleft palate range from 1% to 16% in cases of families with children born with nonsyndromic cleft lip and/or palate.

6. **Name some of the more common syndromes in which cleft lip/palate is a characteristics.**
   - Apert's syndrome
   - Stickler's syndrome
   - Treacher Collins syndrome
   - 22q11 deletion syndrome (previously named velocardiofacial syndrome, Sphrintzen syndrome, or DiGeorge complex syndrome)
   - Van der Woude syndrome
   - Goldenhar syndrome or hemifacial microsomia

7. **What is Pierre Robin or Robin (*pr. Rō-bāń*) sequence?**
Pierre Robin sequence was first described in the early 1800's but bears the name of Robin, a French stomatologist who wrote extensively on and drew attention to the constellation of findings beginning in 1923. It is usually described as micrognathia (small mandible), relative glossoptosis (tongue of normal size, but relatively large compared to the small mandible), and airway obstruction. The constellation of findings is thought to occur from a single embryologic event, which occurs between 6½ to 10 weeks of embryologic development resulting in a small mandible. The relative macroglossia causes the tongue to sit high and posterior in the oropharynx, leading to upper airway obstruction at birth. A wide U-shaped cleft palate is present in most, but not all, patients due to inability of the palate to close normally because the tongue impedes it. Robin sequence is rarely isolated and can occur in a variety of craniofacial syndromes.

8. **What is the ratio of cleft lip to cleft lip and palate?**
Cleft lip and palate is the most common occurrence, accounting for 50% of patients. Left unilateral cleft lip and palate is the most common, followed by right unilateral cleft lip and palate, and then bilateral cleft lip and palate. Cleft palate alone occurs in 35% and is more often syndromic than cleft lip and palate or cleft lip alone. Cleft lip alone occurs in 15%.

9. **Distinguish between complete cleft lip and incomplete cleft lip.**
The distinction between complete and incomplete cleft lip is controversial. Generally, a complete cleft lip is defined as a cleft with muscular diastasis of the orbicularis oris. This condition can usually be best determined by observing nostril symmetry or appearance with facial movement. A complete cleft may be present with a Simonart's band.

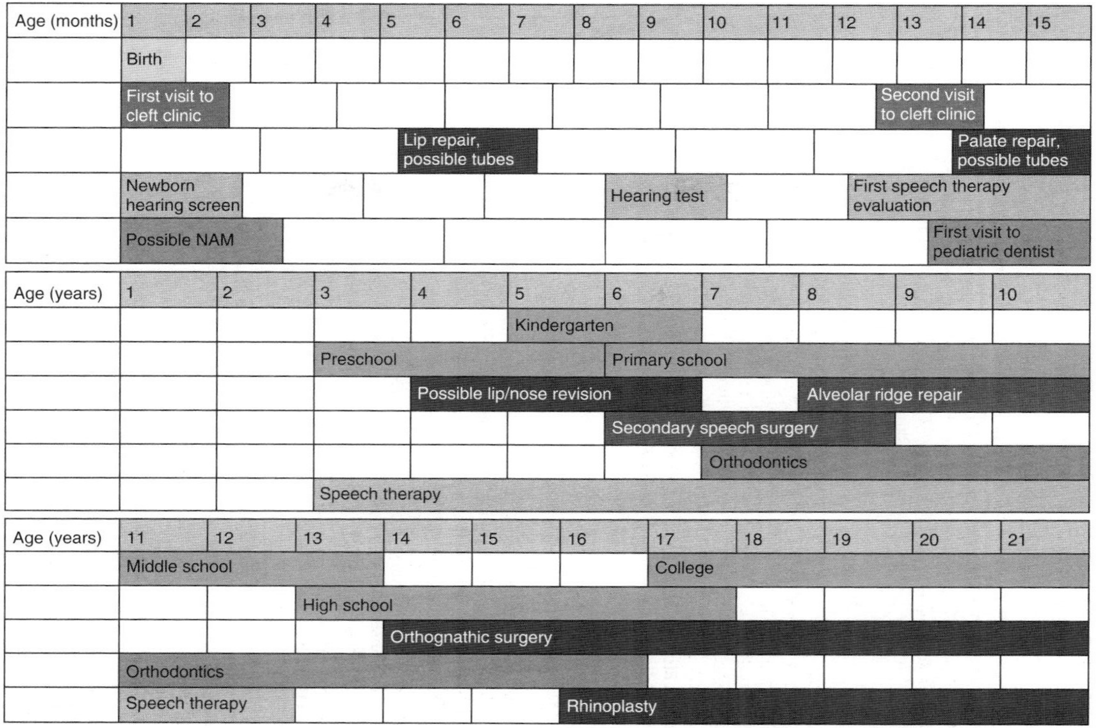

Age (months)	1	2	3	4	5	6	7	8	9	10	11	12	13	14	15
	Birth														
	First visit to cleft clinic												Second visit to cleft clinic		
					Lip repair, possible tubes									Palate repair, possible tubes	
	Newborn hearing screen							Hearing test				First speech therapy evaluation			
	Possible NAM												First visit to pediatric dentist		

Age (years)	1	2	3	4	5	6	7	8	9	10
					Kindergarten					
			Preschool			Primary school				
				Possible lip/nose revision				Alveolar ridge repair		
						Secondary speech surgery				
							Orthodontics			
			Speech therapy							

Age (years)	11	12	13	14	15	16	17	18	19	20	21
	Middle school						College				
			High school								
				Orthognathic surgery							
	Orthodontics										
	Speech therapy					Rhinoplasty					

Figure 51-1. Example timelines for cleft lip and palate care as provided by a multidisciplinary team.

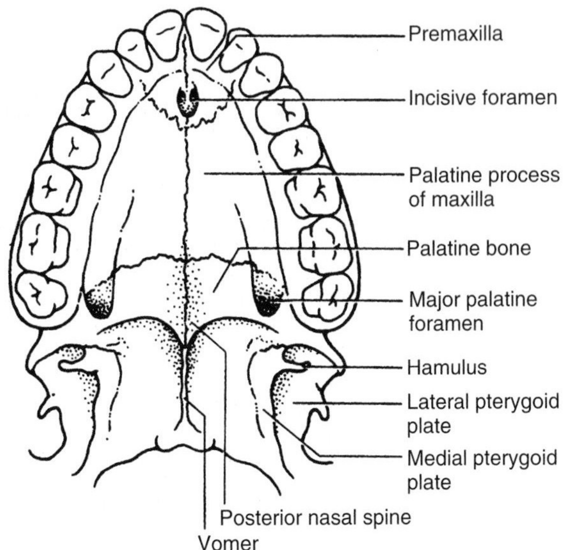

Figure 51-2. Basic anatomy and divisions of the palate. *(From Randall P, LaRossa D: Cleft palate. In McCarthy JG, editor: Plastic Surgery. Philadelphia, 1990, Saunders.)*

10. **What is a Simonart's band?**
    A Simonart's band is a thin remnant of tissue in the floor of the nasal vestibule bridging the medial and lateral lip elements across the cleft. The tissue may consist of skin and/or mucosa and subcutaneous tissue with or without a small amount of muscle fibers. The origin of the term is obscure, but many attribute it to Pierre Joseph Cécilien Simonart, a Belgian obstetrician (1817–1847).

11. **What is the primary palate? The secondary palate?**
    The primary and secondary palates are separated by the incisive foramen. The primary palate consists of the lip, alveolar arch, and palate anterior to the incisive foramen (the premaxilla). The secondary palate consists of the soft palate and the hard palate posterior to the incisive foramen (Figure 51-2).

12. **How is the primary palate formed?**
    Primary palate formation occurs between weeks 4 and 7. The development of the primary palate is largely complete prior to formation of the secondary palate. During week 4 the frontonasal prominence forms, including nasal placodes. The nasal placode consists of ectodermal thickenings located on the lateral aspect of the prominence. By week 5 the frontonasal prominence elevates and forms medial and lateral nasal prominences around the nasal placode. Next, the placode invaginates and forms nasal pits. During weeks 6 and 7, the maxillary prominences enlarge and grow medially. This growth forces the medial nasal prominences toward the midline. With the fusion of both medial nasal prominences, the tip of the nose, central upper lip, and philtrum of the upper lip are formed. The lateral portion of the upper lip and maxilla are formed by fusion of the medial nasal prominence and maxillary prominence. Finally, the nasal alae are formed by fusion of the lateral nasal prominences with the maxillary prominence.

13. **How is the secondary palate formed?**
    Formation of the secondary palate occurs between weeks 6½ and 10 in three stages: growth, shelf elevation, and fusion. First, outgrowths from the maxillary processes extend vertically downward along the tongue. Next, the shelves quickly assume a horizontal position above the tongue. The palatal shelves then fuse, forming an intact secondary palate.

14. **Describe the embryologic failures in regard to the formation of a cleft lip and palate.**
A cleft lip is due to failure of fusion between the medial nasal prominence and the maxillary prominence, lateral nasal prominence, or both. Cleft palate formation is hypothesized to result from one of the following: defects in palatal shelf growth, delayed or failed shelf elevation, defective shelf fusion, failure of medial epithelial seam cell death, or failure of mesenchymal consolidation and differentiation.

15. **What is a submucous cleft? How is it diagnosed?**
A submucous cleft is a muscular diastasis in the palate with intact overlying mucosa. A submucous cleft is classically characterized by the triad of bifid uvula, a midline furrow along the length of the soft palate due to abnormal muscle insertion (zona pellucida), and a notch in the posterior margin of the hard palate. Submucous cleft palate can usually be seen on physical examination or nasopharyngoscopy. A midline furrow of the nasal surface of the posterior palate seen during phonation is a classic endoscopic finding.

16. **List some characteristics of the classic cleft nose deformity.**
- Shortened columella with its base angled to the noncleft side
- Nasal spine deviation to the noncleft side, with a similar deflection of the caudal septum toward the noncleft side and compensatory hypertrophy of the cleft side inferior turbinate
- The lower lateral cartilage of the nose on the cleft side is rotated or displaced laterally in the nasal tip with the medial crura collapsed inferiorly and the lateral crura collapsed and buckled.
- Deflection of the nasal tip toward the cleft side due to the above deficiencies
- Relative stenosis or collapse of the nasal valve on the cleft side
- Hypoplastic maxilla on the cleft side, causing lateralization of the alar base and widening of the nares
- Broad nasal dorsum
- Horizontal as opposed to vertical nostril orientation, as seen on basal view

17. **What specific role does the otolaryngologist play in the care of a child with cleft lip/palate?**
In some institutions, the otolaryngologists perform all surgical procedures involving cleft lip/palate repair, correction of velopharyngeal insufficiency (VPI), alveolar bone grafting, rhinoplasty, and orthognathic surgery. In other institutions, the plastic surgeon performs some or all of the previously listed procedures except for management of ear disease associated with cleft palate. Oral and maxillofacial surgeons may be involved in or perform alveolar bone grafting and orthognathic surgery procedures. A pediatric otolaryngologist should be involved with the complex feeding and airway issues that often occur in children born with cleft lip and/or palate.

18. **List the initial priorities for managing a newborn with cleft lip/palate.**
As in any newborn, airway management is of primary importance. Feeding and achieving adequate nutrition is the second priority for any newborn, including infants with cleft lip/palate (see Question 20).

19. **Discuss airway management in newborns with cleft lip/palate.**
For a child born with Pierre Robin sequence or more complex craniofacial anomalies, airway management is of much greater concern. Such children may have few signs of upper airway obstruction; however, severely affected children may require immediate attention. Intervention may be as simple as prone positioning, which is most effective in nonsyndromic cases. Surgical techniques for management are more often required in syndromic patients and may include glossopexy or tongue-lip adhesion (primarily of historical interest, since its effectiveness is controversial), nasal airway placement, mandibular distraction osteogenesis, or tracheostomy tube placement.

20. **Describe the approach to feeding in infants with cleft lip/palate.**
Patients with cleft lip only may require little or no intervention, and many are able to breast-feed or use regular bottle nipples. Children with cleft palate or cleft lip/cleft palate are at a disadvantage, given the anatomic and functional deficits caused by a cleft. The inability to generate negative pressure within the oral cavity secondary to palatal insufficiency can lead to the expenditure of too much energy for feeding, long feeding times, and subsequent poor weight gain, or even dehydration.

Strategies developed to assist these children include special feeding systems (e.g., Medela Special Needs Feeder, formerly called Haberman feeder, Mead Johnson squeeze bottle, Pigeon feeder, Dr. Brown's nipple/bottle) and the fabrication of a palatal obturator or prosthetic. The obturator not only acts to aid in feeding but can also be used to help reposition the protruded premaxilla, lengthen the columella, reposition lateral maxillary segments, and reshape the nostril (see Question 24).

21. **Discuss the underlying pathophysiology of middle ear disease in a child with cleft lip/palate.**
Studies since the 1960s have implicated eustachian tube dysfunction as the main cause of ear disease. Multiple investigations have supported the hypothesis that the eustachian tube in a cleft child is unable to open properly and ventilate the middle ear because the muscles of the palate are involved in eustachian tube physiology. When these muscles are abnormal, such as in a cleft palate, they cannot function normally to open and close the eustachian tube.

22. **What percentage of children with cleft palate have middle ear disease? How is it treated?**
Virtually all (≥90%) children younger than 2 years of age with an unrepaired cleft have an effusion of the middle ear. Persistence of an effusion in young children leads to variable levels of hearing loss. Hearing loss during early childhood may lead to difficulties in speech and language development. The majority of centers treating children with clefts recommend tube placement during the first year of life or sooner if effusions become infected or hearing is markedly impaired. During either cleft lip or palate repair, the first set of tubes is often placed.

23. **When is the optimal time to perform a cleft lip repair?**
Commonly, the cleft lip is repaired between the ages of 2 and 6 months. After 10 weeks of age (corrected for prematurity if necessary) there is a decrease in respiratory complications following general anesthesia. The classic "rule of 10s" is often used at many centers. This rule requires children to be at least 10 weeks old, to weigh at least 10 pounds, and to have a hemoglobin level of 10 mg/dL. Although these criteria are commonly used, they are largely of historical interest and are not based on scientific data. Efficient feeding, proven weight gain, and good general health are much more important factors in successful surgical repair. Obviously, other congenital anomalies, such as congenital heart disease, must take precedence over cleft repair.

24. **What is presurgical nasoalveolar molding (NAM)?**
Presurgical nasoalveolar molding (NAM or pNAM) is basically presurgical orthodontics. An anterior palatal obturator is fabricated. The obturator may help in feeding. The obturator is then progressively modified to move the lateral maxillary segments. A protuberant premaxilla can be moved posteriorly, and attachments can be added to lengthen the short columella. Nasoalveolar molding is most beneficial in wide complete bilateral clefts of the lip and palate, but increasing use is being seen in unilateral clefts.

25. **What is a cleft lip adhesion?**
In certain cases of wide unilateral or bilateral cleft lip, some surgeons perform a cleft lip adhesion. This procedure is a staged lip repair in which the first stage (adhesion) involves reapproximating medial and lateral lip elements and the orbicularis oris muscle. The first stage converts a complete cleft, either unilateral or bilateral, to a more easily repaired incomplete cleft. The second stage then uses one of the techniques in Question 26 as the formal lip repair.

26. **List the techniques used for formal repair of unilateral cleft lip.**
    - Millard rotation-advancement repair: The medial lip element is rotated inferiorly and the lateral lip element is advanced into the resulting upper lip defect. The columellar flap is then used to lengthen the columella or create the nasal sill.
    - Tennison-Randell repair: The medial lip element is lengthened by introduction of a triangular flap from the inferior portion of the lateral lip element.
    - Hagedorn-LeMesurier repair: A quadrilateral flap developed from the lateral lip element is introduced to lengthen the medial lip element.
    - Rose-Thompson repair: Curved or angled paring of the cleft margins is used to lengthen the lip as a straight-line closure.
    - Skoog repair: The medial lip element is lengthened through the introduction of two small triangular flaps developed from the lateral lip element.

27. **List the techniques used for formal repair of bilateral cleft lip.**
   - Millard's repair involves complete elevation of the prolabium and reconstitution of the orbicularis across the premaxilla. In addition, Millard banked lateral segments of the prolabium as "forked flaps" that were meant to add columellar height at a later stage. The banking of fork flaps has recently fallen out of favor with more emphasis on primary columellar lengthening and rhinoplasty.
   - Veau repair: The Veau operation is a straight-line closure without elevation of the prolabial skin and correspondingly without any attempt to restore the continuity of the orbicularis oris, which is not favored because this results in incompetence of the oral sphincter.
   - Manchester repair: Manchester preferred to maintain the prolabial vermilion to create the cupid's bow and tubercle, but similarly to Veau, Manchester did not repair the orbicularis because he thought it would create an overly tight lip.

28. **Describe recent developments in nasal and lip repair.**
   In recent years, significant contributions by McComb, Mulliken, Nakajima, Nordhoff, and Cutting have integrated the correction of the associated nasal deformity with simultaneous lip repair that appears to achieve adequate primary columellar lengthening and nasal tip projection. Greyson and Cutting have introduced presurgical molding of the nasal tip and columella with acrylic outriggers, orthodontic elastics, and tapes attached to a palatal appliance (see Question 24).

29. **When should cleft palates be repaired?**
   Timing of cleft palate repair is much more controversial than that of cleft lip repair. The goals of cleft palate repair include attaining normal long-term speech and avoiding deleterious effects on future facial growth. Patients with unrepaired clefts have the least amount of abnormal growth, but the speech impact of this approach is unacceptable. Recent research into speech development supports cleft palate repair before the age of 12 months but for optimum outcomes some centers recommend closure much earlier, at 7 to 12 months of age. Early repair avoids compensatory techniques that may impair speech and be difficult to unlearn. Studies have shown that children with clefts repaired before 12 months have improved speech outcomes compared with children who undergo repair closer to 24 months. Long-term follow-up has found no significant impact on growth in children with earlier repaired clefts.

30. **Name the more common methods of cleft palate repair.**
   - Two-flap palatoplasty
   - Wardill-Kilner V-Y advancement
   - Von Langenbeck palatoplasty
   - Furlow double-opposing Z-plasty

31. **List possible postoperative complications of cleft palate repair.**
   - Bleeding
   - Fistula (5% to 35%)
   - VPI
   - Postoperative upper airway obstruction

32. **What is velopharyngeal insufficiency?**
   VPI is hypernasality during speech or reflux of saliva or food into the nasopharynx during swallowing. VPI occurs when the nasopharynx and oropharynx are not successfully separated by complete palatal closure during certain speech sounds or during swallowing. Persistent VPI occurs in about 10% to 40% of children after cleft palate repair.

33. **How is VPI treated?**
   An experienced speech and language pathologist should evaluate the presence, specific cause, and severity of VPI, often in conjunction with an imaging technique such as video nasopharyngoscopy or video fluoroscopy. Both medical and surgical methods for correction of VPI are available. Medical management includes speech therapy and oral appliances that aid in correcting the underlying problem. The majority of children undergo speech therapy before being referred for surgical management. Surgical management includes a variety of procedures aimed at attaining separation of the oropharynx from the nasopharynx during speech. Specific procedures include the pharyngeal flap, sphincter pharyngoplasty, Furlow palatoplasty, and posterior pharyngeal wall augmentation.

34. **What are concerns as children reach older ages?**
As previously stated, the treatment of cleft lip and palate is best directed by a multidisciplinary team. Figure 51-1 demonstrates example times/ages when specific concerns are addressed.
- As children reach elementary school age, dental and speech needs become more of a concern.
- In late elementary school and early middle school, orthodontic and alveolar cleft repair are usually addressed.
- In high school age patients, orthodontics and secondary cosmetic surgical procedures are addressed.
- At skeletal maturity (16 to 18 years in females, 18 to 21 years in males), orthodontics and orthognathic surgical procedures are addressed.

35. **What are adult concerns for patients with cleft lip and palate anomalies?**
It is the goal of team care that the majority of functional and cosmetic concerns will be address by the time a patient reaches adult age. In some instances, other circumstances prevent the address of all concerns by this time. Functional and cosmetic concerns can be addressed at any age, even in adults. Many adults born with cleft and craniofacial disorders will choose medical and/or surgical treatments to address these concerns.

CONTROVERSIES

36. **How is rhinoplasty approached in the child with cleft lip/palate?**
The approach to correction of the cleft nose is controversial. Some experts recommend immediate or primary correction with cleft lip repair, whereas others who are concerned with potential disrupted growth recommend a much later repair when patients are in their late teens. Advocates of primary repair found that early repair creates better symmetry and hence symmetric growth. They also claim there is much less psychological stress with earlier repair. Advocates of later definitive repair claim that they avoid any potential disturbances in growth, produce less scarring, and avoid multiple surgeries due to unexpected changes caused by growth. Recently there has been increased support for limited, primary rhinoplasty at the time of initial lip repair.

37. **What are the advantages of fetal repair of cleft lip/palate?**
Fetal surgery began in 1981 for life-threatening anomalies (e.g., diaphragmatic hernia). As fetal surgical techniques have improved, the scope of fetal surgery has expanded into the head and neck area. Securing the airway in cases of laryngeal atresia and large cervical/facial tumors has garnered the most interest. On the fringe of this interest, and highly controversial, is the desire to correct cleft lip/palate deformities in utero. The proposed advantages of this undertaking include scar-free wound healing if performed at the proper time, as well as interruption and correction of the associated facial maldevelopments that result from cleft lip/palate.

38. **What are the disadvantages of fetal repair?**
The disadvantages involve the risks to fetus and mother during the procedures. Until the limitations of fetal surgery are overcome (e.g., preterm labor, fetal demise, technical limitations), mainstream medicine will not accept such a procedure to repair a nonlethal deformity.

Bibliography

Byrd BH, Jhonny S: Primary correction of unilateral cleft nasal deformity, *Plast Reconstr Surg* 106:1276–1286, 2000.

Clark JM, Skoner JM, Wang TD: Repair of the unilateral cleft lip/nose deformity, *Facial Plast Surg* 19:29–39, 2003.

Matthews MS, Cohen M, Viglione M, et al: Prenatal counseling for cleft lip and palate, *Plast Reconstr Surg* 101:1–5, 1998.

Murray JC: Gene/environment causes of cleft lip and/or palate, *Clin Genet* 61:248–256, 2002.

Randall P, Krogman WM, Jahins S: Pierre Robin and the syndrome that bears his name, *Cleft Palate J* 36:237–246, 1965.

Redford-Badwal DA, Mabry K, Frassinelli JD: Impact of cleft lip and/or palate on nutritional health and oral-motor development, *Dent Clin North Am* 47:305–317, 2003.

Rohrich RJ, Love EJ, Byrd S, et al: Optimal timing of cleft palate closure, *Plast Reconstr Surg* 106:413–421, 2000.

Seibert RW, Weit GJ, Bumsted RM: Cleft lip and palate. In Cummings CW, et al, editors: *Otolaryngology-Head and Neck Surgery*, ed 3, St. Louis, 1998, Mosby, pp 133–173.

Shih CW, Sykes JM: Correction of the cleft-lip nasal deformity, *Facial Plast Surg* 18:253–262, 2002.

Thomas C, Mishra P: Open tip rhinoplasty along with the repair of cleft lip in cleft lip and palate cases, *Br J Plast Surg* 53:1–6, 2000.

CHAPTER 52

PEDIATRIC HEARING LOSS

Allison M. Dobbie, MD

KEY POINTS

1. Early identification of hearing loss, with intervention, is crucial to achieve better outcomes for speech and learning in children.
2. Close evaluation for other physical abnormalities in the presence of congenital hearing loss may lead one to a diagnosis of syndromic hearing loss.
3. Genetic evaluation of hearing loss requires audiologic, otologic, and detailed physical examinations, family history/pedigrees, as well as molecular genetic testing. Genetic testing for hearing loss is rapidly improving, which has begun to provide more frequent identification of hearing loss etiology.

Pearls

1. In developed countries the most common environmental, nongenetic cause of congenital hearing loss is congenital cytomegalovirus infection.
2. Patients with hearing loss and an enlarged vestibular aqueduct or Mondini dysplasia should be tested for mutations in *SLC26A4,* which is associated with Pendred syndrome.
3. Alport syndrome is characterized by glomerulonephritis and progressive SNHL. It has a variable inheritance pattern but 85% of cases are X-linked and 15% are AR.
4. In children with congenital severe to profound hearing presumed AR nonsyndromic hearing loss in whom *GJB2* and *GJB6* testing is normal, Usher syndrome should be considered.

QUESTIONS

1. **How common is pediatric hearing loss?**
Hearing loss is the most common birth defect and most prevalent sensorineural disorder in developed countries. Each year in the United States, 4000 infants are born with bilateral profound hearing loss, and 8000 infants are born with unilateral or bilateral mild-to-moderate hearing loss. Pediatric hearing loss can be categorized into congenital and acquired hearing loss. Congenital hearing loss is one of the most common anomalies present at birth and is estimated to occur in 2 to 4 infants per 1000. The overall prevalence of childhood hearing loss including loss present at birth, progressive, and acquired causes is thought to be 2 cases in 100 children.

2. **What is universal newborn hearing screening?**
In 1993, the National Institutes of Health published a consensus statement endorsing screening of all newborns for hearing loss before hospital discharge. Prior to universal newborn hearing screening programs, testing was only conducted on infants who met the criteria of the high-risk register (see Question 7). Currently, 43 states in the United States mandate newborn hearing screening and all have Early Hearing Detection and Intervention programs. Prior to universal newborn hearing screening, nearly 50% of infant hearing loss cases were identified later, after the critical period for speech and language development. Now, greater than 95% of newborns are tested prior to discharge home from the hospital. It has been recommended that all infants should have hearing screening before one month of age. Infants who do not pass newborn screening should have a follow-up medical and audiologic evaluation prior to three months of age.

3. **How are neonatal hearing screen tests performed?**
There are two methods utilized for hearing screening at birth: otoacoustic emissions (OAE) and automated auditory brainstem response (AABR) testing. Both OAEs and AABR tests are noninvasive

and can be obtained during normal physiologic sleep in the setting of a newborn nursery or neonatal intensive care unit. Newborns who do not pass their hearing screens are referred to audiologists for further workup, typically with complete diagnostic auditory brainstem response testing.

4. **Why is early identification of hearing loss important?**
   Early identification and subsequent treatment of hearing loss has a substantial impact on the development of speech and language skills. Studies have shown that children with hearing loss who began receiving treatment at or before 6 months of age have language skills comparable to their peers regardless of degree of hearing loss. Patients who were treated early had language skills significantly better than those in whom hearing loss was diagnosed after 6 months of age. Delayed diagnosis is known to have negative impacts not only on language skills, but also academic performance, career opportunities, and psychosocial well-being.

5. **Why is it important for physicians to be familiar with the milestones for development of speech and hearing? What is the most critical period?**
   Familiarity with milestones affords an effective initial screening method for children with hearing loss. Hearing loss may be most detrimental during the critical period between birth and 3 years of age when children develop speech, auditory pathways, and emotional bonds to family members. Infants with profound SNHL are unable to obtain auditory feedback, and without this feedback they cannot acquire the motor speech skills necessary for communication.

6. **Summarize the major milestones for development of speech and hearing.**
   Generally, infants younger than 3 months of age are startled by loud sounds and are calmed by familiar voices. At 6 months, infants have the ability to localize sounds, and by 9 months they respond to their names and are able to mimic environmental sounds. By 18 months of age, infants react to sounds from any direction and are capable of following commands to perform simple tasks. Although most infants say "ma-ma" or "da-da" early on, the first obvious speech milestone occurs at about 1 year of age when infants learn their first meaningful words. By age 2, most normally hearing monolingual children have a vocabulary of 20 or more words.

7. **What are risk factors for early childhood hearing loss?**
   - Family history of permanent childhood hearing loss
   - Birth weight less than 1500 grams
   - Congenital craniofacial anomalies
   - In utero infections (ToRCHeS)
   - Maternal diabetes or alcohol/drug use
   - Hyperbilirubinemia requiring exchange transfusion
   - Apgar scores less than 5 at 1 minute and less than 7 at 5 minutes
   - Neonatal exposure to:
     - Ototoxic agents
     - Mechanical ventilation for 5 days or longer
     - Extracorporeal membrane oxygenation (ECMO)
   - Postnatal infections associated with hearing loss
   - Identified syndromes known to cause sensorineural or conductive hearing loss
   - Neurodegenerative disorders or sensorimotor neuropathies
   - Parental or caregiver concerns regarding hearing
   - Head trauma
   - Recurrent or persistent otitis media with effusion lasting for at least 3 months

8. **What are the causes of congenital hearing loss?**
   Approximately 50% of all cases of congenital deafness are inherited, about 30% are considered to be from acquired/environmental causes, and 20% are cause unknown.

9. **How are genetic causes of hearing loss categorized?**
   Genetically influenced hearing loss is believed to be responsible for a major portion of pediatric hearing loss and can be grouped into disorders that are syndromic and nonsyndromic. Disorders that cause syndromic hearing loss are associated with congenital anomalies involving other organ systems. Nonsyndromic hearing loss is isolated to anomalies of the middle or inner ear and does not involve other organ systems or the external ear. Approximately 70% of hereditary hearing loss is nonsyndromic.

10. What are the most common syndromes causing sensorineural hearing loss? Describe their features and modes of inheritance.
    - **Usher syndrome:** This syndrome is inherited in an autosomal recessive (AR) pattern and is responsible for up to 10% of congenital deafness. It is the most common type of AR syndromic hearing loss and the degree of hearing loss may vary. It is also associated with retinitis pigmentosa, which can cause progressive blindness, and vestibular dysfunction. Multiple mutations of genes have been associated with Usher syndrome including MYO7A, USH2A, CDH23 and others.
    - **Pendred syndrome***:* This syndrome is transmitted in an AR pattern and is responsible for 5% to 10% of recessive hearing loss. It is associated with multinodular goiter, inner ear malformations including Mondini deformity, and enlarged vestibular aqueducts and abnormal perchlorate testing. Mutations in the SLC26A4 gene are common.
    - **Jervell and Lange-Nielsen syndrome:** This is the third most common cause of AR syndromic hearing loss and is thought to be responsible for 1% of all cases of recessive hearing loss. This syndrome is associated with congenital severe bilateral hearing loss and a prolonged Q-T interval in ECG, which is associated with sudden death. Mutations in the KCNQ1 and KCNE1 genes are thought to be associated.
    - **Waardenburg syndrome:** This syndrome is the most common cause of autosomal dominant (AD) hearing loss and accounts for 2% of all cases of congenital hearing loss, which can be variable. Other physical findings may include telecanthus, white forelock, hyperplastic high nasal root, hyperplastic medial eyebrows, and heterochromia irides. Multiple genetic mutations exist, most commonly in PAX3 and MITF genes.
    - **Branchio-oto-renal syndrome:** This syndrome is inherited in an AD pattern and includes branchial fistulas, renal abnormalities, and abnormal development of the inner, middle or external ears including preauricular pits. It is associated with mutations in EYA1, SIX1, and SIX5 genes.
    - **Stickler syndrome:** This is an AD inherited syndrome associated with cleft palate, osteoarthritis, myopia, and progressive SNHL. Three types are recognized based on the molecular genetic defect: STL1 (*COL2A1*), STL2 (*COL11A1*), and STL3 (*COL11A2*).

11. How is nonsyndromic hearing loss inherited? What are some nonsyndromic causes of congenital hearing loss?
    Most genetically acquired hearing losses are caused by single-gene Mendelian inheritance in *the absence* of a recognizable syndrome. Nonsyndromic SNHL may be caused by any one of an increasing number of identified genes; currently over 100 SNHL genes have been mapped and over 50% have been identified. Eighty percent of nonsyndromic hearing loss cases follow the autosomal recessive pattern, 15% are autosomal dominant, with the remainder being X-linked or mitochondrial.

    The most common mutation causing congenital profound hearing loss is in the GJB2 gene, which encodes the connexin-26 gap junction protein. This mutation may be responsible for 30% to 50% of all congenital profound hearing loss. SLC26A4 mutations make up the second most common genetic cause of SNHL; this may be present in Pendred syndrome, and patients may also have enlarged vestibular aqueducts.

12. Describe inner and middle ear anomalies that can cause hearing loss.
    Malformations of the inner ear are rare. They can be categorized into malformations of the bony and membranous labyrinth and those limited just to the membranous labyrinth. **Michel's aplasia** is complete failure of inner ear development (labyrinthine aplasia), which typically leads to complete deafness. **Mondini dysplasia** results in an incomplete partition in the cochlea; only the basal turn of the cochlea is developed, and the bony cochlea is restricted to 1.5 turns. This can present in early childhood or later in adult life, with hearing that ranges from complete loss to normal hearing. Mondini dysplasia is inherited in an autosomal dominant pattern.

    Membranous labyrinthine anomalies include **Siebenmann-Bing** (complete membranous labyrinthine) **dysplasia**, **Scheibe** (cochleosaccular) **dysplasia**, and **Alexander** (cochlear basal turn) **dysplasia**. Siebenmann-Bing dysplasia is extremely rare, and has been reported in association with Jervell-Nielsen-Lange and Usher syndromes. Scheibe dysplasia is often noted in autosomal recessive congenital hearing losses. Alexander dysplasia may be related to familial high-frequency sensorineural hearing loss. Diagnosis of dysplasia requires examination of the membranous labyrinth and can only be confirmed by post-mortem histopathologic study.

    Enlarged vestibular aqueduct (EVA) is the most common inner ear anomaly seen on temporal bone imaging in patients with sensorineural hearing loss. It is described as a vestibular aqueduct that measures 1.5 mm or greater. The clinical presentation of enlarged vestibular aqueduct may be sensorineural or mixed, with hearing loss present either at birth, progressive through childhood, or even fluctuating. Sudden hearing loss can occur spontaneously or with mild head trauma. Patients diagnosed with EVA are urged to avoid contact sports and other situations that may result in head trauma to reduce progression of their hearing loss.

Congenital middle ear ossicular anomalies can also occur and often result in varying degrees of conductive hearing loss. These can include malformed or entirely absent ossicles. Malleus head fixation is likely the most common ossicular abnormality, and occurs secondary to incomplete pneumatization of the epitympanic space. Congenital absence of the incus' long process can occur, which leads to a maximal conductive hearing loss. Congenital stapes fixation may also be responsible for stable conductive hearing loss and require stapedectomy for hearing restoration.

13. **What are the most common causes of acquired pediatric hearing loss?**
Acute otitis media and chronic otitis media with effusion are the most common causes of conductive hearing loss in children. Fluid within the middle ear space can inhibit the vibration of the tympanic membrane, reducing sound conduction. Acquired hearing loss can also be caused by cholesteatoma when desquamated epithelium expands into the middle ear and mastoid spaces, which can erode middle ear ossicles or even into the otic capsule.

14. **Which infections can lead to hearing loss in children?**
Toxoplasmosis, rubella, congenital cytomegalovirus (CMV), herpes, and syphilis (ToRCHeS) are infections that can be responsible for hearing loss if contracted in the perinatal period. Congenital CMV is the most common cause of nonhereditary sensorineural hearing loss in children. The prevalence of congenital CMV is 0.58%, and among those newborns infected, 12.8% will experience hearing loss. Among patients with symptomatic CMV infections, the majority have bilateral hearing loss; in those with asymptomatic infection, unilateral loss is more common.

Bacterial meningitis is thought to cause hearing loss in approximately 10% of children infected. Bacterial meningitis is usually caused by *Streptococcus pneumoniae*, *Group B streptococcus*, *Neisseria meningitidis*, and less commonly by *Haemophilus influenzae* type b. Hearing loss is a result of ossification of the cochlea from the inflammatory process. Frequent hearing evaluations are necessary with a CT scan of the temporal bone to look for ossification if hearing loss is found. Cochlear implantation may proceed urgently if ossification is found in order to preserve some membranous cochlear architecture.

15. **What is the role of radiographic imaging in pediatric hearing loss?**
Temporal bone computed tomography (CT) and brain/internal auditory canal magnetic resonance imaging (MRI) are the imaging modalities of choice to evaluate hearing loss. Either CT or MRI is the only way to determine presence of an enlarged vestibular aqueduct, vestibular anomalies, or absent cochlear nerves. Some debate exists as to which modality should be obtained primarily, but in general, weighing the differential diagnosis should drive which study should be ordered. For example, CT has been demonstrated to have a greater yield for identifying enlarged vestibular aqueduct; thus if this is suspected by clinical presentation, obtaining a CT of the temporal bones would be recommended.

16. **What are some other adjunctive tests that may be helpful to obtain after hearing loss is diagnosed?**
In children with profound congenital deafness and absent vestibular function, an electrocardiogram (EKG) and/or cardiology consultation should be obtained to evaluate for prolonged Q-T interval that can be found in Jervell-Nielsen-Lange syndrome. Urinalysis may be obtained to evaluate for microscopic hematuria in Alport syndrome. If hearing loss is present along with cleft palate, ophthalmologic consultation can be important in evaluating for Stickler syndrome.

17. **What are some medications used in the pediatric population that can cause ototoxicity?**
Aminoglycosides, erythromycin, cisplatin and other platinum-derived chemotherapeutics, and loop diuretics (e.g., furosemide) can all have ototoxic effects.

18. **What is auditory neuropathy spectrum disorder (ANSD)?**
Patients with ANSD may display robust OAEs but have either an absent or a markedly dysmorphic AABR response in combination with varying degrees of hearing loss (as demonstrated by behavioral threshold testing).

19. **What role does genetic testing play in the diagnosis of congenital hearing loss?**
Recent advances in genetic testing for hearing loss have drastically improved the feasibility and yield of identifying etiology of congenital hearing loss. If a mutation is found, it may explain why the person has hearing loss. In some cases it may explain how severe a condition may become or other associated problems that may occur in association with the mutation. From a counseling standpoint, finding out about a genetic condition can help families know the chances of having another child with the same condition or of that child passing on the mutation to their own offspring. Not all the genes the cause hearing loss are known, so it may not be possible to find the mutation that causes it. Additionally, since genetic testing provides information about the family as a whole, the wants and concerns of the whole family must be addressed. That is why counseling should be an integral part of the genetic testing process.

20. **What are the treatments for pediatric hearing loss?**
Depending on the type and degree of hearing loss, there are a variety of treatments for hearing loss. Conductive hearing loss caused by otitis media and/or eustachian tube dysfunction may be improved with tympanostomy tube placement. Other causes of conductive hearing loss (middle ear malformations) may require middle ear exploration with ossicular reconstruction or stapedectomy.

Hearing aids are frequently used in children to amplify sound. Behind-the-ear hearing aids are most often used in children as they are more adaptable to a child's growing ear canal.

Bone anchored hearing aids (BAHA) are devices that can be used to restore conductive hearing loss that cannot be treated with traditional hearing aids, such as external auditory canal atresia or in patients with chronic otorrhea. Osseointegrated implants are placed into the skull and a sound processor is attached to provide conducted sound amplification through the bone.

Cochlear implants are a treatment for patients in whom surgical hearing reconstruction or hearing aids are not an option. A cochlear implant bypasses the nonfunctional cochlea and directly stimulates the cochlear nerve. In patients with bilateral profound hearing loss, excellent speech and language outcomes can be achieved with early implantation, often prior to one year of age.

BIBLIOGRAPHY

Cohen M, Phillips JA: Genetic approach to evaluation of hearing loss, *Otolaryngol Clin North Am* 45(1):25–39, 2012.

Force, USPST: Universal screening for hearing loss in newborns: US Preventive Services Task Force recommendation statement, *Pediatrics* 122(1):143–148, 2008.

Goderis J, De Leenheer E, Smets K, et al: Hearing loss and congenital CMV infection: a systematic review, *Pediatrics* 134(5):972–982, 2014.

Kachniarz B, Chen JX, Gilani S, et al: Diagnostic yield of MRI for pediatric hearing loss: a systematic review, *Otolaryngol Head Neck Surg* 152(1):5–22, 2015.

Lasak JM, Allen P, McVay T, et al: Hearing loss: diagnosis and management, *Prim Care* 41(1):19–31, 2014.

Parker M, Bitner-Glindzicz M: Genetic investigations in childhood deafness, *Arch Dis Child* 3:271–278, 2015.

Raveh E, Hu W, Papsin BC, et al: Congenital conductive hearing loss, *J Laryngol Otol* 116(2):92–96, 2002.

Rodriguez K, Shah RK, Kenna M: Anomalies of the middle and inner ear, *Otolaryngol Clin North Am* 40(1):81–96, vi, 2007.

CHAPTER 53

MICROTIA AND OTOPLASTY

Peggy E. Kelley, MD

KEY POINTS

Otoplasty Options

1. Tape and wax reshaping in the neonatal period
2. Incisionless otoplasty for ears that correct easily with finger pressure
3. Open or traditional otoplasty
4. Creative options such as grafting to cover skin defects or slide rotational flaps to borrow cartilage when it is deficient
5. Autologous rib grafting for microtia or traumatic deformities
6. Awareness of and colleagues working with prosthetics and bone anchored hearing aid placement for patients with microtia/atresia

QUESTIONS

1. What is otoplasty?
   Otoplasty is the manipulation of abnormally shaped cartilages to achieve a more natural appearing shape of the external ear. This can be achieved by surgical and nonsurgical methods.

2. What are the indications for otoplasty?
   Otoplasty is not based on the ear shape, but rather the patient's perception of the ear shape. Look at the patient's ears and listen to the patient's concerns. If the ears are asymmetric or if their shape draws attention to the ears instead of the person's face, otoplasty may be indicated. If the patient sees only his or her ears in the mirror or is teased because of their size or shape, otoplasty can improve self-esteem.

3. What anatomic landmarks of the external ear are important in otoplasty? (Figure 53-1)
   The circumference of the external ear is described by the helix, lobule, and tragus. The inner folds of the ear consist of the antihelix and antitragus. The antihelix divides the external ear superiorly into the superior and inferior crus. Between the crura is the fossa triangularis. Between the helical rim and the antihelical fold is the scaphoid fossa. Between the antihelix and the tragus is the conchal bowl, which is divided by the root of the helix into the concha cymba above and the concha cavum below. The tragus overlies the ear canal opening.

4. How are external ear malformations classified?
   Various grading systems have been proposed for congenital malformations of the auricle. Most reliable for documentation or discussion between health care providers is an anatomic description of the abnormality since no staging system is widely recognized. Description of the abnormality can help direct thought about reconstruction or correction. Commonly used terms are *protruding* or *prominent ears, lop ears, Stahl's ears, constricted ears, cryptotia, microtia,* and *anotia.*

5. Describe the dimensions of a normal ear.
   A normal ear is in proportion to the person's face. It blends and looks "natural." Ears are fully grown by 9 years of age. They do not change shape spontaneously beyond 12 months of age. Whereas no one size or shape is normal for all people, some approximate measurements can be helpful in assessing the degree of abnormality of an ear. Ear height is typically 55 to 65 mm, and width is from 30 to 45 mm. Width is usually 50% to 60% of the height. The ear is rotated so that the top is 15° to 30° more posterior than the earlobe. At its midpoint, the ear protrudes from the scalp about 18 to 20 mm. The angle of protrusion of the ear from the head is usually <21° in a female and <25° in a male. The root of the helix is usually 60 to 70 mm posterior to the lateral canthus of the eye.

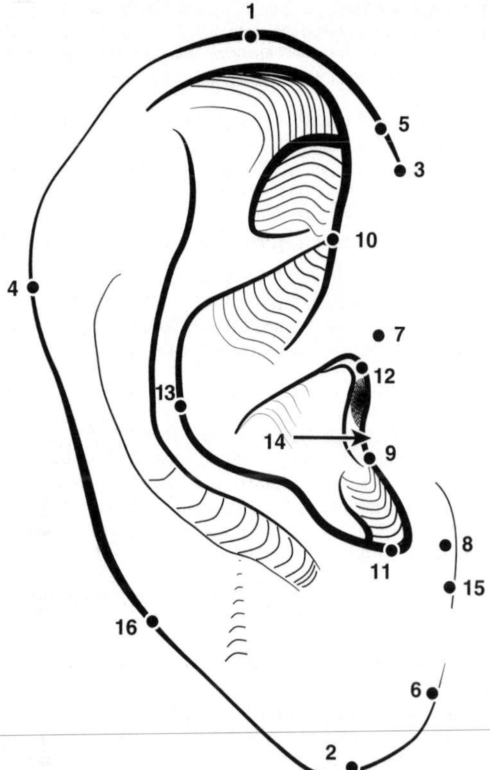

Figure 53-1. Landmarks of the external ear: (1) superaurale, (2) subaurale, (3) preaurale, (4) postaurale, (5) otobasion superius (6) otobasion inferius, (7) deepest point on the notch on upper margin of tragus, (8) lowest point on the lower border of tragus, (9) protragion, (10) concha superior (the intersection of the lower edge of the anterior end of the crus antihelicis inferius and the posterior border of crus helicus, (11) incisura intertragica inferior (the deepest point in the incisura intertragica), (12) incisura anterior auris posterior (the most posterior point on the edge of incisura anterior auris), (13) strongest antihelical curvature, (14) deepest lateral border of external auditory meatus, (15) lobule anterior (ear attachment line is drawn joining the otobasion superior and inferior. The point on this line just below the incisura intertragica where the cartilage ends is the landmark.) and (16) lobule posterior (the most posterior point on the margin of lobule perpendicular to lobule anterior). *(From Purkait R, Singh P: A test of individuality of human external ear pattern: Its application in the field of personal identification. Forensic Sci Int 178(2–3):112–118, 2008.)*

6. What is a prominent or protruding ear deformity?
   This common external malformation is diagnosed when the angle of the ear to the head is >35°. It is most commonly a result of the lack of antihelical fold development. The ear then protrudes more than the 20 mm expected from the scalp. The prominent ear takes over the frontal profile. Instead of seeing a person's face, the eyes of the observer are drawn to the ears. A normal ear shape and angle of protrusion can be attained by gentle repositioning of the ear with finger pressure.
7. What is a constricted or cup ear deformity?
   This ear deformity is characterized by the inability of gentle finger pressure to attain a normal shape or position of the ear. A deficiency of skin, cartilage, or both restricts the "unfolding" of the ear.
8. How is microtia or anotia characterized?
   In the microtic ear, the cartilage shape is not normal The classic description is a cartilage remnant that looks like a rolled "peanut" positioned at the root of the helix. The lower portion of the microtic

remnant is soft fatty tissue—the earlobe remnant. Superiorly, the remnant is composed of crumpled cartilage under the skin. An atypical microtia may have the beginnings of normal ear architecture but with obvious disruption in development. Anotia is absence of the external ear. A small earlobe remnant may be present and is often not in the expected location.

9. **Summarize the goals of otoplasty.**
   The primary goal of otoplasty is to make the patient (and often the parents) happy. The postoperative ear or ears should be symmetric. From the frontal view, you should have a small glimpse of both ears at the same time. On lateral view, the ear should have smooth contours with recognizable major anatomic features: helical rim, antihelical fold with crus, scapha, conchal bowl, and lobule. The posterior view should exhibit appropriate scalp-to-ear distances (<20 mm).

10. **When should otoplasty be offered to a patient?**
    The age at which otoplasty can be performed depends on the type of corrective surgery needed. The goal of timing is to avoid psychological insult to the child by completing the repair as soon as possible while balancing the maturity needed for participation and cooperation in surgical and postoperative care.

11. **What is the youngest patient age at which otoplasty can be performed?**
    The first opportunity for the correction of abnormal ear shapes is within the first several days after birth. Reshaping with wax and tape within the first 96 hours of life can obviate the need for surgery in the future. The splint or molding technique requires 2 weeks of reshaping if applied during the neonatal period. Older infants may require longer periods of shape control. Recently, the use of a splint and double-sided tape for many months was reported in children up to 5 years of age as a means of avoiding surgical correction.

12. **What is the youngest patient age at which more complicated techniques can be done?**
    If the abnormality can be corrected by gentle finger pressure into a desired shape, then a permanent change in shape can be accomplished with the incisionless technique as early as age 2 years when general anesthesia is considered safe for elective procedures. If the abnormality cannot be corrected by gentle finger pressure then the child will need an open procedure and will need to be able to participate in the postoperative care and suture removal. An open otoplasty is typically performed as early as 5–6 years of age for very motivated children and parents but may be delayed until the child is ready. Boys are often slower than girls at being ready for the cooperation needed in the postop care of either an otoplasty or microtia construction. When microtia construction with autologous rib grafting is to be considered, the ribs must be large enough to carve. Some techniques can start as early as age 6–7 years of age but the newer 3D techniques require more rib and most children do not have enough rib stock until age 10–12 years of age.

13. **What is the oldest patient age at which otoplasty can be done?**
    No age is too old for otoplasty. Many adults who did not have the opportunity for ear corrective surgery in childhood still desire a normally shaped ear. Both open and closed procedures may be appropriate.

14. **What are the options for protruding ear otoplasty?**
    Open versus closed: Open techniques begin with skin excision and progress to weakening or thinning the cartilage, reshaping with mattress sutures, or dividing the cartilage with removal of cartilage to reduce the conchal bowl. Closed options include tape and wax or splint application as well as the incisionless otoplasty described by Fritsch. Incisionless otoplasty employs permanent horizontal mattress sutures placed percutaneously.
    Cartilage sparing versus cartilage removal: Surgeons are highly opinionated as to whether cartilage can be reshaped with mattress sutures, scoring, or thinning by drilling, or whether cartilage must be removed to attain a desirable ear shape. Either option can be used successfully, but usually only one option is adopted as "the way" by an individual surgeon.

15. **How long do dressings need to be used after otoplasty?**
    One of the advantages of the incisionless technique is that no dressing is needed. A soft headband can be used at night, if desired, for comfort. When an open technique is used, the dressing is usually kept in place for 2 weeks. This period allows the skin flap to reattach and the cartilage to begin healing if it has been divided or removed. An elastic headband is worn at night for an

additional 4 to 6 weeks to prevent accidental forward displacement of the ear until full healing is complete. This concern is greatest if cartilage is removed or divided.

16. **Describe the early complications of otoplasty for protruding ears.**
Hematoma is the major concern after open otoplasty. If a hematoma goes undiagnosed and untreated, perichondritis and loss of cartilage result. Persistent postoperative pain can be a sign of hematoma. Proper treatment consists of immediate evacuation of the clot and debridement of any necrotic tissue resulting from pressure of the hematoma, followed by reapplication of the compressive dressing. Other early complications include skin necrosis secondary to dressing pressure, skin hypersensitivity to pressure or temperature, and suture spitting. All of these, except suture extrusion, are avoided with the incisionless technique because no dressing is used postoperatively and no dead space for hematoma formation is raised during the procedure.

17. **What are the significant late complications of otoplasty for protruding ears?**
The most common late complication is unhappiness with the postoperative correction, usually because of undercorrection, asymmetry, or cartilage deformation over time. In an open procedure, scar hypertrophy or keloids may result. In an open or closed otoplasty, suture knot protrusion can result over time. Keloids should be considered a possibility at the puncture sites but are rarely encountered.

18. **What is a "telephone ear" deformity?**
A telephone ear deformity describes the shape of an overcorrected midportion of the ear. The resultant shape is reminiscent of the original hand piece of a telephone with a separate receiver and a mouthpiece with a connecting narrower handle. The deformity is best appreciated on frontal view. Such overcorrection can be due to excessive removal of postauricular skin or mastoid soft tissue or by overtightening set-back sutures of the concha to the mastoid.

19. **What historical names should I know if I want to discuss otoplasty for protruding ears?**
Many surgeons have made inroads in the correction of ear shapes. Mustardé is known for the development of the horizontal mattress suture to reshape the antihelical fold (Figure 53-2). This same horizontal mattress suture has been adapted to a percutaneous technique of incisionless otoplasty. Converse and Furness otoplasty techniques use cartilage repositioning and weakening in their otoplasties. Converse uses the cartilage weakening and repositioning to create the appearance of an antihelical fold. The Furness technique does not address the antihelical fold but focuses on the conchal bowl protrusion by suturing the bowl to the mastoid periosteum, rotating the ear posteriorly and thus decreasing protrusion. This technique is often used in conjunction with a technique for reshaping the antihelical fold.

20. **How is correcting a "cup" or constricted ear different from correcting a protruding ear?**
A cup or constricted ear is missing enough skin, cartilage, or both so that a normal shape cannot be attained through the techniques used for protruding surgery. New skin or cartilage or advancement of tissue must be used to release the constricted part of the ear (Figure 53-3).

Each ear is slightly different, and a full armamentarium of reconstructive options must be learned and used to get consistent results. The deficiencies usually lie in the helical rim, scapha, and root of the helix. Techniques to unfurl and fan open have been described, but may fail over time because the skin/soft tissue envelope collapses the new expanded cartilage shape. Rotational or advancement flaps have more stability. A preferred technique is to release the root of the helix as a V-Y advancement flap, incorporating the ridge of cartilage between the concha cavum and concha cymba. Several millimeters of length can be borrowed and advanced into the height of the ear. The donor site is closed primarily. Skin grafts are used if needed in the new fossa triangularis area, and the cartilage is reshaped with horizontal mattress sutures to add strength and stability over time.

21. **When does a lobule need to be corrected?**
The earlobe may angle forward, particularly in a cupped or protruding ear. The upper cartilage can be corrected, but the ear can still look abnormal if the earlobe is not repositioned. The earlobe angles forward if there is an abnormally long or flared caudal helical cartilage. Resecting or repositioning this tail of cartilage will result in less anterior angulation of the lobule. Sometimes skin behind can be removed to assist in earlobe correction. If the earlobe is to be reduced in size, a

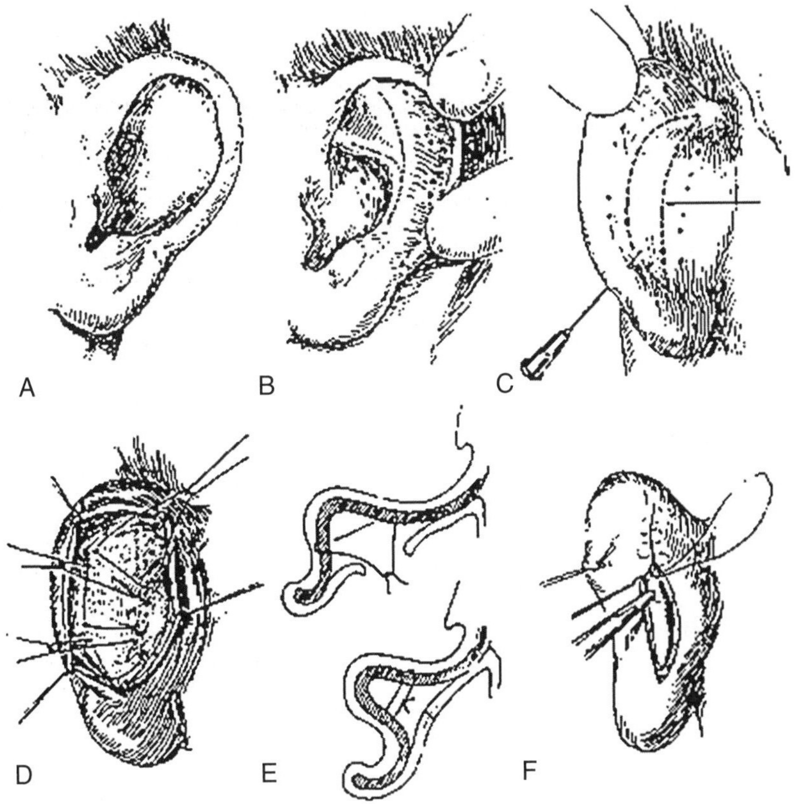

Figure 53-2. The Mustardé technique of otoplasty. *(From Wood-Smith D: Otoplasty. In Rees TD, editor: Aesthetic Plastic Surgery, Philadelphia, 1980, Saunders, p. 851.)*

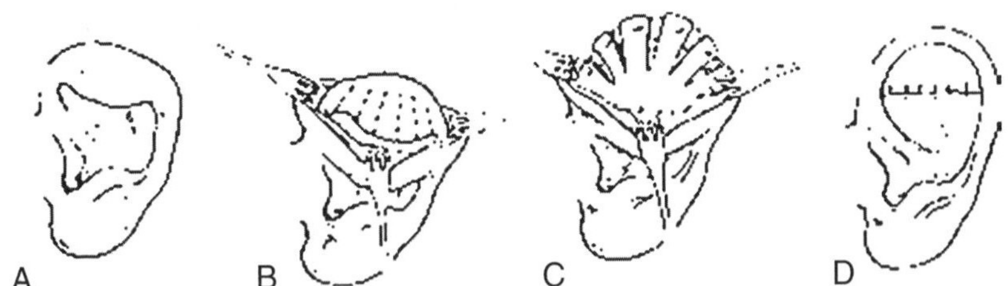

Figure 53-3. Correction of severe cup ear deformity. *(From Converse JH: Congenital deformities of the auricle. In Converse JM, editor: Reconstructive Plastic Surgery, ed 2, Philadelphia, 1977, Saunders, p. 1708.)*

geometric resection with overlapping and, if possible, different anterior and posterior closures, will result in less scar contracture and earlobe notching.

22. **Can a huge ear be reduced in size overall?**
Of course! Auricular reduction may be necessary to attain symmetry with a smaller opposite ear. Sometimes it is easier to reduce the larger ear than to expand the deficient one. All methods of reduction surgery involve geometric excision and closure. This approach decreases the chance of a notched scar along the sweeping helical rim.

23. **What can be done with a microtic ear?**
A person with microtia can be treated with a silicone prosthesis that is made to look like the opposite ear and attached with skin glues or, more recently, with bone-anchored screws or magnets.

Surgical correction can be attained with a buried silicone or Silastic ear mold, but the mold is prone to extrusion and malformation with the trauma of childhood play or sports. The long-term effects of a foreign body in children are also significant; thus, this form of reconstruction should no longer be considered, particularly in children.

Synthetic biocompatible porous polyethylene frameworks can be used with a temporalis fascia flap as a one- or two-stage operation. This procedure was popularized by Reinisch in the early 1990s. Concerns for long-term rejection or trauma have lessened with recent publications on long-term outcomes. This procedure can be done as early as 3 years but an adult sized ear is placed because the ear will not grow over time.

Brent describes a four-stage autologous rib reconstruction. This form of reconstruction has been used for the past 40 years with good results. The first stage is the harvesting, carving, and placement of the autologous rib graft. Portions of 3 or 4 ribs (depending on the need for tragal reconstruction) are used to form the helical rim, antihelical fold, scapha, and fossa triangularis. The second stage rotates the microtic remnant earlobe onto the cartilage framework and attaches it there. The third stage is ear elevation away from the head with a skin graft. The fourth stage, if necessary, involves creation of a tragus and deepening of the conchal bowl. This type of reconstruction is typically begun after age 6, but boys are usually recommended to wait until age 10 for full cooperation. Usually 9 to 12 months are required to complete all 4 stages.

Beginning in the mid-1980s another autologous rib reconstruction method was developed by Nagata. This two-stage operation is performed beginning at age 10 and requires an evaluation for adequate costal cartilage volume. The first stage includes harvesting, fabrication of the three-dimensional costal cartilage framework, and grafting it into place. The second stage elevates the auricle to match projection. Results are more reliable with the topographic method of ear cartilage fabrication as carving is not as dependent on in situ rib width and depth. During the same period, Firman developed a similar three dimensional model of microtia construction from autologous rib. Today many mictrotia surgeons borrow from both Firman and Nagata to create a rib based framework.

24. **What does the future hold for microtia construction?**
Currently the development of a bone anchored hearing aid embedded in a silicone prosthetic ear is being trialed outside the United States. Ongoing research in tissue engineering with the goal of harvesting autologous chondrocytes continues to teach us more and more about cell growth and immunology, but there are no clinical applications available at this time. Currently 3D printing of the opposite ear as model to carve on the operative field is feasible and the hope is that the 3D model will be able to be seeded with live cartilage that will reproduce and hold its shape over time so that the patient is not dependent on cartilage availability, can therefore undergo construction sooner, not have a donor defect and will have an "implant" that will grow with the child proportionally.

Bibliography

Beahm EK, Walton RL: Auricular reconstruction for microtia Part I: anatomy, embryology, and clinical evaluation, *Plast Reconstr Surg* 109(7):2473–2482, 2002.

Brent B: Microtia repair with rib cartilage grafts: a review of personal experience with 1000 cases, *Clin Plast Surg* 29:257–271, vii, 2002.

Kamil SH, Vacanti MP, Vacanti CA, et al: Microtia chondrocytes as a donor source for tissue engineered cartilage, *Laryngoscope* 114(12):2187–2190, 2004.

Nagata S: A new method of total reconstruction of the auricle for microtia, *Plast Reconstr Surg* 92:187–201, 1993.

Romo T 3rd, Reitzen SD: Aesthetic microtia reconstruction with Medpor, *Facial Plast Surg* 24:120–128, 2008.

Sorribes MM, Tos M: Nonsurgical treatment of prominent ears with the Auri method, *Arch Otolaryngol Head Neck Surg* 128:1369–1376, 2002.

Walton RL, Beahm EK: Auricular reconstruction for microtia: Part II. Surgical techniques, *Plast Reconstr Surg* 110(1): 234–249, 2002.

Yotsuyanagi T, Yokoi K, Sawada Y: Nonsurgical treatment of various auricular deformities, *Clin Plast Surg* 29:327–332, ix, 2002.

CHAPTER 54

VASCULAR MALFORMATIONS

Pamela A. Mudd, MD

KEY POINTS

1. The head and neck is the most common site for vascular anomalies.
2. Infantile hemangioma is the most common tumor in infancy.
3. Vascular malformations are classified based on vessel involvement (capillary, venous, arterial, lymphatic, combination).
4. Absolute indication for treatment of vascular anomalies is functional ocular or airway obstruction, ulceration, hemorrhage, or for lesions that may lead to long-term functional or cosmetic problems.
5. Multiple systemic syndromes may be associated with cutaneous vascular lesions.

Pearls

1. GLUT-1 positivity distinguishes hemangiomas from vascular malformations.
2. Propranolol is the first-line treatment for infantile hemangioma.
3. Hemangiomas affecting the beard distribution have a high association of airway hemangioma.
4. Lymphatic malformations are classified as microcystic, macrocystic, and mixed lesions, which affects the treatment of choice.
5. Pulsed-dye laser (PDL) is the treatment of choice for cutaneous capillary malformations such as port-wine stain.

QUESTIONS

1. What are the four major classification schemes for vascular lesions, and what is the most useful and currently used nomenclature?

- Descriptive
- Anatomic-physiologic (microscopic)
- Embryologic
- Biologic behavior

Mulliken and Glowacki published a landmark paper in 1982 simplifying the nomenclature of vascular anomalies by classifying them based on cellular turnover and histology, which is most useful in the diagnosis, management, and prognosis of these lesions.

- **Vascular tumors** or infantile hemangiomas, characterized by rapidly enlarging endothelial proliferations that spontaneously involute.
- **Vascular malformations** are structural anomalies that are subcategorized based on channel type (capillary, venous, arterial, lymphatic, or combinations of these), present at birth and are characterized by growth proportional to the child. Unlike an infantile hemangioma, there is no cellular proliferation and instead there is progressive dilation of vascular channels.

2. What is the most common tumor of infancy and what is the classic presentation?

Hemangioma is the most common tumor of infancy with an incidence of 1% to 2.6% at birth and ≈10% by one year of age. Eighty percent are noted within the first month of life, typically presenting at 2 to 4 weeks of life. The female to male ratio is 3:1 and 60% occur in the head and neck. Superficial lesions are bright red or crimson whereas deeper lesions may have a bluish hue. Hemangiomas have a very characteristic cycle involving a proliferative phase (first 8 to 12 months of life), quiescence, and a slow involution (beginning at about 12 months of age and involute at variable rates, typically over 5 to 8 years).

3. **What is the distinguishing cellular marker for hemangioma?**
GLUT-1 (glucose transporter isoform-1) shares common antigenicity to placental tissue and GLUT-1 positivity distinguishes hemangiomas from vascular malformations. Exceptions are rapid involuting congenital hemangioma (RICH) and non-involuting congenital hemangiomas (NICH), which may be GLUT-1 negative.

4. **What are the indications for treatment for hemangiomas of the head and neck?**
Absolute indications for treatment include functional ocular obstruction or airway compromise. Other indications for intervention include large ulcerated lesions with hemorrhage or infection, those prone to functional compromise (ear/nose) or long-term cosmetic deformity, and those that are a source of psychosocial trauma to the child.

5. **What is the first-line treatment for hemangiomas? What other treatments are available?**
Currently, propranolol is used as the first-line treatment for hemangiomas unless a contraindication exists. Propranalol is a nonselective beta blocker that exerts a vasoconstrictive effect, which may result in reduction of lesion volume, softening, and regression of the lesion. Induction of apoptosis is also a possible mechanism of action for reducing hemangioma lesions. Propranolol has a 97% response rate and is taken orally with possible utility for topical beta blockers such as timolol. Side effects include bronchospasm, hypoglycemia, GERD, hypotension, and somnolence.
Systemic or intralesional steroids were the mainstay of therapy prior to the use of propranolol and exhibit a 50% to 90% response rate. Intralesional injections require multiple treatments at 6- to 8-week intervals. Periorbital lesions should not undergo intralesional injections because this carries a risk of central retinal artery occlusion.
Interferon a-2a is an angiostatic agent indicated if steroids or propranolol are ineffective or for recurrent or refractory cases. It is not commonly used secondary to a 25% risk of spastic diplegia.
Photocoagulation of hemangiomas can be performed with pulsed dye (superficial), argon (ulcerated or active bleedings), and Nd:Yag (deep penetration into dermis) lasers.
Surgical excision is typically timed during the involution phase or during the proliferative phase in cases recalcitrant to medical therapy.

6. **What are the advantages and limitations of medical treatments for hemangiomas?**
See Table 54-1.

7. **What is Kasabach-Merritt syndrome?**
Kasabach-Merritt syndrome is a complication of rapidly enlarging vascular lesions (hemangioma) and is characterized by platelet trapping, hemolytic anemia, thrombocytopenia, and coagulopathy. This is most commonly associated with kaposiform hemangioendothelioma and tufted angioma.

Table 54-1. Medical Treatment of Hemangioma

TREATMENT	MECHANISM OF ACTION	ADVANTAGE	MAJOR SIDE EFFECT
Propranolol	Non-selective beta blocker Vasoconstriction vs. apoptosis effect	High response oral med	Hypotension Hypoglycemia Pulmonary effects
Corticosteroid	Vasoconstriction vs. down regulation of angiogenic factors (VEGF)	High response oral med	Growth retardation Adrenal crisis/Cushing's Gastric effects
Interferon a-2a	Antiviral Angiostatic	Effective in severe resilient cases	Spastic diplegia (severe and nonreversible)
Vincristine	Chemotherapeutic agent Mitotic inhibition	Use in Kasabach-Merritt syndrome	Neurotoxic (also requires central access and 4-6 month treatment)

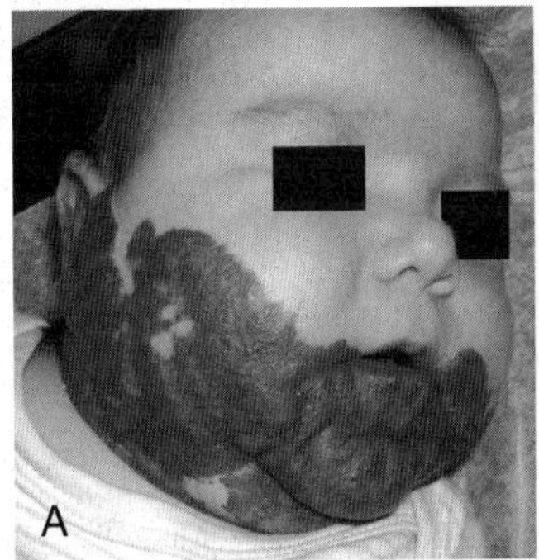

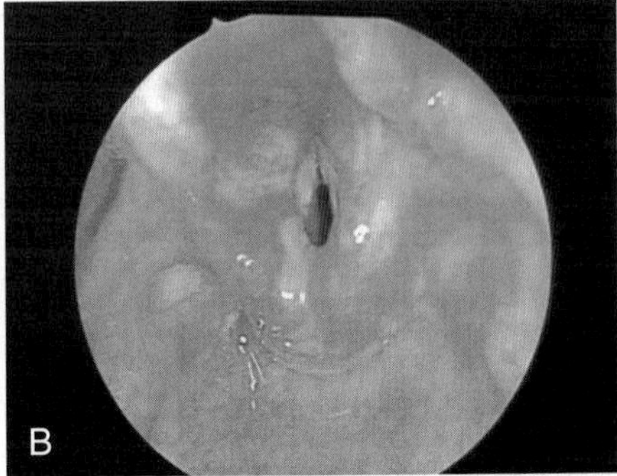

Figure 54-1. A, Infant with beard distribution (V3) cervicofacial hemangioma. **B,** Segmental airway hemangioma as viewed under microlaryngoscopy in an infant with PHACE syndrome with beard distribution cervicofacial hemangioma. *(Courtesy of David Low, MD.)*

8. What is **PHACES** syndrome?
   PHACES is an acronym for Posterior fossa malformation, Hemangiomas, Arterial anomalies, Cardiac defects (coarctation of the aorta), Eye abnormalities (coloboma), and Sternal abnormalities or ventral developmental defect (need 2 of 6 for diagnosis). **PHACES** syndrome is common in patients with segmental (dermatome distribution) hemangioma. Workup should include ophthalmology and cardiology consultation along with brain MRI.

9. Hemangiomas in the beard distribution carry high risk of what related vascular anomaly? (Figure 54-1)
   Hemangiomas in the V3/beard distribution have a high incidence (≈30% to 65%) of airway hemangioma, which may involve the oral cavity, oropharynx, hypopharynx, supraglottis, glottis, or subglottis. The subglottis is the most common location of focal hemangioma in the upper airway. Treatment modalities include systemic therapy with propranolol or steroids and local treatment with laser therapy or surgical excision. A tracheotomy may be required to bypass obstruction in some cases.

10. What is a port-wine stain?
    Port-wine stain is a superficial capillary vascular malformation typically present at birth appearing as a sharply demarcated pink-red patch that darkens over time and grows proportionately to the child. Pulsed-dye laser is the gold standard treatment with improved results if treated early in life.

11. What syndrome is related to this vascular malformation? (Figure 54-2)
    Sturge-Weber syndrome, also known as encephalotrigeminal angiomatosis, is characterized by a facial port-wine stain in the V1 (ophthalmic) distribution, glaucoma, seizures, mental retardation, and dural involvement.

12. How are lymphatic malformations (LM) classified (based on 1996 International Society for the Study of Vascular Anomalies)? (Figure 54-3)
    Classified as macrocystic (e.g., cystic hygroma), microcystic (e.g., lymphangioma), or mixed. Macrocystic LM are comprised of single or multiple cysts >2 cm^3 in size. Microcystic LM are cysts <2 cm^3. Mixed LM contain both macro- and microcystic components.

13. What are the mainstays of treatment for lymphatic malformations?
    Microcystic lesions are more severe and extensively infiltrate tissues; treatment is usually not curative. Treatment goals are to correct deformity and maintain function via surgery, coblation/radiofrequency, or laser excision/reduction. Macrocystic lesions are amenable to treatment with complete surgical excision or sclerosing agents such as doxycycline, bleomycin, ethanol, and OK-432 (picibanil). Acutely infected cysts may be treated with antibiotics and/or steroids.

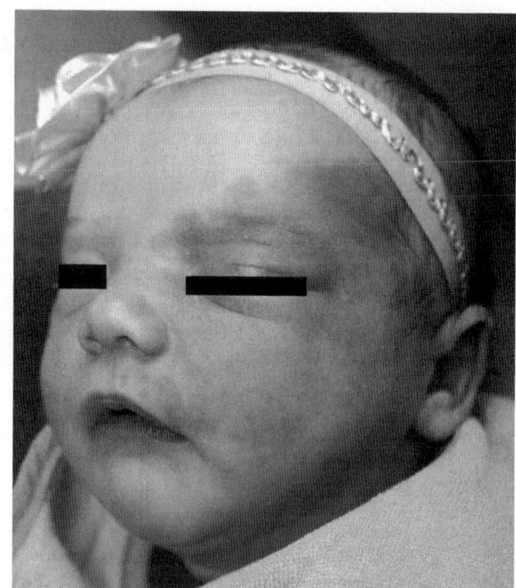

Figure 54-2. Infant with port-wine stain (capillary vascular malformation) in V1/ ophthalmic distributionassociated with Sturge-Weber syndrome. *(Courtesy of David Low, MD.)*

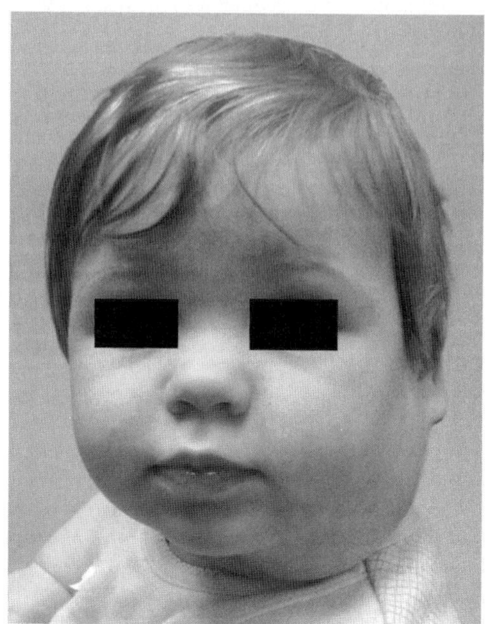

Figure 54-3. Child with left sided macrocytic lymphatic malformation. *(Courtesy of David Low, MD.)*

14. **What is the diagnostic workup for lymphatic malformation? (Figure 54-4)**
MRI with gadolinium and fat suppression, which shows marked high intensity of the lesion on T2 images and fluid/fluid levels suggestive of LM. Ultrasound may be useful, but CT scans are often not helpful.

15. **Which low flow vascular malformation tends to involve muscle such as the tongue? (Figure 54-5)**
Venous malformations tend to involve muscles and may be deep. These lesions tend to swell with activity or in a dependent fashion. They can be painful, may clot, and may have palpable phleboliths (can be identified on US or CT scan) from previous clot resolution.

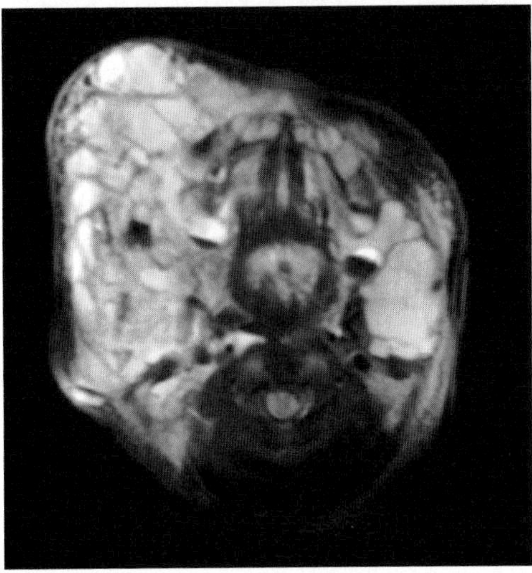

Figure 54-4. T2-weighted MRI scan of a microcystic lymphatic malformation demonstrating fluid layering. *(Courtesy of Children's Hospital of Philadelphia.)*

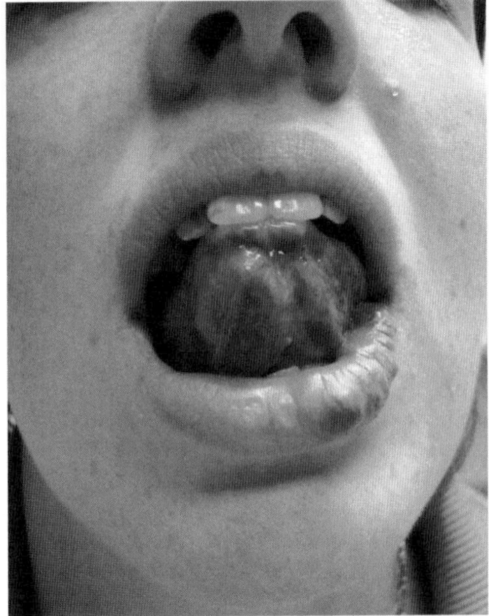

Figure 54-5. Child with venous malformation affecting the tongue, floor of mouth, and lower lip. *(Courtesy of David Low, MD.)*

16. **Which high flow vascular malformation can cause local soft tissue and bony destruction, often presenting in adulthood?**
    Arteriovenous malformations (AVM). These lesions are often mild in childhood and become progressively symptomatic in adulthood with local destruction and functional impairment. Current management is with surgery, endovascular embolization (with onyx), or a combination of embolization and surgery.

Bibliography

Bauman NM, McCarter RJ, Guzzetta PC, et al: Propranolol vs prednisolone for symptomatic proliferating infantile hemangiomas: a randomized clinical trial, *JAMA Otolaryngol Head Neck Surg* 140(4):323–330, 2014.

Blei F: Basic science and clinical aspects of vascular anomalies, *Curr Opin Pediatr* 17(4):501, 2005.

Buckmiller LM, Munson PD, Dyamenahalli U, et al: Propranolol for infantile hemangiomas: early experience at a tertiary vascular anomalies center, *Laryngoscope* 120(4):676, 2010.

Eivazi B, Ardelean M, Bäumler W, et al: Update on hemangiomas and vascular malformations of the head and neck, *Eur Arch Otorhinolaryngol* 266(2):187, 2009.

Eivazi B, Werner JA: Management of vascular malformations and hemangiomas of the head and neck—an update, *Curr Opin Otolaryngol Head Neck Surg* 21(2):157, 2013.

Glade RS, Richter GT, Jame CA, et al: Diagnosis and management of pediatric cervicofacial venous malformations: retrospective review from a vascular anomalies center, *Laryngoscope* 120(2):229, 2010.

Manning SC, Perkins J: Lymphatic malformations, *Curr Opin Otolaryngol Head Neck Surg* 21(6):571, 2013.

Mulliken JB, Glowacki J: Hemangiomas and vascular malformations in infants and children: a classification based on endothelial characteristics, *Plast Reconstructive Surg* 69(3):412, 1982.

Renton JP, Smith RJ: Current treatment paradigms in the management of lymphatic malformations, *Laryngoscope* 12(1):56, 2013.

Sajan JA, Tibesar R, Jabbour N, et al: Assessment of pulsed-dye laser therapy for pediatric cutaneous vascular anomalies, *JAMA Facial Plast Surg* 15(6):434, 2013.

Tlougan BE, Lee MT, Drolet BA, et al: Medical management of tumors associated with Kasabach-Merritt phenomenon: an expert survey, *J Pediatr Hematol Oncol* 35(8):618, 2013.

Wiegand S, Tiburtius J, Zimmermann AP, et al: Localization and treatment of lingual venous and arteriovenous malformations, *Vasc Med* 19(1):49, 2014.

CHAPTER 55

PEDIATRIC HEAD AND NECK TUMORS

Todd M. Wine, MD

KEY POINTS

1. The location of a neck mass is the key to understanding the differential diagnosis.
2. Imaging studies are important in the evaluation of many masses of the head and neck.
3. A neck mass that presents with infectious symptoms may be due to an infected congenital lesion.
4. The choice of treatment of atypical mycobacterial infections of the neck must always consider the risks of the treatment versus the negative quality of life related to a prolonged neck mass and/or drainage.
5. Fine needle aspiration can often identify benign and malignant masses, but many masses will require a core or an open biopsy for definitive diagnosis.

Pearls

1. The most common mass in the neck in children is a reactive lymph node. Lymphomas are the most common malignancy seen in the neck in children.
2. The key to a Sistrunk procedure is not just resecting the central portion of the hyoid bone, but resecting tongue musculature between the hyoid bone and foramen cecum.

QUESTIONS

1. **What are the categories of neck masses in children that are important when creating a differential diagnosis?**
   - *Congenital neck masses* are those that are present at birth and secondary to defects occurring in embryology.
   - *Infectious neck masses* are those that present due to an infection and typically resolve with treatment of the infection. These are most commonly infected or reactive lymph nodes, but can also occur in other tissues in the head and neck such as the salivary glands.
   - *Inflammatory masses* that do not have a known infectious cause, such as those associated with Kawasaki's disease.
   - *Neoplastic lesions* of the neck including benign and malignant processes. These encompass malignant lymphadenopathy, benign and malignant salivary gland tumors, benign and malignant thyroid tumors, and tumors originating from neurologic, muscular, vascular, lymphatic, cartilaginous, or osseus tissues.
   - *Vascular malformations* (see Chapter 54).

2. **What is the most common neck mass in a child?**

   An enlarged lymph node is the most common reason that a child presents with a neck mass. The most common cause of enlarged lymphadenopathy is infection, either viral or bacterial. Viral causes of lymphadenopathy include adenovirus, rhinovirus, and enterovirus, which can all occur with a viral upper respiratory infection. Epstein-Barr virus (EBV) causes mononucleosis, which consists of cervical lymphadenopathy, exudative tonsillitis, and hepatosplenomegaly.

   Bacterial causes of an enlarged lymph node most commonly include infections due to *Staphylococcus aureus* and *Streptococcus pyogenes.* Sometimes, the infected lymph node can suppurate and create a neck abscess. Other significant causes of bacterial lymphadenitis are atypical mycobacterium, *Bartonella henselae* (cat-scratch disease), and tuberculosis.

3. **What presenting features suggest an acute infectious cause of a neck mass?**
Fever, pain, acute swelling, erythema of the overlying skin, decreased neck range of motion, and odynophagia can indicate that a neck mass is secondary to an infectious cause. Concomitant upper respiratory tract symptoms, exposure to sick contacts, foreign travel, exposure to animals (cats, ticks), and the presence of immunodeficiency are all important historical features that can allow better understanding of the etiology of a neck mass.

4. **What other type of neck lesions can present with an acute infection or inflammation?**
Congenital lesions including thyroglossal duct cysts, dermoids, branchial cleft cysts, vascular malformations, and preauricular cysts can often present with acute swelling, erythema, pain, and fevers. The preferred treatment of these infectious exacerbations is antibiotic therapy. Incision and drainage should be performed only if necessary because they may complicate the definitive resection of the congenital mass. The resection of a congenital lesion is more easily accomplished after complete resolution of the infection.

5. **What congenital neck masses occur in the midline neck?**
Thyroglossal duct cyst is the most common congenital neck mass. Thyroglossal duct cysts occur in the midline due to incomplete obliteration of the thyroglossal duct. The median thyroid anlage starts at the foramen cecum of the tongue and migrates caudally in the neck until it reaches its final anatomic position near the cricoid cartilage. The thyroglossal duct should obliterate, but occasionally, this process is incomplete. A cyst can then form at that location with a tract that connects the cyst to the foramen cecum. Ectopic thyroid tissue can occur anywhere from the foramen cecum to the normal position of the thyroid gland.

Dermoid cysts are benign cystic structures that can occur anywhere in the body. They frequently occur in the head and neck and can occur in the midline neck and mimic a thyroglossal duct cyst. Other common locations include the nose, oral cavity, orbit, and nasopharynx. Dermoid cysts arise due to entrapment of epithelial cells along lines of fusion. They usually contain other skin appendages including sebaceous glands, hair, or hair follicles. They can often be adherent to the overlying skin and may even have a small draining sinus.

Teratomas are similar to dermoids, with the exception that they contain cell types of ectodermal, mesodermal, and endodermal origin. They may present as a firm neck mass and can cause respiratory symptoms when they are very large. Treatment requires complete surgical excision.

Laryngoceles occur as midline neck masses when they herniate through the thyrohyoid membrane (external laryngocele). If confined to the larynx, it is an internal laryngocele and will not likely present as a mass. Symptoms include hoarseness, dysphagia, and severe dyspnea, particularly when presenting in a neonate.

6. **What is the significance of the Sistrunk procedure used to resect a thyroglossal duct cyst?**
The earliest reports of thyroglossal duct cyst excision were plagued by a rate of recurrence as high as 50%. Resection of the hyoid bone along with cyst improved recurrence rates to 20%. Walter Sistrunk expanded that technique to include resection of the cyst, hyoid bone, and suprahyoid tongue musculature to ensure that the tract(s) connecting the cyst to the foramen cecum was adequately resected. This decreased the recurrence rate to near 5%. Removal of the cuff of lingual musculature is important because the tract may pass anterior or posterior to the hyoid and may be multiple.

7. **What congenital neck masses occur in the lateral neck?**
Congenital lateral neck masses are most likely to be of branchial origin. Otherwise, congenital lateral neck masses can include vascular malformations and thymic cysts. Branchial anomalies presenting as a mass are most likely to be a cyst with or without a sinus, which may connect it to the skin or to an internal structure. Branchial anomalies are classified by their branchial origin. They can be first, second, third, or fourth branchial anomalies.

The most common branchial anomaly is a second branchial cleft cyst. Second brachial cleft cysts occur in the upper neck and present as a cystic mass anterior to the sternocleidomastoid muscle. They can present as an acute, painful swelling of the neck that follows upper respiratory tract symptoms. It often could be confused with a suppurative lymph node. The differentiation between these two entities can be difficult, but imaging with contrast-enhanced computed tomography may be helpful. The infected cyst will have a circumferential thin wall compared to a thicker wall with more surrounding inflammation of an abscess.

The second most common branchial anomaly is a first branchial cleft cyst. These occur in the infra-auricular region and may occur anterior, inferior, or posterior to the lobule. These can be associated with the facial nerve and resection will require dissection of the facial nerve.

Least common are branchial anomalies of the third and fourth arch which typically present as left sided infections in the lower neck. Thyroiditis may occur in the setting of a fourth branchial cleft cyst as the tract should extend through the thyroid gland. These cysts will often have a connection to the piriform sinus. Proper resection of a fourth arch anomaly requires hemithyroidectomy. Otherwise, recurrence is more likely.

Thymic cysts can occur in the lateral neck as thymic tissue originates from the third branchial arch and descends into the mediastinum via the thymopharyngeal duct. Thymic cysts usually occur in the left neck and can be unilocular or multilocular. The diagnosis is confirmed on pathology with the presence of Hassall corpuscles (concentric epithelioreticular cells and macrophages in the medulla).

Vascular malformations are discussed in greater detail in Chapter 54. These include a range of pathologies that include venous malformation, lymphatic malformation, venolymphatic malformation, and arterovenous malformation. These classically present in the posterior triangle of the neck.

8. **How does an atypical mycobacterial infection present?**

Atypical mycobacterium infections in the neck often present with a mass, which is often firm, nontender, and located in the submandibular or preauricular regions. Classically, there is a violaceous discoloration to the overlying skin. The skin may be thin with areas of fluctuance. Typically, there is no preceding illness, fevers, weight loss, or night sweats. An intradermal tuberculin test will usually be negative or indeterminate. Computed tomography and magnetic resonance imaging may suggest an infectious cause by revealing fat stranding, thick wall of abscess cavity (if present), inflammation of skin, and multiloculated appearance, but they are not diagnostic.

The clinical course may start as a discrete mass in the submandibular or periauricular regions. A course of antibiotics will have no significant effect. The mass may continue to enlarge and it is not uncommon for violaceous skin changes to occur overlying a fluctuant component of the mass. The fluctuant area may progress to the point that the skin breaks down and a draining wound is created. The natural history is that this infection is self-limited and will heal without treatment. Unfortunately, the natural history is not typically expedient and may take many months to a couple of years for resolution.

9. **What are the treatment considerations for atypical mycobacterium?**

Treatment options consist of observation, medical management with antibiotics, surgical curettage, and surgical excision or any combination of the above. The optimal treatment would be one that eradicates the disease quickly and does so with minimal short- and long-term risk to the patient. Prompt eradication is expected if complete surgical excision is performed. As such, many studies have supported complete excision as the optimal treatment for quicker time to resolution and better cosmetic outcomes. Unfortunately, the disease process often closely encounters the facial nerve or its branches. Complete excision can be associated with temporary nerve injury in approximately 20% to 30% and permanent nerve injury in 2% to 5% of cases. Other outcomes include higher incidence of poor scarring (21%), wound infection (14%), and recurrence (9%). While the risk of permanent injury is low, the risk is significant considering that the disease resolves, albeit more slowly, without surgery.

If complete surgical excision is deemed too risky, other treatment options consist of surgical incision and curettage of the purulent portion of the mass. This can help confirm the diagnosis and may help treat a draining or "about to drain" wound.

Medical therapy with various antibiotics (clarithromycin, azithromycin, ethambutol, and rifabutin) may be helpful and antimicrobial therapy can be utilized alone or in combination with surgical treatment. The use of medical therapy is often debated, however, as there has been no research proving its efficacy over observation. Observation alone allows the disease to take its expectant course and most patients will have resolved the infection by one year.

10. **What is the differential for inflammatory, but noninfectious lymphadenopathy?**

Kawasaki disease, also known as mucocutaneous lymph node syndrome, typically occurs in children less than 5 years old. It is considered a vasculitis and presents with high fever for 5 days and four of the following signs: acute cervical adenopathy, nonexudative conjunctivitis, strawberry tongue, lip fissure, rash, erythema of palms and soles, edema of hands and feet, and desquamation. It may cause coronary artery aneurysm and cardiologic evaluation is necessary. Treatment consists of intravenous immunoglobulins and aspirin.

PFAPA (periodic fevers with aphthous stomatitis, pharyngitis, and cervical adenitis) causes recurrent high fever in children typically less than 5 years old without signs of concomitant upper respiratory infections. Between episodes, they are likely asymptomatic. Diagnosis must rule out other causes of recurrent fevers and medical treatment can be helpful (steroids and/or cimetidine). Tonsillectomy is often curative.

Castleman disease is giant lymph node hyperplasia that causes concern due to the large size of lymph nodes. Fortunately, it is benign and excisional biopsy can be both diagnostic and curative.

Rosai-Dorfman disease consists of massive lymphadenopathy due to sinus histiocytosis occurring in patients under 10 years old. Diagnosis is made on biopsy of a lymph node. Treatment can be observational, but surgery, radiation, and chemotherapy may also play roles depending on severity of the disease.

Kikuchi-Fujimoto disease is a histiocytic necrotizing lymphadenitis typically occurring in 20- to 40-year-olds and may be unilateral or bilateral. Biopsy of the lymph node is required for diagnosis and resolution occurs in about 6 months.

11. What are reassuring sonographic findings of lymph nodes?

- Hypoechoic to muscle
- Flat, oval shaped, short axis: long axis <0.5, but submandibular and parotid nodes may be rounder
- Echogenic hilum
- Hilar vascularity seen in reactive or normal node
- Surrounding edema
- Sharp margins

12. What are sonographic features of malignant nodes?

- Markedly hypoechoic to muscle (except if papillary thyroid cancer)
- Round shape
- No echogenic hilus
- Coagulation necrosis
- Eccentric cortical hypertrophy
- Cystic necrosis
- Ill-defined borders
- Peripheral or mixed vascularity
- Calcifications suggest metastatic thyroid cancer
- No surrounding inflammation

13. What is the most likely malignant pathology type to be found in the head and neck?

Lymphomas (Hodgkin and non-Hodgkin) are the most common malignancy in the head and neck. Enlargement of lymph nodes is very common in children and when it is not reactive lymphadenopathy, lymphoma is the primary pathology that must be considered. Ultrasound can be reassuring when a normal appearing fatty hilum is identified. Otherwise, a persistently enlarged lymph node without resolution in time or antibiotic course may warrant biopsy to investigate further. Fine needle aspiration can often diagnose if a malignancy is present, but usually flow cytometry of a lymph node that has been completely excised is required to make the specific diagnosis that can help clarify the treatment of choice.

14. What is the most likely type of thyroid malignancy in a child?

Papillary thyroid carcinoma is the most common thyroid malignancy in adults and children. Papillary thyroid carcinoma will present with a painless, firm thyroid nodule. Usually the nodule will be cystic and nonfunctioning. Fine needle aspiration is recommend to achieve the diagnosis. Suspicious lymph nodes in the central and lateral neck compartments should be biopsied at the same time. Nodal metastasis is quite common, but overall survival remains high (2.5% mortality). Treatment is most often total thyroidectomy with central and/or lateral neck dissections for biopsy for proven or highly suspicious lymph nodes, followed by radioactive iodine ablation.

15. **What are common infectious or inflammatory lesions of salivary glands?**
Acute bacterial sialadenitis, viral sialadenitis, and juvenile recurrent parotitis. Acute bacterial sialadenitis occurs as unilateral, painful swelling with purulent drainage coming from the salivary duct. Treatment is with hydration, warm compress, massage, and sialogogues. Viral sialadenitis can occur due to coxsackievirus, cytomegalovirus, parainfluenza, or mumps.

16. **What pathologies are causes of benign salivary gland tumors?**
In children, the most common benign tumors are pleomorphic adenoma occurring in the parotid, submandibular, and minor salivary glands and hemangioma occurring in the parotid gland. Other benign pathologies exist and include Warthin's tumors (papillary cystadenoma lymphomatosum), basal cell adenoma, myoepithelioma, and lymphoepithelioma.

Hemangioma of the parotid gland, and submandibular gland less commonly, presents at birth or shortly thereafter. Like hemangiomas occurring elsewhere, there is a rapid proliferative phase that occurs in the first few months of life followed by slow involution over a period of one to many years. Treatment of hemangioma classically is to allow involution over time and to medically treat with steroids, interferon, and more recently propranolol for more symptomatic lesions. Surgical resection is also an option, but must be carefully considered due to an increased risk to the facial nerve.

17. **What pathologies are the most common causes of malignant salivary gland tumors?**
Mucoepidermoid, acinic cell, adenocarcinoma, adenoid cystic carcinomas, and carcinoma ex pleomorphic are possible salivary malignancies in childhood. Mucoepidermoid carcinoma is the most common malignant salivary mass in children, typically presenting in adolescence. Like benign tumors, treatment is with complete surgical excision with margins if possible. Neck dissection will be required in some malignancies, particularly if the lesion is of higher grade, lymph nodes are clinically suspicious, or there is evidence that the tumor has extraglandular extension or facial nerve invasion. Adjuvant radiotherapy is used as well if there is significant nodal involvement, extraglandular extension, perineural invasion, or incomplete excision. The risks and benefits of radiotherapy must be carefully considered in children due to the risk of second malignancy and other complications of radiation therapy.

18. **What is the most common type of sarcoma occurring in the head and neck of children?**
Rhabdomyosarcoma (RMS) is the most common sarcoma occurring in the head and neck region of children. Approximately one third of RMS occur in the head and neck and within the head and neck, the orbit is the most common site. The presenting symptoms will depend on the site of origin for the tumor. Tumors can be classified as parameningeal, which implies that they arise either along the anterior or lateral skull base, or nonparameningeal, occurring in oro/hypopharynx, parotid, external ear, or lateral neck. Ideally, complete surgical resection with wide margins results in the best long-term prognosis. Unfortunately, in the head and neck wide margins are rarely possible without major functional impairment. Thus, the initial treatment involves obtaining the tissue diagnosis. Although fine needle aspiration may identify tumor as a sarcoma, more detailed histologic typing by a pathologist experienced in sarcomas is required to allow proper treatment decisions. Therefore, core or open biopsies are often required. Treatment of head and neck sarcomas will often consist of chemotherapy (directed by the Intergroup Rhabdomyosarcoma Studies [IRS] protocols for rhabdomyosarcomas or Children's Oncology Group [COG] protocols for nonrhabdomyosarcomas), surgery, and radiation therapy.

19. **What are other types of sarcomas?**
Fibrosarcoma, onrhabdomyosarcoma, hemangiopericytoma, osteosarcoma, chondrosarcoma, extraskeletal Ewing sarcoma, liposarcoma, and leiomyosarcoma.

20. **What are the types of neuroblastic neck masses?**
Neuroblastic masses include ganglioneuroma, ganglioneuroblastoma, and neuroblastoma. Neuroblastoma is the most common of these lesions and is the third most common malignancy in children. These three pathologies represent different stages of the same disease process, with neuroblastoma being the least differentiated with the most malignant potential and ganglioneuroma being the most differentiated with likely no malignant potential. Typically, these are painless neck

masses and symptoms are related to nerve (cranial nerves, sympathetic chain) or aerodigestive tract compression.

21. **What is the importance of creating a differential diagnosis as it pertains to investigating a neck mass?**
    Creating an appropriate differential diagnosis for each patient presenting with a neck mass allows judicious consideration for the appropriate diagnostic tests to order, whether it be laboratory assessment or radiographic imaging. The history should dictate which imaging modality should be utilized and this is particularly important when considering computed tomography scans. Through the cumulative effects of radiation exposure, two to three computed tomography scans of the head can increase the risk of brain cancer threefold and 5 to 10 head CTs may increase risk of leukemia by threefold. As such, special consideration should be taken when considering each imaging study.

Bibliography

Acierno SP, Waldhausen JH: Congenital cervical cysts, sinuses and fistulae, *Otolaryngol Clin North Am* 40(1):161–176, vii–viii, 2007.

Anne S, Teot LA, Mandell DL: Fine needle aspiration biopsy: role in diagnosis of pediatric head and neck masses, *Int J Pediatr Otorhinolaryngol* 72(10):1547–1553, 2008.

Fang QG, Shi S, Li ZN, et al: Epithelial salivary gland tumors in children: a twenty-five-year experience of 122 patients, *Int J Pediatr Otorhinolaryngol* 77(8):1252–1254, 2013.

Giacomini CP, Jeffrey RB, Shin LK: Ultrasonographic evaluation of malignant and normal cervical lymph nodes, *Semin Ultrasound CT MR* 34(3):236–247, 2013.

Huh WW, Fitzgerald N, Mahajan A, et al: Pediatric sarcomas and related tumors of the head and neck, *Cancer Treat Rev* 37(6):431–439, 2011.

Lee DH, Yoon TM, Lee JK, et al: Clinical utility of fine needle aspiration cytology in pediatric parotid tumors, *Int J Pediatr Otorhinolaryngol* 77(8):1272–1275, 2013.

Lindeboom JA, Kuijper EJ, Bruijnesteijn van Coppenraet ES, et al: Surgical excision versus antibiotic treatment for nontuberculous mycobacterial cervicofacial lymphadenitis in children: a multicenter, randomized, controlled trial, *Clin Infect Dis* 44(8):1057–1064, 2007.

Lindeboom JA, Lindeboom R, Bruijnesteijn van Coppenraet ES, et al: Esthetic outcome of surgical excision versus antibiotic therapy for nontuberculous mycobacterial cervicofacial lymphadenitis in children, *Pediatr Infect Dis J* 28(11):1028–1130, 2009.

Maddalozzo J, Alderfer J, Modi V: Posterior hyoid space as related to excision of the thyroglossal duct cyst, *Laryngoscope* 120(9):1773–1778, 2010.

Moukheiber AK, Nicollas R, Roman S, et al: Primary pediatric neuroblastic tumors of the neck, *Int J Pediatr Otorhinolaryngol* 60(2):155–161, 2001.

Owusu JA, Parker NP, Rimell FL: Postoperative facial nerve function in pediatric parotidectomy: a 12-year review, *Otolaryngol Head Neck Surg* 148(2):249–252, 2013.

Parker NP, Scott AR, Finkelstein M, et al: Predicting surgical outcomes in pediatric cervicofacial nontuberculous mycobacterial lymphadenitis, *Ann Otol Rhinol Laryngol* 121(7):478–484, 2012.

Pearce MS, Salotti JA, Little MP, et al: Radiation exposure from CT scans in childhood and subsequent risk of leukaemia and brain tumours: a retrospective cohort study, *Lancet* 380(9840):499–505, 2012.

Wei JL, Bond J, Sykes KJ, et al: Treatment outcomes for nontuberculous mycobacterial cervicofacial lymphadenitis in children based on the type of surgical intervention, *Otolaryngol Head Neck Surg* 138(5):566–571, 2008.

Whittemore KR Jr, Cunningham MJ: Malignant tumors of the head and neck. In Bluestone C, Healy G, Simons J, editors: *Pediatric Otolaryngology*, China, 2014, Peoples Medical Publishing House, p 1803.

Zeharia A, Eidlitz-Markus T, Haimi-Cohen Y, et al: Management of nontuberculous mycobacteria-induced cervical lymphadenitis with observation alone, *Pediatr Infect Dis J* 27(10):920–922, 2008.

VI
Facial Plastic Surgery, Reconstruction and Trauma

ANATOMY AND EMBRYOLOGY WITH RADIOLOGIC CORRELATES

Mofiyinfolu Sokoya, MD and Adam M. Terella, MD

CHAPTER 56

KEY POINTS

1. Head and neck formation is intimately related to the development of the pharyngeal arches, with each arch carrying an artery, nerve, cartilaginous bar, and muscle.
2. Palate formation requires midline fusion of the medial nasal prominences and palatal shelves. Incomplete fusion results in a spectrum of cleft palate deformities.
3. The superficial muscular aponeurotic system (SMAS) represents a discrete fascial layer that separates the subcutaneous fat from the underlying parotidomasseteric fascia and facial nerve.
4. When operating on the face, if the dissection is kept superficial to the superficially situated musculature the facial nerve should not be harmed.
5. When completing a facial fracture repair it is often necessary to reestablish the vertical buttresses with rigid fixation.

Pearls

1. The forehead is composed of five anatomic layers, described by the mnemonic "SCALP." Identification of these layers is important for both cosmetic and reconstructive procedures in this region.
2. The galea aponeurosis can serve as a tension-bearing layer during scalp reconstruction.
3. The majority of facial mimetic muscles are superficially situated and receive facial nerve innervation from their deep surface.
4. With progressive age, descent of the suborbicularis orbital fat pad (SOOF) structures leads to deepening of the nasolabial crease.

QUESTIONS

Applied Embryology

1. What are the pharyngeal arches? How are they significant to head and neck development?

   Head and neck formation is intimately related to the development of the pharyngeal arches. Formation of these arches begins at approximately 20 days gestation, and by 28 days four arches are visible. Each arch carries an artery, nerve, cartilaginous bar, and muscle. Of note, the first arch cartilage develops into the maxillary process and mandible. The first arch also carries the mandibular branch of the trigeminal nerve and the muscles of mastication. The second arch carries CN 7 (facial nerve) and the muscles of facial expression.

2. What primitive structures contribute to the formation of the face?

   At the end of the fourth embryonic week, neural crest–derived facial prominences appear from the first pair of pharyngeal arches. Maxillary prominences are found laterally. The frontal nasal prominences develop into the forehead and frontal nasal process. On either side of the frontal nasal prominences are local thickenings that form nasal placodes. These placodes invaginate to form nasal pits and ultimately ridges of tissue that can be divided into a lateral nasal prominence and medial nasal prominences (Figure 56-1).

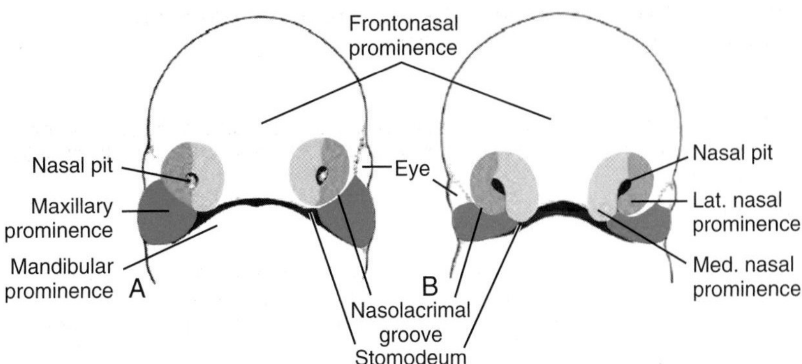

Figure 56-1. Frontal aspect of the face. A, Five-week embryo. B, Six-week embryo. Illustrated is the relationship of the maxillary promince and the nasal placodes, contributing to the lateral and medial nasal promince. *(From Friedman O, Wang TD, Milczuk H: Cleft lip and palate. In Flint PW, Haughey BH, Lund VJ, et al, editors: Cummings Otolaryngology—Head & Neck Surgery, ed 5, Philadelphia, 2010, Mosby Elsevier.)*

3. How and when is the upper lip formed?
At approximately 6 weeks post conception, the paired maxillary prominences grow medially and contact the paired medial nasal prominences. As fusion of these structures occurs, the upper lip is formed. Ultimately, the maxillary prominences form the lateral lip and the medial nasal prominences form the philtrum, medial upper lip, columella, and nasal tip.

4. Discuss the embryology of the nose.
In the 7-week embryo, five facial prominences contribute to the formation of the nose: the frontal nasal prominence, the paired medial nasal prominences, and the paired lateral nasal prominences. The frontal nasal prominence forms the nasal bridge, the medial nasal prominences fuse and form the nasal tip and columella, and the lateral nasal prominence forms the nasal alae.

5. How is the primary palate (intermaxillary segment) formed?
Formation of the palate begins concurrently with formation of the upper lip and nose, at the end of the fifth week. In addition to contributing to the nose and upper lip, fusion of the two medial nasal prominences forms the intermaxillary segment. The *primary palate* includes the hard palate anterior to the incisive foramen.

6. What is the secondary palate, and how is it formed?
The *secondary palate* refers to the portions of the palate posterior to the incisive foramen. It is formed by the medial migration and midline fusion of the two palatine shelves. These shelves are extensions of the maxillary prominences. Midline fusion proceeds from anterior to posterior, ending with creation the uvula.

7. Failed fusion of the intermaxillary segment to the maxillary prominences results in what deformity?
Failure of fusion of the intermaxillary segment and maxillary prominence will result in a cleft lip deformity. There is a wide spectrum of cleft lip deformity including a unilateral versus bilateral cleft lip, and a complete versus incomplete cleft lip.

8. Failure of fusion of the palatal shelves will result in what deformity?
Failed fusion of the palatal shelves, and thus the secondary palate, results in a spectrum of palatal cleft abnormalities. The mildest form of soft palate cleft is a bifid uvula. A submucous cleft occurs when there is midline dehiscence of the palate musculature, but the mucosa remains intact. The most extensive cleft is a bilateral complete cleft of the palate in which the vomer and premaxilla do not fuse with the palatal shelves.

9. Discuss the embryologic development of the pinna.
The pinna develops from the first (mandibular) and second (hyoid) branchial arches. Each arch contributes three *hillocks*. The first hillock gives rise to the tragus. The second and third hillocks

form the crus helicis. The fourth and fifth hillocks become the crura anthelicis and helix, respectively. The sixth hillock forms the antitragus.

10. **Developmental error in hillock formation and/or fusion results in what malformation?**
Microtia is a malformation of the auricle. There can be a wide spectrum of presentation ranging from a small external ear with minimal structural abnormality to an ear with major external, middle, and inner ear structural aberrations.

Applied Anatomy

11. **What are the layers of the forehead and scalp?**
The layers of the forehead are in continuity with layers in the scalp. An effective mnemonic, "SCALP," describes the five anatomic layers: (S) skin, (C) subcutaneous tissue, (A) galea aponeurosis, (L) loose areolar tissue, and (P) pericranium. The galea aponeurosis is a discrete fibrous layer that is important during both cosmetic and reconstructive procedures. This layer surrounds the entire skull and divides to envelope the frontalis and occipitalis muscles. It is continuous with the temporoparietal fascia (TPF) below the temporal line.

12. **What four muscles are responsible for forehead and eyebrow movement?**
The frontalis, procerus, paired corrugator supercilii, and paired orbicularis oculi muscles each independently contributes to brow positioning and forehead/glabellar rhytids. It is useful to classify these muscles as brow elevators or brow depressors. The frontalis muscle is the primary and sole elevator of the brow. The procerus, corrugator supercilii, and orbicularis oculi all act as brow depressors.

13. **What is the superficial muscular aponeurotic system (SMAS)?**
The SMAS represents a discrete fascial layer that separates the subcutaneous fat from the underlying parotidomasseteric fascia and facial nerve. In the temporal region the SMAS is continuous with the temporal parietal fascia (TPF) and in the neck it is continuous with the platysma. This layer has importance in many procedures in facial plastic surgery such as face lifting (rhytidectomy) and soft tissue reconstruction, and represents an important surgical landmark.

14. **Describe the anatomic structures contributing to the malar prominence.**
The malar prominence is formed by the subcutaneous malar fat pad, which overlies the orbicularis oculi muscle. Deep to this muscle is the suborbicularis orbital fat pad (SOOF). With progressive age, descent of these structures leads to deepening of the nasolabial crease.

15. **What is the relationship of the facial mimetic muscles to the facial nerve? Why is this anatomic relationship important?**
The orbicularis oculi, platysma, and zygomaticus major and minor are considered superficially situated facial mimetic muscles and receive innervation from the facial nerve. These superficially situated muscles receive innervation from the deep surface.

16. **What facial mimetic muscles receive innervation from the superficial surface?**
Only the buccinators, levator anguli oris, and mentalis muscle lie in a plane deep to the facial nerve, and thus receive innervation from the superficial surface.

17. **What is the primary blood supply to the face?**
The primary arterial supply to the face consists of branches from the facial artery, which is a branch of the external carotid artery. The facial artery ascends over the body of the mandible anterior to the masseter muscle. It has a tortuous course, which is thought to help accommodate movement of the underlying mandible. As the facial artery passes across the face, branches of the facial nerve cross it superficially. The facial artery gives off several branches, including the superior and inferior labial arteries to the upper and lower lip, and the angular artery to the lateral soft tissue envelope of the nose.

Surface Anatomy

18. **What are the facial aesthetic units?**
The face can be divided into, and evaluated by, individual aesthetic units. These aesthetic units include the forehead and brow, the periorbital region, cheeks, nose, perioral region and chin, and the neck.

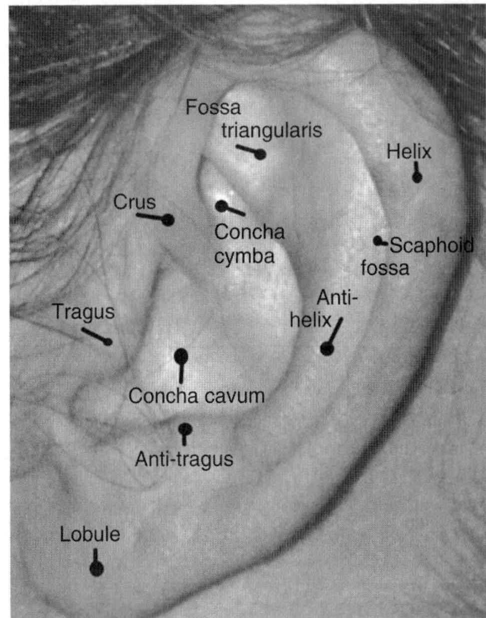

Figure 56-2. The surface anatomy of the pinna is described as a series of prominences and depressions.

19. What are the aesthetic subunits of the nose?

There are nine aesthetic units of the nose, including the nasal tip, dorsum, columella, paired sidewalls, paired alae, and paired soft tissue facets. These aesthetic subunits were proposed based on the observation that the nasal surface is made up of several concave and convex surfaces separated from one another by ridges and valleys.

20. Describe the surface anatomy of the pinna.

The surface anatomy of the pinna can be organized into a series of fossae and prominences or ridges, as illustrated in Figure 56-2. The four fossae include the triangular fossa, concha cymba, concha cavum, and scaphoid fossa. The primary prominences include the helix, antihelix, crus, tragus, antitragus, and lobule.

Bibliography

Baker S: *Local Flaps in Facial Reconstruction*, ed 2, Philadelphia, 2007, Mosby.

Burget GC, Menick FJ: The subunit principle in nasal reconstruction, *Plast Reconstr Surg* 76(2):239–247, 1985. PubMed PMID: 4023097.

Friedman O, Wang TD, Milczuk H: Cleft lip and palate. In Flint PW, Haughey BH, Lund VJ, et al, editors: *Cummings Otolaryngology—Head & Neck Surgery*, ed 5, Philadelphia, 2010, Mosby Elsevier.

Manson PN, Hoopes JE, Su CT: Structural pillars of the facial skeleton: an approach to the management of Le Fort fractures, *Plast Reconstr Surg* 66(1):54–62, 1980. PubMed PMID: 7394047.

Ruder RO: Congenital malformation of the auricle. In Papel ID, et al, editors: *Facial Plastic and Reconstructive Surgery*, ed 2, New York, 2002, Thieme.

Som PM, Naidich TP: Illustrated review of the embryology and development of the facial region, part 1: early face and lateral nasal cavities, *Am J Neuroradiol* 34(12):2233–2240, 2013.

Terella AM, Wang TD: Technical considerations in endoscopic brow lift. In Azizzadeh B, Massry GG, editors: *Clinics in Plastic Surgery. Brow and Upper Eyelid Surgery: Multispecialty Approach*, Philadelphia, 2013, Elsevier.

CHAPTER 57

PRINCIPLES OF WOUND HEALING

Mofiyinfolu Sokoya, MD and Andrew A. Winkler, MD

KEY POINTS

1. The tenets of Halstead are highly important in good surgical wound healing.
2. Wound healing occurs in overlapping phases: inflammatory, proliferative, and remodeling phases.
3. A patient's metabolic issues should always be addressed to promote ideal wound healing. It is wise to prescribe a daily multivitamin.
4. Wounds heal best when kept continually moist (white petrolatum ointment), clean, and protected.
5. Keloid scars grow outside the border of the initial wound.

Pearls

1. Scar revision timing: most scars improve in appearance without revision 1 to 3 years after the inciting event. Patients should be counseled to wait at least 6 to 12 months before undergoing a scar revision surgery, unless there are obvious scar characteristics that aren't expected to improve.
2. Dermabrasion is typically undertaken 8 to 12 weeks after the initial inflammatory phase, taking advantage of the end of the proliferative phase.

QUESTIONS

1. **What are the layers of skin?**
   The epidermis and dermis are the two main layers of skin. The epidermis is further separated into the stratum corneum, stratum lucidum, stratum granulosum, stratum spinosum, and stratum basale (from superficial to deep). The layers of the dermis include the papillary and reticular dermis.

2. **What is a scar?**
   A scar is an area of fibrosis that replaces normal skin after injury. A scar always forms after an injury, as it is the product of a normal wound healing process. Scars can be made less visible with various surgical and nonsurgical techniques.

3. **What is healing by primary intention?**
   Healing by primary intention healing occurs when the edges of the wound are brought together in direct contact, which may involve sutures, staples or other closure methods. This is the most commonly used method of wound closure and results in a minimally visible surgical scar.

4. **What is healing by secondary intention (Figure 57-1)?**
   Healing by secondary intention occurs when wound edges are not approximated, leaving an area of exposed subcutaneous tissue. This may result in greater wound contracture than seen in primary closure. This type of healing works best in concavities (e.g., temporal fossa, medial canthus, alar groove). It can be useful in scalp and forehead wounds. Advantages include low risk of infection, high rate of healing, acceptable cosmesis, and surveillance in cases where cancer may be incompletely excised.

5. **What is healing by tertiary intention?**
   Healing by tertiary intention is delayed primary closure. Wound edges are not closed immediately, but the defect is allowed to undergo the acute inflammatory phase in which phagocytosis of contaminated tissue occurs and the microbial count decreases. The wound edges are then brought together and closed.

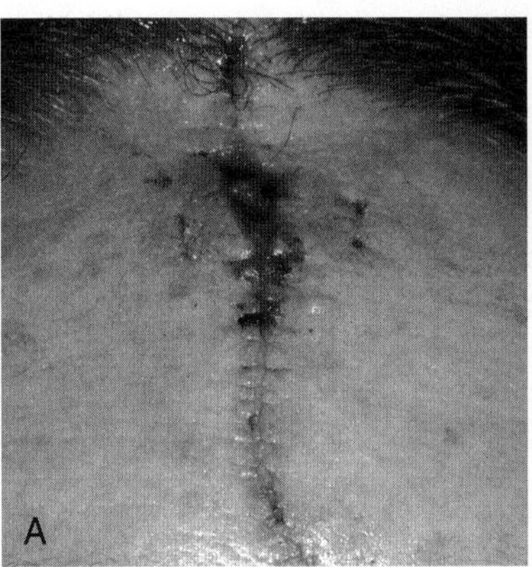

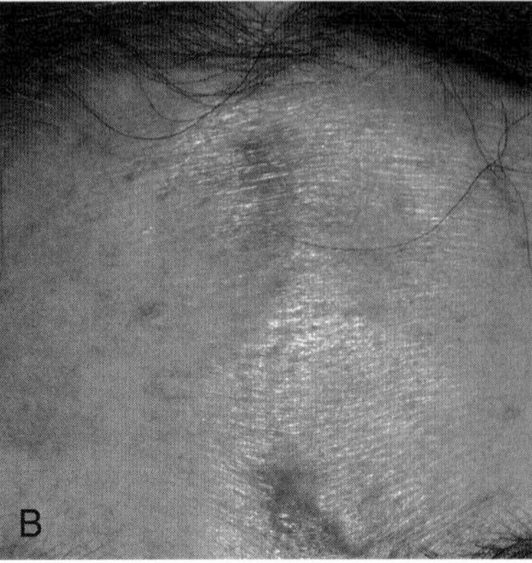

Figure 57-1. A, B. Healing by secondary intention of a forehead wound.

6. What are the three phases of surgical wound healing?
   1. Inflammatory Phase (injury to approximately 1 week)
   2. Proliferative Phase (30 minutes to approximately 1 month)
   3. Remodeling Phase (3 weeks to approximately 1 year)
7. What occurs in a wound during the inflammatory phase?
   Local *vasoconstriction* occurs within the first 5 to 10 minutes; then the coagulation cascade proceeds and a fibrin clot is formed. Activated platelets release several chemotactic factors that affect vascular tone. *Vasodilation* subsequently ensues secondary to histamine release. Next, the *cellular response* begins. Macrophage, neutrophil, and lymphocyte infiltration occurs, hallmarking the inflammatory phase. Importantly, only when inflammation subsides, does collagen deposition begin. Therefore, wounds with excess nonviable debris will experience a prolonged inflammatory phase.
8. What is the proliferative phase?
   The proliferative phase begins with *re-epithelialization* of the wound. This process begins at the time of the injury, and in primary closure is completed in 24 hours. *Collagen synthesis* begins on day 2. Fibroblasts proliferate and produce type III collagen, elastin, and extracellular matrix. The final component of the proliferative phase is *wound contraction*, which is mediated by myofibroblasts. This contraction is centripetal and is maximal at 10 to 15 days. Contraction may be severe in inflamed wounds.
9. What is the remodeling phase?
   Collagen remodeling and vascular maturation occur in the remodeling phase. Scars become pale, soft, and less protruding. Type III collagen initially deposited in the proliferative phase is converted into type I collagen. Collagen fibers become more organized into parallel bundles. Completion of remodeling may take 12 to 18 months and, even then, scars achieve only 70% to 80% of the tensile strength of normal skin.
10. What four local factors influence wound healing?
    1. Oxygenation
    2. Infection
    3. Foreign bodies
    4. Venous sufficiency
11. What chemotactic and proliferative factors are released during wound healing?
    - **Growth Hormone (GH):** Produced by the pituitary gland; promotes fibroblast proliferation
    - **Epidermal Growth Factor (EGF):** Produced by platelets; promotes epithelial cell and fibroblast proliferation and migration; activates fibroblast and vascular formation

- **Platelet Derived Growth Factor (PDGF):** Produced by platelets, macrophages, endothelial cells and keratinocytes; functions as chemoattractant for neutrophils, macrophages, and fibroblasts. Also works as mitogenic agent for fibroblasts, inducing production of collagen and hyaluronic acid.
- **Fibroblast Growth Factor (FGF):** Produced by macrophages, mast cells, lymphocytes, endothelial cells, and fibroblasts; promotes proliferation of vascular endothelial cells; also mitogenic for keratinocytes and fibroblasts
- **Transforming Growth Factor (TGF):** Produced by platelets, fibroblasts, neutrophils, macrophages, and lymphocytes; promotes proliferation of epithelial cell and fibroblasts
- **Insulin-like Growth Factor (IGF-1):** Produced by liver, plasma, and fibroblasts; promotes fibroblast proliferation and synthesis of extracellular matrix
- **Tumor Necrosis Factor (TNF):** Produced by macrophages, mast cells, and lymphocytes; promotes fibroblast proliferation

12. What are the tenets of Halstead?
These tenets address gentle handling of tissue, aseptic technique, sharp anatomic dissection, obliteration of dead space, careful hemostasis, and avoidance of wound tension. These principles are highly important to surgical wound healing.

13. How does wound desiccation affect healing?
A moist environment is essential for wound healing, particularly in re-epithelialization. Dry, scabbed wounds heal more slowly than wounds with adequate humidity. Desiccation increases the energy expenditure of epithelial cells in wound closure, thereby lengthening wound healing time.

14. How are wound healing phases affected by oxygen?
Initial hypoxia by vasoconstriction and vascular disruption actuates the early phases of wound healing by activating platelets and endothelium. However, recovery of tissue oxygenation is required for adequate healing, and chronic hypoxia can disrupt all aspects of wound healing.

15. What are relaxed skin tension lines (RSTLs)?
These are lines of tension that are intrinsic to the skin and determined largely by the underlying collagen matrix. RSTLs typically lie parallel to wrinkles. Incisions made at 90-degree angles to RSTLs will gape open widely, while those lying parallel will close with minimal tension.

16. Describe the differences and similarities between hypertrophic scars and keloids (Figure 57-2).
    - Hypertrophic scars:
        - Remain within the boundaries of original tissue injury.
        - Tend to regress with time.
        - Contain collagen fibers in a wavy, randomly organized pattern, parallel to the epithelial surface.

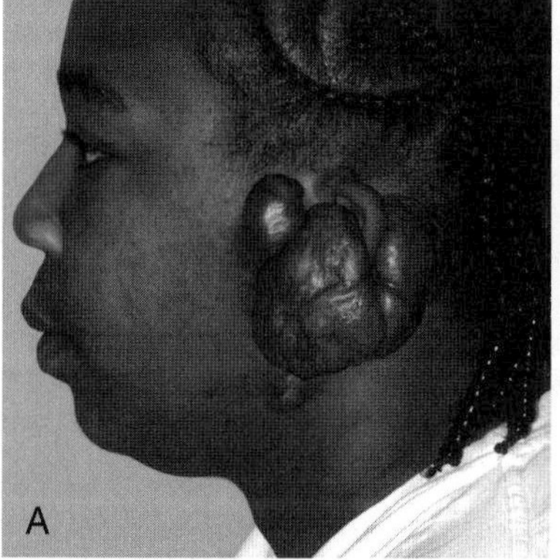

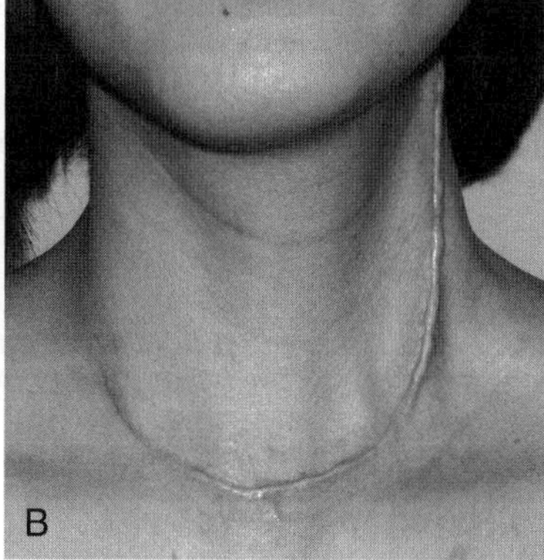

Figure 57-2. A, A profound keloid scar stemming from ear piercings. **B,** A hypertrophic scar of a neck apron incision following thyroidectomy.

- Keloids:
  - Tend to overgrow the boundaries of the initial tissue injury.
  - May continue to enlarge with time.
  - Can be treated with intralesional corticosteroids, interferons, or radiation.
  - Contain thick collagen fibers, closely packed together, haphazardly oriented to the epithelial surface.

17. **How do vitamin deficiencies affect wound healing?**
Vitamin A is important in epithelialization, collagen synthesis, and cross-linking. Vitamin C is an important cofactor in lysine and proline hydroxylation in collagen synthesis. It is also important to neutrophil function and serves as a reductant in free radical formation ("antioxidant"). Vitamin E reduces collagen production, thereby decreasing wound tensile strength. Vitamin K is important to the production of clotting factors II, VII, IX, and X. Zinc is important to wound healing by promoting cell differentiation and fibroplasia.

18. **Which lifestyle factors affect wound healing?**
Smoking, through the effects of nicotine, leads to vascular compromise and causes wound tissue ischemia and delayed healing. Alcoholism is associated with global malnutrition, which is detrimental to the wound healing process.

19. **What is the ideal dressing for a surgical wound?**
An ideal dressing for a surgical wound would have the following characteristics: maintains a moist wound environment, absorbs exudate, and keeps the surgical site protected.

20. **What are the types of collagen?**
Type I collagen: Found in skin, bone, and tendons and supports connective tissue
Type II collagen: Found in cartilage, corneal stroma, and vitreous humor; promotes shock absorption and joint mobility
Type III collagen: Ubiquitous; promotes formation of fibrous elements
Type IV collagen: Found in basement membranes; forms a scaffold for filtration
Type V collagen: Ubiquitous; forms cytoskeleton around cells

21. **How does radiation affect wound healing?**
Radiation leads to diminished fibroblast, myofibroblast, and endothelial cell proliferation. There is also considerable ischemia of tissue due to hyalinization and sclerosis of blood vessels. This leads to overall delay and poor wound healing in radiated patients.

22. **What is the role of vacuum-assisted closure in otolaryngology?**
Vacuum-assisted closure may be used in skin grafts to remove fluid secretions that prevent revascularization and imbibition of the graft. They are also used to promote granulation in infected wounds that are healing by secondary intention. Vacuum-assisted devices must not be used in nasal, oral, tracheal, blood vessels or neoplastic sites.

CONTROVERSIES

23. **What is the role of autologous platelet rich plasma in wound healing?**
The theoretical principle of the use of platelet rich plasma (PRP) in wound healing is that platelets are a potent source of growth factors and a concentrate of these growth factors potentially improves healing. Clinical reports studying the efficacy of PRP in reducing ecchymosis and edema have been mixed and its use remains controversial.

Bibliography

English RS, Shenefelt PD: Keloids and hypertrophic scars, *Dermatol Surg* 25(8):631–638, 1999.

Fisher E, Frodel JL: Wound healing. In Papel ID, Frodel J, editors: *Facial Plastic and Reconstructive Surgery*, New York, 2002, Thieme, pp 15–25.

Gantwerker EA, Hom DB: Skin: histology and physiology of wound healing, *Facial Plast Surg Clin North Am* 19(3): 441–453, 2011.

Guo S, Dipietro LA: Factors affecting wound healing, *J Dent Res* 89(3):219–229, 2010.

Hom DB, Sun GH, Elluru RG: A contemporary review of wound healing in otolaryngology: current state and future promise, *Laryngoscope* 119(11):2099–2110, 2009.

Terris DJ: Dynamics of wound healing. In Bailey BJ, editor: *Otolaryngology: Head and Neck Surgery*, Philadelphia, 1998, Lippincott-Raven.

CHAPTER 58

FACIAL ANALYSIS

Henry H. Chen, MD, MBA and Edwin F. Williams, III, MD

KEY POINTS

1. Symmetry and proportion are important to facial harmony. The individual subunits must balance each other to achieve an aesthetically pleasing result.
2. Ideal relationships have been established based on the relationship of soft tissue landmarks to each other. However, variations exist for different ethnicities.
3. When analyzing the nose, it is important to evaluate its relationship to the rest of the face in addition to its individual characteristics.

Pearls

1. The Frankfort horizontal line allows for standardization in photographs and is a cornerstone for facial analysis.
2. Nasal rotation refers to movement of the tip along an arc from the external auditory canal.
3. Nasal projection refers to how far the tip projects from the face.

QUESTIONS

1. **What are the important soft tissue reference points of the face with regards to facial analysis?**
   Trichion (Tr): anterior hairline at the midline
   Glabella (G): most anterior point of the forehead on profile view
   Nasion (N): point of deepest depression at the root of the nose on profile view
   Nasal tip (T): most anterior point of nasal tip on profile view
   Columellar point (Cm): most anterior point of the columella on profile view
   Subnasale (Sn): point where the nasal columella merges with the upper lip
   Labrale superioris (LS): vermillion border of the upper lip
   Labrale inferiorris (LI): vermillion border of the lower lip
   Pogonion (Pg): most anterior point of the chin on profile view
   Menton (Me): lowest point of the chin
   Cervical point (C): innermost point between the submental area and the neck

   Figure 58-1 illustrates these reference points.

2. **What is the Frankfort horizontal plane?**
   A line drawn from the superior aspect of the external auditory canal to the inferior aspect of the infraorbital rim on a lateral view (Figure 58-2). In photographs, it is approximated by a line drawn from the superior tragus to the lower eyelid-cheek skin junction. This allows standardization for patient positioning in photographs as well as for facial analysis.

3. **What is the facial plane?**
   A line drawn from the glabella to the pogonion. The facial plane should intersect the Frankfurt horizontal plane at an angle of 80 to 95 degrees.

4. **What is the zero meridian of Gonzales-Ulloa?**
   A line perpendicular to the Frankfort horizontal line that goes through the nasion. The pogonion should be within 5 mm of this line.

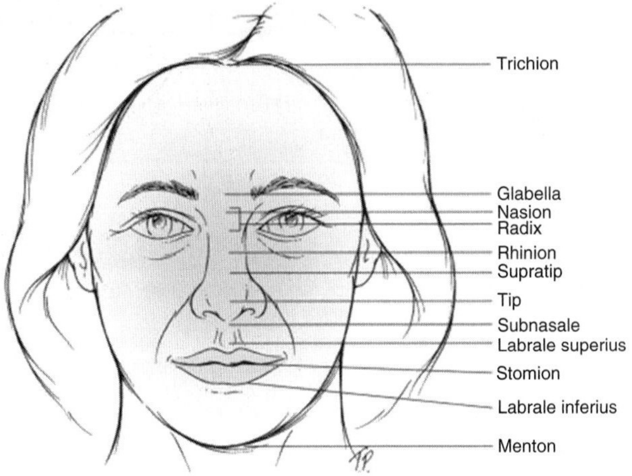

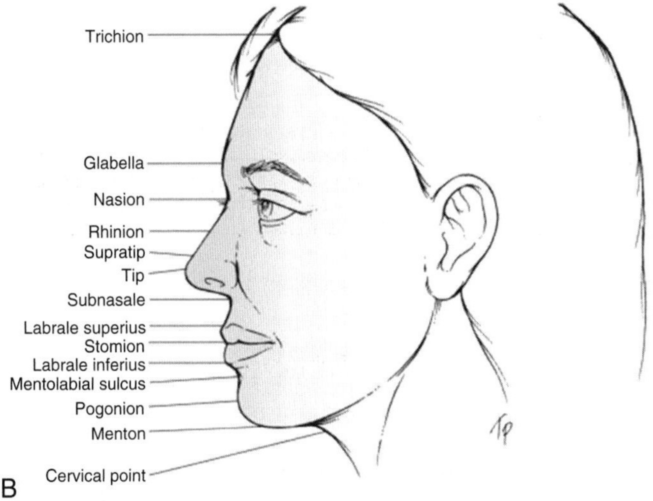

Figure 58-1. Frontal view **(A)** and lateral view **(B)** of soft tissue reference points. *(From Zimbler MS: Cummings Otolaryngology Head & Neck Surgery, p. 269–280 © 2010 Copyright © 2010, 2005, 1998, 1993, 1986 by Mosby, Inc. All Rights Reserved.)*

5. What are some important angles used for facial analysis?

Nasofrontal angle (Figure 58-3A): intercept of glabella (G) to nasion (N) line with nasion (N) to tip (T) line

Nasofacial angle (Figure 58-3B): intercept of glabella (G) to pogonion (Pg) line with nasion (N) to tip (T) line

Nasolabial angle (Figure 58-3C): intercept of columella point (Cm) to subnasale (Sn) line with subnasale (Sn) to labrale superioris (LS) line

Nasomental angle (Figure 58-3D): intercept of nasion (N) to tip (T) line with tip (T) to pogonion (Pg) line

Mentocervical angle (Figure 58-3E): intercept of glabella (G) to pogonion (Pg) line with menton (M) to cervical point (C) line

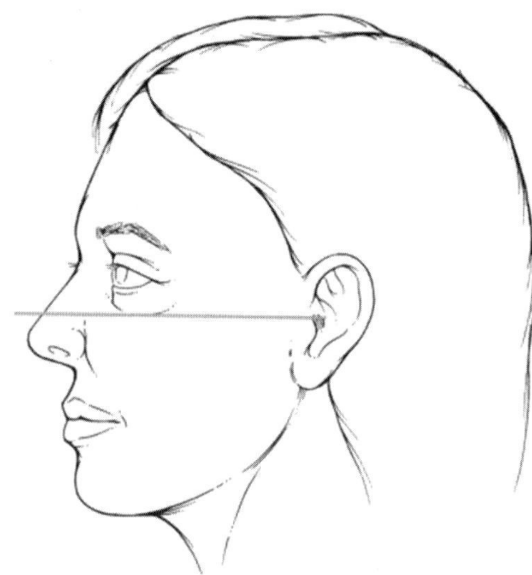

Figure 58-2. Frankfort horizontal plane. *(From Zimbler MS: Cummings Otolaryngology Head & Neck Surgery, p. 269–280 © 2010 Copyright © 2010, 2005, 1998, 1993, 1986 by Mosby, Inc. All Rights Reserved.)*

6. **What is the aesthetic triangle of Powell and Humphreys?**
   This system incorporates the nasofrontal, nasofacial, nasomental, and the mentocervical angles to relate all the major components of the face in the evaluation of facial harmony (Figure 58-4). The nasomental angle is considered the most important measurement because it is dependent upon nasal projection as well as chin position and shows the interdependence of individual facial features.

7. **What are ideal measurements of the angles mentioned above?**
   Nasofrontal angle: 115–130 degrees
   Nasofacial angle: 36–40 degrees
   Nasolabial angle: 90–95 degrees in males and 95–110 degrees in females
   Nasomental angle: 120–132 degrees
   Mentocervical angle: 80–95 degrees

8. **What is the rule of thirds?**
   The face can be divided into thirds of approximate equal vertical height on frontal view (Figure 58-5A). The distance from the trichion to the glabella should equal the length from the glabella to the subnasale, which should equal the length from the subnasale to the menton.

9. **What is the rule of fifths?**
   The face can be divided into fifths of equal width on frontal view (Figure 58-5B). The width of one eye should equal one fifth of the facial width. In other words, the intercanthal distance should approximate the width of the nose as well as the width from lateral canthus to the ear.

10. **What are the subunits of the face?**
    Forehead, periorbital region, cheeks, nose, perioral region and chin, and neck

11. **What are the subunits of the nose?**
    The nose is divided into nine (9) subunits. These are the paired sidewalls, ala, and soft tissue triangles, and the unpaired dorsum, tip, and columellar subunits.

12. **What is the supratip break?**
    The transitional area from the dorsum to the tip where the lower and upper lateral cartilages overlap is called the supratip break. The nasal tip should ideally lead the dorsum by 1 to 2 mm, leading to a break in the line of the dorsum. This is an aesthetic that is more important in women than men.

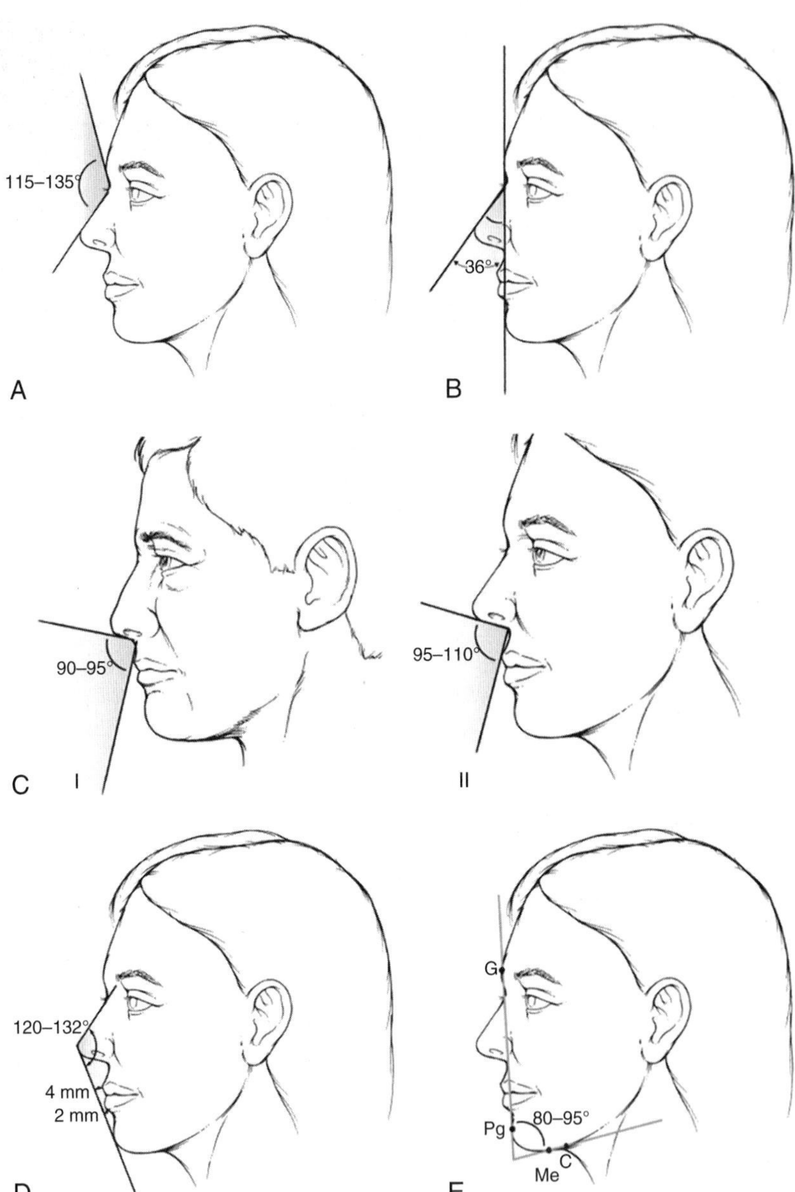

Figure 58-3. A, Nasofrontal angle. **B,** Nasofacial angle. **C,** Nasolabial angle. Male (i) and female (ii). **D,** Nasomental angle. **E,** Mentocervical angle. *(From Zimbler MS: Cummings Otolaryngology Head & Neck Surgery, p. 269–280 © 2010 Copyright © 2010, 2005, 1998, 1993, 1986 by Mosby, Inc. All Rights Reserved.)*

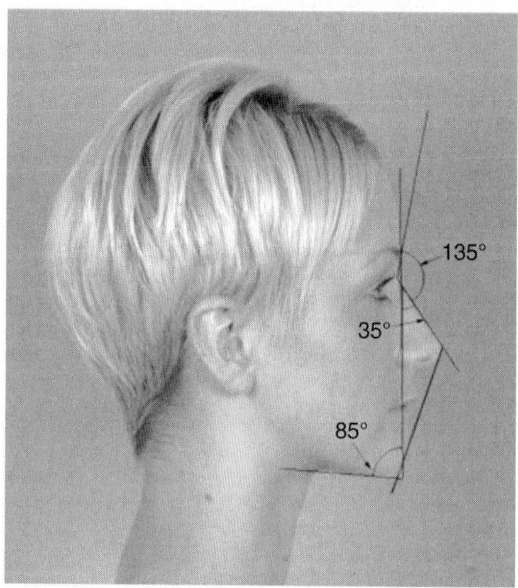

Figure 58-4. Aesthetic triangle of Powell and Humphreys.

13. **What is the double break of the columella?**
As the nasal tip transitions to the columella, it is seen making two breaks. The first break is the point at which the tip turns posteriorly and inferiorly onto the infratip lobule while the second break occurs where the infratip lobule transitions to a flatter and more horizontal columella. The second break corresponds to the junction of the medial and intermediate crura.

14. **Where is the ideal location for the nasion?**
The nasion ideally should lie at the level of the supratarsal crease on profile view. If it is too low, it may lead to overestimation of nasal projection.

15. **What are the characteristics of an ideal nasal base?**
On base view, the nose should approximate an equilateral triangle. The columella should comprise two thirds of the height and the lobule comprises another third, leading to a columella: lobule ratio of 2:1.

    The nostrils should be symmetric and appear pear shaped with the widest portion at the nostril sill. The width of the lobule should be 75% of the width of the nasal base. On lateral view, the alar: lobule ratio should be 1:1 and there should be 2 to 4 mm of columellar show.

16. **What is nasal tip rotation?**
Rotation refers to the movement of the nasal tip along an arc based at the external auditory canal. Increasing rotation refers to cephalic movement of the nasal tip along that arc while caudal movement of the tip leads to derotation.

17. **What is nasal tip projection?**
Projection refers to the distance the nasal tip projects from the face.

18. **What are the methods used to assess nasal projection?**
Joseph: Described nasal projection in relation to the facial plane, defining the nasofacial angle, which is important in describing projection. The more acute the angle, the less the tip projection and vice versa.
Simons: Ratio of nasal projection to length of the upper lip should equal 1:1. The ratio of the length of the vermilion border (LS) to the subnasale (Sn) should equal the length of the nasal tip as measured from the subnasale (Sn) to the tip (T).
Goode: Ratio of tip projection to nasal dorsum length should equal 0.55:1 to 0.6:1. A vertical line is drawn from the nasion (N) to the alar facial groove (A). Tip projection is measured by the

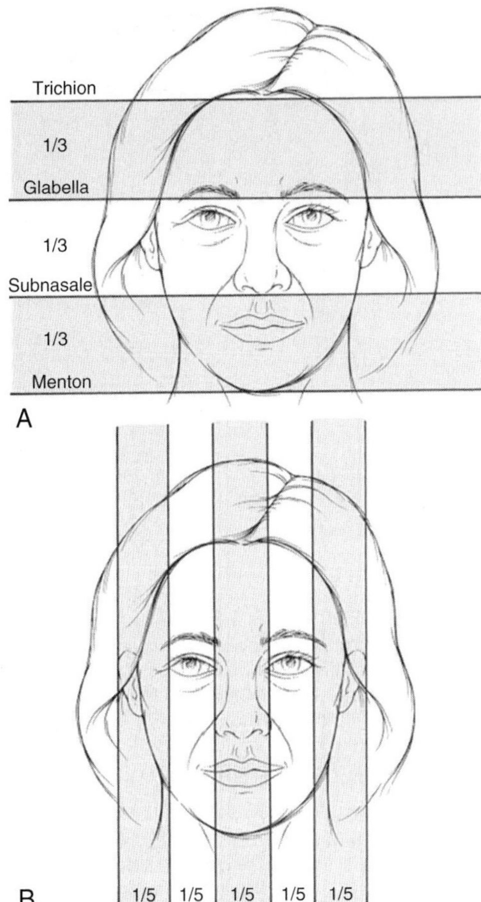

Figure 58-5. **A,** Facial height. The facial height is divided into equal thirds. **B,** Facial width. The facial width is divided into equal fifths. *(From Zimbler MS: Cummings Otolaryngology Head & Neck Surgery, p. 269–280 © 2010 Copyright © 2010, 2005, 1998, 1993, 1986 by Mosby, Inc. All Rights Reserved.)*

length of a horizontal line drawn from the nasal tip (T) perpendicular to the vertical line. Nasal dorsum length is measured from nasion (N) to tip (T) (Figure 58-6).

Crumley: Ratio of tip projection to vertical height to nasal length should equal 3 : 4 : 5. Tip projection, vertical height, and nasal length are measured as described by Goode's method, and these sides should form a right triangle.

Powell and Humphries: Ratio of nasal height to tip projection should equal 2.8 : 1. Height is measured by the length from nasion (N) to subnasale (Sn) and projection is measured by a line drawn perpendicular to the line of nasal height through the tip (T).

19. **What is a simple way to assess chin projection?**
Draw a vertical line from the vermilion border of the lower lip (LI). The pogonion (Pg) should approximate this line in males and should be 2 to 3 mm posterior to this line in females.

20. **How does chin projection affect nasal appearance?**
An underprojected chin leads to a perceived increase in nasal size while an overprojected chin leads to a perceived decrease in nasal size.

21. **How does forehead shape affect nasal appearance?**
A prominent forehead leads to a perceived decrease in nasal size while a retrusive forehead leads to a perceived increase in nasal size.

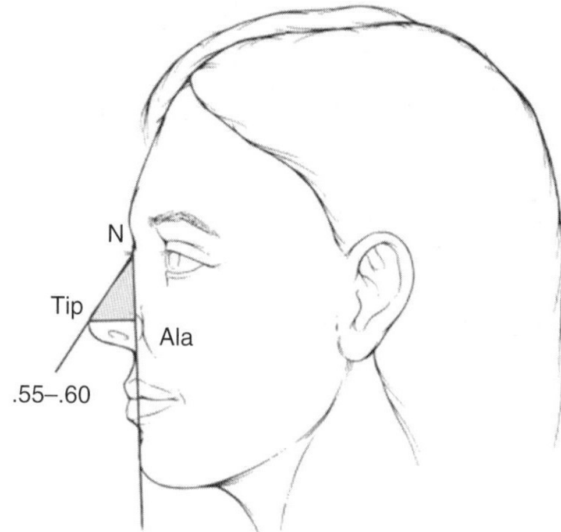

Figure 58-6. Goode's method of tip projection. *(From Zimbler MS: Cummings Otolaryngology Head & Neck Surgery, p. 269–280 © 2010 Copyright © 2010, 2005, 1998, 1993, 1986 by Mosby, Inc. All Rights Reserved.)*

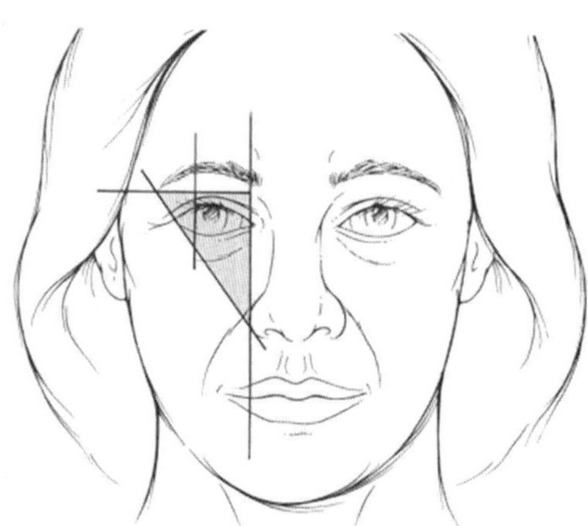

Figure 58-7. Ideal eyebrow position. *(From Zimbler MS: Cummings Otolaryngology Head & Neck Surgery, p. 269–280 © 2010 Copyright © 2010, 2005, 1998, 1993, 1986 by Mosby, Inc. All Rights Reserved.)*

22. What are different ways to assess lip projection?

- A line is drawn from the subnasale (Sn) to the pogonion (Pg). The upper lip should rest 3.5 mm anterior to this line and the lower lip should rest 2.2 mm anterior.
- A line is drawn from the nasal tip (T) to the pogonion (Pg). This line is called the nasomental line. The upper lip ideally falls 2 mm posterior to this line and the lower lip 4 mm posterior.

23. What accounts for an aesthetic eyebrow and what are the differences between the male and female brow?

The female brow ideally should start medially directly above the nasal ala and reach its highest point at the lateral limbus or lateral canthus and should end at an oblique line passing through from the nasal ala to the lateral canthus. The medial and lateral aspects of the brow should be on the same horizontal plane. The medial aspect should be club shaped and gradually taper laterally. Female brows tend to be thinner, more arched, and positioned above the supraorbital rim while male brows tend to be thicker, straighter, and positioned at the supraorbital rim (Figure 58-7).

BIBLIOGRAPHY

Bernstein L: Esthetics in rhinoplasty, *Otolaryngol Clin North Am* 8:705–715, 1975.

Brennan GH: Correction of the ptotic brow, *Otolaryngol Clin North Am* 13:265–273, 1980.

Burstone CJ: Lip posture and its significance in treatment planning, *Am J Orthod* 53:262–284, 1967.

Crumley RL, Lanser M: Quantitative analysis of nasal tip projection, *Laryngoscope* 98:202–208, 1988.

Gonzalez-Ulloa M: Quantitative principles in cosmetic surgery of the face (profileplasty), *Plast Reconstr Surg Transplant Bull* 29:186–198, 1962.

Goode R: A method of tip projection measurement. In Humphries B, Powell N, editors: *Proportions of the Aesthetic Face*, New York, 1984, Thieme-Stratton, pp 15–39.

Powell N, Humphreys B: *Proportions of the aesthetic face*, New York, 1984, Thieme-Stratton.

Simons RL: Adjunctive measures in rhinoplasty, *Otolaryngol Clin North Am* 8:717–742, 1975.

Winkler A, Wudel JM: Preoperative evaluation and facial analysis in facial plastic surgery. In Johnson JT, Rosen CA, editors: *Bailey's Head and Neck Surgery Otolaryngology*, Philadelphia, 2014, Lippincott Williams & Wilkins, pp 2757–2771.

RHINOPLASTY AND NASAL RECONSTRUCTION

Geoffrey R. Ferril, MD and Andrew A. Winkler, MD

CHAPTER 59

KEY POINTS

1. A thorough understanding of the anatomy and physiology of the nose is paramount to successfully perform rhinoplasty surgery.
2. Nasal tip support mechanisms must be respected and preserved and/or addressed in rhinoplasty.
3. Preoperative goals, expected outcomes, and potential complications must be discussed at length between the surgeon and patient.

Pearls

1. Major nasal tip support mechanisms include strength and integrity of lower lateral cartilages, attachments of the lower lateral cartilages to the septum, and the attachments of the lower lateral cartilages to the upper lateral cartilages.
2. The internal nasal valve is comprised of the upper lateral cartilage, nasal septum, and nasal floor. The Cottle maneuver helps to diagnose internal nasal valve collapse.
3. Endonasal (closed) rhinoplasty utilizes transcartilaginous or intercartilaginous incisions with or without hemitransfixion or transfixion incisions. External (open) rhinoplasty utilizes transcolumellar and marginal incisions.
4. A "pollybeak" deformity is a complication of rhinoplasty whereby supratip fullness results in the appearance of a parrot's beak; this can be the result of loss of tip support or supratip scar tissue.
5. A saddle nose deformity is a concavity of the midvault secondary to insufficient cartilage support of the middle third of the nose; this can be a result of rhinoplasty, septal hematoma, septal abscess, autoimmune disease, or cocaine use.

QUESTIONS

1. What is rhinoplasty?
   Rhinoplasty is a challenging surgical operation used to change the functional performance and aesthetic appearance of the nose through manipulation of bone, cartilage, and soft tissue.

2. How common is rhinoplasty?
   Rhinoplasty is the most frequently performed operation in the field of facial plastic and reconstructive surgery. In 2012, approximately 240,000 rhinoplasty surgeries were performed in the United States.

3. Who tends to undergo rhinoplasty?
   An estimated 80% of rhinoplasty surgeries are performed on women, though it is the second most common facial plastic surgery performed in that group (facelift is the most common). Conversely, rhinoplasty is the most common procedure performed in men, though they represent only 20% of all rhinoplasty patients. Rhinoplasty is most common in the 22- to 34-year-old age group (44% of all), followed by the 35- to 60-year-old age group (31% of all).

4. Why is rhinoplasty considered a challenging operation?
   There are few surgical procedures in which the perception of success rests so substantially on the abilities of the surgeon. In cosmetic rhinoplasty, millimeter changes make the difference between a satisfactory and a disappointing outcome. Rhinoplasty, therefore, requires a collaborative exploration

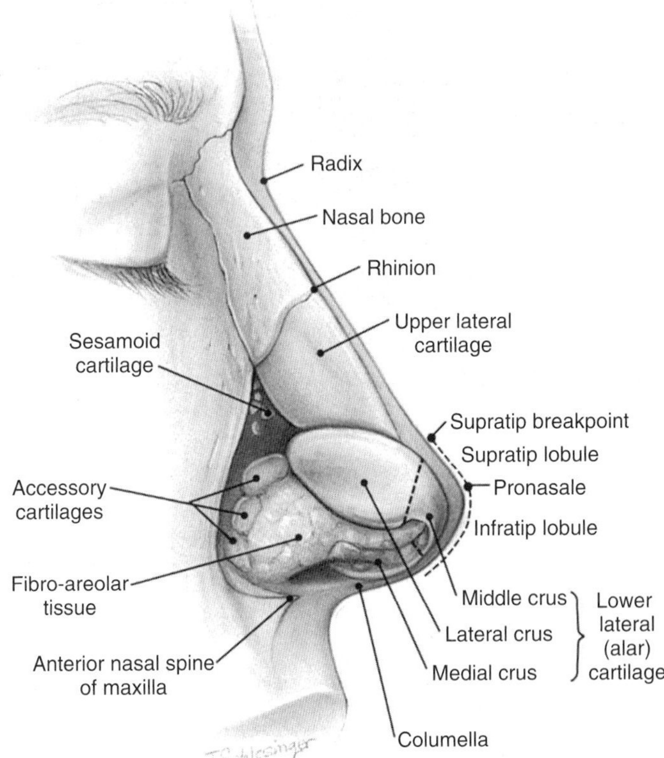

Figure 59-1. Anatomy of the nose, frontal view. *(From Winkler AA: Open Septorhinoplasty: The Complete Operative Guide, ed 1, Cupertino, CA, 2013, Apple, Inc.)*

of what the patient would consider an appropriate result and how his or her expectations match surgical realities. The surgeon must have experience with numerous rhinoplasty techniques and a thorough grasp of nasal anatomy (Figures 59-1 and 59-2). The success or failure of rhinoplasty depends on the interplay of the patient's unique nasal anatomy and comorbidities, the surgeon's experience and ability, and the patient's preparation regarding realistic outcomes.

5. **How does one "analyze" the nose preoperatively for rhinoplasty?**
While a comprehensive discussion of preoperative nasal analysis is beyond the scope of this chapter, there are several general points worth mentioning. Every initial rhinoplasty consultation includes six standard preoperative rhinoplasty photos, which provide a framework to analyze the nose. These views are the frontal, right/left oblique, right/left lateral, and the basal views.
   - **Frontal View:** On frontal view, the nose is divided horizontally into thirds. The upper third is comprised of the nasal bones, which should be symmetric and 75% of the intercanthal distance. The middle third, also called the "midvault" is formed by the upper lateral cartilages and the dorsal septal cartilage. A line connecting the glabella to the ipsilateral tip-defining point is called the brow-tip aesthetic line. It should be curvilinear, symmetric, and smooth along the midvault. Deformities from trauma or prior surgery disrupt the brow-tip aesthetic line. A narrow middle third suggests the presence of nasal valve dysfunction (see Question 9). Nasal tip shape may be characterized as bulbous, narrow, bifid, boxy, or amorphous. The elegant tip forms a diamond shape with two tip-defining points, which are identified by the light reflex they produce. The tip-defining points are ideally separated by less than 1 cm. Finally, the nostril rims should form a "gull-in-flight" relationship with the columella.

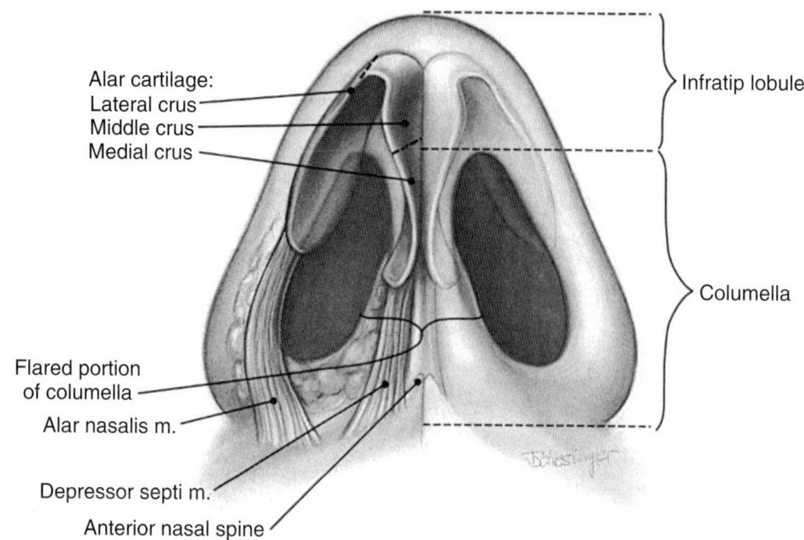

Figure 59-2. Anatomy of the nose, basal view. *(From Winkler AA: Open Septorhinoplasty: The Complete Operative Guide, ed 1, Cupertino, CA, 2013, Apple, Inc.)*

- **Lateral View:** The lateral view provides assessment of the profile of the nose and also the ala-tip complex. On lateral view, the length of the ala and tip should be roughly equal and there should be 2 to 4 mm of columella showing below the level of the nostril rim. The elegant nasal tip profile has a "double break" produced by (1) the tip-defining point and (2) a subtle angulation at the junction of the tip lobule with the columella. Additionally, a supratip break should be present between the nasal tip and the nasal dorsum.
- **Basal View:** The basal view is used to assess nasal base width and nasal tip symmetry. On basal view, the nose should form an equilateral triangle. The width of the columella compared to the width of the lobule should be 2:1. The tip should comprise one third of the total height, while the nostrils make up the remaining two thirds on basal view.

6. How does nasal tip rotation differ from nasal tip projection?
   - **Tip Rotation:** Rotational movement of the position of the tip along an arc formed from a fixed point at the superior tragus
   - **Tip Projection:** The anterior or posterior positioning of the nasal tip relative to the midface
7. On the lateral view, the nasofrontal, nasolabial, and nasofacial aesthetic angles can be created based on the geometry of the nose. Define them (Figure 59-3).
   - **Nasofrontal Angle:** Intersection of a line connecting the glabella and sellion and a line tangent to the nasal dorsum (ideal 115 to 130 degrees)
   - **Nasolabial Angle:** Intersection of a line tangent to the columella and a line tangent to the upper lip, which forms a vertex at the subnasale (ideal 90 to 95 degrees in males and 95° to 110° in females)
   - **Nasofacial Angle:** Intersection of a line tangent to the nasal dorsum with a line from the glabella to the soft tissue pogonion (ideal 36 to 40 degrees)
8. What is Goode's ratio?

   Goode's ratio is a means by which to measure the anterior projection of the nasal tip. Goode's method of assessing tip projection takes into account the relationship between nasal length and the alar groove. On lateral view, a vertical line is drawn from the sellion (the posterior-most soft tissue point at the root of the nose) through the alar groove. The amount of tip projection is determined by then dropping a perpendicular second line from the tip-defining point to the first line. Nasal length is

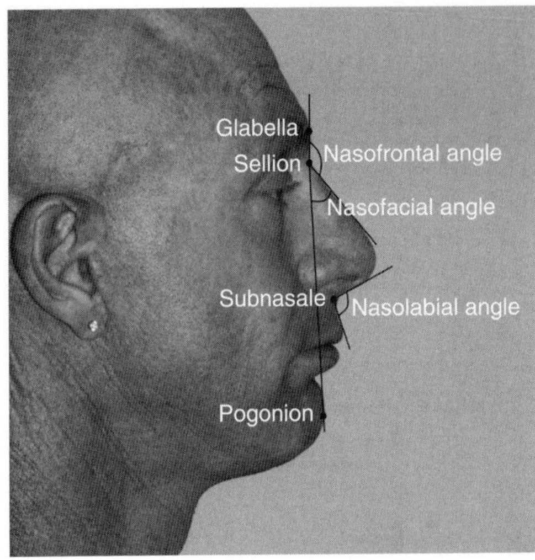

Figure 59-3. Aesthetic angles of the nose from the lateral view.

determined using a line from the sellion to the tip-defining point. The ideal ratio of tip projection to nasal length using the Goode method is 0.55 : 1 to 0.6 : 1.

9. **What is the internal nasal valve and why is it functionally important?**
   The internal nasal valve is approximately 1 cm posterior to the nostril aperture and is comprised of the septum, the upper lateral cartilage, and the nasal floor. The angle between the upper lateral cartilage and the septum is acute at this location and is susceptible to collapse. The anterior head of the inferior turbinate may crowd the internal nasal valve, though it is not strictly part of this structure. This internal nasal valve behaves like a Starling resistor in that it shuts once a threshold flow rate is reached. If the triggering flow rate is relatively low, the patient perceives difficulty breathing through the nose.

10. **What is external nasal valve collapse?**
    The lower lateral cartilages form incomplete rings around the nostril openings called the external nasal valve. They are designed to prevent the collapse of the soft tissue of the nose during nasal inspiration. External nasal valve collapse occurs when these cartilages provide insufficient soft tissue support during inspiration.

11. **What is the Cottle maneuver?**
    The Cottle maneuver is a dynamic nasal examination tool whereby the cheeks are distracted laterally, assessing for any subjective improvement in nasal airflow. This tool aids in diagnosing nasal valve incompetence.

12. **How are internal and external valve collapse corrected?**
    Cartilage spreader grafts are classically used to correct internal nasal valve incompetence. Spreader grafts are rectangular cartilage grafts that are sutured to either side of the dorsal septum to lateralize the upper lateral cartilages. External nasal valve collapse is characteristically corrected with alar batten grafts, which are cartilage grafts placed over or under the lateral crus cartilages to provide greater stability.

13. **What are the major and minor support mechanisms for the nasal tip?**
    - Major (3)
      - Size, strength, and resiliency of the lower lateral cartilages
      - Attachments of the lower lateral cartilages to the septum at the medial crural footplate
      - Attachments of the lateral crura of the lower lateral cartilages to the upper lateral cartilages, known as the scroll region

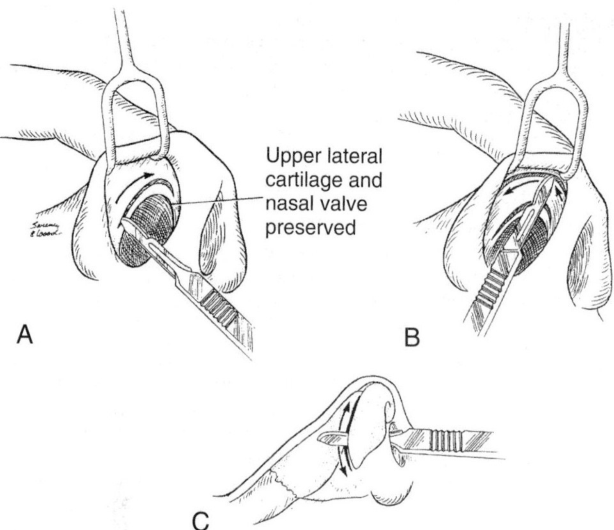

Figure 59-4. The intercartilaginous incision **(A)** and marginal rim incision **(B)** are made on either side of the lateral crura of the alar cartilage. The intercartilaginous incision permits good access to the nasal dorsum **(C)**. *(From Tardy ME Jr: Rhinoplasty. In Cummings C, et al, editors: Otolaryngology—Head and Neck Surgery, ed 3, St. Louis, 1998, Mosby.)*

- Minor (6)
  - Interdomal ligament
  - Cartilaginous dorsal septum (anterior septal angle)
  - Sesamoid complex
  - Attachment of the lower lateral cartilage to the overlying superficial musculoaponeurotic system
  - Nasal spine
  - Membranous septum

14. Describe the incisions used in open (external) rhinoplasty.
    - **Transcolumellar:** A horizontal incision made at the narrowest, most convex portion of the columella. To prevent a straight-line scar, this incision is broken up with an "inverted V" at the midline.
    - **Marginal:** A curvilinear incision that follows the caudal margin of the lower lateral cartilages. When combined with the transcolumellar incision, this allows the nasal tip to be degloved (Figure 59-4).

15. Describe the incisions used in closed (endonasal) rhinoplasty.
    - **Intercartilaginous:** Placed between the lower lateral and upper lateral cartilage to gain access to the nasal dorsum (Figure 59-4). These incisions may be extended medially to the septum and continued as a hemitransfixion or full transfixion incision for access to the septum.
    - **Transcartilaginous:** A variant of the intercartilaginous incision. The transcartilaginous incision is made several millimeters caudal to the junction of the upper and lower lateral cartilages. The incision is carried through the overlying cartilage, which is then removed as a cephalic trim (see Question 19). The transcartilaginous incision allows for a conservative volume reduction of the lateral crus of the lower lateral cartilage.

16. What are the advantages and disadvantages of the two standard rhinoplasty approaches?
    - Endonasal/Closed:
      - Advantages: no external incisions, less operative time, less edema
      - Disadvantages: compromised exposure, compromised tip support

- External/Open:
  - Advantages: maximum exposure, accurate placement and suturing of grafts, greater accuracy in establishing relationships between the various parts of the nose, greater visualization helpful in surgeon training
  - Disadvantages: longer operative time, more postoperative edema, external scar

17. **What is the tripod concept of the nasal tip?**
The tripod concept is a simplified way to depict the structures that control the position of the domes of the nasal tip (see Figures 59-1 and 59-2). The tripod consists of:
   - The paired medial crura of the lower lateral cartilages
   - The left lateral crus of the lower lateral cartilage
   - The right lateral crus of the lower lateral cartilage
   In this model, lengthening or shortening any of the members of the tripod will alter tip position.

18. **How is upward tip rotation achieved?**
Upward tip rotation can be achieved using tip suspension sutures to pull the domes or lateral crus cartilage in the cephalic direction. More subtle rotation is achieved by simply resecting cartilage from the cephalic portion of the lateral crus. Postoperative scar tissue forms in the resected void and scar contraction causes tip rotation in the cephalic direction. Cephalic rotation may also be accomplished by repositioning the lower lateral cartilages onto a graft that is attached to the caudal septum, known as a caudal septal extension graft. This nonanatomic cartilage graft provides a support structure between the medial crura, which may then be sutured in the desired position to provide increased rotation (or projection if necessary). Another method is to transect, overlap, and suture the lateral crura. This shortens these two limbs of the "tripod" and causes the domes to rotate upward. Finally, the illusion of upward tip rotation can be achieved through the blunting of the nasolabial angle using diced cartilage "plumping" grafts.

19. **What is done to correct the bulbous nasal tip?**
Volume reduction of the lobules typically requires the excision of some portion of the cephalic border of the alar cartilage, known commonly as a "cephalic trim." The strip of lateral crus cartilage left behind is ideally kept entirely intact; that is, a "complete strip" is maintained. However, the intact strip may be cut and strategically resutured or intentionally weakened, as long as its integrity is ultimately restored. The more that the complete strip is weakened, the more severe is the potential for loss of tip support and postoperative tip asymmetry. Most surgeons believe that a minimum of 4 to 8 mm of complete strip must be preserved to avoid a significant loss of tip support. A useful and cosmetically appealing adjunct is the lateral crural strut graft, which is a 1-cm by 0.5-cm rectangular cartilage graft placed into a pocket beneath the lateral crus. This flattens the lateral crus, providing less bulbosity, and also strengthens the cartilage, which limits postoperative complications.

20. **What is a dorsal hump and how is it removed, and what is an "open-roof" deformity?**
Both the nasal bones and the midvault cartilages contribute to dorsal humps, though the latter typically comprises more of the hump. A variety of techniques and tools have been developed to treat dorsal humps. In the case of a small dorsal hump, rasps are used to reduce the hump with fine control. Larger humps are taken down using straight osteotomes. However, removing large portions of the dorsum may lead to an "open-roof" deformity. This deformity is analogous to cutting the peak off of an A-frame house. The nasal dorsum appears widened on frontal view and the cut edges of the nasal bones may be visible through the skin. To correct an open-roof deformity, osteotomies are made at the lateral aspect of the nasal bones. The mobile nasal bones are then pushed together medially, closing the open-roof.

21. **What potential complications should be discussed with the patient prior to rhinoplasty surgery?**
Bleeding, infection, scarring, septal perforation, need for further procedures, failure to improve symptoms, poor cosmetic result

22. **What is a "pollybeak" deformity and how does it occur?**
The pollybeak deformity is a complication of rhinoplasty in which the postoperative appearance resembles the curved beak of a parrot because of supratip fullness. Pollybeaks are categorized by

their cartilaginous or soft tissue etiologies. Cartilaginous pollybeak deformity results from loss of nasal tip support. This causes the nasal tip to descend, which allows the anterior septal angle to produce a convexity in the supratip. Soft tissue pollybeak occurs when scar tissue fills the supratip break. This may occur following overresection of the nasal dorsum with resultant dead space, especially in the patient with thick or inelastic skin. The treatment of a pollybeak depends on the etiology. Intralesional steroids may improve soft tissue pollybeak whereas tip support reconstruction may be necessary for cartilaginous pollybeak deformity.

23. **What is a saddle nose deformity?**
    The saddle nose deformity is a concave depression of the midvault resulting from insufficient cartilage support in the middle third of the nose. This can be caused by an untreated septal infection, septal hematoma, cocaine abuse, inflammatory or autoimmune disease, and prior surgery.

24. **What is the inverted V deformity?**
    An inverted V deformity occurs when the upper lateral cartilages lose their attachments to the nasal bones and/or septum. This allows the cartilage to fall away from the nasal bones. The caudal edge of the nasal bones can then be seen in relief through the skin. Placement of spreader grafts resuspends the upper lateral cartilages to the septum and improves the inverted V.

25. **How long does it take to heal following rhinoplasty surgery?**
    The majority of the healing following primary rhinoplasty takes place in the first 8 weeks. However, a small amount of healing takes place for up to 18 months. Soft tissue swelling may take months to resolve completely, especially following open rhinoplasty. Patients must be made aware of this fact preoperatively so that they are not disappointed by their immediate postoperative results. Numbness or sensitivity of the nasal tip skin is commonplace following rhinoplasty due to neuropraxia of the nasopalatine nerve as it travels through the incisive canal. This typically resolves over 3 to 6 months. In addition, the nasal tip will feel very stiff after surgery due to scar tissue formation. However, as the scar tissue remodels over the first 3 to 6 months the nasal tip becomes more mobile. If revisions are necessary, it is wise to wait at least 6 months between operations.

CONTROVERSIES

26. **Which approach is superior: open or closed?**
    Open rhinoplasty involves degloving the nasal tip and provides optimal exposure of the nasal skeleton. Although exposure is improved, it is at the expense of greater postoperative edema. Open rhinoplasty also produces a small external columellar scar, though this is typically very well tolerated. Closed rhinoplasty involves intranasal incisions to gain access to the nasal structures through the nostrils. Exposure is limited and tip work requires "delivery" of the lower lateral cartilages for direct visualization. Although closed rhinoplasty does not produce an external scar, it disrupts more of the nasal tip support mechanisms than the open approach.

    The approach utilized depends on the goals of the surgery and expertise of the surgeon. Most experienced rhinoplastic surgeons prefer and advocate one approach over the other for general rhinoplasty, but few surgeons would argue against using the closed approach for addressing minimal defects and the open approach for correcting significant, severe nasal deformities.

27. **Do alloplastic implants have a role in rhinoplasty surgery?**
    In many situations, the availability of cartilage for grafts is limited. Alloplastic implants, though not without inherent problems, can serve an important role. The most common implants used include polymeric silicone, expanded polytetrafluoroethylene (ePTFE; Gore-Tex, W.L. Gore and Associates Inc., Flagstaff, AZ), porous high-density polyethylene (pHDPE; Mepor, Porex Technologies, Fairburn, GA), polydioxanone plate (PDS Flexible Plate, Johnson & Johnson Company, Langhorne, PA), and acellular human dermis (AlloDerm®, LifeCell Corporation, Branchburg, NJ). The surgeon must counsel patients on the increased incidence of infection and extrusion with their use when compared to autologous grafts in preoperative discussions.

CHAPTER 60

PERIORBITAL SURGERY

Brett W. Davies, MD, MS and Vikram D. Durairaj, MD, FACS

KEY POINTS

1. Detailed knowledge of eyelid and orbital anatomy is crucial for any physician working in the periocular area.
2. There are a variety of surgical approaches to the orbit. The best choice depends on the size and location of the pathologic process.
3. Rejuvenation of the periocular area is best accomplished using a combination of injectables, fillers, and surgical procedures.
4. The Asian eyelid differs from the western eyelid. When performing blepharoplasty, careful surgical planning and clear patient expectations are necessary to have a good outcome.

Pearls

1. Know the seven bones that make up the orbit: sphenoid, maxillary, ethmoid, lacrimal, zygoma, palantine, and frontal.
2. Know the layers of the eyelid. The layers from anterior to posterior are the skin, orbicularis oculi, orbital septum, preaponeurotic fat, levator aponeurosis, Müller's muscle, and conjunctiva.
3. Levator function is the most important variable in determining what type of ptosis surgery to perform.
4. When closing a full thickness eyelid defect, only one lamella should be repaired with a free graft.

QUESTIONS

1. **Name the seven bones that make up the orbit.**
   Sphenoid, maxillary, ethmoid, lacrimal, zygoma, palantine, and frontal.

2. **What are the distances of the anterior ethmoid artery, posterior ethmoid artery, and optic canal from the orbital rim?**
   This can be remembered by the mnemonic 24-12-6. The anterior ethmoid is approximately 24 mm from the orbital rim, the posterior ethmoid is another 12 mm posterior to that, and the optic canal is another 6 mm.

3. **An object travels through the upper eyelid 12 mm superior to the lid margin. What structures does it travel through?**
   In the upper eyelid, the tarsus is typically not taller than 10 mm. So at 12 mm, the object will travel above the tarsus. The layers from anterior to posterior are the skin, orbicularis oculi, orbital septum, preaponeurotic fat, levator aponeurosis, Müller's muscle, and conjunctiva.

4. **What are the eyelid lamellae?**
   The eyelid is sometimes conceptualized as consisting of an anterior and a posterior lamella. The anterior lamella consists of the skin, and the layer of striated muscle fibers of the orbicularis muscle. The posterior lamella consists of the tarsal plates, a layer of smooth muscle (Müller's palpebral muscle), and the palpebral conjunctiva. The anterior and posterior lamellae are separated by the orbital septum.

5. **What is the difference between dermatochalasis and blepharoptosis?**
   Dermatochalasis refers to excess skin on the upper eyelid. When severe, it can hang down over the upper eyelid lashes and block the superior visual field. Blepharoptosis refers to drooping of the eyelid, often due to levator dysfunction.

6. **How is dermatochalasis repaired?**
By performing a blepharoplasty. In this procedure, excess skin, and occasionally orbicularis muscle, is excised. If there is excessive preaponeurotic or orbital fat, it can be judiciously excised by opening the septum.

7. **How is blepharoptosis repaired?**
The two most common methods to repair blepharoptosis are external levator advancement (ELA) and Müller's muscle conjunctiva resection (MMCR). ELA involves a skin incision at the lid crease, whereas MMCR is performed on the conjunctival side of the upper lid. When levator function is poor, such as in congenital ptosis, the upper eyelid can be tethered to the frontalis muscle to assist in eyelid elevation. This is known as a frontalis sling.

8. **The contralateral eyelid occasionally falls after ipsilateral blepharoptosis repair. Why does this happen?**
Hering's law of equal innervation postulates that yoke muscles receive equal innervation. More specifically, when one eyelid is ptotic, the brain increases innervation to both levator palpebrae muscles in an attempt to clear the visual axis. The increased innervation to the contralateral eyelid can result in pseudoretraction. After repair of unilateral blepharoptosis, the innervation to the levator palpebrae is decreased and a drop of the contralateral eyelid may occur.

9. **What is the best treatment a patient with biopsy-proven basal cell carcinoma of the lower eyelid?**
Complete excision with frozen sections. Alternatively, they can be referred to a Mohs surgeon for excision.

10. **What principles should be kept in mind when planning reconstruction of an eyelid defect?**
Important principles include avoiding vertical tension and maintaining a good vascular supply. Minimizing vertical tension avoids eyelid retraction. When a full thickness defect is present, only one lamella can be repaired with a free graft. If both anterior and posterior lamella are replaced with free grafts, the rate of failure is high due to lack of blood supply.

11. **What is ectropion? What are the causes?**
Ectropion is outward turning of the eyelid. Causes can be involutional, paralytic, mechanical, cicatricial, and congenital in nature.

12. **What is entropion? What are the causes?**
Entropion is an inward turning of the eyelid. Causes can be involutional, acute spastic, cicatricial, and congenital in nature.

13. **How does repair of involutional ectropion and entropion differ?**
Both involve horizontal shortening of the eyelid. For ectropion, this is usually sufficient. For entropion, the surgeon must also reattach the lower lid retractors to the tarsus to avoid recurrence.

14. **If a patient with thyroid eye disease has proptosis, strabismus, and eyelid retraction, what is the order of surgeries to correct their issues?**
They should first have a decompression, followed by strabismus surgery, then correction of eyelid retraction. This is because decompression can alter strabismus, and strabismus surgery can alter eyelid position.

15. **Name five surgical incisions to approach the orbit.**
Transconjunctival, lateral canthotomy, upper lid skin crease, transcaruncular, vertical lid split.

16. **During decompression of the orbital floor, what should be preserved to minimize dystopia and diplopia?**
The inferomedial orbital strut.

17. **What choices are available to fill an anophthalmic socket after enucleation or evisceration?**
Orbital implants can be autologous or alloplastic. A dermis fat graft is an example of an autologous implant. Alloplastic implants can be divided into porous and nonporous implants. Porous materials allow fibrovascular ingrowth and include hydroxyapatite (HA), porous polyethylene, and aluminum oxide. Nonporous materials include polymethylmethacrylate (PMMA) and silicone.

18. What are the signs of an orbital compartment syndrome due to retrobulbar hemorrhage? What is the treatment?
Symptoms can include decreased vision, afferent pupillary defect, and increased intraocular pressure. Diagnosis is clinical, not radiographic. Treatment involves lateral canthotomy and cantholysis to relieve orbital pressure.

19. When biopsy of the lacrimal gland is indicated, what lobe should be biopsied?
The lacrimal gland is made up of an orbital lobe and a palpebral lobe. The orbital lobe drains into the palpebral lobe, which then drains onto the ocular surface. Biopsy of the palpebral lobe can cause injury to the tear outflow apparatus. Therefore, biopsy should be taken from the orbital lobe.

20. What is a DCR? What approaches are available?
DCR stands for dacryocystorhinostomy. It is a surgery used to treat nasolacrimal duct obstruction. The procedure creates a new passage from the nasolacrimal system into the nasal cavity above the level of obstruction. It can be accomplished by an external approach through the skin or by an internal approach through the nose.

21. What are the most common reasons for DCR failure?
Common canalicular obstruction and closure of the osteotomy secondary to fibrosis or scarring.

22. What lies between the lower eyelid medial and central fat pads?
The inferior oblique muscle.

23. What factors contribute to periorbital aging?
Involutional changes in the upper face include descent of tissues, loss of subcutaneous fat, and deepening of skin wrinkles. Specific findings include static rhytids, dynamic rhytids, brow ptosis, upper eyelid dermatochalasis, and orbital fat prolapse secondary to weakening of the orbital septum.

24. Name some nonsurgical treatments for periorbital aging.
Botulinum toxin injections, dermal fillers, laser resurfacing, and chemical peels.

25. What is the lethal dose of botulinum toxin in an average sized adult?
Approximately 3000 units.

26. Name some of the common filler materials used in the face?
Autologous fat
Collagen materials
Hyaluronic acid: Juvederm (Allergan) Restylane, Perlane (Medicis Aesthetics)
Poly-L-lactic acid (PLLA): Sculptra (Valeant Aesthetics)
Calcium hydroxylapatite: Radiesse (Merz)
Polymethylmethacrylate (PMMA): Artefill (Suneva Medical)

27. What is the advantage of using hyaluronic acid fillers?
Hyaluronic acid has represented the largest market share for dermal filling products. This is partly because these fillers are reversible with the application of hyaluronidase.

28. List some of the complications of filler injection.
The most serious reported complications of dermal filler injection include infection, tissue necrosis, and blindness from direct intravascular injection. Other complications include migration of filler, erythema, bruising, pain, and visible nodules due to injection technique or granulomatous inflammation.

29. List the major and minor complications of blepharoplasty.
Major complications include retrobulbar hemorrhage, globe perforation, diplopia, and severe dry eyes. Minor complications include eyelid malposition, eyelid hematoma, wound dehiscence, milia, and chemosis.

30. Name the different techniques to lift the brow.
Transblepharoplasty, direct, midforehead, temporal, pretrichial, coronal, and endoscopic brow lifts have all been described. These approaches vary with respect to incision site, dissection plane, and fixation method.

31. How is the Asian eyelid different from the western eyelid?
The insertion point of the septum into the levator aponeurosis is lower in Asians. As a result, the fat behind the septum can move lower on the eyelid. This causes the eyelid crease to be lower or nonexistent, and gives the appearance of a fuller lid. If a crease is present, it usually runs parallel to the lid margin, as opposed to the semilunar shape of the western lid. Asian eyelids are also more likely to have an epicanthal fold.

Bibliography

Baroody M, Holds JB, Vick VL: Advances in the diagnosis and treatment of ptosis, *Curr Opin Ophthalmol* 16(6):351–355, 2005.

Bray D, Hopkins C, Roberts DN: A review of dermal fillers in facial plastic surgery, *Curr Opin Otolaryngol Head Neck Surg* 18(4):295–302, 2010.

Chen WP, Park JD: Asian upper lid blepharoplasty: an update on indications and technique, *Facial Plast Surg* 29(1): 26–31, 2013.

Custer PL, Kennedy RH, Woog JJ, et al: Orbital implants in enucleation surgery: a report by the American Academy of Ophthalmology, *Ophthalmology* 110(10):2054–2061, 2003.

Kahn DM, Shaw RB: Overview of current thoughts on facial volume and aging, *Facial Plast Surg* 26(5):350–355, 2010.

Knoll BI, Attkiss KJ, Persing JA, et al: The influence of forehead, brow, and periorbital aesthetics on perceived expression in the youthful face, *Plast Reconstr Surg* 121:1793–1802, 2008.

Levy LL, Emer JJ: Complications of minimally invasive cosmetic procedures: prevention and management, *J Cutan Aesthet Surg* 5(2):121–132, 2012.

Pedroza F, dos Anjos GC, Bedoya M, et al: Update on brow and forehead lifting, *Curr Opin Otolaryngol Head Neck Surg* 14(4):283–288, 2006.

Ramakrishnan VR, Hink EM, Durairaj VD, et al: Outcomes after endoscopic dacryocystorhinostomy without mucosal flap preservation, *Am J Rhinol* 21:753–757, 2007.

CHAPTER 61

LASERS, SKIN RESURFACING, AND ALOPECIA

Marcelo B. Antunes, MD

KEY POINTS

1. Skin resurfacing modalities and methods of action
   - Chemical peels: caustic injury
   - Dermabrasion: mechanical injury
   - Laser: thermal injury
2. Different types of chemical peels
   - Superficial chemical peels (epidermis): TCA 10% to 30%, Jessner's solution, glycolic acid 40% to 70%, and salicylic acid 5% to 15%
   - Medium chemical peels (superficial dermis): TCA 35% to 40%, combination of 35% TCA with other agents and phenol 88%
   - Deep chemical peels (deep dermis): TCA 50% and the Baker-Gordon phenol peel
3. Contraindications of skin resurfacing with chemical peels, dermabrasion, and lasers
   - Facelift surgery, medium or deep chemical peel or laser resurfacing in the previous 6 months
   - Isotretinoin in the past 1 year
   - Active herpes simplex virus infection
   - Active skin disorders
4. Ablative lasers
   - CO_2 laser (10,600 nm) targets water
   - Er-YAG laser (2940 nm) targets water
5. Nonablative lasers
   - Vascular lasers: pulsed KTP (532 nm) and pulsed dye (585 nm) target hemoglobin
   - Infrared laser: Nd-YAG (1064 nm)
   - Intense Pulsed Light: IPL (550 to 1200 nm) laser targets melanin and hemoglobin
   - Fractionated CO_2 laser (1500 nm)

Pearls

1. The most important consideration prior to skin resurfacing is proper patient selection, especially in respect to the Fitzpatrick skin type (types I and II are the best candidates).
2. The Baker-Gordon formula's (phenol 88%, croton oil, septisol, and distilled water) depth of penetration is more dependent on the croton oil than on the concentration of phenol.
3. Pigmentary changes can result from any skin resurfacing modality (chemical peels, lasers or dermabrasion). Hyperpigmentation tends to occur sooner and can be successfully treated with topical therapy, while hypopigmentation tends to be a delayed phenomenon and is often permanent.
4. Ablative laser resurfacing is comparable to medium and deep chemical peels and dermabrasion.
5. Phenol chemical peels are associated with cardiac toxicity, and should be applied to individual facial subunits in 15-minute intervals.
6. Follicular unit transplantation consists of the transfer of the individual follicular unit, maximizing the amount of hair and minimizing the amount of scarring. When evaluating the patient for hair restoration, the patient's age, medical history, family pattern of hair loss, and the amount of donor area on the posterior scalp needs to be determined.
7. Know the Norwood classification scheme for androgenic alopecia.

QUESTIONS

Skin Resurfacing

1. **Describe age-related changes of the skin.**
The skin changes in the aging process include: thinning of the dermis and epidermis, effacement of the epidermal-dermal junction (most consistent change), thinning of the subcutaneous fat, and loss of organization of elastic fibers and collagen. These changes contribute to increased skin laxity and wrinkling characteristics of the aged face.

2. **Describe the Fitzpatrick skin type classification system.**
The Fitzpatrick skin type classifies the degrees of skin pigmentation and ability to tan. It is graded from I to VI and forecasts sun sensitivity, susceptibility to photodamage, and ability for melanogenesis (Table 61-1). It also provides important information related to risk factors for complications during skin resurfacing procedures. Types III through VI have a higher risk for pigmentary dyschromia (hypo- or hyperpigmentation) after skin resurfacing procedures.

3. **What are the different methods of skin resurfacing and how do they promote rejuvenation?**
The different methods are chemical peels, dermabrasion, and laser photothermolysis. Superficial resurfacing (microdermabrasion and superficial chemical peels) exfoliate the epidermis only and stimulate regeneration and thickening of the epidermis. Medium and deep resurfacing (medium and deep chemical peels, dermabrasion, and lasers) penetrate into the superficial and deep dermis, inducing the production of collagen.

4. **What are the main indications for chemical peels and dermabrasion?**
Photodamage, fine wrinkles, pigmentary dyschromia, and acne scars.

5. **What are the agents used for superficial chemical peels?**
Superficial chemical peels (epidermis) can be done with: trichloroacetic acid (TCA) 10% to 30% solution, Jessner's solution (resorcinol, salicylic acid, lactic acid, and ethanol), glycolic acid 40% to 70% solution, and salicylic acid 5% to 15% solution.

6. **What are the agents used for medium-depth chemical peels?**
The medium-depth peel (papillary dermis) agents are: trichloroacetic acid (TCA) 35% to 40% solution, the combination of 35% TCA with other agents (35% TCA + solid CO_2, 35% TCA + Jessner's solution, 35% TCA + 70% glycolic acid), and phenol 88% solution.

7. **What are the agents used for deep chemical peels?**
The deep chemical peel (reticular dermis) agents are: trichloroacetic acid (TCA) 50% and the Baker-Gordon phenol peel (phenol 88%, croton oil, septisol, and distilled water). The addition of croton oil, an epidermolytic agent, increases the penetration of phenol into the dermis.

8. **What are the limitations associated with the use of phenol?**
The use of phenol is associated with cardiotoxicity (mostly premature ventricular contractions), hepatotoxicity, and nephrotoxicity. Phenol application requires intravenous hydration and cardiac

Table 61-1. Fitzpatrick Skin Classification System

SKIN TYPE	SKIN COLOR	SUN REACTION
I	White or freckled	Always burns
II	White	Usually burns
III	White to olive	Sometimes burns
IV	Brown	Rarely burns
V	Dark brown	Very rarely burns
VI	Black	Never burns

monitoring for the development of arrhythmias. The facial subunits should be treated in 15-minute intervals to avoid toxicity.

9. **Describe the complications related to chemical peels.**
   The complications associated with chemical peel resurfacing include milia formation (most common complication with all resurfacing procedures), hyper- or hypopigmentation, scar formation, allergic or irritant dermatitis, bacterial or fungal (most commonly *Candida*) infection, and reactivation of herpes simplex virus (which could lead to scarring).

10. **What is dermabrasion?**
    Dermabrasion is a method for skin resurfacing that uses a mechanical injury to the skin. It is usually performed using an abrasive wheel that is attached to a drill motor and a hand-piece.

Lasers

11. **What is a laser?**
    Laser stands for Light Amplification by Stimulated Emission of Radiation. It's a light that is collimated (parallel), coherent (same frequency and periodicity), and monochromatic (single wavelength).

12. **What is selective photodermolysis?**
    Selective photothermolysis is the property of maximal absorbance of the laser by the targeted tissue cromophore with minimal damage of surrounding tissues.

13. **What is ablative laser resurfacing?**
    Ablative laser resurfacing involves the principle of selective photothermolysis with the target tissue (cromophore) being water. The most common lasers used for ablation are CO_2 and Erbium-YAG.

14. **What is the difference between CO_2 and Erbium-YAG lasers?**
    Er-YAG energy is absorbed more efficiently the skin (tenfold greater absorption) than is energy from the CO_2 laser. This leads to a more precise tissue ablation with less adjacent thermal injury. This, in turn, leads to a shorter recovery time, less erythema, and a lower risk of hypo- or hyperpigmentation. On the other hand, it produces less tissue tightening.

15. **What is nonablative and fractional laser resurfacing?**
    Nonablative resurfacing produces dermal thermal injury to improve rhytids and photodamage while preserving the epidermis. Fractional resurfacing thermally ablates microscopic columns of epidermal and dermal tissue in regularly spaced arrays over a fraction of the skin surface.

16. **How do nonablative lasers produce photorejuvenation?**
    They work by the induction of proliferation of fibroblasts with new collagen (types I and III) and elastin deposition in the papillary dermis. Infrared and visible light lasers are used with cooling mechanisms to protect the overlying epidermis.

17. **Is there a need for any preoperative treatment?**
    Yes. All patients undergoing laser resurfacing should take antiviral prophylaxis and avoid sun exposure prior to resurfacing. The use of hydroquinone, isotretinoin, glycolic acid, and antibiotics is less established.

18. **What are important considerations in patient selection for laser resurfacing?**
    One of the most important considerations is the patient's skin type. The safest skin types are Fitzpatrick I and II. Types III through VI are more susceptible to complications.

19. **What are the most common complications associated with laser skin resurfacing?**
    Milia, hypopigmentation, hyperpigmentation, scar formation, infection (viral, fungal and bacterial), and contact dermatitis.

Alopecia and Hair Restoriation

20. **What are follicular units?**
    Hair follicles grow together in groups, the follicular unit (FU). This unit, which is considered the fundamental component of hair transplantation, consists of one to four terminal hair follicles with its associated sebaceous gland, arrector pili muscle, blood supply, and neural plexus surrounded by a

fine adventitial collagen sheath. The FU is considered not only an anatomic unit but also a physiologic one.

21. **Describe the hair cycle.**
Hair growth is a cyclical phenomenon with a period of growth (anagen), involution (catagen), and rest (telogen). In the normal scalp, 90 to 95% of the hairs are in anagen, about 1% in catagen, and 5% to 10% in the telogen phase. Each hair goes through this process 10 to 20 times during a lifetime. This cycle is regulated by a complex signaling system, which is not yet fully understood.

22. **What is androgenic alopecia?**
Androgenic alopecia (AGA) affects males and females. Its onset is extremely variable and seems to be determined by the presence of circulating androgens. The prevalence of AGA is extremely variable, affecting about 30% of males at 30 years of age and about 50% of the 50-year-old males. This type of alopecia is nonscarring and has a characteristic pattern with variation in hair shaft diameter and the presence of miniaturized hair leading to their transformation into vellus-like follicles. The exact mechanism by which the androgens cause hair loss remains unclear. It is likely that, in susceptible follicles in the scalp, dihydrotestosterone (DHT) binds to the androgen receptor and the hormone-receptor complex activates genes that gradually transform large terminal hairs into miniaturized hairs.

23. **How is androgenic alopecia is classified?**
Androgenic hair loss in males, or male pattern baldness (MPB), often follows a characteristic pattern beginning with temporal recession followed by diffuse thinning of the crown area, eventually leading to complete hair loss in this region. Balding in this area enlarges and eventually meets the temporal recession. On the final stages of progression the parietal and occipital fringes thin and recede. This step-wise progression was classified by Norwood, with a grading scale ranging from I to VII (Figure 61-1).

24. **Describe female pattern baldness.**
Because the role of androgens on alopecia in women remains uncertain, female pattern hair loss (FPHL) became the preferred term for AGA in women. It affects about 20% of all women, with the onset being as early as the third decade with a steady progression until acceleration during menopause. Diagnosis of FPHL is clinical, based on the characteristic appearance of the scalp. It normally does not require further workup, but patients should be asked about signs of hirsutism, acne, menstrual and hormonal abnormalities. The most widely used classification system for FPHL was proposed by Ludwig (Figure 61-2). The frontal hairline usually remains intact and the hair loss occurs on the top of the scalp and is arbitrarily divided into three degrees of severity.

25. **What are the nonsurgical treatment options for alopecia?**
Without treatment, AGA advances at a rate of about 5% a year. There are currently two drugs available foe treatment of AGA, Minoxidil and Finasteride. Minoxidil is a vasodilator and its mechanism of action to promote hair growth is not well understood, but seems to be independent of vasodilation. It causes an initial surge in hair growth, which quickly stops when the medication is stopped. Adverse effects include scalp irritation, dryness, itching, and redness. Finasteride is a competitive inhibitor of type 2 5α-reductase that inhibits the conversion of testosterone into DHT. It lowers the levels of DHT but has no affinity for other androgen receptors, therefore does not interfere with metabolic actions of testosterone. The adverse effects include decreased libido, erectile dysfunction, and ejaculatory dysfunction, which are reversible with discontinuation of the medication.

26. **Describe follicular unit transplantation.**
Follicular unit transplantation (FUT) consists of the transfer of the individual FU, maximizing the amount of hair and minimizing the amount of scarring.

Its starts by dissecting the FUs and setting them apart into individual units of one, two, three, or four hairs. They are then transferred to the recipient site and inserted in small openings, which minimizes recipient site scarring and trauma to the local blood vessels, but more importantly, creates a snug fit for the FU. The main advantage of FUT, and one of the reasons for its popularity, is the remarkably natural appearance that it provides the patient.

27. **How are the FUs obtained?**
The FUs can be obtained through a single strip harvest or through follicular unit extraction (FUE). The strip technique starts by determining and marking the donor area on the occipital scalp. With a

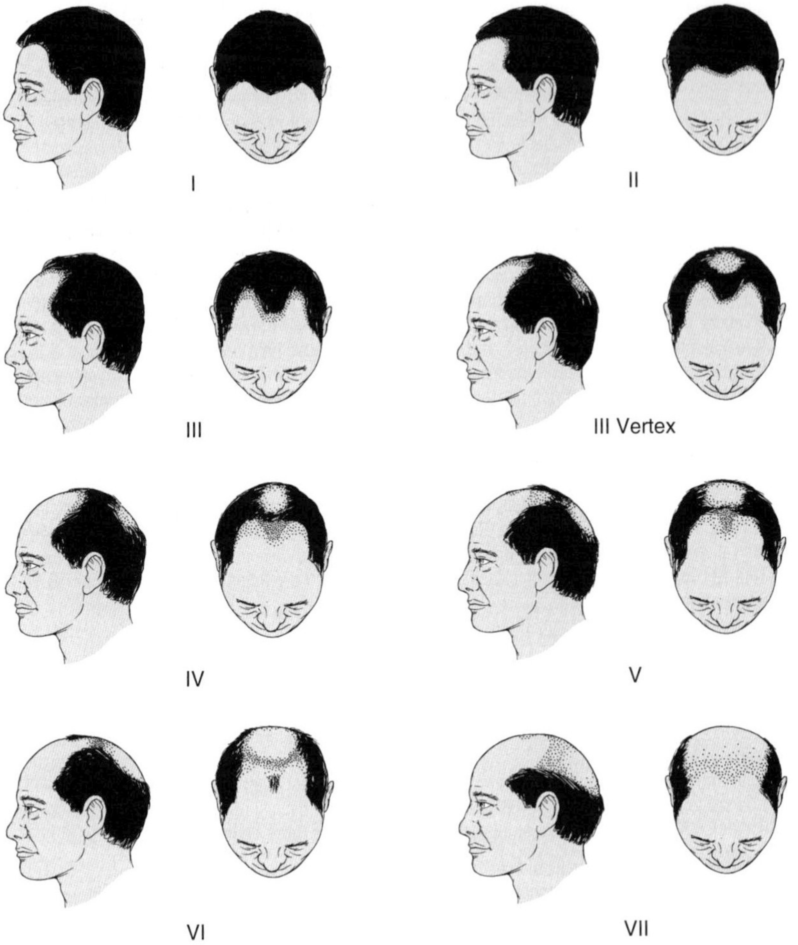

I
II
III
III Vertex
IV
V
VI
VII

Figure 61-1. Norwood classification of male pattern baldness. *(Previously published in Flint PW, Haughey BH, Lund VJ, et al, eds: Cummings Otolaryngology—Head and Neck Surgery, ed 5, Philadelphia, 2010, Mosby Elsevier, Figure 26-4, p. 377.)*

Grade I
Grade II
Grade III

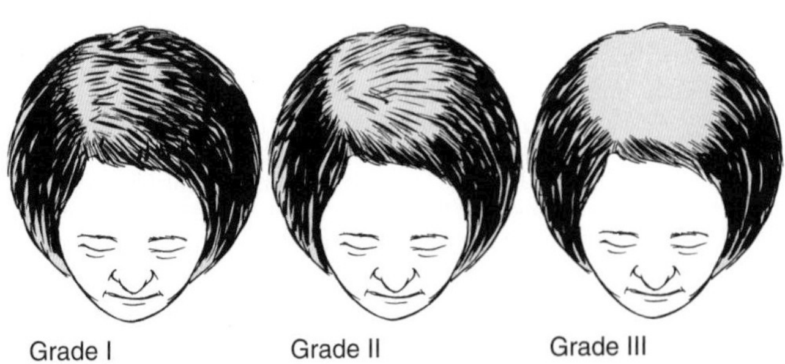

Figure 61-2. Ludwig classification of female pattern baldness. *(Previously published in Flint PW, Haughey BH, Lund VJ, et al, eds, Cummings Otolaryngology—Head and Neck Surgery, ed 5, Philadelphia, 2010, Mosby Elsevier, Figure 26-5, p. 377.)*

scalpel, the incision is made, beveling the knife along the axis of the follicles to avoid transection. The FUs are then dissected from the scalp strip, and the donor area is closed with sutures. In the FUE technique, a sharp 1-mm punch is used to incise into the midreticular dermis, stopping just above the subcutaneous tissue. This is done observing the angle of the hair shaft in the scalp and using the punch on the same axis to avoid transection. Then using a forceps or a suction-assisted device, the top of the graft is firmly grasped and pulled out.

28. **What is postsurgical effluvium?**
Postsurgical effluvium is the loss of preexisting hair in the FU following transplant and occurs to a small degree in some patients. This loss happens at any point from the first 3 weeks to 3 months after surgery and is usually minor and unnoticed by the patient. Significant postsurgical effluvium happens when a large number of transplanted grafts are placed in an area that contains a large proportion of miniaturized hairs. The degree of effluvium is unpredictable and can affect any patient, although it occurs more frequently in women. The patient needs to be reassured that hair will start growing again in the following 3 to 6 months.

Bibliography

Alexiades-Armenakas MR, Dover JS, Arndt KA: The spectrum of laser skin resurfacing: nonablative, fractional, and ablative laser resurfacing. *J Am Acad Dermatol* 58(5):719–737, 2008.

Bernstein RM, Rassman WR: Follicular unit transplantation: 2005. *Dermatol Clin* 23(3):393–414, 2005.

Carniol PJ, Harmon CB: Laser facial resurfacing. In Papel ID, editor: *Facial Plastic and Reconstructive Surgery*, New York, 2002, Thieme Medical, pp 241–246.

Fitzpatrick TB: The validity and practicality of sun-reactive skin types I through VI. *Arch Dermatol* 124(6):869–871, 1988.

Jackson A: Chemical peels. *Facial Plast Surg* 30(1):26–34, 2014.

Ludwig E: Classification of the types of androgenetic alopecia (common baldness) occurring in the female sex. *Br J Dermatol* 97(3):247–254, 1977.

Norwood OT: Male pattern baldness: classification and incidence. *South Med J* 68(11):1359–1365, 1975.

Smith JE. Dermabrasion. *Facial Plast Surg* 30(1):35–39, 2014.

CHAPTER 62

COSMETIC SURGERY FOR THE AGING NECK AND FACE

Andrew A. Winkler, MD

KEY POINTS

1. Facelift is a cosmetic procedure that involves elevating the tissues of the lower face and neck into a more youthful position.
2. There are several possible complications from facelift, including hematoma, nerve injury, skin necrosis, and contour irregularities.
3. Numerous facelift techniques have been described, each with its own risks and benefits.

Pearls

1. The most common complication from facelift surgery is hematoma. It occurs in up to 10% of cases and is more common in men.
2. The rate limiting anatomy in facelift surgery is the position of the hyoid bone. A congenitally anterior hyoid bone relative to the chin forces the MCA and LFTA to be more obtuse.
3. The most commonly injured nerve in facelift surgery is the great auricular nerve. The most commonly injured motor nerve in facelift surgery is the marginal mandibular.
4. The superficial musculoaponeurotic system (SMAS) contains the muscles of facial expression and is the tissue layer that is lifted in most facelift techniques.

QUESTIONS

1. What is a facelift?
Facelift, or cervicofacial rhytidectomy is a surgery that elevates the skin and soft tissues of the lower third of the face and neck. The procedure involves elevating a skin flap around the ear, drawing the deeper tissues up superiorly and fixating them to strong fascia. This is generally considered a cosmetic procedure and is performed in the outpatient setting.

2. What type of anesthesia is required?
Facelift can be performed under general anesthesia, IV sedation, or with local anesthesia only.

3. What aging stigmata are addressed with facelift?
When examining the aging-face patient interested in facelift, it is useful to know what areas can be corrected with this procedure. The following aging issues can be addressed (Figure 62-1):

- Sagging neck skin
- Platysmal bands
- Jowls
- Excess cervical fat

A combination of facelift, liposuction, and platysmaplasty (see later) are used to correct these problems. Fine wrinkles are not treated by facelift.

4. What is the SMAS?
The superficial musculoaponeurotic system (SMAS) is a continuous layer of the face that contains the muscles of facial expression. The SMAS layer is connected to the dermis, which allows these muscles to move the skin and convey emotion. These are the only muscles in the body that attach directly to skin, which highlights the importance of facial expression in social species such as our own.

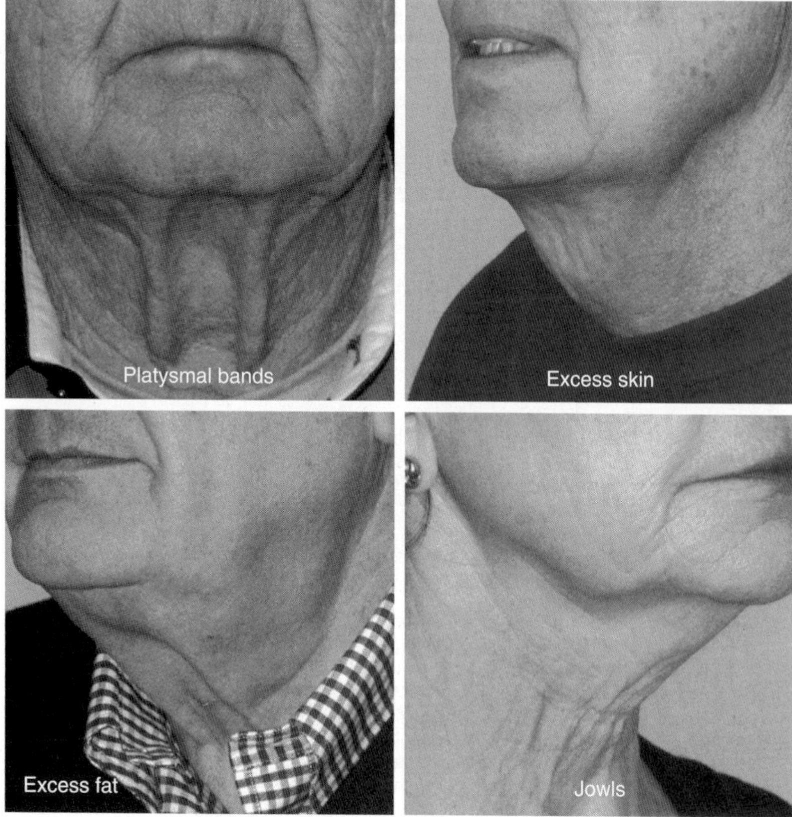

Figure 62-1. Areas of the lower face and neck that can be improved with facelift surgery.

5. **What is the most common complication of facelift and what are some risk factors?**
The most common complication is hematoma and the reported incidence is 5% to 10%. This can range from major postoperative hematoma requiring emergent surgical evacuation to minor hematomas that are aspirated in clinic. Hematoma is more common in men due to differences in skin vascular perfusion around facial hair. Another significant risk factor is uncontrolled hypertension. When blood pressure is above 150/100 mmHg at admission, hematoma is 2.6 times more likely than in normotensive patients.

6. **What is the most commonly injured nerve in facelift surgery?**
The great auricular nerve—a sensory nerve originating from spinal levels C2 and C3—is the most commonly injured nerve. It innervates to the lower ear and periauricular skin and is found 6.5 cm below the external ear canal on the belly of the sternocleidomastoid muscle. Injury to this nerve occurs in around 7% of cases.

7. **What is the most commonly injured motor nerve in facelift surgery?**
The marginal mandibular nerve—a motor nerve to the depressors of the oral commissure. Injury to the marginal mandibular nerve is thought to occur in less than 1% of cases and depends greatly on the facelift technique utilized.

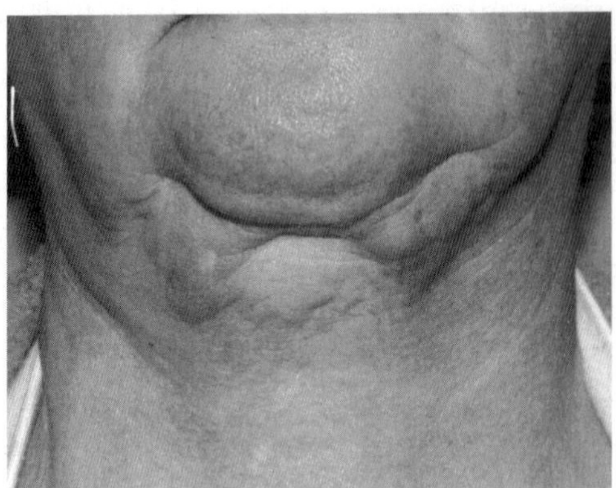

Figure 62-2. Contour irregularities, such as the cobra-neck deformity pictured here, are possible complications of facelift surgery.

8. What are other complications of facelift surgery?
   - Skin necrosis can occur in the preauricular (most common) and postauricular (second most common) skin.
   - Cobra-neck deformity describes over-prominence of the platysmal bands due to overly aggressive removal of submental fat (Figure 62-2).

9. What are the some popular facelift techniques?
   - **Skin-only:** The skin-only facelift technique is the earliest described technique, and is safe and reliable for the beginning surgeon. This technique employs subcutaneous dissection only. The skin is elevated off the underlying SMAS to a variable extent around the ear. Excess skin is trimmed and the incision is closed. The skin-only technique has the advantage of having minimal risk to the facial nerve. The main drawback of this technique is a lack of longevity, which is greatly improved with the SMAS techniques described below.
   - **SMAS plication:** Plication describes folding the SMAS over on itself near the ear and securing it with sutures. A subcutaneous flap is elevated, but no sub-SMAS dissection is performed. The SMAS plication is performed with resorbable or permanent sutures.
   - **MACS lift:** The minimal access cranial suspension (MACS) lift is a plication technique that utilizes only a preauricular incision and a limited skin flap dissection. Suspension sutures are used to elevate the underlying SMAS tissue vertically. These sutures pass down to the neck, jowls, and malar fat pad in a purse-string manner to achieve elevation. The main difficulty with this technique is contour irregularities from the bunching of the SMAS, though these typically flatten with time.
   - **Extended SMAS:** Extended SMAS dissection has been purported to improve facelift results at the nasolabial fold. The SMAS is incised near the ear and elevated off of the parotid gland, where the facial nerve is protected. The SMAS is released from the upper lateral border of the zygomaticus muscle and medially to release the zygomatic retaining ligaments. As the facial nerve branches exit at the anterior border of the parotid gland, they course directly beneath the SMAS. An increased risk of facial nerve paresis has been reported with this technique.
   - **Deep plane:** The deep plane technique is perhaps the most invasive facelift technique. It was developed to further improve the results at the nasolabial fold and the ptotic malar fat pad. This procedure begins with an extended SMAS procedure. Dissection then continues anteriorly and the surgical plane is transitioned from a sub-SMAS plane to a supra-SMAS plane to avoid injuring the facial nerve. The anterior extent of the sub-SMAS dissection is the facial artery. In the deep plane technique, the facial nerve branches are protected because they enter muscles on their undersurface.

10. What are some important reference angles and points with regards to facelift?
    - **Lower Face-Throat Angle (90–105 degrees):** The lower face-throat angle (LFTA) describes the extent to which the submental tissues are tucked beneath the chin. It is the angle formed by connecting a line from the cervical point (posterior most point in the submental area) to the

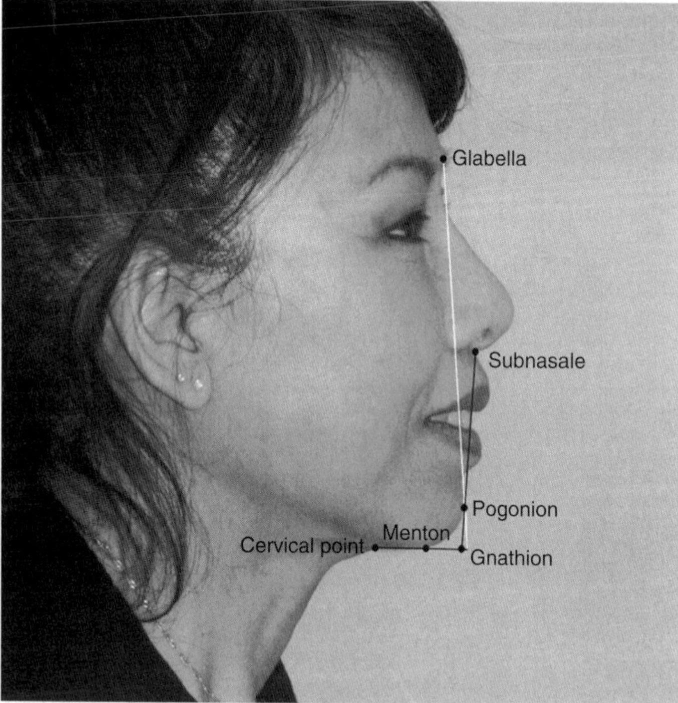

Figure 62-3. The lower face-throat angle *(black)* and mentocervical angle *(white)* are useful to take note of in the pre- and postoperative period.

menton (inferior most point of the chin), with a line from the subnasale (junction of the columella and upper lip) to the pogonion (anterior most point of the chin in the midline). The intersection of these lines is a virtual point called the gnathion (Figure 62-3).

- **Mentocervical Angle (80–90 degrees):** The mentocervical angle (MCA) takes into account a broader area of the face and therefore better describes the relationship of the neck to the face. The MCA is formed by the intersection of a line from the cervical point to the menton with a line from the glabella (anterior most point between the eyebrows) to the pogonion (Figure 62-4).

11. What anatomic structures limit the improvement of the LFTA and the MCA?
The values of the MCA and LFTA are reliant on the relationship of the hyoid bone to the mandible. The relative position of these two entities to one another represents the limiting factor in any attempt to surgically manipulate the neckline.

12. What can be done about platysmal bands?
The "corset platysmaplasty" is the most popular technique to address plastysmal bands. The medial bands of the platysma are identified via a submental crease incision. They are then trimmed, incised at the hyoid bone, and imbricated together across the midline.

CONTROVERSIES

13. SMAS plication versus deep plane facelifts?
In recent years, the pendulum has swung back toward less invasive facelift techniques. This is in part due to less risk of complications, but perhaps more to a failure to realize the improved results touted by more extensive dissection techniques. Certainly, excellent results can be seen with any technique in the hands of an experienced surgeon. However, many very experienced surgeons

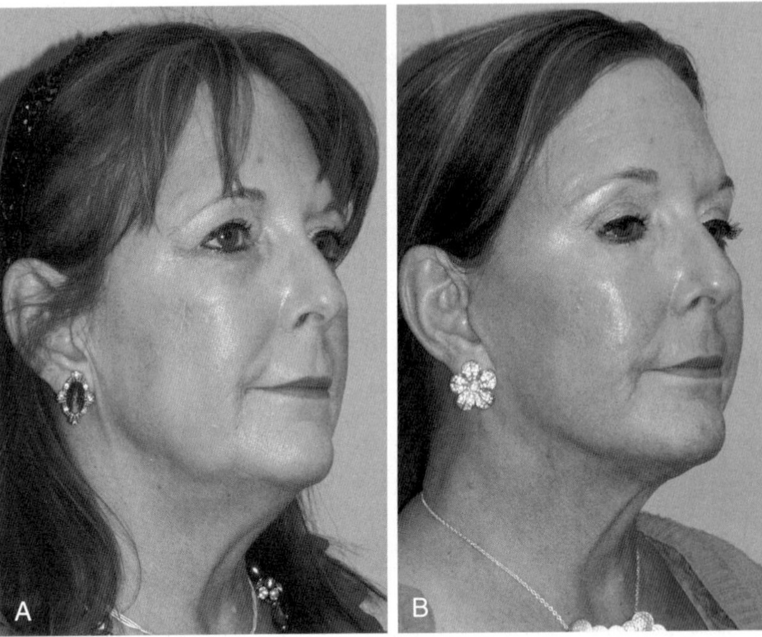

Figure 62-4. **(A)** Before and **(B)** after images of a happy patient who underwent a modified MACS facelift (with additional procedures).

now perform limited SMAS elevating techniques or plication in favor of extensive deep plane dissection.

14. Drains and/or compression dressings?
    The use of subcutaneous drains is controversial. Hematoma is the most common complication of this surgery and can even be life-threatening. Preventing this complication is foremost in the surgeon's mind. However, drains are uncomfortable and not necessary in the majority of patients. Compression dressings wrapped around the head may reduce the risk of hematoma, but they increase the risk of focal skin necrosis. Also to be considered is gender as well as the particular facelift technique employed, as more skin undermining tends to increase bleeding.

Bibliography

Daane SP, Owsley JQ: Incidence of cervical branch injury with "marginal mandibular nerve pseudo-paralysis" in patients undergoing face lift, *Plast Reconstr Surg* 111(7):2414–2418, 2003.

Feldman JJ: Corset platysmaplasty, *Plast Reconstr Surg* 85(3):333–343, 1990.

Griffin JE, Jo C: Complications after superficial plane cervicofacial rhytidectomy: a retrospective analysis of 178 consecutive facelifts and review of the literature, *J Oral Maxillofac Surg* 65(11):2227–2234, 2007.

Mayrovitz HN, Regan MB: Gender differences in facial skin blood perfusion during basal and heated conditions determined by laser Doppler flowmetry, *Microvasc Res* 45(2):211–218, 1993.

McCollough EG, Perkins S, Thomas JR: Facelift: panel discussion, controversies, and techniques, *Facial Plast Surg Clin North Am* 20(3):279–325, 2012.

McKinney P, Katrana DJ: Prevention of injury to the great auricular nerve during rhytidectomy, *Plast Reconstr Surg* 66(5):675–679, 1980.

Rees TD, Aston SJ: Complications of rhytidectomy, *Clin Plast Surg* 5(1):109–119, 1978.

Straith RE, Raju DR, Hipps CJ: The study of hematomas in 500 consecutive face lifts, *Plast Reconstr Surg* 59(5): 694–698, 1977.

Tanna N, Lindsey WH: Review of 1,000 consecutive short-scar rhytidectomies, *Dermatol Surg* 34(2):196–202, discussion 202–203, 2008.

Winkler AA, Wudel JM: Preoperative evaluation and facial analysis in facial plastic surgery. In Johnson J, editor: *Bailey's Head and Neck Surgery Otolaryngology*, ed 5, Philadelphia, 2013, Lippincott Williams & Wilkins.

BOTULINUM TOXIN AND FILLERS

Henry H. Chen, MD, MBA and Edwin F. Williams, III, MD

CHAPTER 63

KEY POINTS

1. Of the botulinum toxins available, Botox® has the longest record of safety and efficacy as well as the most FDA-approved indications. However, due to similar mechanism of action and widespread off-label use, Dysport® and Xeomin® can be used interchangeably for cosmetic purposes.
2. Hyaluronic acids are by far the most commonly used facial filler.
3. Major adverse reactions to injection with facial fillers are rare and can largely be prevented through meticulous technique and injection into the right plane.

Pearls

1. Botulinum toxin works at the presynaptic neuromuscular junction preventing acetylcholine release leading to temporary muscle paralysis.
2. Ptosis secondary to botulinum toxin injection can be treated with α-adrenergic ophthalmic drops.
3. Hyaluronic acid fillers exert their effects by tightly binding water leading to volumization and hydration of the skin.
4. Sculptra's® mechanism of action is through gradual neocollagenesis.

QUESTIONS

1. **What is botulinum toxin and what is its mechanism of action?**
   Clostridium botulinum produces botulinum exotoxin (BTX), of which there are seven serotypes (A-G). These potent neurotoxins cause flaccid paralysis by preventing the release of acetylcholine from presynaptic vesicles at the neuromuscular junction. This is accomplished by cleaving the SNARE complex of proteins (SNAP-25, synaptobrevin, and syntaxin) that allows the vesicles containing acetylcholine to fuse with the plasmalemma of the nerve terminal leading to exocytosis. By preventing muscle contraction, BTX prevents the formation of facial rhytids from dynamic muscle movement.

2. **What are the formulations of botulinum toxin that are available in the United States?**
   There are currently three FDA-approved formulations of BTX-A:
   - Botox and Botox Cosmetic (onabotulinumtoxinA, Allergan, Irvine, CA)
   - Dysport (abobotulinumtoxinA, Valeant, Laval, Quebec)
   - Xeomin (incobotulinutoxinA, Merz, Frankfurt, Germany)

   Botox and Xeomin have an equivalent strength of activity per unit. Dysport has less strength per unit, and it takes on average 2 to 3 units of Dysport to equal the strength of 1 unit of Botox.

   The only BTX-B formulation available is Myobloc (rimabotulinumtoxinB, Solstice Neurosciences, Louisville, KY).

3. **What is botulinum toxin used for?**
   From a cosmetic standpoint, Botox Cosmetic, Dysport, and Xeomin are all FDA approved for the temporary improvement of glabellar lines. Botox Cosmetic also has an additional cosmetic indication for the temporary improvement of lateral canthal lines, otherwise known as crow's feet. Use of these products in other locations for aesthetic purposes is considered off-label.

From a medical standpoint, Botox, Dysport, and Xeomin also have FDA approval for the treatment of cervical dystonia. Botox and Xeomin are also approved for the treatment of blepharospasm. Botox, because it has been around the longest and has the longest record of safety, is also FDA approved for the treatment of strabismus, upper limb spasticity, chronic migraines, urinary incontinence in patients with overactive bladder due to neurologic disease, and severe primary axillary hyperhidrosis.

Other common off-label uses for botulinum toxin include facial tics, spasmodic dysphonia, myofascial pain syndrome, and sialorrhea.

4. What is the onset and duration of botulinum toxin?

For cosmetic injections in the face, it takes 3 to 7 days for the effects of botulinum toxin to be seen, reaching maximal efficacy around 2 weeks after injection. This effect lasts for approximately 3 months. However, with repeated injection, the duration could extend to 4 to 6 months as the facial muscles atrophy.

The return of normal muscle function occurs through axonal sprouting and production of new neuromuscular junctions.

5. What is the lethal dose of Botox and what is a common dose for cosmetic purposes?

The LD_{50} (lethal to 50% of those injected) is 2500 to 3000 units in humans. For cosmetic purposes, use of 40 to 60 units per treatment is common.

6. What are typical doses of Botox for facial rhytids?

- Glabella: 20–40 units divided in 5 sites
- Forehead: 10–30 units divided in 4–8 sites; inject at least 2 cm above eyebrow
- Crow's feet: 8–12 units on each side divided in 3–4 sites
- Perioral area: 4–10 units divided in 2–6 sites
- Chin: 2–8 units divided in 1–2 sites
- Neck (platysmal banding): 10–40 units divided in 2–4 sites per band

7. What are the depressors and elevators of the brow?

- Depressors: corrugators supercilii, procerus, depressor supercilii (part of the orbicularis muscle), procerus
- Elevators: frontalis

These muscles are demonstrated in Figure 63-1.

8. What is the "Mr. Spock" look and how do you treat it?

The "Mr. Spock" look is caused by excessive elevation of the lateral brow while the medial brow remains relatively fixed. The look is due to overactivity of the lateral aspect of the frontalis and is easily treated by injecting botulinum toxin in that area to weaken its activity.

9. What is a chemical brow lift?

Botox is injected in the superolateral orbicularis oculi muscle just below the eyebrow to weaken the orbicularis oculi's depressor function. This results in a 1 to 2 mm elevation of the brow.

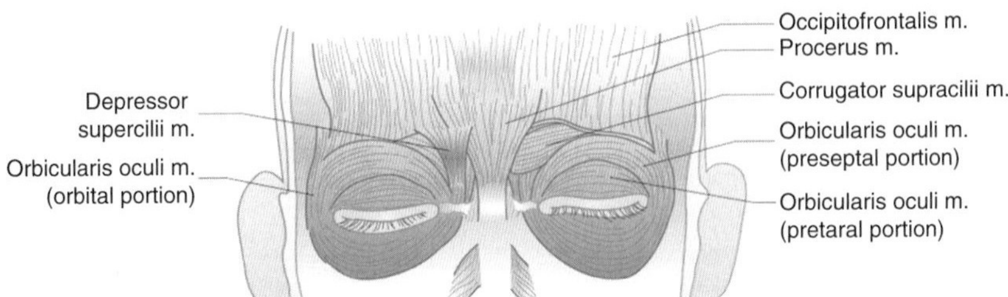

Figure 63-1. Depressors and elevators of the brow. *(From Biesman B: Atlas of Cosmetic Surgery. Philadelphia, SAUNDERS An imprint of Elsevier Limited, © 2009, p. 483–503.)*

10. **What are some common side effects of botulinum toxin?**
Pain and bruising at the injection site are most common. Headache, dry mouth, tiredness, neck pain, and eye problems can also occur.

11. **What are some serious potential side effects of botulinum toxin?**
Serious, potentially fatal, side effects include difficulty breathing, difficulty swallowing, dysphonia, dysarthria, loss of bladder control, and generalized weakness. This is most likely due to spread of the toxin from the injection site to other parts of the body. At usual cosmetic doses, these side effects are very unlikely.

12. **How does eyelid ptosis occur after botulinum toxin injection and how do you treat it?**
Ptosis occurs by diffusion of the botulinum toxin to the levator palpebrae superioris or levator aponeurosis, usually by injection of botulinum toxin too close to the upper eyelid. It can best be prevented by injecting at least 1 cm above the orbital rim.
Apraclonidine (lopidine) and phenylephrine (Mydfrin) eye drops will selectively target $\alpha 2$ and $\alpha 1$ adrenergic receptors, respectively, leading to contraction of Müller muscle which will decrease the ptosis.

13. **Can a patient be resistant to botulinum toxin?**
Yes. While rare, there are reports of patients developing resistance to botulinum toxin. This is felt to be due to the formation of antibodies either to the neurotoxin or the complexing proteins that accompany it. To avoid this possibility, it is recommended to use the smallest possible doses to achieve the desired effect and to wait at least 3 months between treatments.

14. **What precautions should patients take after botulinum toxin injection?**
The patient should avoid massaging or rubbing the injected areas as well as any skin treatments on the day of the procedure. Additionally, the patient should avoid any vibrational therapy such as the whirlpool or hydrotherapy. The patient ideally should avoid vigorous sports for a week after injection.

15. **What are some different types of fillers available for facial aesthetics?**
Broadly, fillers can be classified as absorbable or nonabsorbable. The only nonabsorbable filler available is Artefill (Suneva Medical, San Diego, CA), composed of polymethylmethacrylate microspheres. Its use has largely fallen out of favor due to the widespread success of absorbable fillers.
Absorbables can be divided into synthetic or natural products. Synthetic fillers include Radiesse (Merz, Frankfurt, Germany), composed of calcium hydroxylapatite and Sculptra (Valeant, Laval, Quebec), composed of poly-L-lactic acid.
Natural absorbable fillers account for the most commonly used facial fillers, with hyaluronic acid (HA) products comprising the bulk of this category. Other options include autologous fat and collagen, but collagen products are no longer used due to superiority of the HA products and fat.

16. **What is hyaluronic acid?**
Hyaluronic acid is the most common glycosaminoglycan in the skin. It is potently hydrophilic and binds to water leading to volumization and hydration of the skin. Interestingly, hyaluronic acid is identical across all species, making it extremely unlikely to lead to allergic reaction. As such, no skin testing is needed prior to injection. Hyaluronic acid products are by far the most commonly used type of facial filler.
Hyaluronic acid fillers available include Restylane and Perlane (Valeant, Laval, Quebec), Juvéderm (Allergan, Irvine, CA), Prevelle Silk (Mentor, Santa Barbara, CA), Belotero (Merz, Frankfurt, Germany), and Elevess (Anika Therapeutics, Bedford, MA). The main differences between products are due to particle size and concentration of hyaluronic acid, which determine how soft and pliable the product is.

17. **How long do hyaluronic acid fillers last?**
Anywhere from 6 to 12 months.

18. **What are different methods of injection of facial fillers?**
- Serial puncture: Injecting a series of small boluses
- Threading: Tunneling the needle beneath the area of concern and injecting as the needle is withdrawn

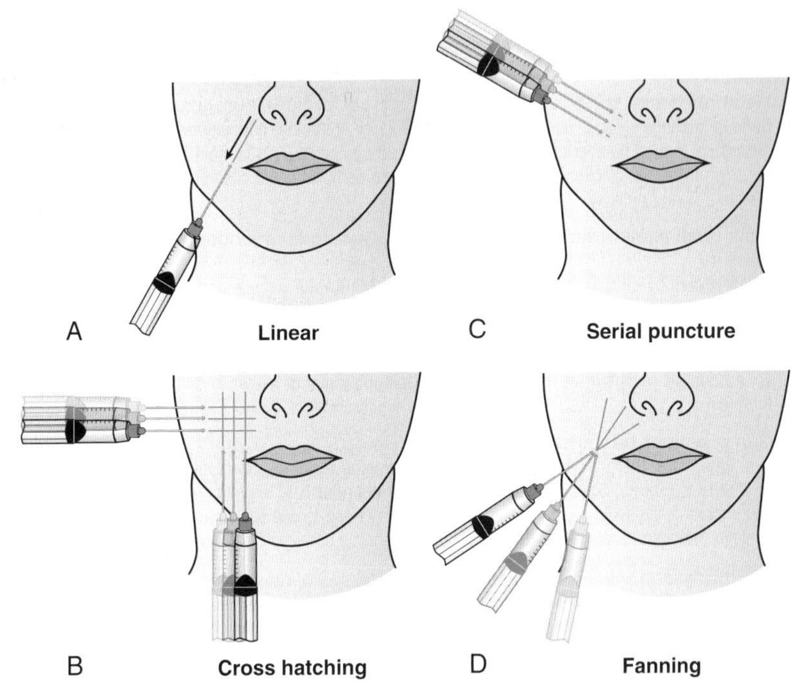

Figure 63-2. Injection techniques for facial fillers.

- Fanning: Injection of multiple threads radially by changing direction without withdrawing the needle
- Crosshatching: Injection of multiple threads perpendicular to one another in a grid

These techniques are demonstrated in Figure 63-2.

Threading is useful for lip and nasolabial fold augmentation. Fanning and crosshatching are particularly useful for filling in larger defects.

19. **What is the mechanism of action of Sculptra?**
Sculptra works through the process of neocollagenesis wherein the body gradually builds collagen over time in the areas where the product is injected. This leads to a gradual increase in volume over time as opposed to an immediate effect. Effects of Sculptra have been reported up to 3 years after treatment.

20. **What are complications that can result from injection of facial fillers?**
Common complications include ecchymosis, erythema, and edema at the site of injection. Asymmetry from over- or undercorrection can also be seen. Nodules and granulomas can form as a result of the inflammatory response to the filler but are usually rare. Nodules specifically have been reported for Sculptra but can be avoided by the depth and technique of injection. Finally, serious, even fatal complications have been reported including skin necrosis, blindness, and even death. These are due to accidental intravascular injection leading to occlusion of blood flow.

21. **What is the Tyndall effect?**
A complication of injecting hyaluronic acid too superficially, leading to a visible bump under the skin with a bluish discoloration. This can be prevented by deeper injection as well as beveling the needle away from the skin.

22. **What is hyaluronidase and how is it used?**
Hyaluronidase causes hydrolysis and breakdown of hyaluronic acid, allowing areas of overcorrection to be dissolved away. Its effect is usually seen within 24 hours.

CONTROVERSIES

23. **Should blunt tip cannulas or needles be used for the injection of facial fillers?**
Because of the risk of puncture of blood vessels due to needles, which can lead to bruising or other intravascular complications associated with the injection of fillers, some practitioners prefer using blunt tip cannulas to minimize this risk. However, others feel it is still possible to puncture vessels with blunt tip cannulas due to their small caliber.

BIBLIOGRAPHY

Carruthers J, Fagien S, Matarasso SL, et al: Consensus recommendations on the use of botulinum toxin type a in facial aesthetics, *Plast Reconstr Surg* 114(6 Suppl):1S–22S, 2004.

Carruthers A, Kane MA, Flynn TC, et al: The convergence of medicine and neurotoxins: a focus on botulinum toxin type A and its application in aesthetic medicine—a global, evidence-based botulinum toxin consensus education initiative: part I: botulinum toxin in clinical and cosmetic practice, *Dermatol Surg* 39:493–509, 2013.

Cohen JL: Understanding, avoiding, and managing dermal filler complications, *Dermatol Surg* 34(Suppl 1):S92–S99, 2008.

Flynn TC: Advances in the use of botulinum neurotoxins in facial esthetics, *J Cosmet Dermatol* 11:42–50, 2012.

Gilman GS: Cosmetic uses of neurotoxins and injectable fillers. In Johnson JT, Rosen CA, editors: *Bailey's Head and Neck Surgery Otolaryngology*, Philadelphia, 2014, Lippincott Williams & Wilkins, pp 3239–3251.

Kontis TC: Contemporary review of injectable facial fillers, *JAMA Facial Plast Surg* 15:58–64, 2013.

Kim JE, Sykes JM: Hyaluronic acid fillers: history and overview, *Facial Plast Surg* 27:523–528, 2011.

Vleggaar D: Facial volumetric correction with injectable poly-L-lactic acid, *Dermatol Surg* 31:1511–1517, 2005.

Walker TJ, Dayan SH: Comparison and overview of currently available neurotoxins, *J Clin Aesthet Dermatol* 7:31–39, 2014.

CHAPTER 64

FACIAL REANIMATION

Geoffrey R. Ferril, MD and Adam M. Terella, MD

KEY POINTS

1. The patient with facial nerve paralysis necessitates a thorough workup to delineate timing of the injury, mechanism of paralysis, and extent of injury.
2. Ophthalmologic care, be it medical and/or surgical, is crucial in the management of facial nerve paralysis and should be instituted as early as possible.
3. Facial reanimation procedures are classified as static or dynamic, depending on whether or not facial movement may be achieved. Patient expectations must be discussed, as few reanimation procedures fully approximate the pre-injury state.
4. The elapsed time period since nerve injury affects the viability of distal nerve fibers and, in turn, influences the appropriate type of reanimation procedure (neural reinnervation versus muscle transposition or static).

Pearls

1. In the setting of denervation, there is nerve and motor endplate fibrosis that leads to muscle atrophy. Thus, reinnervation procedures must be completed by 12 to 18 months post injury before atrophic changes for best results.
2. Electromyographic testing (EMG) is an invaluable tool to help determine if spontaneous recovery is occurring.
3. Address paralytic lagophthalmos early and aggressively with medical and surgical management to prevent dry eye and exposure keratitis.

QUESTIONS

1. **Briefly describe the course of the facial nerve.**
   The facial nerve exits the brainstem, courses through the cerebellopontine angle, and then enters the temporal bone. After a complex course through the temporal bone, it exits the stylomastoid foramen and branches within the parotid gland into two main branches, the temporofacial and cervicofacial, at the pes anserinus. Traditionally, five terminal branches are present, including the temporal, zygomatic, buccal, marginal mandibular, and cervical.

2. **What is the most commonly used classification of facial nerve injury?**
   The House-Brackmann Grading Scale is the most commonly used in the literature. House and Brackmann staged injury from grade 1 to 6 (Table 64-1). Increasing grade corresponds to a decreasing likelihood of spontaneous recovery.

3. **What is synkinesis, and what is the first-line treatment for this disorder?**
   Synkinesis is the hyperkinetic, uncoordinated mass facial movement seen with aberrant regeneration of nerve fibers after facial nerve injury. This involuntary synkinesia often occurs between the orbicularis oculi and orbicularis oris muscles, or presents as increased lacrimation of the affected eye. Currently, botulinum toxin injection is the first-line therapy. Botulinum toxin blocks the presynaptic release of acetylcholine causing a temporary functional denervation, thus limiting the synkinesis.

4. **What key elements of the history and physical exam must be taken into account when approaching the patient with facial nerve paralysis?**
   It is important to consider the patient's medical history, mechanism of injury, presumed site of injury, timing of injury, vestibulocochlear function, eye closure, and individual expectations.

Table 64-1. Facial Nerve Grading Scale

GRADE	DESCRIPTION	CHARACTERISTICS
I	Normal	
II	Mild dysfunction	Slight weakness or synkinesis; symmetry at rest
III	Moderate dysfunction	Noticeable weakness or synkinesis; symmetry at rest; complete eye closure with maximal effort
IV	Moderately severe dysfunction	Obvious weakness; symmetry at rest; incomplete eye closure
V	Severe dysfunction	Only perceptible movement; asymmetry at rest
VI	Total paralysis	

Adapted from House JW, Brackmann DE: Facial nerve grading system. Otolaryngol Head Neck Surg 93(2): 146–147, 1985.

5. **What is the role of electrodiagnostic testing following facial paralysis?**
The goal of electrodiagnostic testing is to evaluate the degree of facial nerve injury and the functionality of the facial musculature. Commonly utilized electrical tests are the maximum stimulation test (MST), the nerve excitability test (NET), electroneuronography (ENOG), and electromyography (EMG).

6. **Discuss electromyography (EMG) testing and how it is useful in the setting of facial reanimation.**
EMG is the study of depolarization potentials in a muscle fiber. In the patient with facial paralysis, an EMG provides important information that can help determine appropriate treatment options. Typically, resting muscle exhibits no spontaneous electrical activity. In the setting of denervation from facial nerve injury, electrical activity may be increased, and *spontaneous fibrillation potentials* develop. Fibrillation potentials are strong evidence that denervation has occurred. Conversely, *polyphasic action potentials* indicate that regeneration is occurring.

7. **Is there a role for physical therapy in facial reanimation?**
Yes. Physical therapy is often underutilized in the setting of facial nerve paralysis. Facial neuromuscular reeducation using surface EMG and biofeedback techniques has demonstrated improvements in facial movement in randomized trials.

8. **What is a potential sequela of paralysis of the orbicularis oculi?**
Paralysis of the orbicularis oculi muscle may result in incomplete eye closure, or *lagophthalmos*. Left untreated, paralytic lagophthalmos can lead to exposure keratitis, corneal ulceration, and blindness.

9. **Describe broadly the types of surgical rehabilitation utilized for facial paralysis.**
Surgical techniques for the management of facial paralysis can be classified as either *static* or *dynamic*. Static procedures serve to restore symmetry and limit functional sequela, but generally do not restore facial movement or tone. Dynamic procedures aim to restore movement and can be subdivided into *neural procedures* (cable grafting, cross-facial nerve grafting, XII to VII, V to VII), *microvascular free flaps* (gracilis flap), or other dynamic procedures (transposition of the temporalis or masseter, and temporalis tendon transfer).

10. **Discuss treatment of the lower eyelid in the setting of facial paralysis.**
The decision to treat or not largely depends on lower lid laxity, which can be assessed by the snap test. Medial lower lid laxity can cause the inferior punctum to evert from the globe and result in epiphora. Correction is with a medial canthoplasty. For excess lateral lower lid laxity, producing scleral show or ectropion, a horizontal lid shortening procedure is indicated.

11. **What is ectropion?**
Ectropion is the abnormal eversion of the lower eyelid in relation to the globe and can be associated with lower eyelid paralysis.

12. **Discuss treatment of the paralyzed upper eyelid.**
    Gold weight implantation is the most popular procedure for managing upper eyelid paralytic lagophthalmos. Gold or platinum are often used because of their low reactivity and high density. The procedure can often be performed under local anesthesia, and is reversible. Since the procedure results in lid loading and is gravity dependent, it can lead to undesirable lid closure when lying supine.

13. **In situations where the facial nerve was transected or resected, what is the technique of choice for repair?**
    Regardless of cause, primary nerve anastomosis, in the acute setting, is the technique of choice for repair of a completely disrupted facial nerve. Repair should occur as early as possible, ideally prior to Wallerian degeneration (within 72 hours). Success is largely dependent on the ability to reapproximate the disrupted segments without tension. Obtaining a tensionless repair may require mobilization or rerouting of the adjacent facial nerve segments.

14. **What are some alternative options to repair a transected facial nerve when a tension-free reapproximation is not possible?**
    For situations in which a tension-free reapproximation is not possible, one can utilize an interposition nerve graft. The two most popular nerves utilized for this purpose are the great auricular and sural nerves.

15. **When counseling patients in terms of House-Brackmann score after a primary neurorrhaphy or interposition graft facial nerve repair, what is the best possible outcome?**
    House-Brackmann Grade III (see Table 64-1).

16. **What is cross-facial nerve grafting?**
    Cross-facial nerve grafting is a two-stage procedure whereby the functioning facial nerve and its branches are used to innervate contralateral paralyzed nerve branches by way of an interposition graft. The first stage involves identifying distal facial nerve branches (buccal and zygomatic) on the normally functioning side and coapting a sural nerve graft to these. The second stage, undertaken 9 to 12 months later, is comprised of secondary neurorraphies between selected paralyzed facial nerve branches and the cross-face nerve graft. This procedure relies on a contralateral, normal-functioning nerve, and functional motor endplates on the paralyzed side. For this reason the period of degeneration ideally should be less than 6 months (Figure 64-1).

17. **What is meant by the term "nerve transposition"? What is the most common nerve transposition procedure?**
    A nerve transposition procedure involves coapting to the facial nerve trunk or distal branches to another cranial nerve. This technique is utilized when a proximal facial nerve stump is not available or viable, but distal nerve and motor endplates on the paralyzed side are viable. Several cranial nerves have been utilized for nerve transpositions, but the hypoglossal nerve (CN XII) remains the most commonly utilized due to relatively low donor site morbidity and close anatomic proximity to the facial nerve.

18. **What is the role of muscle transposition in the setting of facial paralysis?**
    Muscle transposition is usually used when nerve grafting is not possible due to degradation of distal nerve fibers. In this setting, transposition of the temporalis or masseter muscles can provide tone and dynamic reanimation to the lower face.

19. **What are the advantages of temporalis tendon transfer versus temporalis muscle transposition?**
    The original temporalis muscle transfer described the transfer of the temporalis muscle belly over the zygomatic arch. This technique resulted in a significant cosmetic deformity in the temporal and zygoma region. The orthodromic temporalis tendon transfer technique prevents this deformity by avoiding transfer of the muscle over the arch. Instead the temporalis tendon is disinserted from its attachment to the coronoid and transferred to the lateral commissure or melolabial fold.

20. **Discuss the role of microneurovascular free flaps in facial reanimation.**
    Microneurovascular free flaps utilize free tissue transfer, including soft tissue and corresponding nerve and vascular supply, to rehabilitate a paralyzed face. They have the potential to offer

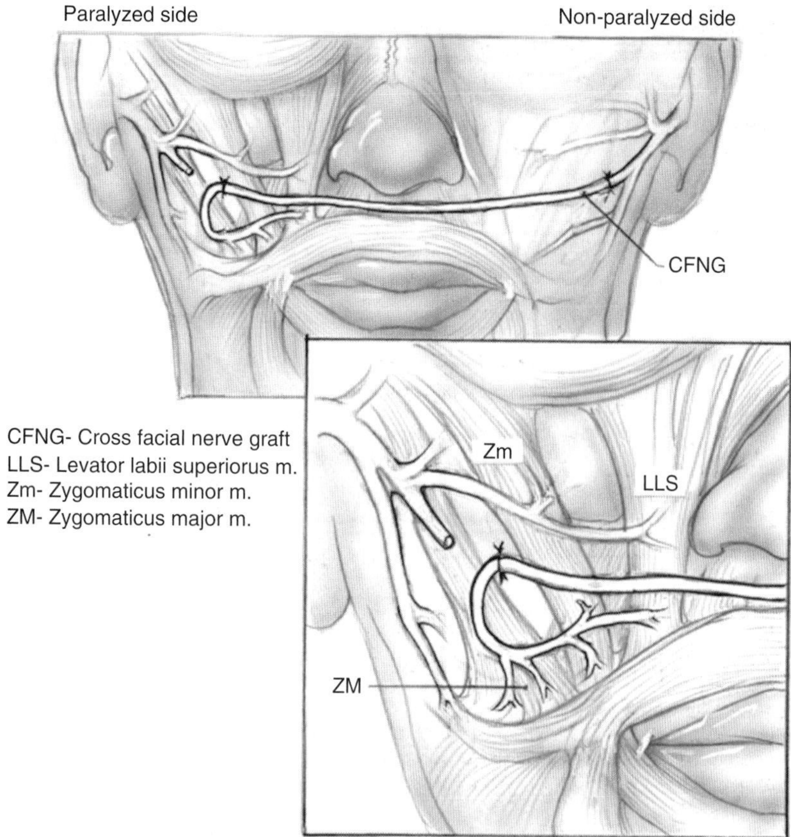

Figure 64-1. Illustration of the cross-facial nerve graft from a buccal branch on the nonparalyzed left side to a buccal branch on the paralyzed side. *(From Collar RM, Byrne PJ, Boahene KD: Cross-facial nerve grafting. Oper Techn Otolaryngol-Head Neck Surg 23(4): 258–261, 2012.)*

emotional animation in addition to good tone. They typically involve a two-stage procedure in which a cross-facial nerve graft is performed approximately 9 to 12 months prior to the flap. The microneurovascular flap is then anastomosed to the cross-facial graft and the facial artery and vein.

21. **What is the most commonly utilized microneurovascular flap in facial reanimation?**
The most commonly utilized microneurovascular free flap is the gracilis flap. This muscle is found in the medial thigh and is innervated by the anterior branch of the obturator nerve. The vascular supply is by way of the adductor branch of the profunda femoris artery and accompanying paired venae comitantes.

22. **What is the role of static procedures in the facial paralysis patient?**
Static procedures are commonly utlized to address asymmetry in the facial paralysis patient. They do not provide restoration of facial movement. Such procedures are frequently applied to the brow. Static sling procedures to suspend the midface, help recreate a melolabial fold, or address nasal obstruction due to valve collapse have also been utilized when dynamic procedures are not an option.

BIBLIOGRAPHY

Bergeron CM, Moe KS: The evaluation and treatment of lower eyelid paralysis, *Facial Plast Surg* 24:231–241, 2008.

Catalano PJ, Bergstein MJ, Biller HF: Comprehensive management of the eye in facial paralysis, *Arch Otolaryngol Head Neck Surg* 121(1):81–86, 1995.

Clark JM, Shockley WW: Management and reanimation of the paralyzed face. In Papel ID, Frodel J, Holt GR, et al, editors: *Facial Plastic and Reconstructive Surgery*, ed 2, New York, 2002, Thieme Medical Publishers.

House JW, Brackmann DE: Facial nerve grading system, *Otolaryngol Head Neck Surg* 93(2):146–147, 1985.

Meltzer NE, Alam DS: Facial paralysis rehabilitation: state of the art, *Curr Opin Otolaryngol Head Neck Surg* 18(4): 232–237, 2010.

SKIN GRAFTS AND LOCAL FLAPS

Adam M. Terella, MD

CHAPTER 65

KEY POINTS

1. Apply the concept of the "reconstructive ladder" when assessing the complexity of the reconstructive method required. The more problematic the wound, the more complex the reconstruction.
2. Cutaneous flaps are classified according to their blood supply, configuration, location, or method of transfer.
3. Orienting a skin excision, wound closure, or local flap parallel to relaxed skin tension lines (RSTLs) will serve to camouflage the resulting scar, limit closure tension, and result in an optimal aesthetic outcome.
4. When utilizing a skin graft, the reconstructive surgeon must consider the vascularity of the recipient site, and develop a strategy to optimize contact between graft and recipient bed.

Pearls

1. Utilization of a full-thickness skin graft, when possible, will limit graft contraction, and usually result in an improved texture and color match.
2. Avoiding injury to the dermal and subdermal plexus is critical to preserving the blood supply to random flaps.
3. Orient local flaps such that the final scar orientation and tension vector is away from distortable structures such as the lower eyelids.
4. In designing a rotational flap, the arc of rotation (flap length) should be approximately four times the diameter of the defect.

QUESTIONS

Skin Grafting

1. Describe the concept of the "reconstructive ladder."
   The goal of surgical management of a wound aims to obtain rapid wound closure utilizing the simplest method, while creating the best functional and cosmetic outcome. The "reconstructive ladder" concept helps the reconstructive surgeon assess the complexity of the treatment required, beginning with the simplest modality and progressing in difficulty from there (Box 65-1).

2. What are the three histologic layers of the skin?
   The skin is composed of the epidermis, the dermis, and the subcutaneous connective tissue. The epidermis is composed of keratinizing stratified squamous epithelium and is separated from the dermis by a basement membrane. The dermis is subdivided into a thin papillary dermis overlying a thicker reticular dermis.

3. What is a skin graft?
   A skin graft is an island of epidermis with varying thicknesses of dermis, which has been surgically removed from a donor site and transferred to a recipient site. The blood supply to the skin graft is dependent on the vascularity of the recipient site.

Box 65-1. The Reconstructive Ladder

Secondary intention/granulation
Primary closure
Split-thickness skin graft
Full-thickness skin graft
Local flaps
Regional flaps
Free flaps

4. **When should a skin graft be utilized?**
Skin grafts are best utilized to address wounds that cannot reasonably be reconstructed with primary closure or a local flap. Wound size or location may often prohibit primary closure or the use of local flaps. To obtain the best cosmetic outcome the graft should be harvested from a site closely matching the color and texture of the skin surrounding the wound.

5. **What two ways can be used for harvesting skin grafts?**
Skin grafts are harvested as full thickness or split thickness. Full-thickness skin grafts (FTSG) consist of epidermis and the full thickness of dermis. They are usually harvested deep to the dermis and within the superficial subcutaneous plane. Split-thickness skin grafts (STSG) consist of epidermis and a variable portion of underlying dermis. They are usually harvested utilizing a dermatome.

6. **What factors will most affect skin graft viability?**
Several factors directly influence skin graft viability. These include the vascularity of the recipient site, vascularity of donor graft tissue, contact between graft and recipient site, and certain systemic illness. Irradiated tissue, exposed bone or cartilage, infected tissue, or bleeding wounds, tend to be unfavorable for skin graft take.

7. **What are the phases of skin graft survival?**
Skin grafts initially survive by the diffusion of nutrition from serum at the recipient site through a process termed *plasma imbibition.* Between days three and seven, there is reestablishment of blood flow between preexisting graft capillaries and recipient end capillaries, in a phase termed *inosculation. Revascularization* begins at approximately day 4 and is characterized by the ingrowth of new vessels into the graft.

8. **What are the advantages and disadvantages of a full-thickness skin graft?**
Full-thickness grafts provide a better color match, better texture match, and will undergo less contraction than split-thickness grafts. The disadvantage is reduced survival rate and longer healing time.

9. **What are the advantages and disadvantages of a split-thickness skin graft?**
A split-thickness skin graft will have increased viability due to greater capillary exposure on the undersurface of the graft. This permits greater absorption of nutrients from the wound bed. Also, because STSGs contain less tissue, revascularization occurs more quickly. The main disadvantage is that STSGs often result in poor texture and color match.

10. **What are the important points for postoperative care of skin grafts?**
Skin graft dressings should aim to immobilize the graft on the recipient bed. Often this immobilization is accomplished with bolsters, made of Xeroform™ or petroleum gauze. The dressing should remain in place for 5 to 7 days to enable adequate graft adherence to take place and help prevent desiccation.

11. **How should a skin graft donor site be managed?**
Full-thickness donor sites are closed primarily, when possible. Split-thickness skin graft donor sites are best treated with an occlusive dressing. Studies have shown that a moist, clean, healing environment allows wounds to heal more quickly.

12. **What are the four main mechanisms by which skin grafts fail?**
The most common mechanisms of failure include: (1) inadequate wound bed vascularity, (2) shearing forces that separate the graft from the bed and prevent revascularization, (3) hematoma or seroma formation that prevents contact of the graft to the bed, and (4) infection.

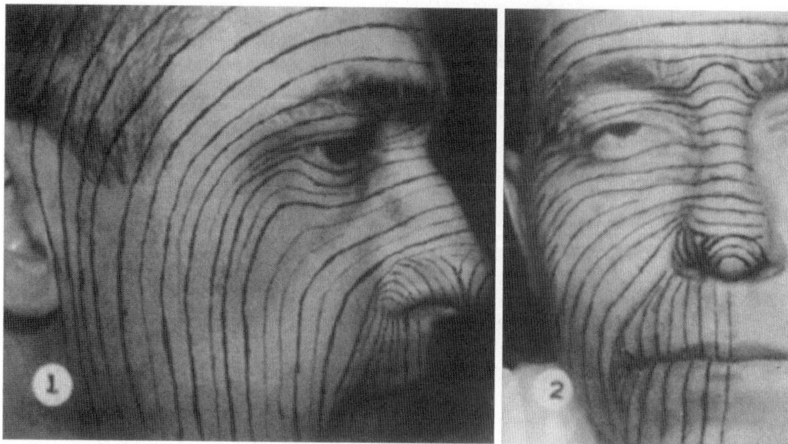

Figure 65-1. Lateral and frontal view of the face illustrating relaxed skin tension lines. *(From Borges AF, Alexander JE: Relaxed skin tension lines, Z-plasties on scars, and fusiform excision of lesions. Br J Plast Surg 15:242–254, 1962.)*

Local Flaps

13. What is a local cutaneous flap?
A local cutaneous flap is an area of skin and subcutaneous tissue with direct vascular supply that is transferred to a site located adjacent to or near the flap. By contrast, a graft does not carry its own blood supply.

14. What are relaxed skin tension lines, and why are they important?
Relaxed skin tension lines (RSTL) are lines intrinsic to aging skin. They manifest as creases and wrinkles orientated perpendicular to the underlying facial mimetic musculature (Figure 65-1). In planning skin excisions, wound closures, or local flaps, it is desirable to orient the resulting closure or scar parallel to RSTLs. Wounds oriented parallel to RSTLs will camouflage nicely, and have minimal wound closure tension, thus resulting in a less apparent scar.

15. How and why would a surgeon perform undermining?
Undermining the skin reduces wound closure tension by distributing skin deformation. During undermining, the skin and some portion of subcutaneous fat are released from the underlying fascia. The lysis and release of vertical attachments between the dermis and subcutaneous tissue allows the skin to slide more freely over the subcutaneous tissue.

16. What is the concept of facial aesthetic regions? Why is this concept important to the design of local flaps?
The face can be divided into specific "primary aesthetic regions," including the forehead, eyelids, cheeks, nose, lips, mentum, and auricles. Valleys, troughs, and creases represent the boundaries between facial aesthetic regions. It is preferable to design flaps within the same aesthetic region. Additionally, it is desirable to orient incisions, and thus scars, along the borders of aesthetic units because this will improve scar camouflage.

17. How are cutaneous flaps classified?
Cutaneous flaps are commonly classified according to their blood supply, configuration, location, or method of transfer. When characterizing by blood supply, local flaps can be based on a random or an axial pattern. Random flaps are based on the subdermal plexus and do not include a named blood vessel. An axial flap utilizes a dominant and named vessel for its primary vascularity.
The paramedian forehead flap, based on the supratrochlear artery, is a commonly utilized axial pattern flap.

18. How are local flaps classified by method of transfer?
Pivotal flaps and advancement flaps are commonly utilized local flaps. An advancement flap has a linear configuration, and is advanced into a defect (Figure 65-2A). Because they involve stretching

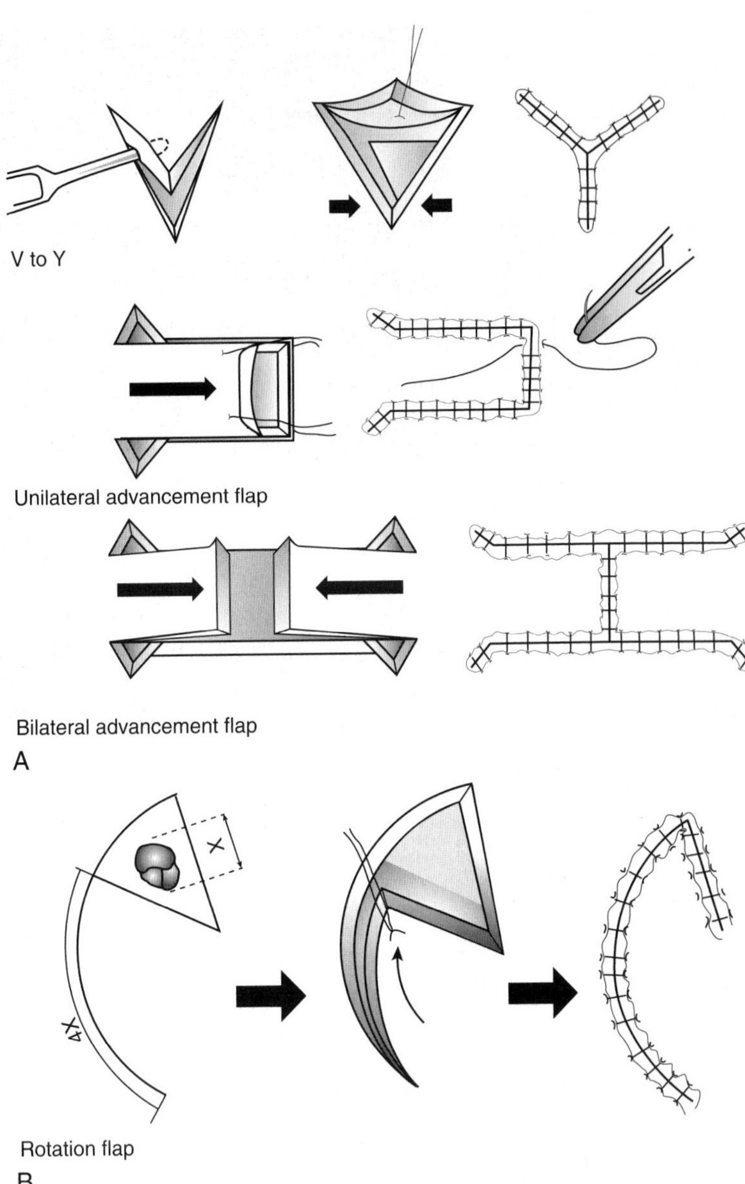

Figure 65-2. A, B. Schematic representation of local flaps. Illustrated are the unilateral advancement, bilateral advancement, and rotational flaps. The flap length should be approximately 4 times the diameter of the defect. *(From Patel KG, Sykes J: Concepts in local flap design and classification. Operative Techniques Otolaryngol 22:13–23, 2011.)*

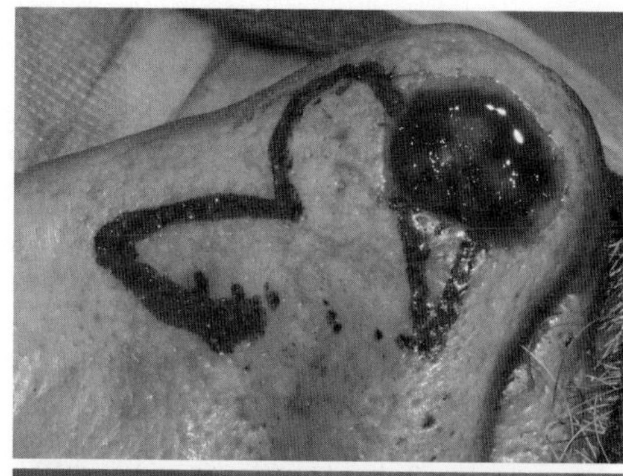

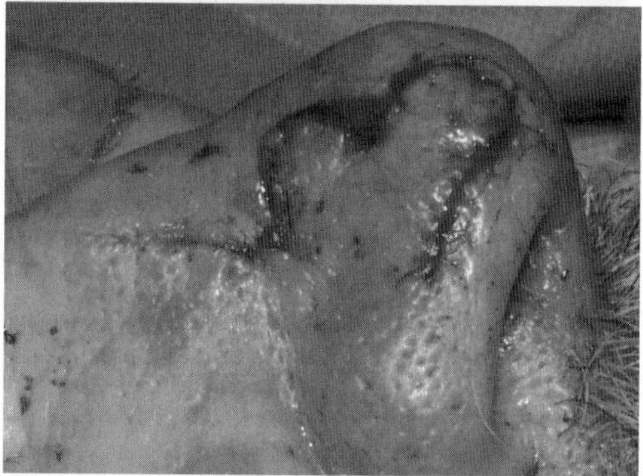

Figure 65-3. Bilobed transposition flap used to close a nasal defect.

the skin of the flap, they work best in areas of significant skin laxity. Pivotal flaps involve pivoting the tissue around a fixed point at the base of the pedicle (Figure 65-2B). Examples of pivotal flaps include rotation, transposition, and interpolated style flaps.

19. How does a transposition flap differ from an interpolated flap?
A transposition flap is rotated over a segment of normal skin to be placed at an adjacent recipient site. Two commonly utilized transposition flaps are the rhombic flap and the bilobed flap (Figure 65-3). By contrast, the base of an interpolated flap is not contiguous with the defect. This arrangement creates a pedicle that crosses over intervening tissue. A second-stage procedure is needed for division and inset of the pedicle. An example of an interpolated flap is the paramedian forehead flap.

20. Describe the concept of a V-Y advancement flap.
The V-Y flap achieves advancement of tissue into a defect. A V-shaped incision is made, and the secondary triangular donor defect is closed primarily. This primary closure serves to push the tissue into the defect. In closing the donor site primarily, the wound closure suture line assumes a Y configuration (see Figure 65-2A).

21. What three changes will a Z-plasty create in a scar contracture?
A Z-plasty (Figure 65-4) is designed with three limbs of equal length that form two triangular flaps. The two triangular flaps represent transposition flaps. The tips of the triangles represent angular flaps that are transposed with each other. This technique is useful to: (1) interrupt the scar linearity, (2) lengthen a scar contracture, and (3) change the orientation of a scar/contracture.

22. What is the theoretical increase in scar length created by a 45-45 degree Z-plasty? A 60-60 degree Z-plasty?
A 45-45 degree Z-plasty will lengthen a scar by 50%. A 60-60 degree Z-plasty will lengthen a scar by 75%.

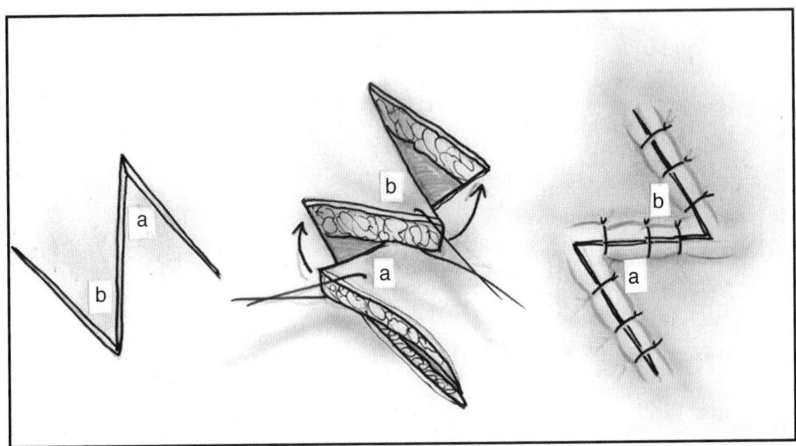

Figure 65-4. A vertical scar is depicted on the left; 60° Z-plasty flaps are designed (a and b). After transposition, the central limb is lengthened and redirected, and the final scar is broken into three limbs (right). *(From Frodel Jr JL: Creative uses of the Z-plasty technique. Operative Techniques Otolaryngol-Head Neck Surg 22(1):30–34, 2011.)*

Bibliography

Baker S: *Local Flaps in Facial Reconstruction*, ed 2, Philadelphia, 2007, Mosby.

Borges AF: Pitfalls in flap design, *Ann Plast Surg* 9(3):201–210, 1982. PubMed PMID: 7137816.

Greer SE: *Handbook of Plastic Surgery*, New York, 2006, Marcel Dekker.

Hudson DA: Some thoughts on choosing a Z-plasty: the Z made simple, *Plast Reconstr Surg* 106(3):665–671, 2000. Review. PubMed PMID: 10987477.

Kaplan B, Moy RL: Flaps and grafts for facial reconstruction, *Dermatol Surg* 21(5):431–440, 1995. PubMed PMID: 7743106.

Kilinç H, Sensöz O, Ozdemir R, et al: Which dressing for split-thickness skin graft donor sites?, *Ann Plast Surg* 46(4):409–414, 2001. PubMed PMID: 11324884.

Papel ID: *Facial Plastic and Reconstructive Surgery*, ed 2, New York, 2002, Thieme.

CHAPTER 66

REGIONAL AND FREE FLAPS

Justin M. Wudel, MD and Sarah J. Novis, MD

KEY POINTS

1. Always consider the tissue defect as well as patient comorbidities, nutritional status, tobacco and alcohol use, and functional status when deciding between reconstruction with regional flaps and microvascular free tissue transfer.
2. Reconstruction should be performed with tissue that most closely replicates the appearance and function of the resected tissue.
3. Microvascular free flaps require close monitoring and clinical inspection to evaluate for flap viability, especially in the first 48 hours when the vascular supply is most prone to thrombosis.
4. Advantages of free flaps
   - Can customize the reconstruction to optimize functional and aesthetic outcomes
   - Not tethered by regional flap pedicle
5. Advantages of regional pedicled flaps
   - Shorter operating time
   - Do not require microsurgical training or second team

Pearls

1. Delayed harvest of flaps creates improved pressure gradient and viability of the distal angiosomes of the flap.
2. In addition to routine preoperative labs, patients undergoing microvascular free tissue transfer may require further vascular studies in the form of angiography and Doppler studies.

QUESTIONS

1. **What is the difference between a regional flap and microvascular free tissue transfer?**
   Regional flaps are based on a main blood vessel known as the pedicle, which nourishes the muscle and skin in the distribution of the flap. Regional flaps are elevated and rotated into place with care to preserve attachment to the pedicle and integrity of this vessel. Microvascular free flaps are also based on tissues supplied by a single vascular pedicle known as the donor vessels, which are usually a single artery and vein. The donor vessels are ligated at the donor site and the entire flap is transferred to the recipient site where the donor vessels are anastomosed to recipient vessels in the face or neck using a microvascular technique to restore blood flow.

2. **What patient considerations are important when deciding between regional and microvascular reconstruction options?**
   Previous radiation treatment causes fibrosis of tissues with decreased blood flow and poor healing, and thus necessitates reconstruction with well-vascularized tissue. Free tissue reconstruction requires longer operative times and may not be ideal for ill patients with multiple medical comorbidities who cannot tolerate a long general anesthetic. It is also important to consider a patient's comorbidities including vascular, cardiac, renal, and pulmonary issues. A patient's nutritional status and dependence on tobacco and alcohol need to be investigated. These factors can greatly affect a patient's recovery and surgical outcome.

3. **How is the angiosome concept important to flap design?**
   An angiosome is the tissue volume supplied by a single source artery and vein. Arteries that connect neighboring angiosomes are known as "choke" vessels. Two or more neighboring angiosomes can

be harvested together on one pedicle by interrupting subsequent pedicles and relying on choke vessels to perfuse the distal angiosomes. More angiosomes connected in a series results in a decreased pressure gradient across the flap and raises the likelihood of distal necrosis.

4. **What is delayed elevation of a flap and how does it work to improve flap viability?**
Delayed harvest of a flap involves elevation of the distal portion of the flap from its underlying vasculature and replacing it into the defect to be utilized later. This allows for dilation of the choke vessels between angiosomes and creates a more favorable pressure gradient for viability of distal angiosomes when the flap is transferred to its recipient site a few weeks later.

5. **What is the difference between fasciocutaneous, myocutaneous, and osteocutaneous flaps?**
Fasciocutaneous flaps include the skin and underlying superficial fascia and are based on a pedicled vessel perfusing one or more angiosomes. Myocutaneous flaps include muscle and are also based on a singular arterovenous system (pedicle) perfusing the muscle and are harvested with a cutaneous portion. A small branch of the vascular pedicle, which perforates the muscle and travels to the skin to supply an angiosome, perfuses the cutaneous portion of the flap. Given the less robust blood supply to the skin portion of the flap, necrosis of the skin flap can occur while the underlying muscle flap remains well perfused. Osteocutaneous flaps are composite flaps that include bone, skin, and sometimes muscle or tendon, which are based on a singular arteriovenous system.

6. **What are the common regional pedicled flaps used in head and neck reconstruction?**
(Table 66-1)

7. **What flap considerations are important in selecting which microvascular reconstruction option to use?**
It is important to consider the surgical defect carefully. Reconstruction should be performed with tissue that replicates the appearance and function of resected tissue, using epithelium for mucosal and skin defects, muscle for bulk, and bone for skeletal reconstruction. The length of the pedicle must be considered as well as the donor vasculature available for anastomosis.

8. **What are the vascular pedicles of common free flaps used in head and neck reconstruction?**
(Table 66-2)

9. **What is the Allen test, how is it performed, and why is it important in the preoperative evaluation of a candidate for a radial forearm free flap?**
The most feared complication of a radial forearm free flap is ischemia of the hand. This complication could result if a patient has both an incomplete superficial palmar arch and a lack of communicating vessels between the deep and superficial arch. This test is used prior to procedures that will compromise the radial artery and assesses the adequacy of ulnar collateral circulation of the hand. The Allen test is performed by having the patient clench his or her fist followed by the examiner digitally occluding the radial and ulnar arteries at the wrist. The patient opens the hand to approximately 10 degrees of flexion. The examiner releases the ulnar artery and capillary refill in the thumb and index finger is assessed. If the results are equivocal or show inadequate ulnar collateral flow, the opposite arm or an alternate flap is used.

10. **How is the donor site of a radial forearm free flap closed?**
The cutaneous defect of the forearm requires coverage with a skin graft to provide coverage of the flexor tendons. This is usually performed with a split-thickness skin graft from the thigh. It is important to preserve the paratenon over the flexor tendons so that the skin graft will survive. The hand and forearm are immobilized postoperatively, as movement can lead to shearing forces and graft failure.

11. **What is the normal "three vessel" blood flow to the foot and why is this important in patients being considered for fibular free flap?**
The popliteal artery provides branches into the anterior tibial artery, posterior tibial artery, and the peroneal artery. Harvest of the peroneal artery with a fibular free flap can lead to ischemia of the

Table 66-1. Common Regional Flaps in Head and Neck Reconstruction

	TYPE	VASCULAR PEDICLE	PROPERTIES AND USES	DISADVANTAGES
Pectoralis major	Myocutaneous	Thoracoacromial artery	• Easy to raise and requires a single-stage procedure • Provides coverage of the carotid after ipsilateral radical neck dissection, numerous head and neck applications	• Excess bulk from adipose tissue between the skin and muscle • Shearing of skin paddle and muscle may lead to damage to perforating vessels an skin paddle loss
Deltopectoral	Fasciocutaneous	Internal mammary artery, perforating branches (2nd and 3rd)	• Used for constructing external cutaneous defects of the neck	• Requires skin graft to close donor site • Distal portions of the flap are unreliable when extended over deltoid
Latissimus	Myocutaneous	Thoracodorsal artery	• Used for cutaneous defects of the neck and scalp	• Patient must be positioned in semidecubitus position during surgery
Trapezius	Myocutaneous	Transverse cervical artery	• Used to resurface cutaneous defects of the posterior and lateral neck	• Short arc of rotation and variable vascular anatomy • Need for lateral decubitus positioning
Supraclavicular	Fasciocutaneous	Supraclavicular artery	• Good color match for facial defects • Used for cutaneous defects of the neck, temporal area, and face.	• Risk of dehiscence and partial flap loss
Temporoparietal fascia (TPF)	Fascia	Superficial temporal artery	• Very thin, durable, and highly vascular • Used in facial and skull base defects	• Risk of damage to the frontal branch of facial nerve and alopecia due to hair follicle damage
Sternocleidomastoid	Myocutaneous	• Occipital (superior third) • Superior thyroid (middle third) • Transverse cervical (inferior third) • 2 of 3 vessels need to be preserved	• Can be pedicled superiorly or inferiorly • Used for oral and pharyngeal defects and cutaneous defects of the neck and face	• Often has poor viability of the skin flap due to variable vessel anatomy • Donor site contour abnormality

Table 66-2. Common Microvascular Free Flaps

	TYPE	VASCULAR PEDICLE	PROPERTIES AND USES	DISADVANTAGES
Radial forearm	Fasciocutaneous or osteocutaneous	Radial artery, venae comitantes or cephalic vein	• Thin and pliable with a long pedicle • Versatile, with numerous uses including oral cavity, tongue, palate, face, pharynx and larynx	• Need for skin graft at the donor site • Risk of vascular compromise to the hand
Anterolateral thigh	Myocutaneous or septocutaneous	Lateral circumflex femoral artery, descending branch, and venae comitantes	• Pliable with a long pedicle • Large surface area • Versatile	• Variable pedicle makes flap volume unpredictable
Rectus abdominis	Myocutaneous or muscle	Deep inferior epigastric artery and vein	• Bulky and good for large volume reconstructions • Used for glossectomy and skull base defects	• Risk of abdominal hernia at the donor site
Fibula	Osteocutaneous	Peroneal artery and vein	• Provides a long segment of bone • Ideal for mandible reconstruction	• Risk of ankle pain and instability • Risk of vascular compromise to the foot
Scapular/ Parascapsular	Fasciocutaneous or osteocutaneous	Circumflex scapular artery and vein	• Ability to include muscle, skin, and bone gives flexibility for 3D reconstruction • Used for closing complex midface and oromandibular defects	• Lateral decubitus positioning during surgery puts patient at risk of brachial plexus injury • Risk of shoulder weakness if musculature not reapproximated
Lateral arm	Fasciocutaneous	Profunda brachii artery and its venae comitantes	• Thickness depends on patient BMI • Used for oropharyngeal and low volume facial defects	• Has a small caliber pedicle • Radial nerve palsy can occur with tight wound closures
Latissimus	Myocutaneous or muscle	Thoracodorsal artery and vein	Used for skull base and scalp defects	• Patient must be positioned in semidecubitus position during surgery
Jejunum	Enteral	Branches of the superior mesenteric artery and vein	Used for circumferential pharyngoesophageal defects	• Peristalsis affects swallowing • Production of succus entericus causes dysgeusia and affects voice rehabilitation

foot if there is inadequate collateral circulation. Preoperative evaluation is critical to ensure adequate blood supply, especially in patients with peripheral vascular disease, heart disease, and history of tobacco use. Commonly used studies include magnetic resonance angiography, standard angiography, or ankle-brachial index screening, and Doppler studies.

12. **How does the abdominal wall anatomy above and below the arcuate line affect closure of a rectus abdominis donor site?**
Above the arcuate line the posterior sheath is composed of contributions from the transversus abdominis and internal oblique muscle and closure of just the posterior sheath is necessary, though the anterior sheath is often also closed for additional strength. Below the arcuate line, the posterior sheath is comprised of only transversalis fascia, which is inadequate to prevent an abdominal hernia in itself. Both anterior and posterior abdominal sheaths must be closed below the arcuate line.

13. **When would a microvascular free tissue latissimus dorsi flap be used as compared to a pedicled regional latissimus dorsi flap?**
The latissimus dorsi flap can be used as either a pedicled or free flap depending on the location and availability of vessels for anastomosis. In a radical neck dissection, when there are few vessels available for microvascular anastomosis, a pedicled flap would be preferred. In scalp and skull base defects, a free tissue transfer is often preferred as it gives more flexibility in flap positioning and allows for placement over more superior defects, such as the vertex scalp, which is difficult with a pedicled flap.

14. **How are microvascular free tissue flaps monitored?**
It is essential to closely monitor free tissue flaps for signs of arterial and venous compromise, as these can quickly lead to loss of the flap and require emergent surgical exploration. Clinical examination is the gold standard for monitoring free tissue flaps. The tissue should be examined for color, temperature, and capillary refill. A Doppler probe is used to monitor arterial and venous blood flow through the vascular pedicle. Some surgeons place an implantable Doppler intraoperatively for monitoring. A pinprick can also be used to assess the color of the blood and how quickly it bleeds. Rapid bleeding of dark blood suggests venous congestion. Lack of bleeding or slow bleeding may indicate arterial compromise.

15. **What are the signs of a failing flap?**
    - Venous Congestion
        - Bluish discoloration
        - Increased warmth and swelling
        - Bounding Doppler
        - Rapid bleeding of dark blood on pinprick
    - Arterial Compromise
        - Pale discoloration
        - Cool temperature
        - Weak or absent Doppler
        - Slow or no bleeding on pinprick

16. **What is the most common cause of microvascular free flap failure?**
Studies have shown that venous thrombus alone is more common than either arterial or combined arterial and venous thrombosis. Thrombosis typically occurs in the first two days in 80% of patients. When recognized early and managed promptly (<6 hrs) the salvage success rate is 75%. Thus, good monitoring and evaluation of these flaps is critical to their success.

17. **How are leeches used in the salvage of compromised microvascular flaps?**
When flap failure occurs, usually due to venous outflow obstruction, and the flap is not otherwise surgically salvageable, leeches may be used as an alternative method to establish venous outflow until inosculation occurs. The effectiveness of leech therapy is due to both the action of the leech extracting congested blood from the flap and coagulation inhibitors in the saliva of the leeches (including hirudin, a factor Xa inhibitor). Patients require close hemodynamic monitoring, frequent hemoglobin evaluations, and often transfusions during leech therapy. Leeches are also colonized with *Aeromonas hydrophilia* and patients require prophylactic antibiotic coverage during and after leech therapy.

CONTROVERSIES

18. **How long can a flap survive ischemia?**
    All flaps undergo a period of primary ischemia during excision at the donor site until blood flow is reestablished at the recipient site. Most flaps can tolerate up to 4 hours of ischemia (enteric flaps can tolerate only a maximum of 2 hours). Once a flap has reached its ischemic limit, reperfusion will result in the "no flow" phenomenon where arterovenous shunting prevents perfusion of the flap despite blood flowing through the pedicle. Reperfusion after a period of ischemia can cause "reperfusion injury" due to activation of neutrophils and release of oxygen free radicals.

19. **Should patients with microvascular free flaps be placed on anticoagulation?**
    Flap failures can result from microvascular thrombosis and it has been suggested that anticoagulation may lead to decreased failure rate. This question has been difficult to study as it would require a large number of flap failures, which are overall uncommon. Existing studies have suggested no significant difference in outcomes or complications between the use of aspirin, heparin, and no anticoagulation.

20. **What is the cost associated with reconstructing head and neck defects with microvascular free flaps versus regional flaps?**
    Longer operative time, increased length of hospital stay, increased use of monitoring in the ICU, and increased use of drugs result in a higher cost of free flaps when compared to pedicled flaps. However, some justify the increase costs of free tissue transfer because of the perceived benefit of improved long-term functional and aesthetic outcomes.

Bibliography

Carroll WR, Esclamado RM: Ischemia/reperfusion injury in microvascular surgery, *Head Neck* 22:700–713, 2000.

Chepeha DB, Nussenbaum B, Bradford CR, et al: Leech therapy for patients with surgically unsalvageable venous obstruction after revascularized free tissue transfer, *Arch Otolaryngol Head Neck Surg* 128:960–965, 2002.

Chepeha DB, Teknos TN: Microvascular free flaps in head and neck reconstruction. In Bailey BJ, Johnson JT, Newlands SD, editors: *Bailey's Head and Neck Surgery: Otolaryngology*, ed 4, Philadelphia, 2006, Lippincott Williams & Wilkins.

Chien W, Varvares MA, Hadlock T, et al: Effects of aspirin and low-dose heparin in head and neck reconstruction using microvascular free flaps, *Laryngoscope* 115:973–976, 2005.

Lighthall JG, Cain R, Ghanem TA, et al: Effect of postoperative aspirin on microvascular free tissue transfer surgery, *Otolaryngol Head Neck Surg* 148(1):40–46, 2013.

McCory AL, Magnuson JS: Free tissue transfer versus pedicled flap in head and neck reconstruction, *Laryngoscope* 112:2161–2165, 2002.

Pertruzzelli GJ, Brockenbrough JM, Vandevender D, et al: The influence of reconstructive modality on cost of care in head and neck oncology, *Arch Otolaryngol Head Neck Surg* 128(12):1377–1380, 2002.

Shestak KC, Myers EN, Ramasastry SS, et al: Microvascular free tissue transfer for reconstruction of head and neck cancer defects, *Oncology (Williston Park)* 6:101–110, discussion 10, 15–16, 21, 1992.

Taylor GI, Palmer JH: The vascular territories (angiosomes) of the body: experimental study and clinical applications, *Br J Plast Surg* 40:113–141, 1987.

Urken M, Cheney M, Blackwell K: *Atlas of Regional and Free Flaps for Head and Neck Reconstruction: Flap Harvest and Insetting*, ed 2, Baltimore, 2011, Lippincott Williams & Wilkins.

PRINCIPLES OF TRAUMA

Paul Montero, MD and Erik Peltz, DO

CHAPTER 67

QUESTIONS

Initial Evaluation of the Trauma Patient

1. Describe the primary assessment of the trauma patient (ABCs).
   - **Airway:** Assess the patient's airway by observation and listening. If the patient is talking, airway and breathing are essentially sufficient. Assess for bleeding, loose teeth, inhalation injury (in case of burn), and level of consciousness. Decreased level of consciousness (GCS 8 or less) is an indication of potential inability to protect the airway and need for elective intubation. Orotracheal intubation with in-line cervical stabilization is the method of choice; however, orofacial trauma or a difficult airway may require a surgical airway (see Chapter 77). In the setting of blunt or penetrating tracheal injury, intubation should ideally be performed in the OR. This is done with adequate equipment for a surgical airway open and readily available and with the neck prepped and draped prior to intubation attempts. Manipulation of the traumatically injured airway during intubation attempts may lead to critical decompensation, which requires immediate, emergent surgical airway.
   - **Breathing:** Assess by looking, listening, and feeling. Look for equal chest rise bilaterally. Auscultation can be difficult in the trauma bay but should be performed to evaluate for absence of breath sounds suggesting pneumothorax or hemothorax. Palpate for crepitus of the chest wall suggesting rib fracture with potential underlying pneumothorax. Evaluate for "flail chest"—three or more ribs with fractures in two or more locations. Paradoxical respiration of this segment and impaired pulmonary mechanics can lead to both life-threatening hypoxia and hypercapnia. Additionally, this substantial injury mechanism is often associated with refractory, life-threatening hypoxia even with mechanical ventilator support.
   - **Circulation:** Assess circulation with frequent vital sign assessments, pulse exam (all extremities), skin color/capillary refill, and mentation. Circulatory assessment may be challenging in the extremes of age, with concomitant heart disease, in athletes and pregnant women, and with medications, hypothermia, and pacemakers.
   - **Disability:** A brief neurologic exam and assessment based on the Glasgow Coma Scale is essential, particularly if the patient requires therapeutic paralysis for intubation (recognize if patient is moving extremities and document facial nerve function prior to administering paralytic agents).
   - **Exposure/Environmental Control:** Perform a full physical examination for injury, especially in the nonalert patient, while minimizing hypothermia.

2. What is an AMPLE history?
   An AMPLE history involves the key elements that can rapidly be obtained by the patient or patient's friends or family when the patient has a limited ability to provide medical history. It consists of: **A**llergies, **M**edications, **P**ast Medical History, **L**ast PO Intake, and the **E**vents leading to the trauma.

3. What are the methods of verifying a secure airway after intubation or surgical airway procedure?
   A secured airway must always be verified, including patients who are intubated in the field. The intubation itself should involve direct visualization of the vocal cords. Observation of equal chest rise/fall should occur. Auscultate for bilateral breath sounds, with consideration of the possibility of right main stem intubation. Capnography should be rapidly used to assess proper position; a small plastic insert is placed onto the endotracheal tube and is assessed over the duration of several breaths. Return of carbon dioxide confirms endotracheal positioning, and is indicated by a color change from purple to yellow on the capnography insert. Persistent purple coloration indicates no

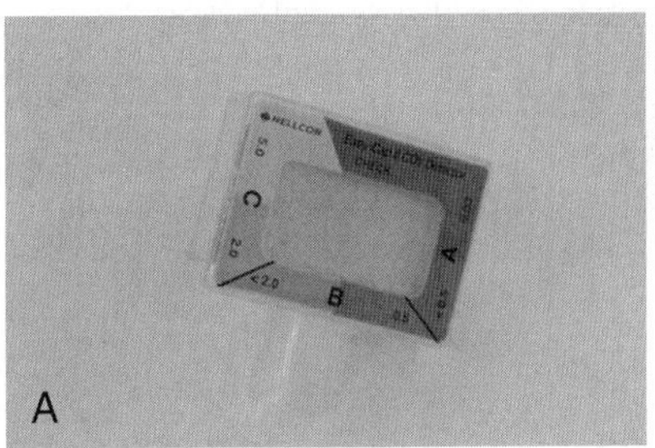

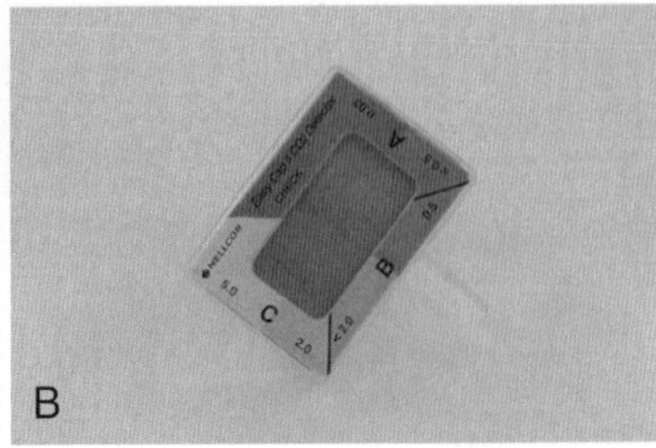

Figure 67-1. A, Capnograph has turned yellow, indicating return of CO_2. This device attaches to an endotracheal tube and changes color from purple to yellow with CO_2 return. **B.** Capnograph remains purple, indicating no return of CO_2.

CO_2 return (Yellow = mellow, Purple = problem) (Figure 67-1). A chest radiograph can demonstrate the position of the endotracheal tube above the carina, but does not necessarily rule out the possibility of esophageal intubation. Bronchoscopic confirmation of endotracheal tube placement is generally not feasible in the trauma bay setting.

4. **What are the indications for chest tube placement?**
   A patient with hypotension and decreased breath sounds in the trauma bay should be presumed to have a tension pneumothorax. Decompression should be immediately performed. Needle decompression can rapidly be performed with a 14-gauge needle catheter in the midclavicular second intercostal space just above the rib. Rapid decompression can also be performed with an incision in the anterior axillary fifth intercostal space (generally the level of the nipple). Entry into the pleural space will decompress the tension pneumothorax; the chest tube can then be placed through this incision (immediate intervention involves the incision; do not wait for a chest tube to be ready if tension pneumothorax is suspected). A chest tube is also placed when hemothorax is suspected by exam or imaging. The initial chest tube output will dictate further management; greater than 1500 cc of blood is an indication for exploratory thoracotomy. Follow-up chest radiograph should occur after chest tube placement. Open chest wounds ("sucking chest wounds") occur where the pleural space/pulmonary circuit directly communicates with the external environment. Large tidal volumes are lost through this open pulmonary wound. Initial management can include "three-sided" occlusive dressing. However, optimal initial management would include chest tube placement on that side of the thorax with a three-sided occlusive dressing to allow decompression and prevent tension pneumothorax.

5. **What are the five locations of blood loss in a trauma patient?**
   - Scalp/Street: The scalp and face are highly vascularized areas and scalp bleeding should promptly be addressed with pressure, sutures, clips, or staples in the significantly injured patient. The prehospital care should include a rapid report that describes any significant blood loss at the scene of the trauma or en route.
   - Chest: Rib fractures (up to 100 ml each), lung laceration, or injury to the great vessels or heart can result in significant thoracic hemorrhage and should be assessed for by examination (observation, palpation, auscultation) and imaging (radiograph, ultrasound, computed tomography).
   - Abdomen: Solid organ or mesenteric injury may result in hemoperitoneum and should be assessed for by examination (observation, palpation) and imaging (ultrasound, CT).
   - Pelvis/retroperitoneum: Bleeding here may occur from pelvic fractures, vascular injury, or solid organ injury (kidney, pancreas) and can be assessed for by examination, pelvis radiograph, and CT.
   - Bones: Blood loss from a pelvic fracture can be as much as 2000 ml, femur fracture 1000 ml, tibia 250 to 500 ml, and rib fracture 100 ml each. Evaluate by physical examination and imaging (radiographs) when injury is suspected.

6. **Define shock.**
   Shock simply means inadequate tissue perfusion. In trauma, the most common cause is *hemorrhagic* shock, which requires immediate hemorrhage control and resuscitation with blood

Table 67-1. Classes of Hemorrhagic Shock

	CLASS I	CLASS II	CLASS III	CLASS IV
Blood Loss (ml)	<750	750–1500	1500–2000	>2000
Blood Loss (%)	<15	15–30	30–40	>40%
Heart Rate	Normal	↑	↑↑	↑↑↑
Blood Pressure	Normal	Normal	↓	↓↓
Respiratory Rate	Normal	↑	↑↑	↑↑↑

Note that HR and RR are the first to change, rather than drop in BP.

products and/or intravenous fluids. Shock may also result from spinal cord injury (spinal shock or neurogenic shock). Cardiogenic shock may occur from tension physiology such as tension pneumothorax or cardiac tamponade. Cardiogenic shock from direct myocardial injury is less common in the trauma setting but should be considered for patients with a history of heart disease (i.e., syncopal episode leading to motor vehicle collision) or significant anterior chest wall trauma or sternal fractures. Septic shock should be considered for patients with a significantly delayed presentation such as extremely prolonged extrication or time-consuming transfer from remote locations.

7. **What are the classes of hemorrhagic shock?**
   See Table 67-1. Patients may display normal vital signs despite significant blood loss, as depicted in Table 67-1, warranting thorough evaluation for all trauma patients.

8. **What are the key elements of the neurologic evaluation of a trauma patient?**
   Traumatic brain injury is very common in the blunt trauma patient. The Glascow Coma Scale is used to rapidly evaluate eye (4 points), verbal (5 points), and motor responses (6 points). A score ranges from 3 (worst) to 15 (normal) and is used to help classify brain injury (13–15 = minor, 9–12 = moderate, 3–8 = severe). At a minimum, the patient should also be assessed for movement in all four extremities. Stable patients should have motor and sensory evaluation of extremities during the secondary survey. Based on identified injuries, further neurologic assessment may be warranted (spine injury, extremity fracture). Imaging (CT brain) in stable patients or immediate intervention with intracranial pressure monitoring by neurosurgery (patients unstable for imaging evaluation) should be considered for all altered trauma patients.

9. **How are spinal cord injuries assessed?**
   All patients suspected of having spinal cord injury should be properly immobilized. A neurologic exam assesses extremity movement, strength, sensation, and reflexes. A rectal exam is performed to evaluate for tone. Palpation of the entire spinal column for step-offs or tenderness is performed. In the absence of abnormalities on exam, distracting injuries, or intoxication, a gentle assessment of range of motion is then performed. Imaging is warranted for continued suspicion and may include cervical spine radiographs (lateral, anterior-posterior, and odontoid views, including C7 and T1 vertebrae) or computed tomography of the cervical spine (T, L-spine dependent on injury mechanism and exam findings). Magnetic resonance imaging is useful for neurologic deficits not explained by CT imaging, and may also be useful for clearing the cervical spine in an obtunded patient who otherwise may suffer from skin breakdown resulting from prolonged preemptive collar placement. MRI is most useful to exclude cervical spine ligamentous injury in the first 24 hours following trauma prior to nonspecific edema development, which MRI can later identify as a false positive.

Initial Management of the Trauma Patient

10. **What are the vascular access options for a trauma patient?**
    An ideal vascular access for the trauma patient is a large-bore peripheral intravenous catheter (14 or 16 gauge). This short length, large-diameter catheter can allow rapid infusion of blood or fluid, but may be difficult to place in an acute setting. Additional options in order of ease of placement and rate of fluid delivery possible include: intraosseus access in the tibia/sternum, saphenous vein cutdown with large-bore peripheral IV placement, or central venous access (femoral, subclavian, or jugular vein).

11. **When is blood transfusion indicated in a trauma patient?**
A trauma patient who displays hemodynamic instability (HR >100, SBP <90) despite a fluid challenge (2 L crystalloid) and is suspected to have ongoing hemorrhage should receive uncrossed, O-negative packed red blood cells while patient specific type and crossmatch are performed.

12. **What is the "Bloody Vicious Cycle"?**
Coagulopathy, acidosis, and hypothermia all contribute to each other, resulting in ongoing bleeding that cannot be controlled surgically and is uniformly fatal if not reversed. Aggressive patient and fluid warming and correction of coagulopathy with blood product resuscitation is warranted and may necessitate quick, basic surgery ("damage control surgery" to halt surgical hemorrhage and prevent ongoing contamination) to allow for more optimal resuscitation including correction of temperature, acidosis, and coagulopathy to continue in the intensive care unit setting.

13. **What is a massive transfusion protocol?**
Massive transfusion protocols are designed to facilitate transfusion of an appropriate ratio of blood products including packed red cells, fresh frozen plasma, platelets, and cryoprecipitate. Such protocols facilitate rapid preparation from the blood bank and help ensure appropriate ratios of product are given.

Imaging of the Trauma Patient

14. **What are the key aspects of the chest radiograph for the trauma patient?**
The chest radiograph in a trauma patient allows for rapid assessment for airway deviation, subcutaneous emphysema, pneumothorax, hemothorax, rib fractures, or mediastinal widening that may be indicative of great vessel injury. It can also assess the positioning of an endotracheal tube, central venous catheter or nasogastric tube.

15. **What is the FAST?**
Focused Abdominal Sonography for Trauma (FAST) is a rapid bedside test that assesses for fluid (presumed to be blood in setting of trauma) in various spaces. When performed and repeated during evaluation, it is a sensitive indicator of abdominal bleeding. Prior surgery (adhesions), ascites, body habitus, and user error are pitfalls. It entails four views:
    1. Pericardial view assesses for cardiac activity and blood in pericardial space
    2. Spleno-renal view assesses for blood loss in left upper quadrant
    3. Morrison's pouch is the most dependent portion of the abdomen, right upper quadrant
    4. Pelvis view assesses for blood in perivesicular space/pelvis/lower abdomen

16. **When is CT angiography of the neck performed?**
CT angiography of the neck is used to evaluate for blunt carotid or vertebral artery injury and is obtained when suggestive signs, symptoms, or head and neck radiographic findings are present. CT angiography of the neck is indicated for patients with injuries including: cervical seat-belt sign, blunt anterior neck trauma, displaced midface fracture, basilar skull fractures involving the carotid canal, diffuse axonal injury, near hanging injury with anoxia, cervical vertebral body or transverse foramen fracture, any cervical spine fracture involving C1 to C3, any ligamentous injury to the cervical spine, or a bruit in a young patient (<50). Mechanisms for high energy transfer across the cervical spine including facial fractures with associated upper thoracic or clavicle fracture or patients with scapular fractures should be considered for CTA of the neck. Any neck injury resulting from direct force that causes significant swelling, pain, or altered mental status should also be evaluated with CT angiography of the neck. Hard signs concerning for vascular injury (pulsatile bleeding, expanding neck hematoma, penetrating trauma through the platysma) in surgically accessible zones of the neck should be operatively explored. Inaccessible injuries in Zone I/Zone III of the neck in the stable patient may necessitate CTA imaging.

Special Considerations in Trauma

17. **What are the key aspects of evaluation of a burn patient?**
The burn patient should be rapidly assessed for associated inhalation injury with a low threshold for airway stabilization (intubation) if suspected. Aggressive fluid resuscitation is vital and should be protocol driven with the Parkland formula or other similar protocols. Urine output monitoring is a good adjunctive resuscitative endpoint. The total body surface area burned should be evaluated. Circumferential burns may require escharotomy to prevent ischemia (extremity) or hypoventilation (chest).

18. What are the indications for referral of a burn patient to a specialty burn center?

1. Partial thickness burns greater than 10% total body surface area (TBSA)
2. Burns that involve the face, hands, feet, genitalia, perineum, or major joints
3. Third-degree burns in any age group
4. Electrical burns, including lightning injury
5. Chemical burns
6. Inhalation injury
7. Burn injury in patients with preexisting medical disorders that could complicate management, prolong recovery, or affect mortality
8. Any patients with burns and concomitant trauma (such as fractures) in which the burn injury poses the greatest risk of morbidity or mortality. In such cases, if the trauma poses the greater immediate risk, the patient may be initially stabilized in a trauma center before being transferred to a burn unit. Physician judgment will be necessary in such situations and should be in concert with the regional medical control plan and triage protocols.
9. Burned children in hospitals without qualified personnel or equipment for the care of children
10. Burn injury in patients who will require special social, emotional, or long-term rehabilitative intervention

19. What are the basic elements of triage for a mass casualty event?

Patients involved in a mass casualty should be rapidly assessed for degree of injury. The ability to walk, airway compromise, respiratory rate, and pulse or capillary refill are signs used in the field to assess severity of injury. Patients with serious but survivable injuries are transported/addressed first; the "walking wounded" require less acute attention, and the patient in extremis should not direct limited resources, attention, or time in the setting of a mass casualty event. Life-saving maneuvers such as decompression of a tension pneumothorax or direct pressure or tourniquet application of hemorrhage are carried out in the field.

20. Describe the evaluation of an extremity injury.

Assess for pulses, sensation, function, and range of motion. Pulse exam should be accompanied by measuring the Ankle-Brachial Index using a Doppler device. Comparison to the uninjured side is made (A:A gradient). A difference of 10% or more warrants further investigation, such as CT angiogram or arteriogram, which can be done intraoperatively. In the acute setting, significant hemorrhage should be controlled with direct pressure or application of a tourniquet. In a complex extremity trauma, a mangled extremity severity score (MESS) can be calculated and is useful for predicting limb viability. This score incorporates the patient's age, degree of shock, perfusion status, and length of time sustaining ischemia.

21. What considerations are reviewed when "clearing" a polytrauma patient for elective or semi-elective procedures?

Prior to nonurgent procedures, the multisystem trauma patient should be hemodynamically stable and fully resuscitated (as evidenced by normalized lactate or base deficit). Life-threatening injuries should be stabilized. Injuries undergoing observation must be considered as well (such as a splenic laceration, which may bleed with BP lability, or an observed pneumothorax, which can blossom under positive pressure ventilation). Patient position should be considered (unstable fractures are fixated; patient can tolerate supine positioning, such as with severe head injury with increased intracranial pressure). Coagulopathy must be reversed or controlled (some injuries require anticoagulation).

Bibliography

American College of Surgeons: *Advanced Trauma Life Support*, ed 7, Chicago, 2004, American College of Surgeons.

Biffl WL, Cothren CC, Moore EE, et al: Western Trauma Association critical decisions in trauma: screening for and treatment of blunt cerebrovascular injuries, *J Trauma* 67(6):1150–1153, 2009.

Brunicardi F, Andersen D, Billiar T, et al: *Schwartz's Principles of Surgery*, ed 9, New York, 2010, McGraw Hill.

Feliciano D, Moore E, Mattox K: *Trauma*, ed 6, New York, 2008, McGraw Hill.

CHAPTER 68

FACIAL TRAUMA

Vincent Eusterman, MD, DDS

KEY POINTS

1. Panfacial fractures require a comprehensive timing and treatment plan for each fracture.
2. Muscle pull can affect a fracture and must be considered to prevent complications.
3. Failure to diagnose and repair a medial canthal tendon injury can lead to functional and cosmetic complications that are difficult to repair secondarily.
4. The quickest way to decompress the eye is by lateral canthotomy with inferior cantholysis.
5. Nasal fractures are best treated by closed reduction immediately following the fracture or after swelling has subsided in 5 to 10 days.

Pearls

1. The edentulous mandible has no cross-sectional stability and is too weak to "load share" the fracture site with a small bone plate and requires a load-bearing reconstruction.
2. An early clinical finding of optic nerve injury in the traumatized eye is loss of red color vision.
3. All Le Fort fractures traverse the pterygomaxillary fissure, interrupting the pterygoid plates and resulting in a mobile palate.
4. A "white-eye blowout fracture" is considered a surgical emergency.
5. The most common facial bone fractured is the nasal bone.
6. The most common sites of mandible fracture are the angle and condyle.

QUESTIONS

1. What important elements of the physical exam are considered in facial trauma?

1. Airway, breathing, and circulation (ATLS)
2. Disability: cervical spine and brain injury (ATLS)
3. Cranial nerves: motor (CN VII) and sensory (CN V_1, V_2, V_3)
4. Eyes: vision (CN II), pupils, movement (CN IV, VI) fields, pressure, globe injury, globe position
5. Ears: hearing, hemotympanum, ear canal fracture, temporal bone fracture (CN VII, VIII)
6. Bones: calvarium, midface, and mandible for deformity and dysfunction
7. Throat: occlusion, TMJ function, bleeding, hematoma, airway, speech and swallow (CN IX, X)

2. What type of imaging should be ordered to evaluate facial trauma?

High-resolution (fine cut) axial computed tomography (CT) with coronal and sagittal reconstruction is ideal. Cervical spine imaging should be included in facial fractures caused by high-energy impacts such as motor vehicle accidents (MVA). Coronal and sagittal reconstructions are helpful in evaluating the orbital floor, frontal sinus outflow tracts, and mandibular condyles. Three-dimensional CT scans are very helpful in surgical planning when multiple fractures are present. *Direct radiographic* signs of facial fractures are nonanatomic linear lucency, cortical defects or suture diastasis, overlapping bone fragments causing "double density," and facial asymmetry. *Indirect radiographic* signs include soft tissue swelling, periorbital or intracranial air and fluid in the paranasal sinus.

3. What characteristics of the mechanism of trauma are considered important?

Facial fracture results when the tolerance of facial bone is overcome by the kinetic energy ($KE = \frac{1}{2}mv^2$) transfer from blunt or penetrating trauma. Mechanisms have variable energy from low (fall from standing) to high (MVA). Understanding the mechanism of injury can help predict the extent of facial injury and the risk of associated cervical or brain injuries. High-impact and low-impact forces are defined as greater or lesser than 50 times the force of gravity (g). Facial bones differ in ability to withstand force: nasal bones can resist 30 g, zygoma 50 g, mandible angle 70 g, frontal-glabella

80 g, midline maxilla and mandible 100 g, and supraorbital rim 200 g. The most common facial fracture is the nasal bone.

4. **How is the facial trauma patient evaluated?**
Each patient must be evaluated and treated according to the ATLS guidelines. Once the patient is medically stable, definitive facial fracture assessment and management can proceed. Facial trauma can range from a minimally displaced nasal fracture to a highly comminuted compound panfacial fracture involving the orbit, brain, and cervical spine. Facial trauma evaluation is best done by dividing the face anatomically into three sections as each has its own unique characteristics. The **upper third** assesses frontal bone, frontal sinus, and frontal lobe injury. The **middle third** or "midface" contains nasal, nasal-orbital-ethmoid (NOE), orbit, zygomaticomaxillary complex (ZMC), and maxillary structures. The **lower third** includes the mandible and temporomandibular joint.

Upper Third (Frontal Bone)

5. **How would you evaluate a suspected frontal sinus injury?**
High-resolution thin cut computed tomography (CT) is best to evaluate anterior and posterior table fractures and outflow tract injury. In addition to the standard axial and coronal images, sagittal reconstructions of the paranasal sinuses can enhance visualization of the frontal outflow tract. Additional findings such as NOE complex fractures and anterior skull base injury near the junction of the posterior table and the cribiform plate strongly suggest injury to the frontal outflow tract.

6. **What are the treatment goals of frontal sinus repair?**
   - Protection of intracranial structures
   - Stopping CSF leak
   - Prevention of posttraumatic infection or mucocele (late complications)
   - Restoration of facial aesthetics

7. **What are the surgical indications for anterior and posterior table frontal sinus fractures?**
Surgical indications for anterior table fractures include bony displacement causing a deformity or frontal sinus outflow tract impairment. Surgical indications for posterior table fracture include displacement of the posterior table greater than one table width, dural injury, CSF rhinorrhea, or frontal sinus outflow impairment.

8. **How do you treat a frontal sinus fracture of the anterior table?**
Isolated, nondisplaced, or minimally displaced anterior table fractures are not treated. Displaced fractures are treated by open reduction and internal fixation. Management options include osteoplastic flap with open reduction and internal fixation of anterior table fracture with or without obliteration, or an attempt at outflow tract reconstruction. Observation and medical management with future endoscopic surgery if needed is also an option.

9. **How would you treat a posterior table frontal sinus fracture?**
Uncomplicated nondisplaced posterior table fractures are generally not treated, but nondisplaced posterior table fractures with continued CSF leakage despite initial conservative measures require repair. Surgery is generally recommended for displaced posterior table fractures greater than one posterior table width, or severely comminuted fractures. The risk of dural injury in these cases is high and consultation with a neurosurgeon is recommended for possible dural repair. Mucosal removal and obliteration with abdominal fat or cranialization of the frontal sinus may be considered.

10. **What is the "osteoplastic flap with frontal sinus obliteration" procedure?**
The osteoplastic bone flap is created by a frontal sinus outline marked on the cranium classically using a template from a 6 ft. Caldwell radiograph. Osteotomies are performed and the sinus is opened. The mucosa of the sinus is completely removed, the frontal recess is occluded with temporalis fascia or muscle, abdominal fat is used to fill the sinus, and the bony flap is replaced. Postoperative CT/MR surveillance imaging is used for detection of postoperative mucocele formation; however, imaging is often difficult to interpret.

11. **What is "frontal sinus cranialization"?**
The posterior wall of the frontal sinus is removed and the sinus mucosa is stripped away from the remaining bone. The brain and dura are evaluated by a neurosurgeon for possible debridement and dural closure. A previously mobilized anterior pericranial flap is inserted beneath the brain to

separate it from the paranasal sinuses. The brain and dura are permitted to rest against the repaired anterior wall in the area originally occupied by the frontal sinus, which no longer exists.

12. What are the complications of frontal sinus fractures?
Early complications include wound infection, CSF leak, meningitis, acute sinusitis, deformity, pain, hypesthesia, and brain abscess. Late complications include mucocele, mucopyocele, osteomyelitis, cosmetic defect, brain abscess, and headache.

13. What are the surgical approaches to repair the frontal sinus?
    1. Frontal sinus trephination and elevation of the anterior wall with limited exposure
    2. Frontoethmoidectomy using a Lynch incision or endoscopic repair of the outflow tract
    3. Open reduction and internal fixation through the laceration or by coronal flap
    4. Frontal sinus obliteration
    5. Frontal sinus cranialization
    6. Frontal sinus ablation (Reidel) with removal of the anterior wall (rarely used today)
    7. Endoscopic frontal sinus surgery (delayed)

14. What are the dangers of raising a bicoronal flap for facial fracture repair and how are they avoided?
    1. Injury to the frontal branch of the facial nerve can be avoided by incising the superficial layer of the deep temporal fascia at the temporal line of fusion so elevation can be deep to this layer.
    2. Injury to the supraorbital and supratrochlear nerves at the supraorbital rims is prevented by removing the inferior lip of the nerve foramen with an osteotome to allow the nerve to move inferiorly.
    3. Laxity of the midface soft tissues occurs if the fascia is not resuspended at the time of closure.

15. What endoscopic procedure is used to treat severe chronic frontonasal outflow obstruction?
The *modified Lothrop procedure (Draf III procedure)* may be used to restore severely obstructed frontal outflow pathways after trauma.

MIDDLE THIRD (NOSE, ORBIT, ZYGOMA, MAXILLA)

16. What key features are evaluated in nasal trauma?
Nasal fractures are commonly identified by epistaxis and bony nasal deformity. Often the patient complains of nasal obstruction. The *external exam* should include evaluation of deformity, mobility, step-offs, and telecanthus. The *internal exam* should examine for septal deviation, mucosal tears, or septal hematoma. Clear rhinorrhea may indicate cerebrospinal fluid (CSF) leak. Epistaxis in severe facial trauma may be life threatening and require surgery or embolization of the feeding arteries if packing fails.

17. What are the dangers of a nasal septal hematoma and how is it treated?
A septal hematoma is a collection of blood under the nasal septal perichondrium following trauma. The lack of blood supply to the cartilage can lead to cartilage necrosis or septal abscess and can produce a saddle nose deformity. Urgent treatment is required to evacuate the clot or purulence.

18. How is a nasal fracture treated?
Timing is critical. *Acute nasal fractures* are treated best by closed reduction immediately following the fracture (1 to 2 hours) or after swelling has subsided (5 to 10 days). The bones are repositioned and splinted for 7 to 14 days. *Chronic nasal fractures* (>10 days) may be more difficult to treat and often require complete healing (3 to 6 months) followed by formal septorhinoplasty.

19. What is an NOE fracture?
The nasal-orbital-ethmoid (NOE) complex is the confluence of the frontal sinus, ethmoid sinuses, anterior cranial fossa, orbits, frontal bone, and nasal bones. An NOE fracture is a telescoping fracture of the nasal, lacrimal, and ethmoid bones, which occurs from blunt trauma at the nasal bridge. Injury to the bony septal attachment at the cribiform plate can produce a CSF leak and anosmia. NOE fractures involve the attachment of the medial canthal tendons (MCT) and can produce telecanthus. Failure to diagnose and repair an MCT can lead to functional and cosmetic complications that are difficult to repair secondarily. Long-term sequelae of NOE fractures include blindness, telecanthus, enophthalmos, midface retrusion, cerebrospinal fluid (CSF) fistula, anosmia, epiphora, sinusitis, and nasal deformity.

20. **How are medial canthal tendon injuries classified?**
Markowitz classified NOE fractures based on the status of the MCT and the degree of comminution of the "central fragment" of bone to which it remains attached. In *Type I* fractures the fracture lines leave a single noncomminuted central fragment with MCT attached. In *Type II* the central fragment gets comminuted but the MCT stays attached to its fragments. In *Type III* fractures there is severe central fragment comminution and the MCT is detached. Type II and III are the most difficult to repair and require transnasal wiring in a posterior superior direction to keep medial orbit deformity to a minimum.

21. **What is a blowout fracture?**
An orbital blowout fracture results from hydraulic compression of the orbital contents into the paranasal sinuses through the weakest portions of the orbit. This usually occurs through the thin portion of the orbital floor (0.5 mm) and less frequently through the thin lamina papyracea (0.25 mm), which is supported by the honeycomb structure of the ethmoid sinuses. The *pure* form is purely hydraulic without rim injury; the *impure* form is caused by rim deformation and fracture extending posteriorly to create the blowout fracture.

22. **What are the indications for surgery of the blowout fracture of the orbital floor?**
Surgery is indicated for: (1) enophthalmos greater than 2 mm, (2) double vision on primary or inferior gaze, (3) entrapment of extraocular muscles on forced duction testing, or (4) fracture greater than 50% of the orbital floor on CT imaging.

23. **What is a "white-eyed blowout fracture"? Why is it treated emergently?**
This is a trapdoor or greenstick fracture of the orbital floor, most commonly in children. The orbital floor opens under hydraulic pressure from the compressed globe, forcing the orbital fat and muscle into the maxillary sinus. The elastic bony floor will immediately close on these contents and trap them tightly. Under these circumstances the sclera remains white without hemorrhage, and the child is often nauseated and in severe pain. Careful examination of the irritated child may be difficult and CT scanning of the orbit should be considered for the diagnosis. Urgent surgery is required to preserve the entrapped ischemic inferior rectus muscle.

24. **What are the surgical approaches to repair orbit wall fractures?**
The *orbital floor* is approached through the lower lid, which includes infraorbital, subciliary, and transconjunctival (preseptal or postseptal) routes. The *medial wall* is accessed through a transcaruncular incision, an endonasal endoscopic approach through the ethmoid sinuses, or by an external ethmoidectomy (Lynch) incision. The *lateral wall* is approached through an infrabrow incision, an upper lid skin crease (blepharoplasty) incision or through an extended lower lid transconjunctival incision with a lateral canthotomy. *Orbital roof* approaches include the external ethmoidectomy (Lynch), transbrow, or coronal incisions.

25. **What structures can be damaged using a Lynch approach to the orbit?**
The Lynch orbitotomy is used to access the medial wall using a curved skin incision half-way between the medial canthus and the bridge of the nose. Disadvantages of the Lynch incision are skin scarring, disinsertion of the medial canthal tendon, damage to the lacrimal sac, diplopia caused by trauma to the trochlea of the superior oblique muscle, and scarring of adjacent structures.

26. **Describe the transcaruncular approach to the medial orbit. Why is it used?**
The caruncle is divided to access a plane between Horner's muscle and the medial orbital septum to expose the medial extraperiosteal space. Advantages include rapid entry into the orbit, less damage to skin and muscle layers, better cosmetic result, and less manipulation of the medial canthal tendon and lacrimal sac.

27. **What are common complications of orbital fracture repair?**
- **Diplopia:** double vision from paresis of an extraocular muscle (usually due to the initial injury) or fibrosis of an extraocular muscle causing restriction
- **Enophthalmos:** posterior displacement of the eye within the orbit from changes in orbit volume in the setting of fat atrophy or wall malposition
- **Entropion:** inversion of the eyelid toward the globe
- **Ectropion:** eversion of the lid margin away from the globe
- **Proptosis:** forward displacement of the eye from overcorrection of a blowout fracture
- **Hypoglobus:** downward displacement of the eye in the orbit

- **Telecanthus:** intercanthal distance is bigger than the width of the eye
- **Dacryocystitis:** inflammation of the lacrimal sac related to nasolacrimal duct obstruction
- **Orbital cellulitis:** infections in the orbit or from orbital implants

28. **What is the quickest way to decompress the eye with increased intraocular pressure?**
Orbital compartment syndrome (OCS) is an ocular emergency requiring prompt diagnosis and treatment to prevent blindness from ischemia of the optic nerve and retina. Orbital pressure can be relieved with an emergent *lateral canthotomy with inferior cantholysis.* Absolute indications for lateral canthotomy include retrobulbar hemorrhage resulting in acute loss of visual acuity, increased IOP, and proptosis. In the unconscious or uncooperative patient, an IOP greater than 40 mm Hg is an indication for lateral canthotomy (normal IOP is 10 to 21 mm Hg).

29. **What is the first indication that the optic nerve is injured following orbital trauma?**
Traumatic optic neuropathy (TON) is a condition of acute injury to the optic nerve from direct or indirect trauma. TON is thought to result from shearing injury to the intracanalicular portion of optic nerve, which can cause axonal injury or disturb the blood supply of the optic nerve. The optic nerve may swell in the optic canal after trauma, resulting in increased luminal pressure and secondary ischemic injury. Patients with TON may have decreased central visual acuity, decreased color vision, an afferent pupillary defect or visual field deficits. An early clinical finding of optic nerve injury in the traumatized eye is *loss of red color vision.* Treatment is with high-dose corticosteroids or surgical decompression.

30. **What is the difference between a forced duction test and a traction test?**
The *forced duction test* is an upward tug on the anesthetized sclera to test for inferior rectus muscular entrapment after blowout fracture. The *traction test* is the grasping of the lower eyelid and pulling laterally against its medial attachment to determine if there is abnormal laxity indicating a disruption of the medial canthal tendon following NOE fracture.

31. **How is an open globe injury treated?**
A ruptured globe should be protected from any pressure or contact by placing a rigid eye shield without an eye patch on the patient. Foreign bodies should be left undisturbed. Medications should include antiemetics, sedation, analgesics, and prophylactic antibiotics to prevent endophthalmitis. Tetanus immunity should be updated, as open globe lacerations are considered tetanus prone. The patient should be kept NPO and definitive surgical repair by an ophthalmologist should be expedited.

32. **What is a zygomatic arch fracture and how is it treated?**
A zygomatic arch fracture is usually a medially displaced deformity in the zygomatic arch from an external blow. The defect can be seen and palpated; the indented bone can impinge on the coronoid process of the mandible and cause pain with jaw movement. Treatment is via fracture reduction often without fixation through a (1) *direct cutaneous approach* using a hook or suture, (2) a *Gilles approach*—an incision behind the hairline over the temporalis muscle to reach the fracture, or by (3) a *transoral approach* through a gingivobuccal sulcus incision. Comminuted arch fractures may require a coronal flap and ORIF.

33. **What is a tripod fracture?**
A tripod or malar fracture is officially known as the zygomaticomaxillary complex (ZMC) fracture. The zygoma is separated from the face at the (1) zygomaticomaxillary (ZM) suture (infraorbital rim); (2) zygomatic arch, and (3) zygomaticofrontal (ZF) suture (lateral orbital rim). A fourth sphenozygomatic (SZ) suture is at the lateral orbital wall, which when counted makes the ZMC fracture technically a "tetrapod" rather than a tripod fracture.

34. **What are the midfacial buttresses and why are they important in fracture treatment?**
The midface is reinforced by strong vertical and weaker horizontal buttresses. Three vertical buttresses resist the forces of mastication; the *medial* (nasomaxillary) *buttress* extends from the nasomaxillary region to the frontal bone. The *lateral* (zygomaticomaxillary) *buttress* extends from the molar region superiorly to the zygomaticomaxillary complex along the lateral orbital rim to the frontal bone. The *posterior* (pterygomaxillary) *buttress* is from the pterygoid plates to the skull base. The medial and lateral vertical buttresses are accessible for repair while the pterygoid sites are not. Four

horizontal buttresses are bridging supports between the vertical buttresses and consist of the palate, a central facial buttress from malar to malar interrupted by the piriform aperture, the frontal bar, and the anterior-posterior zygomatic arch.

35. **How are middle third (midface) facial fractures classified?**
In 1901, French military surgeon René Le Fort published a classification of midface fractures that is still in use today. All three fracture types traverse the pterygomaxillary fissure to interrupt the pterygoid plates (Figure 68-1). **Le Fort I fracture** is a horizontal fracture above the maxillary alveolus producing a floating palate. The fracture usually involves the nasal aperture and extends above the apices of the teeth, causing the maxilla and hard palate to move separately. **Le Fort II fracture** is a pyramidal fracture that usually involves the inferior orbital rim. It extends from the nasion through the lacrimal bones and inferior orbital floor and rim through or near the inferior orbital foramen, and inferiorly through the anterior wall of the maxillary sinus. The **Le Fort III fracture** is a transverse fracture that separates the face from the skull, which is known as craniofacial dissociation. It includes fractures through the zygomatic bone, nasofrontal and frontomaxillary sutures, and orbit. The thick greater wing of the sphenoid bone usually prevents the continuation of the fracture into the optic canal thus preserving vision. Le Fort fractures often present in "mixed combinations" and should be reported as such (Figure 68-2).

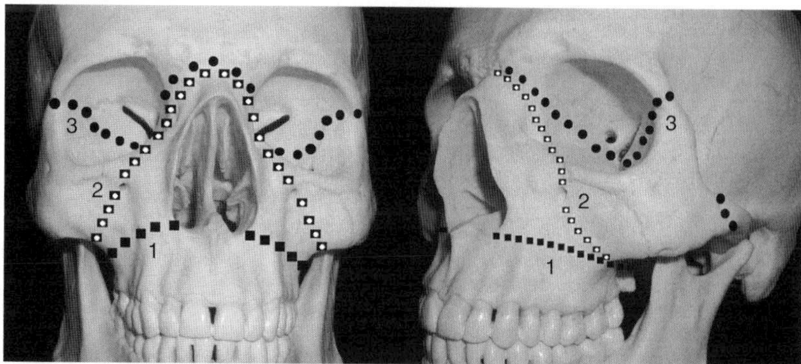

Figure 68-1. Le Fort fractures. Le Fort I fracture (1) is a horizontal fracture above the maxillary alveolus. Lefort II fracture (2) is pyramidal and usually includes the infraorbital rim. Le Fort III fracture (3) includes the zygoma and orbit and is considered a craniofacial dissociation when present bilaterally.

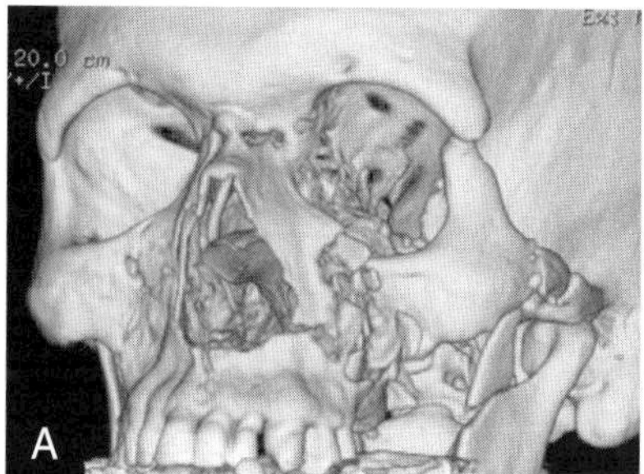

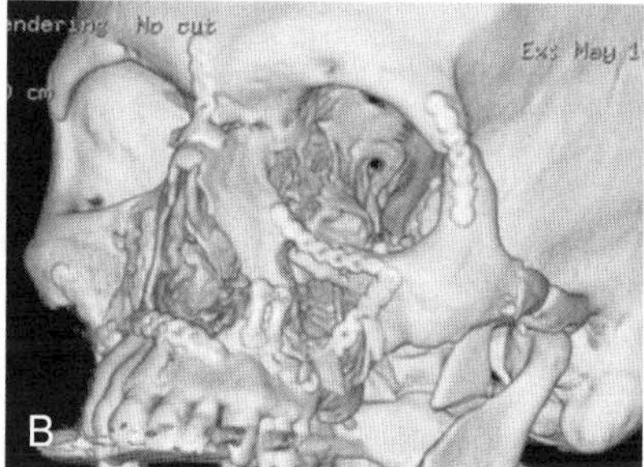

Figure 68-2. A, Left photo is a preoperative 3DCT of a patient with a right Le Fort II, left Le Fort I-II-III, and a palate fracture and left coronoid fracture. **B,** Right is a postoperative 3DCT showing the nose and zygoma repositioned and fixed to the skull base. The maxillary buttresses were repaired in relation to **both** the upper stabilized segments and the mandibular occlusion. Note the untreated coronoid fracture in correct position following zygoma repositioning.

36. **How are midface fractures treated?**
The goal of midface fracture repair is to restore form (cosmesis) and function. It must be done in concert with the nose, orbit, zygoma, and maxilla in relation to the mandible. In treating the patient in Figure 68-2, the upper portions of the midface were treated by stabilizing the nose and ZF suture fractures first with titanium plates. The maxilla was then aligned with the mandible and the remaining right Le Fort II and left Le Fort I-II-III fractures could be repaired in an accurate and functional way to restore the patient's occlusion and facial cosmesis. Facial lacerations and minimally invasive soft tissue access techniques aid in the final cosmetic result.

37. **What is a panfacial fracture and how are panfacial fractures treated?**
Panfacial fractures are defined as fractures involving the lower, middle, and upper face. Treatment is challenging and requires an individualized treatment plan utilizing treatment principles for each individual fracture. Reconstruction should be performed from the stable to the unstable (see Figure 68-2). The mobile zygomatic bone and nasal bones are secured in their correct anatomic position to solid cranial bone. Occlusion and facial height are reestablished first by reconstruction of the mandible to the maxilla, which is then secured to the nasal and zygomatic bones and cranium.

38. **What are surgical complications associated with midface fracture repair?**
    1. Inadequate reduction: malocclusion (maxilla) and facial deformity (zygoma)
    2. Imprecise reconstruction of the orbit: globe malposition
    3. Diplopia: from globe malposition, residual entrapment, muscle or nerve injury
    4. Eyelid malposition: eyelid incision/dissection trauma, orbital septum injury
    5. Reduced vision and blindness: rare, preoperative vision evaluation required
    6. Scars and hair loss: irregular coronal incisions, avoid with careful design and preoperative counseling
    7. Numbness: traumatic versus surgical
    8. Nonunion: chronic implant infection/extrusion, rare in midface fractures
    9. Dental injury: avoid tooth roots when placing screws, tooth and gum care with arch bar use
    10. CSF leaks: recognize early and treat to keep intracranial cavity separate from nose/sinuses

Lower Third (Mandible)

39. **What are the clinical signs of mandibular fracture and how is the mandible assessed in a patient with facial trauma?**
The head and neck exam may show lacerations, swelling, and hematoma in the area of the fracture. Bimanual palpation of the inferior border may identify swelling, step-off deformity or tenderness. Lip numbness occurs in mandibular fractures distal to the mandibular foramen. Oral exam may show deviation of the mouth on opening, limited opening (trismus), TMJ pain, coronoid impingement, occlusal changes, and floor of mouth ecchymosis from periosteal or gingival tearing. Occlusal evaluation may show obvious or subtle malocclusion. Imaging studies are necessary, as mandibular fractures usually occur in pairs—parasymphyseal and condyle fractures often occur together.

40. **What are the best imaging studies for mandibular trauma?**
An axial computed tomography (CT) with coronal and sagittal reconstruction is ideal when visualization is difficult and is the preferred method of imaging for multiple mandibular fractures. Three-dimensional CT is very helpful for treatment planning of complex mandibular fractures. A *Panorex film* of the mandible is an excellent screening study involving low cost, low radiation, and excellent for follow-up evaluation. Other studies include mandible series, occlusal films, and periapical films.

41. **How are mandibular fractures classified?**
Mandibular fractures are classified by anatomic region and by an additional descriptor. Each anatomic region has unique characteristics that require specialized treatment considerations. The additional descriptors describe *severity* (greenstick, simple, compound, comminuted), *displacement* by muscle pull (favorable or unfavorable), and *malocclusion* (open bite, cross bite). Each of these considerations will factor into the treatment plan.

42. **What are the anatomic regions of the mandible?**
The mandible is divided into horizontal and vertical parts. The *horizontal mandible* has four anatomic regions: the dense basal bone consisting of the symphysis, parasymphysis, body, and less dense alveolar bone which holds the dentition. The *vertical mandible* has four anatomic regions: the angle,

ramus, condyle, and coronoid. Fractures can occur in any of these regions but more frequently in the angle and condyle regions (Figure 68-3).

43. **How are condylar fractures classified and why are they considered difficult to treat?**
Condyle fractures are classified by three sites: head, neck, and subcondylar (see Figure 68-3). Condyle fractures are difficult to treat because (1) condyle fractures occur *under the facial nerve* (CN VII), which can be injured in the approach; (2) the condyle is often *malpositioned* by pull of the lateral pterygoid muscle or by traumatic dislocation and are difficult to reduce; (3) the *bone quality* is often inadequate to support hardware. Subcondylar fractures are generally the only site considered for ORIF, while the other regions are often treated without operative intervention. The malocclusion that occurs from condyle fractures creates an open bite deformity.

44. **What are the indications for open reduction and internal fixation (ORIF) of a condyle fracture?**
Absolute and relative indications for surgery are discussed by Zide and Kent (Table 68-1). Unfortunately there is no consensus on the treatment of condylar fractures in adults. The type of

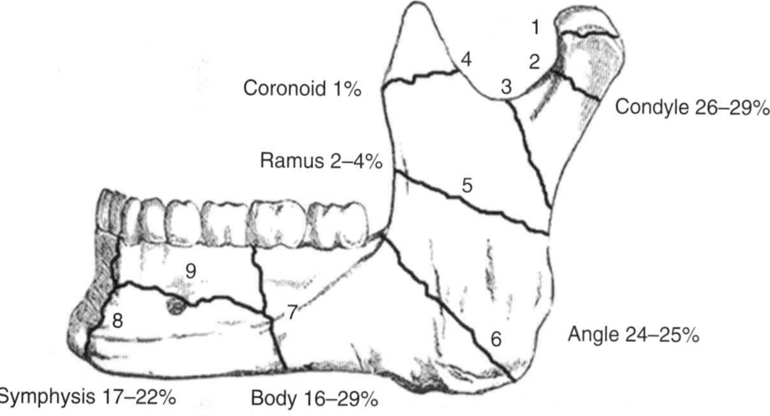

Figure 68-3. Common mandibular fracture sites: (1) condylar head, (2) condylar neck, (3) subcondylar, (4) coronoid, (5) ramus, (6) angle, (7) body, (8) symphysis (symphysis and parasymphysis), (9) and alveolar.

Table 68-1. Indications for Open Reduction and Internal Fixation (ORIF) of a Condyle Fracture

Absolute Indications

1. Displacement of the condyle into the middle cranial fossa or EAC
2. Inability to obtain adequate occlusion
3. Lateral extracapsular dislocation
4. Contaminated open joint wound

Relative Indications

1. Bilateral condylar fractures in an edentulous patient when splints are unavailable or impossible because of alveolar ridge atrophy
2. Bilateral or unilateral condylar fractures when splinting is not recommended because of concomitant medical conditions or when physiotherapy is not possible
3. Bilateral fractures associated with comminuted midface fractures
4. Bilateral subcondylar fractures with associated: (a) retrognathia or prognathia, (b) open bite with periodontal problems or lack of posterior support, (c) loss of multiple teeth and later need for reconstruction, (d) unstable occlusion due to orthodontics, (e) unilateral condylar fracture with unstable fracture base

treatment must be chosen on a case by case basis and by professional experience. Functional therapy (early jaw mobilization) is essential to avoid ankylosis of the TMJ. Three treatments advocated for adults with condylar process fractures include: (1) a period of maxillomandibular fixation (MMF) followed by functional therapy, (2) functional therapy without a period of MMF and, (3) open reduction with or without internal fixation. ORIF in children is becoming more accepted due to technical experience and improvements in rigid fixation.

45. **Why is the mandibular angle subject to high fracture rates?**
First, the angle has a thinner cross-sectional area relative to the neighboring segments of the mandible and second is the presence of third molars which weaken the region. The thin bone and tooth socket creates a pathologic fracture site by weakening the junction between the vertical and horizontal segments. Unfavorable angle fractures are subject to displacement by pull from the masseter and medial pterygoid muscles. Mandibular angle fractures pose a unique challenge for surgeons because they have the highest reported postoperative complication rate of any mandibular region.

46. **How is tension and compression related to mandibular healing?**
During chewing, a functional load creates *tension* which separates the superior border of the mandible (Figure 68-4). This opens the fracture site and will allow bacteria and food to enter and produce a poor result. *Compression* occurs on the inferior border at the same time and closes the fracture. During repair it is important to place a tension plate on the superior border to reduce separation. This fixes the fracture and reduces risks of nonunion and infection.

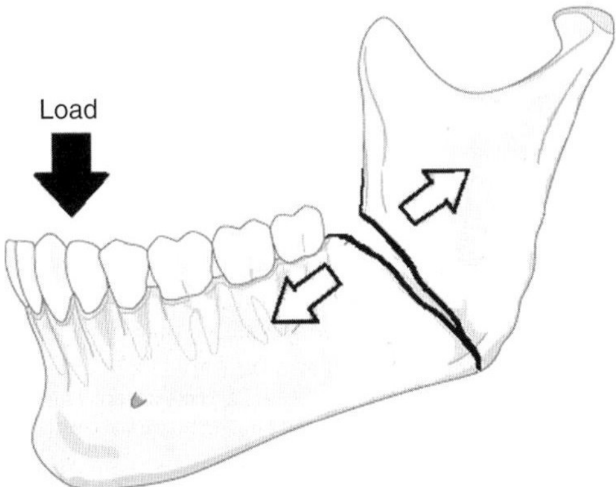

Figure 68-4. Under chewing load a mandibular angle fracture opens at the superior border *(open arrows)*. This is considered the "tension" or distracting site, which can be held together with a lightweight mini-plate. "Compression" or closure occurs on the inferior border during loading and needs no plate to keep the fracture reduced. Some surgeons feel additional help on the inferior border may be necessary.

47. **What do fractures of the mandibular body and parasymphyseal region have in common?**
Both are regions of the horizontal mandible that bear teeth and require adequate occlusal reconstruction to prevent malocclusion. Patients who sustain bilateral parasymphyseal fractures can have a "flail mandible," which can result in the fragment and tongue moving posteriorly and producing airway obstruction.

48. **Explain the angle classification of occlusion.**
Class I is considered normal and the mesiobuccal cusp (MBC) of the permanent maxillary first molar occludes in the buccal groove (BG) of the permanent mandibular first molar. *Class II* (retrognathia) is a posterior mandible, so the upper MBC is now in front of (mesial) the lower BG. *Class III* (prognathia) is an anterior mandible in which the upper MBC is behind (distal) the lower BG (Figure 68-5).

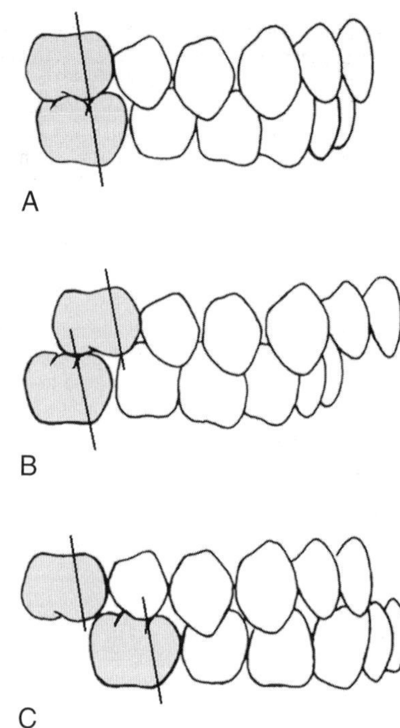

Figure 68-5. Angle classification of occlusion. **A,** Class I, normal occlusion. **B,** Class II, malocclusion. **C,** Class III, malocclusion.

49. **What are the indications for closed verses open reduction of mandible fractures?**
Closed reduction and fixation is considered for nondisplaced favorable fractures, pediatric fractures, grossly comminuted fractures, coronoid fractures, and adult condyle fractures. This is accomplished by maxillomandibular fixation (MMF) using Arch Bars, Ivy loops, Risdon wires, dental splints, and dentures. ORIF is considered for displaced unfavorable fractures, atrophic edentulous mandible fractures, complex facial fractures, and condylar fractures that can't be treated with closed techniques. This is done by exposing and reducing the fracture, and fixating with wires, lag screws, or plates and screws.

50. **How should the edentulous mandible fracture be treated?**
Mandibular atrophy occurs with the loss of teeth, resulting in a smaller fragile bone. This remaining "basal bone" is dense cortical bone that has decreased osteogenesis, reduced blood supply, and depends on the periosteum for nourishment. *Closed treatment* using Gunning splints, dentures, and external pin fixation is done to preserve the blood supply in a noncontaminated environment to promote fracture healing. *Open treatment* requires the placement of heavy load-bearing reconstructive plates using bicortical screws. Edentulous bone has no cross-sectional stability and is too weak to "load-share" the fracture with a small bone plate and monocortical screws. Failure to recognize this important concept when treating with ORIF can lead to serious complications.

51. **How are pediatric mandibular fractures different from adult fractures?**
Pediatric mandible fractures are more difficult to treat than adult fractures. The teeth are conical in shape and have short roots that are not amenable to MMF. Tooth buds and growth centers can be damaged during the fracture treatment. Children 6 years of age and younger are generally treated with closed reduction techniques to avoid injury to developing teeth. Children 12 and older should have their permanent teeth in place and can be treated with ORIF using mini-plates. Mandible growth occurs because of elongation in the condylar region and remodeling and growth in the ramus and body. Injuries in the condylar region during fracture repair may lead to facial asymmetry.

CONTROVERSIES

52. **Posterior table fracture management.**
Management of posterior wall fractures is most controversial of all fracture sites. The issue is assessing whether the fragments are displaced. Fine cut CT scans are helpful in determining if the fracture is linear or displaced. Linear fractures require no treatment. Nondisplaced fractures with CSF leak may be observed for 5 to 7 days. According to the current treatment algorithm, if the wall is displaced, frontal sinus exploration is indicated. The result of the exploration can result in doing nothing, doing a simple posterior table repair, doing a complete mucosal drill out and abdominal fat obliteration, or doing a frontal sinus cranialization procedure.

53. **Outflow obstruction and frontal sinus obliteration verses sinus sparing techniques.**
The question as to whether the frontal outflow tract obstruction can be successfully preserved in selected patient populations (sinus preserving) in contrast to sinus obliteration procedures is a controversial topic. There are no head-to-head comparisons of these two techniques. All agree that the consequences of nasofrontal outflow tract obstruction require treatment.

54. **Use of prophylactic antibiotics in the management of facial fracture.**
There is considerable variability in the management of patients with frontal sinus fractures in the use of prophylactic antibiotics. Prophylactic antibiotics are used to prevent infections; however, they also may inadvertently increase the risk of postoperative infections with opportunistic pathogens. Antibiotics may also alter the physiologic local flora and eliminate the reliability of microbiological analysis of CSF samples when meningitis is suspected. The efficacy of antibiotics is difficult to study given the heterogeneity in injury pattern, patient characteristics, and study designs.

BIBLIOGRAPHY

AAO Resident Manual of Trauma to the Face: Head, and Neck. Available at http://www.entnet.org/mktplace/upload/ResidentTraumaFINALlowres.pdf.

Biller JA, Pletcher SD, Goldberg AN, et al: Complications and the time to repair of mandible fractures, *Laryngoscope* 115(5):769–772, 2005.

Bowerman JE: The superior orbital fissure syndrome complicating fractures of the facial skeleton, *Br J Oral Surg* 7:1–6, 1969.

Castro B, Walcott BP, Redial N, et al: Cerebrospinal fluid fistula prevention and treatment following frontal sinus fractures: a review of initial management and outcomes, *Neurosurg Focus* 32(6):E1, 2012.

Champy M, Loddé JP, Schmitt R, et al: Mandibular osteosynthesis by miniature screwed plates via a buccal approach, *J Maxillofac Surg* 6(1):14–21, 1978.

Daudia A, Biswas D, Jones NS: Risk of meningitis with cerebrospinal fluid rhinorrhea, *Ann Otol Rhinol Laryngol* 116: 902–905, 2007.

Ellis E 3rd, Zide MF: Transfacial approaches to the mandible. In Ellis E 3rd, Zide MF, editors: *Surgical Approaches to the Facial Skeleton*, ed 2, Philadelphia, 2005, Lippincott Williams & Wilkins, pp 151–189.

Ellis E 3rd, Price C: Treatment protocol for fractures of the atrophic mandible, *J Oral Maxillofac Surg* 66(3):421–435, 2008.

Ellis E 3rd: Management of fractures through the angle of the mandible, *Oral Maxillofac Surg Clin North Am* 21(2): 163–174, 2009.

Ellis IIIE, Throckmorton GS: Treatment of mandibular condylar process fractures: biological considerations, *J Oral Maxillofac Surg* 63:115–134, 2005.

Gillies HD, Kilner TP, Stone D: Fractures of the malar-zygomatic compound: with a description of a new x-ray position, *Br J Surg* 14:651–656, 1927.

Hegab A: Management of mandibular fractures in children with a split acrylic splint: a case series, *Br J Oral Maxillofac Surg* 50(6):e93–e95, 2012.

Keen WW: *Surgery: Its Principles and Practice*, Philadelphia, 1909, WB Saunders.

Kellman RA: Maxillofacial trauma. In *Cummings/Otolaryngology: Head and Neck Surgery*, ed 5, Philadelphia, 2010, Mosby Elsevier, pp 318–341.

Kellman RM, Cienfuegos R: Endoscopic approaches to subcondylar fractures of the mandible, *Facial Plast Surg* 25(1): 23–28, 2009.

Liu P, Wu S, Li Z, et al: Surgical strategy for cerebrospinal fluid rhinorrhea repair, *Neurosurgery* 66(6 Suppl Operative): 281–286, 2010.

Markowitz BL, Manson PN, Sargent L, et al: Management of the medial canthal tendon in nasoethmoid orbital fractures: the importance of the central fragment in classification and treatment, *Plast Reconstr Surg* 87(5):843–853, 1991.

Perez R, Oeltien JC, Thaller S: A review of mandibular angle fractures, *Craniomaxillofac Trauma Reconstr* 4(2):69–72, 2011.

Scholsem M, Scholtes F, Collignon F, et al: Surgical management of anterior cranial base fractures with cerebrospinal fluid fistulae: a single-institution experience, *Neurosurgery* 62:463–471, 2008.
Shetty V, Atchison K, Leathers R, et al: Do the benefits of rigid internal fixation of mandible fractures justify the added costs? Results from a randomized controlled trial, *J Oral Maxillofac Surg* 66(11):2203–2212, 2008.
Shorr N, Baylis HI, Goldberg RA: Transcaruncular approach to the medial orbit and orbital apex, *Ophthalmology* 107:1459–1463, 2000.
Smith B, Regan WF: Blowout fracture of the orbit: mechanism and correction of internal orbital fracture, *Am J Ophthalmol* 44(6):733–739, 1957.
Valerie JL, Muriel ER: Ophthalmic considerations in fronto-ethmoid mucoceles, *J Laryngol Otol* 103:667–669, 1989.
Valiati R, Ibrahim D, Abreu ME, et al: The treatment of condylar fractures: to open or not to open? A critical review of this controversy, *Int J Med Sci* 5(6):313–318, 2008.
Winegar BA, Murillo H: Tantiwongkosi B: Spectrum of critical imaging findings in complex facial skeletal trauma, *Radiographics* 33(1):3–19, 2013.
Winkler AA, Smith TL, Meyer TK, et al: The management of frontal sinus fractures. In Kountakis SE, Onerci TM, editors: *Rhinologic and Sleep Apnea Surgical Techniques*, Berlin Heidelberg, 2007, Springer, pp 149–158.
Zide MF, Kent JN: Indications for open reduction of mandibular condyle fractures, *J Oral Maxillofac Surg* 41(2):89–98, 1983.

VII

Laryngology and Swallowing Disorders

AERODIGESTIVE ANATOMY AND EMBRYOLOGY WITH RADIOLOGIC CORRELATES

CHAPTER 69

Craig R. Villari, MD and Matthew S. Clary, MD

KEY POINTS

1. Two unpaired cartilages and three sets of paired cartilages make up the laryngeal framework.
2. Extrinsic laryngeal musculature is primarily associated with swallowing while the intrinsic musculature is responsible for respiration and phonation.
3. The true vocal folds are covered in squamous epithelium that is supported by a gelatinous matrix, the superficial lamina propria, which allows the unique vibratory properties necessary for phonation.
4. The larynx is primarily formed from the third, fourth, and sixth branchial arches.
5. Aberrations from normal embryologic development can lead to common congenital pathologies like laryngeal clefts and glottic webs.

Pearls

1. The hyoid bone is not ossified at birth, but it is the first component of the laryngeal framework to ossify followed by the thyroid cartilage, then the cricoid cartilage.
2. The cricoarytenoid joints are ball-and-socket joints, allowing three-dimensional movement to achieve the complex functions required of the larynx.
3. The posterior cricoarytenoid muscle is the only abductor muscle of the true vocal folds.
4. The cricothyroid muscle is the only intrinsic laryngeal muscle *not* innervated by the recurrent laryngeal nerve; it is innervated by the superior laryngeal nerve.
5. The interarytenoid muscle is the only intrinsic laryngeal muscle with bilateral innervation.

QUESTIONS

ANATOMY

1. What are the three primary subunits of the larynx?

The larynx serves three main and incredibly important functions: airway protection, phonation, and swallowing. Given the complexity of tasks it must complete, it stands to reason that is has equally complex anatomy. It is sometimes easier to compartmentalize the larynx to help better focus discussion and study. Laryngeal cancer staging has helped do that by breaking the larynx into three subsections: the supraglottis, the glottis, and the subglottis.

The supraglottis extends from the rostral edge of the epiglottis to the middle of the laryngeal ventricle. This subsection of the larynx includes the laryngeal surface of the epiglottis, the false vocal folds (also known as the vestibular folds), the aryepiglottic folds, and the most superior portions of the arytenoid cartilages. The glottis extends superiorly from the midventricle to 1 cm below the true vocal folds. This subsection contains the true vocal folds and the majority of the arytenoid cartilages. The subglottis extends from 1 cm below the true vocal folds to the most caudal edge of the cricoid cartilage.

2. **What cartilages compose the larynx?**
The larynx is composed of two unpaired cartilages and three paired cartilages (Figure 69-1). The unpaired cartilages—the thyroid and cricoid cartilages—are palpable externally and serve as excellent surgical landmarks. The paired cartilages—the arytenoid, cuneiform, and corniculate cartilages—are internal to the larynx. The cuneiform and corniculate cartilages are sometimes jointly referred to as sesamoid cartilages and serve as minor structural elements. The hyoid bone is the most superior aspect of the larynx and serves as an important insertion site of several extrinsic laryngeal muscles. These cartilages are all seen on modified barium swallow studies used to assess dysphagia (Figure 69-2).

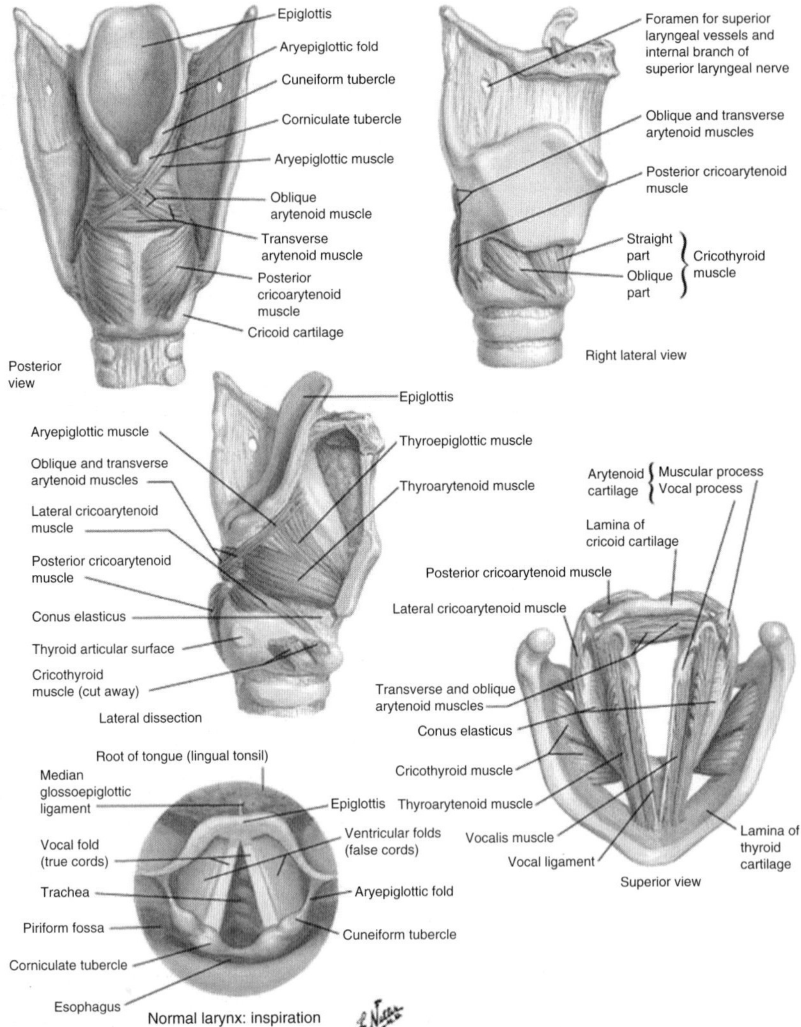

Figure 69-1. Musculature of the larynx. *(Source Netter FH: Atlas of Human Anatomy, Professional Edition, ed 5, Philadelphia, 2011, Saunders Elsevier, Plate 78.)*

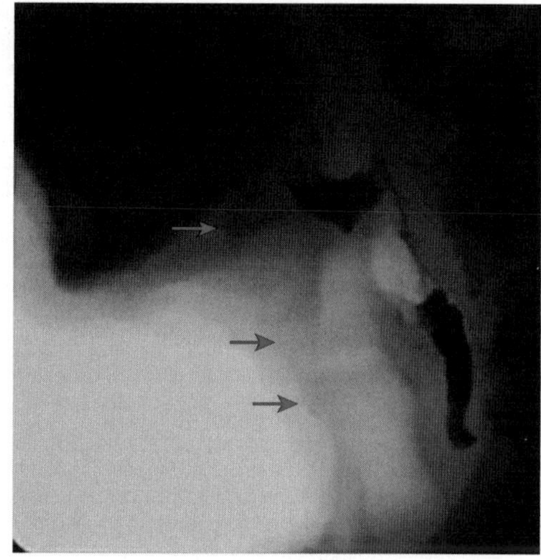

Figure 69-2. Modified barium swallow showing the hyoid bone, thyroid cartilage, and cricoid cartilage (*arrows*, respectively, from top to bottom).

The thyroid cartilage is formed by two ala that fuse in the midline. Each ala contains both superior and inferior cornua, the former tethering to the hyoid via the lateral thyrohyoid ligament and the latter serving as an articulating joint with cricoid cartilage. At the midline, there is a small notch that helps define the Adam's apple; this serves as a second connection to the hyoid via the median thyrohyoid ligament.

The cricoid cartilage is the only complete cartilage ring of the trachea. It has a characteristic three-dimensional shape often referred to as a signet ring, meaning the cricoid cartilage has the shape of many common high school class rings. The ring is oriented such that the larger plate sits posteriorly, allowing a relatively narrow craniocaudal profile anteriorly, while offering additional height posteriorly upon which the arytenoid cartilages sit. The cricoid articulates with the arytenoid cartilages at ball-and-socket joints along the superior surface of the ring.

3. **What muscles are found within the larynx?**
The larynx utilizes two separate groups of muscles—the extrinsic and intrinsic laryngeal muscles—to perform tasks related to phonation, airway protection, and swallowing. The extrinsic musculature connects one structural element of the larynx to another structural element outside of the larynx; conversely, the intrinsic musculature connects one structural element inside of the larynx to another.

4. **Describe the extrinsic musculature.**
The extrinsic musculature includes muscles that elevate and depress the laryngeal suprastructure within the neck, and while they have a small role in phonation they are primarily utilized in swallowing. A combination of the activation of the geniohyoid, digastric, mylohyoid, thyrohyoid or stylohyoid muscles will result in laryngeal elevation while laryngeal depression can be achieved with activation of the strap muscles (sternohyoid, sternothyroid, omohyoid). The extrinsic musculature has various innervations including cervical rootlets and cranial nerves V and VII. The final extrinsic muscle group to discuss is the pharyngeal constrictors. The constrictors, all innervated by the pharyngeal plexus, help advance food bolus distally. The superior constrictor does not insert on the larynx but the middle and inferior constrictors do, resulting in elevation and posterior translation with swallows.

5. **Describe the intrinsic musculature.**
The intrinsic musculature is primarily associated with airway protection and phonation. They are all paired muscles with the exception of the interarytenoid muscle (see Figure 69-1). These muscles can be classified as abductors or adductors based on how they move the vocal folds with activation. The adductors include the thyroarytenoid, the lateral cricoarytenoid, and the interarytenoid muscle. The lone abductor is the posterior cricoarytenoid muscle. The cricothyroid muscle is considered an intrinsic laryngeal muscle, but it does not directly cause adduction or abduction of the vocal folds.

The cricothyroid muscle works to pivot the thyroid cartilage anteriorly along the axis created by the cricothyroid joint, lengthening and tensing the vocal fold to allow a higher register of phonation.

6. **What type of mucosa is found in the larynx?**

The majority of the mucosa is columnar respiratory epithelium. However, stratified squamous epithelium overlies the vibratory portions of the true vocal fold. The transition points from respiratory epithelium to squamous epithelium occur at the superior and inferior arcuate lines; the former is within the laryngeal ventricle while the latter rests just below the true vocal fold.

This stratified squamous epithelium is thought to be protective against trauma caused by high-frequency collisions of the vocal folds against each other during phonation. Despite this protective quality, this existence of different epithelia and transitions between epithelial types is important in understanding both malignant and benign pathologies. Understanding epithelial types in the larynx can help understand likely locations for malignancies (squamous cell carcinoma of the glottis) and benign pathologies (recurrent respiratory papillomatosis usually only occurs at the transition points between respiratory and squamous epithelia).

7. **What is the laryngeal ventricle?**

The ventricle is a unique anatomic outpouching split between the supraglottic and glottic larynx. The inferior extent is the true vocal folds. The superior limit is not straightforward given the three-dimensional nature of the ventricle. When looking down the airway from above, the superior extent appears to be the false vocal fold. However, on anatomic dissection, one finds that the ventricle extends laterally and then superiorly beyond the false fold, allowing a potential space to form that is not easily examined on nasolaryngeal endoscopy. This potential space can collapse on itself and is known as the laryngeal saccule. The saccule can become important in discussions of saccular cysts and must be examined thoroughly when performing direct laryngoscopy for cancer diagnosis/surveillance (Figure 69-3).

8. **What are the quadrangular membrane and the conus elasticus?**

The quadrangular membrane is a fibroelastic membrane extending from the epiglottis to the false vocal fold, terminating in the ventricular ligament. It roughly comprises the aryepiglottic folds but has no definitive structural integrity. The conus elasticus is also a fibroelastic membrane but it extends from the superior aspect of the cricoid cartilage and spans superiorly to interdigitate with the vocal ligament within the true vocal folds.

Both the quadrangular membrane and the conus elasticus serve as potential barriers for the spread of malignancy.

9. **What is the significance of the cricoarytenoid joint? How does the arytenoid cartilage's shape help specialize the joint?**

The cricoarytenoid joint is a specialized ball-and-socket joint that is integral in allowing the larynx to perform its vital functions. The joint allows the arytenoids to both rotate on a vertical axis while also allowing them the freedom to glide and tip anteromedially.

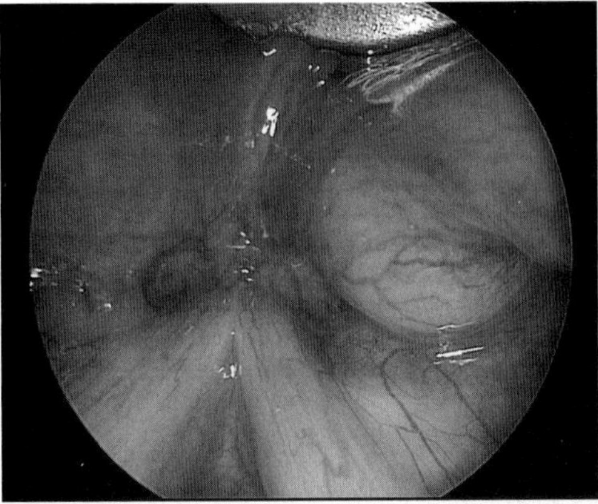

Figure 69-3. Endoscopic view of anterior commissure with 70-degree rigid endoscope showing saccular cyst.

The arytenoid has a pyramidal shape with the base serving as the socket for the cricoarytenoid joint. The arytenoid, however, has two important appendages known as the vocal process and the muscular process. The vocal process serves as the insertion point of the vocal ligament while the muscular process, as the name implies, serves as the insertion point for several intrinsic laryngeal muscles. The muscles insert in several vectors, allowing the arytenoid to rotate on the cricoarytenoid joint facet, in turn abducting or adducting the vocal ligament and vocal folds. This coordinated, highly specialized activation of laryngeal musculature allows for airway protection and phonation.

10. What laryngeal muscles are used for respiration?
Any muscle that helps to adduct or abduct the vocal folds is technically utilized during respiration. For optimal airflow, the vocal folds should be in an abducted position for respiration. Therefore the most important muscle is the posterior cricoarytenoid muscle, the lone abductor of the vocal folds. It is innervated by the recurrent laryngeal nerve (RLN).

11. What muscles are used for phonation?
As with respiration, any muscle that helps to adduct or abduct the vocal folds is technically utilized during phonation. Converse to respiration, optimal phonation occurs when the vocal folds are adducted to the midline. The muscles responsible for this motion are the thyroarytenoid, the interarytenoid, and the lateral cricoarytenoid muscles. These muscles are primarily innervated by the RLN.

While optimal phonation occurs with adducted vocal folds, as stated above, the laryngeal framework can pivot along the cricothyroid joint. This movement allows for tensing of the vocal ligament as it is stretched between the vocal process of the arytenoid cartilage and the insertion of the ligament on the thyroid cartilage. The cricothyroid muscle is responsible for this anterior pivoting and its activation will lead to higher pitched phonation. This muscle is the lone intrinsic muscle innervated by the superior laryngeal nerve (SLN).

12. Can phonation occur through alternative neurolaryngeal pathways?
The innervation detailed in the previous question is the dominant pathway; however, there are other variations. While most of the intrinsic musculature responsible for adduction of the vocal folds (a key element necessary for phonation) is innervated by the RLN, there is a named anastamosis between the RLN and SLN. This anastamosis is the nerve of Galen and can lead to some phonatory activation from the SLN.

13. What muscles are used for swallowing?
Swallowing is an incredibly complex task that involves multiple muscle groups inside and outside of the larynx. From a laryngeal standpoint, airway protection must occur to minimize risk of aspiration. This involves two separate tasks: first, the glottis must be closed to protect from frank aspiration so the vocal folds must be adducted to the midline (see above). Simultaneously, the extrinsic musculature is activated. This results in laryngeal elevation, inversion of the epiglottis, and proximal pharyngeal constriction to help direct the food bolus towards the esophagus.

14. Do any of the intrinsic laryngeal muscles have bilateral innervation?
Only one—the interarytenoid muscle receives bilateral innervation. This can result in an interesting clinical finding when there is known denervation of one side of the larynx (from a RLN injury during thyroidectomy, for example). With such an injury, one would expect immobility of the ipsilateral hemilarynx; however, one may see a slight adducting motion of the ipsilateral arytenoid cartilage. This can sometimes be confused for residual ipsilateral innervation but is more likely innervation of the interarytenoid muscle from the contralateral RLN.

15. What are the layers of the vibratory vocal fold?
From histologic studies, we now have a great understanding of vocal composition. While once thought to be a solid layer of muscle with a thin overlying epithelial layer, we now understand there are several integral layers all of which contribute to the unique vibratory function of the vocal folds (Figure 69-4).

The deepest portion of the vocal fold is the thyroarytenoid muscle and the most superficial is the squamous epithelium. Between them is a tri-layered level known as the lamina propria. The intermediate and deep layers fuse together and integrate to form the vocal ligament. The superficial layer of the lamina propria is a gelatinous matrix that is incredibly important for the unique vibratory qualities necessary for phonation.

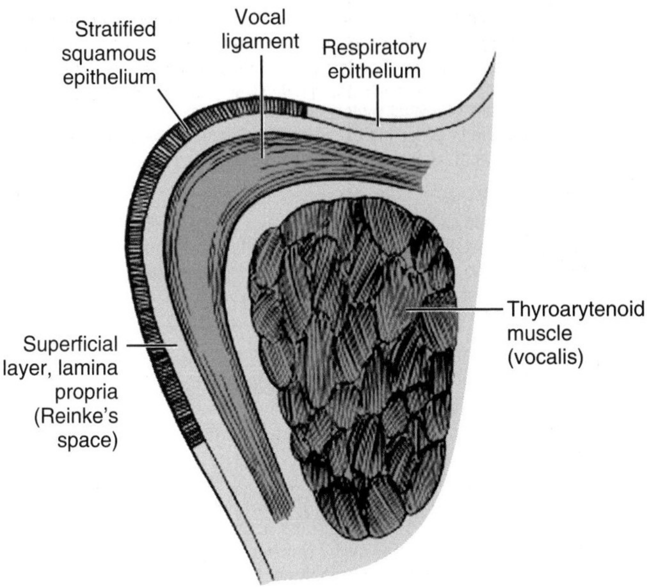

Figure 69-4. Cross-section of true vocal fold. *(From Bastian RW: Benign vocal fold mucosal disorders. In Flint PW, Haughey BH, Lund VJ, et al, editors: Cummings Otolaryngology: Head & Neck Surgery, ed 5, Philadelphia, 2010, Mosby Elsevier.)*

Table 69-1. Branchial Arch Contributions to the Larynx

BRANCHIAL ARCH	ASSOCIATED NERVE	CARTILAGE/OSSEOUS DERIVATION	MUSCLES DERIVATION
Third	Cranial Nerve IX	Greater Cornu of Hyoid* Epiglottis*	None in larynx
Fourth	Superior Laryngeal Nerve	Thyroid cartilage Cuneiform cartilage Epiglottis*	Cricopharyngeus Cricothyroid muscle
Sixth	Recurrent Laryngeal Nerve	Cricoid cartilage Arytenoid cartilages Corniculate cartilages	Intrinsic musculature of larynx

(* indicates composition from multiple branchial arches)

EMBRYOLOGY

16. **How does the larynx form in utero?**

The larynx begins to form during the fourth week of gestation with the emergence of the laryngotracheal groove. This groove begins just caudal to the fourth branchial arch and forms the beginning of the unified upper aerodigestive tract. As the groove deepens, it begins to separate from the primitive esophagus in a coronal plane with the formation of the esophagotracheal septum. Lung buds will eventually descend from the resultant laryngotracheal diverticulum while the most cranial aspect is destined to form the larynx.

The larynx forms with contributions from the third, fourth, and sixth branchial arches as detailed in Table 69-1 with a few exceptions. The hyoid bone forms with contributions from both the second and third branchial arches. The epiglottis originates from the hypobranchial eminence with contributions from both the third and fourth branchial arches.

Understanding the branchial origins of these structures also helps give insight to laryngeal sensory innervation. As the SLN derives from the same branchial arch as the epiglottis and thyroid cartilages, it follows that the supraglottis and superior aspect of the glottis contain afferent SLN innervation. A similar relationship is found with the RLN carrying sensory innervation from the inferior glottis and subglottis.

The laryngeal framework begins to form around week five of gestation and continues through week nine. Early within that timeframe the epithelium of the larynx fuses and obliterates the previously present lumen. This lumen must reform to allow for proper tracheal and lung development; it does so between weeks seven and ten of gestation. The laryngeal ventricles form as the lumen recanalizes but manages to leave the tissue that ultimately becomes the false and true vocal folds.

17. What in vivo pathologies exist because of derangements of laryngeal embryologic formations?

Two relatively common pathologies can occur secondary to abnormal embryologic development. Laryngeal webbing occurs with failure to recanalize the lumen of the airway. Laryngeal clefts form because of incomplete cleavage of the laryngotracheal diverticulum from the primitive esophagus. As the esophagotracheal septum forms in a cranial direction, the progression may stall. The earlier the stall occurs during embryologic development, the more severe the laryngeal cleft.

While they are explained in depth elsewhere, branchial cleft abnormalities can also involve the hypopharynx. Both third and fourth branchial cleft cysts can originate in the piriform sinus and, in select cases, cautery of the orifice within the sinus or excision can be curative.

18. Are any portions of the laryngeal framework ossified at birth?

No. The hyoid is the earliest structural aspect of the larynx to ossify, occurring around the child's second birthday. The thyroid cartilage begins to ossify in the teenage years and the cricoid cartilage starts to ossify in the third or fourth decade of life. Complete ossification may not occur in all portions of the laryngeal framework but almost always occurs in the hyoid. This lack of ossification may serve as a protective mechanism against laryngeal fracture during childhood.

Bibliography

Bastian RW: Benign vocal fold mucosal disorders. In Flint PW, Haughey BH, Lund VJ, et al, editors: *Cummings Otolaryngology: Head & Neck Surgery*, ed 5, Philadelphia, 2010, Mosby Elsevier.

Hirano M: Structure and vibratory behavior of the vocal folds. In Sawashima M, Cooper FS, editors: *Dynamic Aspects of Speech Production*, Tokyo, 1977, University of Tokyo Press, pp 13–27.

Lee KJ: *Essential Otolaryngology*, ed 9, New York City, 2008, McGraw-Hill.

Netter FH: *Atlas of Human Anatomy, Professional Edition*, ed 5, Philadelphia, 2011, Saunders Elsevier.

Pansky B: *Review of Medical Embryology*, New York, 1982, Macmillian.

Rosen C, Simpson CB: *Operative Techniques in Laryngology*, New York, 2008, Springer.

Sulica L: Voice: anatomy, physiology, and clinical evaluation. In Johnson JT, Rosen CA, editors: *Bailey's Head & Neck Surgery: Otolaryngology*, ed 5, Baltimore, MD, 2014, Lippincott Williams & Wilkins.

Tucker HM: *The Larynx*, Cleveland, OH, 1993, Thieme.

Woodson GE: Laryngeal and pharyngeal function. In Cummings CW, Robbins KT, Schuller DE, editors: *Cummings Otolaryngology: Head and Neck Surgery*, ed 4, Philadelphia, 2005, Elsevier.

CHAPTER 70

LARYNGOSCOPY, BRONCHOSCOPY, AND ESOPHAGOSCOPY

Todd M. Wine, MD

KEY POINTS

1. Laryngoscopy is integral to otolaryngology and is required for both diagnosis and treatment in clinic and in the operating theater.
2. Rigid bronchoscopy is not only diagnostic but also therapeutic, and can be the key tool in an airway emergency.
3. Communication with the anesthesiologist is of utmost importance during laryngoscopy and bronchoscopy to prevent complications.
4. The narrowest part of the pediatric airway is the subglottis, which should be remembered during intubation so that iatrogenic injury can be avoided.
5. Food impaction assessment should be accompanied by esophageal biopsies to rule out eosinophilic esophagitis.
6. Esophageal button battery foreign bodies are true emergencies requiring prompt removal due to the rapid damage that can occur in just 2 to 3 hours.
7. Using a shoulder roll during rigid esophagoscopy can be helpful in achieving a better angle for the esophagoscope to be advanced into the distal esophagus.

Pearls

1. Correct direct laryngoscopy technique greatly enhances visualization of the vocal cords. Always ensure that there are no contraindications to proper neck flexion and head extension (i.e., unstable cervical spine, Down syndrome).
2. Sizing the airway is inaccurate when acute soft tissue edema is present.
3. The proper depth of anesthesia and spontaneous respiration can be assessed in children by watching the abdomen prior to rigid bronchoscopy.

QUESTIONS

1. What are laryngoscopy, bronchoscopy, and esophagoscopy?
   Laryngoscopy is the examination of the larynx. This can be performed indirectly using a head light and mirror and directly using rigid or flexible laryngoscopes. Bronchoscopy is examination of the trachea, bronchi, and its branches performed using either rigid or flexible bronchoscopes. Esophagoscopy is the endoscopic examination of the esophagus and this too may be performed using either flexible or rigid esophagoscopes.
2. When is office laryngoscopy indicated in adults?
   Examination of the larynx in adults is part of the complete physical examination of the head and neck and can be performed using indirect or flexible laryngoscopy. In examining the larynx in an adult, the supraglottis, oropharynx, and hypopharynx are often visualized as well. Examination of the larynx and surrounding anatomic areas are indicated for complaints of dysphonia, chronic cough,

globus sensation, chronic throat discomfort or pain, stridor, neck mass, thyroid mass, and obstructive sleep apnea.

3. **When is office laryngoscopy indicated in children?**
Examining the larynx in children is indicated for stridor, voice abnormalities, and obstructive sleep apnea status post adenotonsillectomy.

4. **What are different types of laryngoscopy?**
Direct laryngoscopy is visualization of the larynx achieved by direct line-of-sight. This requires the use of a laryngoscope to achieve the proper view. The patient usually will be anesthetized, although some patients may tolerate laryngoscopy performed with the use of local and/or regional blocks. Direct laryngoscopy is performed to allow insertion of an endotracheal tube, inspect the larynx in its entirely, and to properly expose a portion of the larynx that requires biopsy or excision of a mass.
Indirect laryngoscopy is visualization of the larynx that involves instruments to achieve an "indirect" view of the larynx. The laryngeal mirror was the first instrument to be used to indirectly direct light from an external source into the larynx providing illumination and visualization of the structures. Indirect laryngoscopy can be limited by a patient's gag reflex. Other forms of indirect laryngoscopy involve the use of angled telescopes (70 or 90 degree) or flexible laryngoscopes to visualize the larynx. Rigid endoscopic evaluation with an angled telescope can achieve a high-definition view of the larynx.
Flexible laryngoscopy is often performed in clinic using a flexible fiber-optic endoscope. The nasal cavity can be treated with a topical decongestant/anesthetic mixture to improve visualization and comfort of the examination. Lubrication of the telescope may aid in comfort as well. Flexible laryngoscopy can also be used to evaluate swallowing in a procedure termed flexible endoscopic evaluation of swallowing (FEES). This procedure involves visualization of the larynx while feeding the patient various consistencies to determine if there is aspiration or penetration of the food bolus into the larynx.
Videolaryngoscopy involves attaching a camera to an angled rigid endoscope or a flexible endoscope to project the image onto a monitor. Digital recording devices can record the video and allow storage of the examination for later visualization or review.
Videolaryngostroboscopy is videolaryngoscopy with the addition of a stroboscope. The stroboscope uses a microphone or EMG activity to detect the fundamental frequency of the vibrating vocal cords. The stroboscope flashes the light source based on the fundamental frequency creating the appearance of vocal cord wave in slow motion. This allows assessment of the mucosal wave of the vocal cord, which can help differentiate various pathologies of the vocal cord.

5. **What are laryngoscopes and how do they differ?**
Laryngoscopes are instruments used to achieve visualization of the larynx while the patient is in the supine position. There are multiple types of laryngoscopes and their designs differ to achieve certain goals. Examples of laryngoscopes optimized for specific functions include an anterior commissure scope (has anterior flare and shorter interdental dimension allowing better view of anterior commissure), bivalved laryngoscopes to approach supraglottic and hypopharyngeal tumors, and slotted laryngoscopes, which allow intubation more easily. Many different types of laryngoscopes are capable of being suspended so that the surgeon may perform surgical procedures using a two-handed technique.

6. **How is flexible laryngoscopy performed?**
Prior to performing this procedure, the patient is counseled on this procedure. Usually, the nose is topically prepared with a combination of a local anesthetic and topical decongestant. Lubrication can be applied to the scope to allow added comfort for the patient. The scope is inserted into the nasal cavity and advanced posteriorly, allowing visualization of the nasopharynx. The scope is directed inferiorly to allow assessment of the oropharynx and then advanced to a position that allows proper assessment of the supraglottis and glottis. Voluntary vocalization and inspiration can confirm normal vocal cord mobility.

7. **What are the proper positions for direct laryngoscopy?**
The proper patient positioning for rigid direct laryngoscopy is the sniffing position with the head extended on the neck and the neck flexed. A shoulder roll is not needed for direct laryngoscopy. To get adequate anterior exposure, sometimes it is necessary to increase the neck flexion further by lifting the head off of the table.

8. **What makes laryngoscopy difficult?**
   Difficult laryngoscopy entails not being able to visualize the larynx well. Factors contributing to this are usually anatomic factors. Trismus (inability to open mouth widely), micrognathia, tumors, infections, and trauma of the oropharynx and supraglottis can make laryngoscopy difficult.

9. **How is the laryngoscopic view of the larynx classified?**
   When using an intubating laryngoscope, the view of the glottic opening should be reported. The grade of the view is important to communicate to other medical providers for future care of the patient to minimize risk involved for patients with known difficult laryngeal exposures. Grade I view occurs when the entirety of the vocal cords can be seen. Grade II occurs with a partial view of the true vocal cords. Grade III view occurs when only the arytenoids are viewed. Grade IV occurs when no laryngeal structures are visualized.

10. **What should be reported while doing direct laryngoscopy that is part of the head and neck examination?**
    As otolaryngologists we are trained to examine the larynx in its entirety. This is most important in our head and neck cancer patients. A thorough examination includes visualization of the base of tongue, vallecula, epiglottis (remarking on the lingual and laryngeal surfaces), supraglottis, glottis, and hypopharynx.

11. **What are the potential complications of direct laryngoscopy?**
    Injury to anything from the lips to the larynx can occur. Care must be used to not pinch the lips between the laryngoscope and the teeth. Teeth can be inadvertently chipped, loosened, fractured, or avulsed. A tooth guard is used to help minimize dental injury. Difficult exposure of the larynx increases the chance of tooth injury. Should dental injury be recognized intraoperatively, immediate dental consultation should be sought. Other risks include injury to the vocal cords. Additionally, laryngospasm can occur, which inhibits adequate ventilation and, if not treated properly, and can lead to a respiratory arrest.

12. **What is the narrowest portion of the airway in adults and children?**
    In adults the narrowest portion of the airway occurs at the glottis, whereas in children the narrowest portion is the subglottis. The significance of this is that as the airway grows in children, different sizes of endotracheal tubes are appropriate and knowing how to estimate and measure this becomes critical.

13. **How is the appropriate endotracheal tube estimated?**
    In children, the appropriate size endotracheal tube can be estimated by age. In children 2 years old and above, the formula $(4 + \text{age})/4$ can estimate the appropriate size. In children under 2 years of age, it must be remembered that a newborn should be intubated with a 3.5 ETT. As an infant approaches one year of age, a 4.0 ETT becomes appropriate. By 2 years of age, a 4.5 ETT is appropriate. In adults, most men can accept an 8.0 ETT and women can tolerate a 7.5 ETT.

14. **How is subglottic airway size measured?**
    Subglottic airway sizing is determined by performing a leak test. Performing a leak test requires insertion of a series of uncuffed ETTs and viewing and/or listening for a leak to occur around the endotracheal tubes. This is meant to determine the degree of narrowing of a firm stenosis of the subglottic airway. Usually, the first tube is 0.5 size smaller than what is expected for the patient's age. There should be a free leak around the tube if the airway is an appropriate diameter. Progressively larger tubes are placed until there is no leak of air at 25 cm H_2O or less. The largest tube that allows a leak is considered the size of the airway. Based on the patient's age and corresponding ETT that fits, the degree of stenosis can be determined using the scale created by Dr. Myer and Cotton (Table 70-1).

15. **When is bronchoscopy indicated?**
    Bronchoscopy is indicated whenever symptoms suggest that disease or evidence of disease may be present in the tracheobronchial tree. The symptoms present will determine the goals of the procedure. In infants and children, indications for bronchoscopy are usually related to stridor, suspected foreign body aspiration, and other diseases of the lower airway and lung parenchyma. In adults, bronchoscopy is most often performed when there is hemoptysis, concern for neoplasm, and any other prolonged respiratory disease. In both children and adults, rigid bronchoscopy is vital to achieving success in difficult airway situations when direct laryngoscopy fails. The rigid

Table 70-1. Percent Subglottic Stenosis by Endotracheal Tube Size

Patient Age		Endotracheal Tube Size 2	2.5	3	3.5	4	4.5	5	5.5	6
Premature	No Detectable Lumen	40								
		58	30			No Obstruction				
0–3/12		68	48	26						
3/12–9/12		75	59	41	22					
9/12–2		80	67	53	38	20				
2		84	74	62	50	35	19			
4		86	78	68	57	45	32	17		
6		89	81	73	64	54	43	30	16	
Grade	**IV**	**III**			**II**		**I**			

With permission, table from Myer CM, O'Connor DM, Cotton RT: Proposed grading system for subglottic stenosis based on endotracheal tube sizes. Ann Otol Rhinol Laryngol 103:319–323, 1994.

bronchoscope can be used as a tool to bypass sites of obstruction. If rigid bronchoscopy cannot obtain an airway, a surgical airway is needed in the form of emergent tracheotomy or cricothyrotomy.

16. **What are different types of bronchoscopy?**
Bronchoscopy can be performed using a rigid or a flexible bronchoscope. Historically, rigid bronchoscopy is the older of the two techniques and was formerly termed open bronchoscopy. Rigid bronchoscopes are usually equipped with ventilation ports and also can be termed ventilating bronchoscopes. Compared with a flexible bronchoscope, use of a rigid bronchoscope is potentially more traumatic and usually requires a deeper plane of anesthesia. When coupled with a Hopkins rod telescope, rigid bronchoscopy allows a more high-definition view of the airway compared to flexible bronchoscopy. In addition to this advantage, rigid bronchoscopy allows ventilation (can be used in emergency situations to secure airway) and a larger working port, which can allow more efficient removal of foreign bodies or mucosal plugs. Flexible bronchoscopy is performed with a flexible endoscope that can be inserted into the airway under light sedation. Thus, a primary advantage is improved assessment of dynamic airway function, allowing a better assessment of conditions such as tracheobronchomalacia. Another advantage is the ability to assess smaller and more distal bronchi. *Bronchoalveoloar lavage* consists of instilling sterile sodium chloride into a terminal bronchus and suctioning it out to assess the biochemical nature of the distal airways and alveoli. This fluid can be used to assess for presence of chronic aspiration and the microbiology of the lung. Biopsies and dilations are other procedures that can be performed during both types of bronchoscopy.

17. **What abnormalities can be seen during bronchoscopy?**
Masses of the trachea or bronchi are readily noted during bronchoscopy. Other abnormalities include stenosis, cobblestoning, thick secretions, compression of the airway from an external source, and malacia. In adults, stenosis is most likely posttraumatic in origin. Whereas the same is true in children, other possibilities of stenosis include congenital subglottic stenosis and long segment tracheal stenosis due to complete tracheal rings,

18. **How do tracheal dimensions vary with age?**
At 0 to 2 years of age the trachea averages 5.4 cm in length. By 16 to 18 years of age, it has more than doubled in length at 12.2 cm. During that time, the diameter increases threefold, while the cross-sectional area increases by sixfold.

19. **What are embryologic abnormalities of the trachea?**
Innominate artery compression is an anterior vascular compression that can severely limit the size of the airway. It can cause reflex apnea and recurrent respiratory infections. When severe, it can be treated with aortopexy or reimplantation of the innominate artery. Complete tracheal rings can occur at an isolated ring or may include anything up to the entire length of the trachea. Usually, there is a long segment tracheal stenosis and surgical treatment is necessary.

20. **What are the keys to rigid bronchoscopy removal of airway foreign bodies?**
Being prepared is of utmost importance in airway foreign body cases. Proper communication must occur between the operating room staff, anesthesiologist, and surgeon at all times to assure the optimal outcome. Having the appropriately sized rigid bronchoscope and a backup that is one size smaller is essential. The instruments to retrieve the foreign body (endoscopic peanut grasper, alligator forceps, etc.) must be tested to ensure they can fit through the age-appropriate bronchoscope.

21. **What are indications for esophagoscopy?**
Espophagoscopy is indicated to investigate symptoms pertaining to the esophagus. In children, dysphagia for solids, refractory reflux, food impaction, and foreign bodies are the main indications for esophagoscopy. In adults, dysphagia, gastroesophageal reflux disease, hematemesis, and atypical chest pain are indications for esophagoscopy.

22. **What are different types of esophagoscopy?**
Flexible esophagoscopy is performed with a flexible endoscope that usually has a port for insufflation of air (helps aid visualization via distension), suction, and irrigation. It can be used to biopsy, cauterize bleeding, dilate stenosis using a balloon catheter, and remove foreign bodies. Flexible transnasal esophagoscopy is similar to traditional flexible esophagoscopy except that the scope is thinner (to allow transnasal insertion) and can be tolerated by the awake patient. This has been increasingly used in the office setting for adult patients primarily. Rigid esophagoscopy is a rigid hollow tube that is inserted into the esophagus to visualize the mucosa of the esophagus. The visualization can occur unaided or with the help of a Hopkins rod telescope, which greatly enhances the view. Like flexible esophagoscopy, biopsies, dilation, and foreign body removal can occur using this modality.

23. **What are potential complications of esophagoscopy?**
Trauma to lips, tongue, throat, and esophagus, fracture or avulsed teeth, aspiration pneumonia, hypotension, arrhythmia, pneumothorax, bleeding, and esophageal perforation. Esophageal perforation can be particularly dangerous if not recognized promptly and can lead to a life-threatening mediastinitis. Symptoms of chest pain and fever should be taken seriously and perforation of the esophagus should be ruled out. If present, prompt treatment is the key to a successful outcome.

24. **When should esophagoscopy be performed after a caustic ingestion?**
Most often, mucosal damage caused by caustic ingestions may continue to occur for some time after the exposure. Esophagoscopy immediately after the ingestion may underestimate the degree of injury. Esophagoscopy after 48 hours may increase the risk of iatrogenic esophageal perforation. Therefore, most sources recommend delaying esophagoscopy until 12 to 48 hours after the ingestion to allow the most accurate identification of degree of injury.

25. **What type of necrosis do acidic and alkaline ingestions induce?**
Acidic caustic ingestion induces a coagulation necrosis. Coagulation necrosis may be helpful in that it creates a coagulum, which actually protects deeper tissues from injury. *Alkaline caustic ingestion causes liquefaction necrosis.* Liquefaction necrosis causes disintegration of tissue, which allows deeper penetration through tissues and therefore is usually associated with more extensive esophageal damage.

26. **What is the grading system used to stage esophageal corrosive injuries?**
Esophageal corrosive injuries are graded on a scale of 0 through IV (Table 70-2). The scale is based on extent of mucosal damage. In general, patients with grade 0 to IIa lesions are able to have oral intake, while IIb to IV require total esophageal rest. No complications are usually associated with Grade 0 to IIa injuries. Frequent complications are noted for Grade IIb to IV lesions including esophageal strictures and full-thickness necrosis.

27. **How do button batteries cause soft tissue injury?**
The primary way that button batteries cause injury is through their ability to conduct an electrolytic current that produces hydroxide. Leakage of alkaline substances can occur in alkaline button batteries, but does not occur with newer lithium button batteries. Lithium button batteries are 3V cells and are more dangerous because they can conduct greater current. Last, the battery can exert physical pressure and mild injury on adjacent tissue. Button battery ingestion is an emergency that

Table 70-2. Grading System for Caustic Injuries of the Esophagus

GRADE	ENDOSCOPIC FINDINGS
0	Normal
1	Edema and hyperemia of mucosa
2a	Friable, hemorrhage, ulcers, erosions, blisters, exudates, membranes
2b	2a + deep or circumferential ulceration
3a	Small scattered necrosis
3b	Extensive necrosis
4	Perforation

From Zargar SA, Kochhar R, Mehta S, et al: The role of fiberoptic endoscopy in the management of corrosive ingestion and modified endoscopic classification of burns. Gastrointest Endosc 37(2):165–9, 1991.

requires immediate removal because severe injury and subsequent mortality can occur with very short exposures.

28. What needs to be ruled out when food impaction occurs in a child?
Food impaction in a child is highly associated with eosinophilic esophagitis. Therefore, while treating the food impaction, esophageal biopsies should be taken to investigate for the possibility of eosinophilic esophagitis.

29. How is eosinophilic esophagitis diagnosed?
Currently, the diagnosis requires 15 eosinophils per high-power field in a tissue sample. Furthermore, the patient should still exhibit this severe eosinphilic infiltrate after being treated with a proton pump inhibitor.

30. Esophageal foreign bodies are most likely to occur at what location in the esophagus?
Most often foreign bodies occur in the region immediately distal to the cricopharyngeus. The cricopharyngeus is a strong concentric muscle and is capable of forcing a foreign body distal to it. The esophagus is often not capable of passing it any further.

31. What is a Zenker's diverticulum?
A pseudo-herniation through a natural weakness in the posterior hypopharyngeal wall, between the oblique and fusiform fibers of the cricopharyngeus or the inferior pharyngeal constrictor and cricopharyngeus, known as the Killian triangle. When small, this pulsion-type diverticulum is asymptomatic. In time, it gradually enlarges and causes progressive dysphagia. Not only do patients complain of food getting stuck, they complain of regurgitation of food products. The diagnosis is confirmed on barium swallow depicting a posterior herniation from the proximal esophagus.

32. How is Zenker's diverticulum treated?
Historically, treatment has consisted of open techniques used to resect, suspend or ligate the diverticulum along with a cricopharyngeal myotomy. Contemporary treatment is an endoscopic Zenker's diverticulectomy. The cricopharyngeal bar is isolated between the blades of a bivalved esophagoscope and the cricopharyngeal bar is divided using an endoscopic stapling device (if the pouch is large enough), laser, LigaSure, or electrocautery.

Bibliography

Contini S, Scarpignato C: Caustic injury of the upper gastrointestinal tract: a comprehensive review, *World J Gastroenterol* 19(25):3918–3930, 2013.

Griscom NT, Wohl EB: Dimensions of the growing trachea related to age and gender, *AJR Am J Roentgenol* 146: 233–237, 1986.

Griscom NT, Wohl EB, Fenton T: Dimensions of the trachea to age 6 years related to height, *Pediatr Pulmonol* 5:186–190, 1989.

Litovitz T, Whitaker N, Clark L, et al: Emerging battery-ingestion hazard: clinical implications, *Pediatrics* 125(6): 1168–1177, 2010.

Myer CM, O'Connor DM, Cotton RT: Proposed grading system for subglottic stenosis based on endotracheal tube sizes, *Ann Otol Rhinol Laryngol* 103(4 Pt 1):319–323, 1994.

Nielsen HU, Trolle W, Rubek N, et al: New technique using Ligasure for endoscopic mucomyotomy of Zenker's diverticulum: diverticulotomy made easier, *Laryngoscope* 124(9):2039–2042, 2014.

Papadopoulou A, Koletzko S, Heuschkel R, et al: Management guidelines of eosinophilic esophagitis in childhood, *J Pediatr Gastroenterol Nutr* 58(1):107–118, 2014.

Zargar SA, Kochhar R, Mehta S, et al: The role of fiberoptic endoscopy in the management of corrosive ingestion and modified endoscopic classification of burns, *Gastrointest Endosc* 37(2):165–169, 1991.

CHAPTER 71

HOARSENESS AND DYSPHONIA

Anju K. Patel, MD and Thomas L. Carroll, MD

KEY POINTS

1. The recurrent laryngeal nerve (RLN) innervates all intrinsic laryngeal muscles except the cricothyroid (innervated by the superior laryngeal nerve (SLN)).
2. The posterior cricoarytenoid muscle (PCA) is the only muscle that actively abducts the true vocal folds.
3. Acute laryngitis is often associated with a viral upper respiratory tract infection and resolves within 1 to 2 weeks without antibiotic therapy.
4. Laryngopharyngeal reflux (LPR) may often coexist with other laryngeal pathologies and rarely is the sole cause of dysphonia. Pepsin, possibly in a non-acid environment, is actively involved with the inflammation caused by LPR.
5. Systemic inflammatory disorders associated with the larynx can be recalled using the acronym "SAW": sarcoidosis (supraglottic), amyloidosis (glottic), and Wegener granulomatosis (subglottic).

Pearls

1. During phonation, the glottis should be in the closed phase for approximately 45% to 50% or more of each vibratory cycle at the most comfortable pitch and loudness. If the closed phase is less than 45% to 50%, glottic insufficiency (GI) exists and causes of GI should be considered.
2. Vocal nodules, often overdiagnosed, are by definition bilateral, symmetric, and occur at the junction of the anterior and middle thirds of the true vocal folds. More likely, when bilateral lesions are seen, a dominant, subepithelial lesion (cyst, polyp, fibrous mass) on one vocal fold opposes a reactive lesion on the other side.
3. Recurrent respiratory papillomatosis (RRP) is primarily caused by HPV types 6 and 11.
4. Muscle tension dysphonia is typically associated with compensation for underlying glottic insufficiency and is unusual as a stand-alone, primary diagnosis.
5. LPR often requires higher, more prolonged courses of acid suppression than does typical GERD. If suspected LPR does not respond to acid suppression, specific testing to rule out nonacid reflux is required to exclude the diagnosis.

QUESTIONS

1. Describe the function of the larynx.
The larynx plays a role in aspiration prevention, respiration, Valsalva, and phonation. The larynx is a complex three-dimensional structure shaped as a triangle anteriorly and transitioning to a circular appearance posteriorly. It consists of numerous cartilages that support both extrinsic and intrinsic muscles as described below and is divided into the supraglottis, glottis, and subglottis (Figure 71-1).

2. What is the mechanism of phonation including the physiology of vocal fold vibration?
There are three phases to phonation: pulmonary, laryngeal, and supraglottic/oral. The pulmonary phase is akin to the motor that drives the voice and creates this via inhalation and exhalation of air. This activity provides the larynx with a column of air for the laryngeal phase. In the laryngeal phase, the vocal folds approximate either voluntarily or involuntarily and then vibrate at certain frequencies as the air rushes past to create a sound that is then modified in the supraglottic/oral phase. Bernoulli's effect is responsible for the passive vibration of the actively approximated vocal folds.

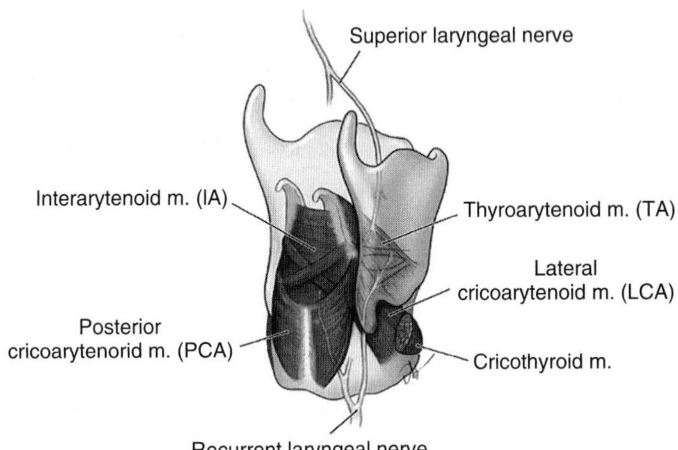

Figure 71-1. Right posterolateral view of cartilages and intrinsic muscles of the larynx with RLN and SLN (internal branch). *(Rosen CA and CB Simpson. Operative Techniques in Laryngology. Berlin: Springer, 2008.)*

When the column of air stops, vibration ceases. Changes in vocal fold length and changes in the tension of the thyroarytenoid (TA) muscle affect pitch. The supraglottis, pharynx and sinonasal cavity resonate the sound produced to create a unique individual voice. Articulation of words is formed by the action of the palate, tongue, lips, and teeth. Dysfunction in any of these levels can lead to voice changes, which may be interpreted as hoarseness by the patient.

3. **What is the difference between hoarseness and dysphonia? What is aphonia?**
Hoarseness is a nonspecific term for change in voice quality, typically associated with a rough or harsh sound. Hoarseness is regarded as a symptom of an underlying pathology, and is not a diagnosis. Dysphonia, also a symptom, is an all encompassing term to describe any problem with voice production including the quality of the sound produced, an increase in vocal effort or fatigue, or pain or discomfort with speaking or singing, among others. Aphonia is the inability to produce a voice. Patients with aphonia often speak in a whisper or just move their lips without sound.

4. **How is the underlying cause of a patient's dysphonia complaint diagnosed?**
Clinical history and physical exam including a complete head and neck exam are all part of the initial workup to evaluate a dysphonic patient. In addition, a voice evaluation by a speech-language pathologist (SLP) including acoustic and aerodynamic measures, laryngeal function studies, and stimulability testing (to determine if a patient is a candidate for voice therapy) is routinely performed in most voice centers before or after visualization of the larynx.

The larynx can be visualized with a mirror, a rigid endoscope or a flexible endoscope in the clinic setting. With the exception of a gross mass on the vocal folds, a mirror is typically inadequate to evaluate the larynx in a dysphonic patient. Laryngovideostroboscopy (LVS) is required in the dysphonic patient to rule in or out various pathologies and can be performed with either a rigid or flexible laryngoscope. LVS uniquely allows for analysis of vocal fold vibration including phase closure pattern, amplitude of vibration, symmetry of vibration, periodicity of vibration, and other mucosal wave abnormalities if present. The LVS exam should be recorded and saved for future comparisons.

When the cause of dysphonia is not obvious during a static white light endoscopy, LVS should be performed because structure may be seen but function is not completely evaluated. Rigid LVS allows for high-resolution visualization of the larynx. However, phonation is limited to sustained vowels due to anterior displacement of the tongue, and the ability to assess vocal fold motion is often suboptimal. Flexible LVS allows dynamic visualization of the larynx in its normal position during all forms of speech and singing. With the recent addition of chip-tip camera technology, flexible LVS is becoming the preferred modality to complete all portions of the laryngeal exam: structural, neurologic, and videostroboscopic.

5. **What are pertinent questions in the clinical history of a dysphonic patient? (Include associated laryngeal complaints such as breathing and dysphagia.)**
   - When was the onset of symptoms? What is the duration of symptoms, and is there any progression? Such questions determine whether the process is acute or chronic.
   - Were there any associated events, such as an upper respiratory infection, a trauma, a recent surgery of the head, neck or chest, an intubation, a period of increased demand or overuse of the voice, or an emotional stressor?
   - How has the quality of voice changed? (Raspy, rough, breathy, weak, tightness, change in pitch.) A rough voice may indicate pathology affecting the vocal fold edge while a breathy voice may suggest hypoadduction of the vocal folds due to vocal cord paresis or paralysis. Tightness or pain in the tongue or strap muscles may point to muscle tension dysphonia (MTD) that is primary or, more likely, as a compensation for an underlying pathology (secondary MTD).
   - Is there dysphagia or odynophagia? If present, these symptoms may indicate a problem with the pharynx, esophagus, and/or larynx.
   - Is there a cough? Cough may be associated with laryngopharyngeal reflux (LPR), asthma, allergy, infection or postviral vagal neuropathy. Cancer of the lung with vocal fold paralysis (secondary to recurrent laryngeal nerve involvement) often presents with dysphonia and cough.
   - Is there hemoptysis? This potentially serious symptom may indicate malignancy.
   - Are symptoms of typical allergy (sneezing, itchy or watery eyes, cat sensitivity), LPR (throat clearing, mucus sensation, cough, globus sensation), or gastroesophageal reflux (GERD; heartburn, regurgitation/acid brash, dyspepsia) present?
   - What is the timing of the complaint (i.e., AM or PM)? Does the voice get better or worse as the day goes on? Does the voice fatigue with use?
   - What other medical problems exist? Hoarseness may be associated with underlying hypothyroidism, an autoimmune disorder, and medications that cause drying of the laryngeal mucosa.
   - What are the occupation and habits of the patient? Singers, teachers, other professional voice users, sports fanatics (shouting), and people who eat a diet contributing to LPR are more likely to suffer from benign causes of dysphonia. Smoking and LPR are risk factors for developing laryngeal and esophageal cancer.

6. **Which laryngeal functions are evaluated with the flexible laryngoscopy portion of the exam?**
   Flexible laryngoscopy allows for visualization of the larynx in its physiologic position and when compared to indirect laryngoscopy can provide a more comprehensive dynamic voice evaluation in the office setting. Patients are asked to sit in the sniffing position with the neck flexed and head extended. This position minimizes unnecessary touching and gagging and brings the larynx into ideal position for visualization. Topical decongestants and anesthetics are applied to the nasal cavity prior to the exam to minimize discomfort. The flexible laryngoscope is advanced through the nasal cavity and in addition to the nasal cavity, the nasopharynx, oropharynx, and hypopharynx are evaluated prior to the larynx. The larynx is first observed with the patient breathing quietly, making note of abnormalities in adduction. Next, the patient is asked to produce a sustained "EE" sound and the larynx is evaluated for any lesions, vocal fold abnormality, or atrophy. Continuing the "EE" sound, the patient is asked to slide from low to high pitch and back down. The vocal folds lengthen when moving to a high pitch and shorten when moving to low pitch. SLN palsies present themselves as abnormalities with vocal fold lengthening maneuvers. The patient then alternates between "EE" and a sniff through the nose. These portions of the exam allow better evaluation of vocal fold paralysis. To complete the laryngeal exam, stroboscopy is then performed to evaluate vocal fold motion.

7. **How does stroboscopy generate a slow-motion image of vocal fold vibration?**
   Stroboscopy requires extraction of the frequency of vocal fold vibration via a flat microphone typically held to the patient's neck. The strobe light then shines on the larynx and flashes at specific points in the glottic cycle that are slightly out of phase with the vibration to create the appearance of slow-motion imaging of the vocal folds. Historically, stroboscopy was thought to rely on the phenomenon termed Talbot's Law, which states that images linger on the retina for 0.2 seconds and only five distinct images can be viewed per second. However, it is now accepted that the phenomenon of *flicker-free perception of light intensity*, in which the perception of apparent motion is obtained from sampled images along the glottic cycle, provides the image seen in LVS.

8. **Can you confidently diagnose the etiology of dysphonia without laryngovideostroboscopy?**
Not really, except in cases of gross abnormality. Even in the case of gross abnormality there are often additional findings that are missed without LVS such as subtle motion abnormalities or reactive subepithelial lesions of the opposite vocal fold. It is often difficult to reliably assess anything less than gross motion abnormalities of the vocal folds, such as supraglottic hyperfunction, without LVS. LVS improves diagnostic abilities by over 25% when compared to isolated flexible laryngoscopy and can alter treatment regimens based on these findings.

9. **What are common causes of dysphonia?**
   - **Glottic insufficiency (GI) with secondary, compensatory muscle tension dysphonia (MTD):** gross, incomplete, or complete but short phase closure of the true vocal folds during phonation with resultant loss of air during phonation. Causes for GI include:
     - Paresis or paralysis of one or both true vocal folds with resultant secondary MTD
     - Atrophy of the true vocal folds with resultant secondary MTD
     - Scar of the true vocal fold epithelium/vibratory layer leading to secondary MTD. Sulcus vocalis is a type of TVF scar where the epithelium is scarred to the vocal ligament, thus creating a void of vibration in that area from loss of superficial lamina propria.
   - **Benign phonotraumatic lesions** of the vocal folds: nodules, polyps, cysts, granulomas, and hemorrhage
   - **Malignant and premalignant exophytic epithelial lesions:** leukoplakia (hyperkeratosis, metaplasia, dysplasia), and squamous cell carcinoma. When comparing leukoplakia to erythroplakia, erythroplakia has a higher probability of showing signs of dysplasia or malignancy because it represents a hypervascular lesion (as malignancies often are).
   - **Neurologic disorders:** spasmodic dysphonia, essential tremor, Parkinson's disease
   - **Inflammatory conditions:** laryngopharyngeal reflux, allergy, irritants, and autoimmune diseases
   - **Recurrent respiratory papillomatosis** from incomplete closure and/or scarring of the vocal folds after intervention
   - **Primary MTD:** no underlying glottic insufficiency or other pathology is appreciated on LVS but significant supraglottic hyperfunction is present

10. **What is the difference between acute and chronic laryngitis?**
Acute laryngitis is classically associated with a viral upper respiratory tract infection (URTI) and is one of the most common causes of hoarseness. It is self-limiting and resolves with the URTI symptoms within 1 to 2 weeks. Patients typically do not require antibiotics and improve with hydration and voice rest. Chronic laryngitis is general inflammation of the larynx lasting longer than 4 weeks and is often caused by smoking, voice abuse, fungal infections, or laryngopharyngeal reflux (reflux that causes irritation to the larynx, pharynx, and pulmonary system). The voice usually improves if the irritating factors are removed or treated. This may involve smoking cessation, medical or surgical reflux management, antifungal medications, and voice rest.

11. **What is glottic insufficiency?**
Glottic insufficiency (GI) is the inappropriate escape of air during phonation that leads to incomplete or a complete but short phase closure pattern (approximately 40% to 45% or less of each vibratory cycle in the closed position) as seen on LVS. GI may be gross or subtle and secondary to vocal fold scar, atrophy, paresis or paralysis. Therapeutic goals seek to augment the affected vocal fold(s) to allow for complete, long phase closure during phonation (approximately 45% to 50% or more of the vibratory cycle in closed phase). The presence of benign lesions of the vocal folds often leads to GI.

12. **What are the different treatments for glottic insufficiency?**
   - Voice therapy (often tried first for many causes of dysphonia)
   - Injection augmentation: Office-based injections versus OR injections. Different substances may be injected into the vocal folds including autologous fat, human acellular dermis, hyaluronic acid gel, carboxymethylcellulose gel, and calcium hydroxyapatite gel.
   - Medialization laryngoplasty with insertion of an implant lateral to the vocal fold comprised of a synthetic material such as silastic or Gore-Tex®

13. **What is muscle tension dysphonia (MTD)?**
Muscle tension dysphonia (MTD) is a pathologic condition whereby excessive tension in the extrinsic laryngeal muscles (Figure 71-2) results in an abnormality with physiology/function of the phonatory

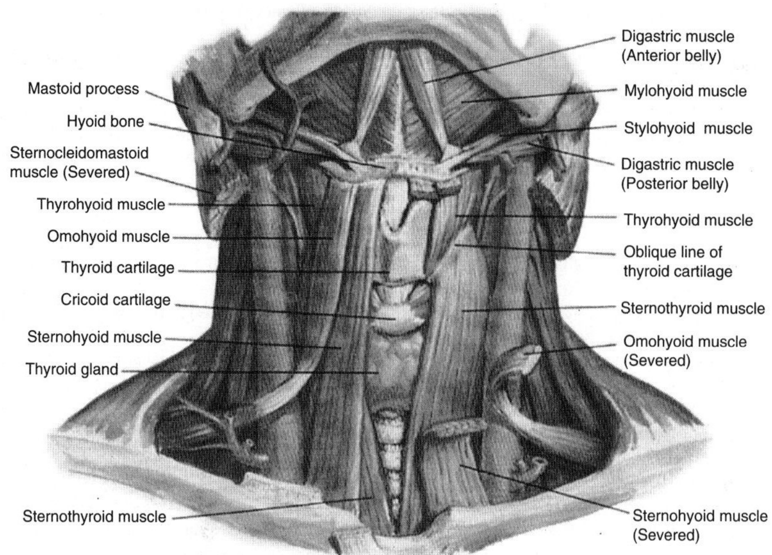

Figure 71-2. Anterior view of extrinsic laryngeal musculature. *(Netter FH. Atlas of Human Anatomy. 5 ed. Philadelphia, PA: Saunders, 2010.)*

mechanism involving the intrinsic laryngeal muscles and/or vocal fold mucosa. The supraglottic laryngeal tissues are often observed to be hyperfunctional in cases of MTD. MTD is divided into primary and secondary types.

14. What is the difference between primary and secondary MTD?

Primary MTD is dysphonia in the absence of organic vocal fold pathology and is associated with excessive supraglottic hyperfunction often in the setting of atypical or abnormal TVF movements during phonation. Secondary MTD occurs in the setting of and as compensation for underlying glottic insufficiency.

15. What is spasmodic dysphonia (SD)?

SD is a focal dystonia affecting the laryngeal muscles during speech. There are two types of SD: **adductor SD** (voice breaks during voiced vowels), where the patient describes a strangled quality to the voice; and **abductor SD** (voice breaks during voiceless consonants such as P and F) where the patient describes an unintentional breathy quality. Symptoms of SD typically improve with singing and when making a "cartoon" voice (ask patient to speak like Mickey Mouse). The treatment of choice for SD is periodic percutaneous botulinum toxin injection into the affected muscle groups under laryngeal electromyographic guidance. In adductor SD the TA/LCA muscle complex is injected, and in abductor SD the PCA is injected.

16. What are systemic diseases associated with hoarseness?

- Neurologic:
  - Hypofunctional disorders: characterized by weak voice, hoarseness, and dysphagia. Examples include Parkinson's disease, motor neuron diseases (amyotrophic lateral sclerosis or ALS, primary lateral sclerosis, postpolio syndrome), neuromuscular junction disorders (myasthenia gravis, Eaton-Lambert disease), and multiple sclerosis
  - Hyperfunctional disorders: commonly have irregular loudness or pitch and straining of the voice, examples include dystonia, essential tremor, and pseudobulbar palsy.
- Inflammatory:
  - Rheumatoid arthritis: cricoarytenoid joint involvement with ankylosis and submucosal vocal fold nodules

- Sarcoidosis: supraglottic (epiglottis most commonly affected) nodular and "turban-like" thickening
- Amyloidosis: laryngeal amyloid deposition most commonly near the glottic level in the true and false vocal folds
- Wegener granulomatosis: classically manifests as subglottic stenosis but may also have glottic changes

17. What benign vocal fold lesions may cause hoarseness?

- **Polyps:** usually unilateral, broad based or pedunculated; found at junction of the anterior and middle thirds of the membranous TVFs with an opposing reactive lesion (fibrous callous on the opposite TVF). They can be hemorrhagic due to acute trauma (Figure 71-3A).
- **Nodules:** always bilateral, symmetric; found at the junction of the anterior and middle thirds of the membranous TVFs (Figure 71-3B).
- **Cysts:** fluid-filled (mucus retention cysts) or cellular (epidermoid cysts); found within the superficial lamina propria with an opposing reactive lesion.
- **Fibrous masses:** Often firm, unilateral, broad based lesions; found at junction of the anterior and middle thirds of the membranous TVF with an opposing reactive lesion
- **Varices and ectasias:** abnormal enlarged or tortuous blood vessels; found primarily on the superior aspect of the middle of the membranous TVFs. The common pathology to identify in singers with intermittent acute dysphonia.
- **Granulomas:** Fleshy masses due to either trauma such as intubation or persistent contact pressure from glottis insufficiency and secondary MTD in the setting of LPR; classically found on the vocal process of the arytenoids, but may appear on the membranous TVF.

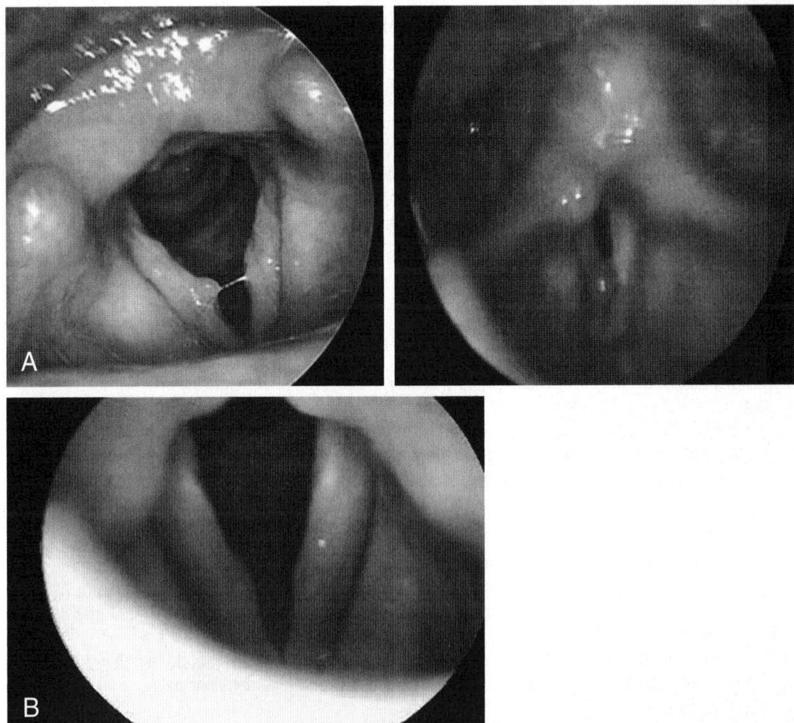

Figure 71-3. A, Right true vocal fold polyp with left reactive lesion: abducted and adducted views. **B,** Nodules.

- **Polypoid corditis/Reinke's edema:** swelling of the superficial lamina propria, associated with smokers and hypothyroidism
- **Recurrent respiratory papillomatosis:** exophytic epithelial lesions caused by HPV (typically types 6 and 11); located anywhere in the larynx, favoring the TVF. Malignant transformation is seen in 1% to 2%.

18. How are nodules different from other benign vocal fold lesions and how are they differentiated?
Nodules are small and discrete lesions located in the membranous portion of the vocal fold, one third the distance from the anterior commissure. Vocal nodules are easily identified because they are paired and symmetric. Seeing bilateral lesions of the vocal folds should not lead to the diagnosis of nodules. Vigilance should be employed during LVS to identify a unilateral dominant phonotraumatic lesion (polyp, cyst or fibrous mass) with an opposing reactive lesion rather than assuming the diagnosis of nodules as the treatment may warrant surgical intervention. Polyps are exophytic, asymmetric, and appear soft and smooth, often coexisting with a reactive lesion of the opposite vocal fold. Vocal fold cysts are mucous retention or epidermoid cysts located in the superficial layer of the lamina propria, usually at the middle third of the vocal fold in the medial and superior aspect and are also found in coordination with a reactive lesion of the opposing vocal fold. Fibrous masses are often firm and broad, significantly limiting the mucosal wave and are seen in the presence of a reactive lesion of the opposing TVF. Vocal process granulomas (VPG) are not actually found on the membranous vocal fold as compared to the other benign lesions presented; VPGs form on the high-pressure contact area of the vocal processes of the arytenoid cartilage. They have a pathognomonic appearance and typically do not require removal/biopsy, but rather regress and become asymptomatic with voice therapy and acid reflux suppressive medications.

19. How do you treat benign vocal fold lesions?
For benign, overuse/phonotraumatic lesions such as nodules, polyps, and cysts, the patient typically undergoes a course of voice therapy and rests the voice when possible. If voice therapy is not successful, or the lesion is too large to have any potential for success, surgical excision of the lesion followed by voice therapy is offered (see below for technique). For RRP, KTP laser excision has emerged as an effective method to preserve voice and avoid injury to the vibratory layer. KTP ablation is typically offered in the OR or in the office depending on the disease burden. Other methods to remove RRP include cold knife excision, CO_2 laser excision, and microdebrider excision. KTP laser is also used successfully in the treatment of TVF ectasias and Reinke's edema. Reinke's edema, when excessive, often requires surgical excision.

20. What is voice therapy and what is the role of voice therapy in the treatment of dysphonia?
Voice therapy consists of vocal and breathing techniques that retrain the patient to produce the best sound with the least injury. It is designed to relieve or "unload" the larynx of hyperfunctional behaviors and instills new muscle memory techniques (akin to a baseball pitcher recovering from an arm injury). It is performed over 4 to 6 weeks by a speech-language pathologist, or voice pathologist, who specializes in voice therapy. It is offered as first-line therapy for anyone with benign laryngeal pathology who is deemed a candidate for voice therapy by a voice pathologist.

21. What are the surgical treatments for benign phonotraumatic vocal fold lesions?
- Microsuspension laryngoscopy (MSL, or suspension microlaryngoscopy) with excision of the offending lesion via medial microflap technique. The incision for the microflap can be made with cold steel or with the CO_2 laser. Dissection then ensues with microinstruments. In some instances the lesion is densely adherent to the overlying epithelium (typical with fibrous mass) or is pedunculated (some polyps) and a microflap cannot be separated from the benign lesion. In these cases the epithelium is removed with the lesion (Figure 71-4).
- Office-based or operative steroid injections for scar, nodules or fibrous masses
- Office-based or operative KTP laser photoangiolysis for vascular lesions (ectasias or hemorrhagic polyps) or deep fibrous masses that are adherent to the epithelium and would result in a significant TVF defect if excised.

22. What is laryngopharyngeal reflux disease?
Laryngopharyngeal reflux (LPR) is the backflow of stomach contents including acid and pepsin into the laryngopharynx. This causes vocal fold and laryngeal inflammation and, in some cases, voice

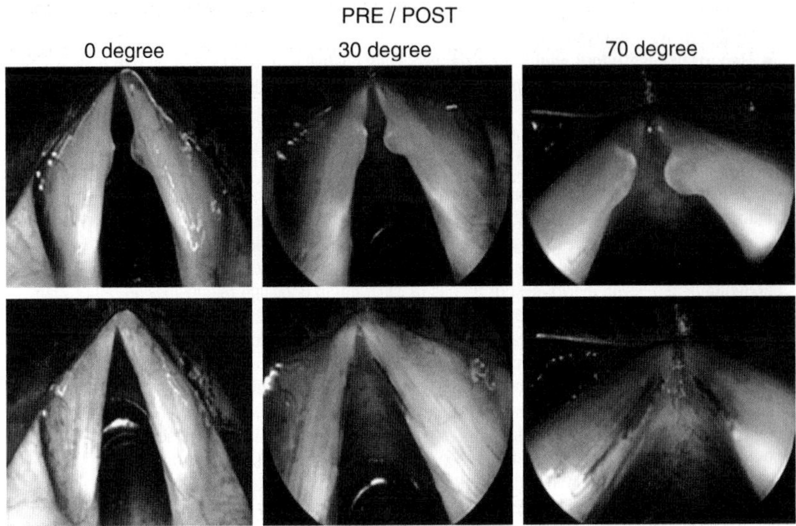

Figure 71-4. MSL view pre/post microflap excision of right TVF polyp and left reactive lesion with three different telescopic views.

change due to exposure of the glottic mucosa to gastric contents. It differs from GERD because it affects a different target end organ, the laryngopharynx as opposed to the esophagus, and presents and is treated differently. LPR is often "silent" because patients don't have typical GERD symptoms like heartburn or feelings of regurgitation. Acid is likely the cofactor that activates pepsin, and therefore LPR should not be considered an acid-only issue.

23. How do you diagnose and treat laryngopharyngeal reflux?

Patients with LPR-induced laryngitis present with symptoms of chronic hoarseness, chronic cough, throat irritation, frequent throat clearing, a mucus sensation in the throat, and globus sensation (a feeling of a lump in the throat and often increased effort with swallowing). All of these symptoms are attributed to LPR, but they overlap dramatically with other laryngeal pathologies that lead to glottic insufficiency and secondary MTD. History alone without an LVS exam is usually insufficient to rule out another etiology for the dysphonia. LPR is often diagnosed too quickly when LVS is not available and studies have shown the high likelihood of an alternative or concurrent diagnosis for the dysphonia that requires intervention. If no other pathology is identified on LVS, a presumed diagnosis is made and empiric PPI trials remain the mainstay of therapy. Most patients respond to diet and lifestyle changes along with acid suppression in the form of high-dose, twice-daily proton pump inhibitors because this removes the acid cofactor. Because the nonacid components of reflux, primarily pepsin, have been demonstrated active even at neutral pH, not all patients will respond to acid suppressive medications. Without dietary changes to avoid acidic foods, dietary acids likely reactivate pepsin that remains in the throat despite medical acid suppression. As with GERD, LPR patients may benefit from sleeping with the head of the bed elevated, avoiding tomato based, spicy or fatty fried foods, and waiting 3 to 4 hours after eating before going to bed.

Bibliography

Altman KW, Atkinson C, Lazarus C: Current and emerging concepts in muscle tension dysphonia: a 30-month review, *J Voice* 19(2):261–267, 2005.

Belafsky PC, Postma GN, Reulbach TR, et al: Muscle tension dysphonia as a sign of underlying glottic insufficiency, *Otolaryngol Head Neck Surg* 127:448–450, 2002.

Carroll TL, Gartner-Schmidt J, Statham MM, et al: Vocal process granuloma and glottal insufficiency: an overlooked etiology?, *Laryngoscope* 120(1):114–120, 2010.

Chang JI, Bevans SE, Schwartz SR: Evidence-based practice management of hoarseness/dysphonia, *Otolaryngol Clin North Am* 45:1109–1126, 2012.

Damrose EJ, Berke GS: Advances in the management of glottic insufficiency, *Curr Opin Otolaryngol Head Neck Surg* 11:480–484, 2003.

Davids K, Klein AM, Johns MM: Current dysphonia trends in patients over the age of 65: is vocal atrophy becoming more prevalent?, *Laryngoscope* 122:332–335, 2012.

Flint PW, Haughey BH, Lund VJ, et al: *Cummings Otolaryngology: Head and Neck Surgery*, ed 5, Philadelphia, 2010, Mosby Elsevier, pp 805–893.

Mau T: Diagnostic evaluation and management of hoarseness, *Med Clin North Am* 94:945–960, 2010.

Mehta DD, Deliyski DD, Hillman RE: Commentary on why laryngeal stroboscopy really works: clarifying misconceptions surrounding Talbot's law and the persistence of vision, *J Speech Lang Hear Res* 53:1263–1267, 2010.

Rosen CA, Lombard LE, Murry T: Acoustic, aerodynamic, and videostroboscopic features of bilateral vocal fold lesions, *Ann Otol Rhinol Laryngol* 109:823–828, 2000.

CHAPTER 72

VOICE DISORDERS AND VOICE THERAPY

Kristina L. Johnston, MA, CCC-SLP and Carly Bergey, MA, CCC-SLP

KEY POINTS

1. Most voice disorders have more than one etiologic factor and medical, surgical, and behavioral therapies may be warranted singly or in combination at any time.
2. Therapists should not apply the "cookie cutter" therapy style. Speech language pathologists (SLPs) should use all management techniques that are appropriate to obtain optimal treatment outcomes.
3. A multidisciplinary team may include otolaryngologists, gastroenterologists, neurologists, speech-language pathologists, and singing/vocal coaches. Additionally, for people who use their voice professionally, you may need to work with managers and producers to provide the best care possible.
4. The voice evaluation includes observation of patients' respiratory, phonatory, and resonance functions. When possible, these functions are quantified with instrumentation. Perceptual judgments are included in the speech-language pathologist's voice evaluation as are patient perceptions of their disorder.
5. Management of paradoxical vocal fold motion (PVFM)/vocal cord dysfunction (VCD) requires a multidisciplinary approach necessitating ongoing communication between the speech-language pathologist, otolaryngologist, and other relevant medical professionals. The speech-language pathologist is an integral member of this team and provides respiratory retraining, counseling, and voice therapy, when appropriate.

Pearls

1. Although the otolaryngologist has the responsibility to provide medical diagnosis and pharmaceutical/surgical intervention of laryngeal pathologies, a speech pathologist knowledgeable in voice can increase the efficaciousness of voice evaluation and treatment.
2. When surgical management of a voice disorder is necessary for a patient, voice therapy should be considered pre- and post surgery to address maladaptive voice production or phonotraumatic behaviors that may delay recovery or result in relapse.

QUESTIONS

1. What pathologies/conditions are appropriate for a referral to a speech-language pathologist?

Voice therapy can be successful for those patients with the following *functional* etiologies: muscle tension dysphonia, diplophonia, phonation breaks, pitch breaks, falsetto, and functional aphonia.

Voice therapy can be beneficial after medical and/or surgical intervention with the following organic etiologies: vocal nodules or polyps, Reinke's edema, sulcus vocalis, contact ulcers, granuloma, papilloma, spasmodic dysphonia, and leukoplakia. Voice therapy would focus on elimination of any unhealthy vocal compensation such as hard glottal attacks or hyperfunction, elimination of coughing or throat clearing habits, and promotion of improved vocal hygiene and reflux management.

In neurogenic etiologies such as myasthenia gravis and Guillain-Barre, the speech-language pathologist can provide education for compensatory techniques and caregiver education of optimal voicing. Unilateral vocal fold paralysis may improve with voice therapy intervention and can act as a bridge in the case of a spontaneous recovery.

Those patients with hypokinetic dysarthria as seen in Parkinson's disease (PD) are appropriate for therapeutic intervention provided by a speech-language pathologist. Surgical intervention such as deep brain stimulation (DBS) may provide the patient with relief from other symptoms related to PD but it typically does not improve vocal quality. Therefore, voice therapy should be recommended prior to DBS surgery.

Hyperkinetic dysarthria seen in essential tremor and ataxic dysarthria may benefit from trials of voice therapy while spasmodic dysphonia (SD) has seen little evidence that voice therapy is the optimal treatment to improve voice quality. While botulinum toxin injections are the primary approach for treating SD, those patients who follow up with voice therapy have significantly better voice outcomes compared to those who just received injections secondary to retraining of poor compensatory behaviors that developed as a result of the SD.

Mixed dysarthrias can be seen in patients with amyotrophic lateral sclerosis, multiple sclerosis, and traumatic brain injury. The dysarthrias may benefit from voice therapy intervention, recommendations for augmentative or alternative communications, oral prostheses, and dysphagia recommendations as the disease progresses.

2. What medical documentation should a speech-language pathologist have to complete an optimal voice assessment?

Prior to initiation of an evaluation of voice, the patient should complete an otolaryngologic examination. Reports and findings including the following are essential to complete an optimal voice assessment: detailed medical and surgical history, current medication list, past and current laryngeal diagnosis, still images or videos of larynx, results of hearing screening or evaluation, radiologic image interpretation of the head and neck, and results of any swallowing evaluations.

3. What intake information is collected during a speech-language pathologist voice evaluation?

Speech-language pathologists comprehensively evaluate patients with voice utilizing a combination of methods. The main goals of the speech-language pathologist voice evaluation are to:

1. Determine etiologic factors relating to voice disorder
2. Determine severity of voice disorder
3. Determine the clinical plan of care and the expected prognosis

Case history, instrumental and physical assessment, acoustic analysis, and perceptual ratings are typically collected during a speech-language pathology voice evaluation. Speech-language pathologists aim to discover behaviors, environmental factors, patterns of occupational and social voice use, and relevant medical and surgical history that impact the patient's voice. The timing and nature of a patient's voice complaints, for example, are extremely valuable pieces of information that help determine the nature of the patient's disorder. Was onset gradual or sudden? Is the problem consistent or intermittent in nature? The patient's vocal hygiene is also evaluated and discussed.

In addition to collecting a case history, a physical examination of the head and neck and cranial nerve examination are usually conducted by the referring physician and provide valuable information to the evaluating speech-language pathologist. Speech-language pathologists may also conduct an oral mechanism exam, such as the Oral Speech Mechanism Screening Examination, or OSMSE-3 (see chart). This standardized protocol is used to assess the appearance and function of the oral mechanism including the lips, tongue, jaw, teeth, palate, pharynx, velopharyngeal mechanism, breathing, and diadochokinetic rates. The larynx may also be palpated for assessment of range of motion.

Singing voice assessment in vocal performers will also be included when indicated. From amateur singers to professional opera stars, the vocal production of a vocal performer requires additional assessment. Special attention is given to reported vocal effort, voice production across pitch range, and vocal demands of the patient's performing schedule, among other factors.

4. Describe objective measures/evaluation completed during a speech-language pathologist voice evaluation.

Rigid Videostroboscopy or Transnasal Flexible Laryngoscopy: Laryngoscopic evaluation allows the structure and function of the vocal folds to be assessed, imaged, and digitally recorded. In most states, speech-language pathologists with expertise in voice can complete either rigid videostroboscopy or transnasal flexible laryngoscopy with stroboscopy with proper training and physician supervision. The AAO-HNS and American Speech Language and Hearing Association have created a joint position statement outlining the roles of physicians and speech-language pathologists completing this procedure. In that statement it is noted that "physicians are the only professionals qualified and licensed to render medical diagnoses related to the identification of laryngeal pathology as it affects voice." Speech-language pathologists with expertise in voice and specialized training can use laryngoscopy "for the purpose of assessing voice production and vocal function." Laryngoscopy also can be an important tool in helping determine the presence of compensatory vocal behaviors and can be used as a biofeedback tool. Direct observation of vocal folds and vocal fold vibration is an essential component of evaluation, as the laryngeal mechanism can be observed and described.

Quantification of other vocal parameters can be performed using advanced equipment to measure aerodynamic and acoustic properties of voice. As equipment cost and time can be prohibitive for some speech-language pathologists, acoustic analysis of voice offers speech-language pathologists a noninvasive and low-cost method for obtaining a significant amount of patient data. For example, fundamental frequency, pitch range, and vocal intensity can be evaluated. These parameters are, in most cases, clinically significant in voice therapy and are therefore often measured throughout treatment, helping to measure patient progress.

5. **What patient-centered assessments are used during a voice evaluation?**
Throughout voice evaluation, the speech-language pathologist listens and forms an impression regarding the patient's vocal quality, pitch, and vocal intensity (loudness) as a way of describing the patient's voice and to set a baseline of the patient's vocal presentation. The use of digital recording equipment to collect patient speech samples is recommended. Because clinician perception can vary, standardized perceptual rating scales are used to help standardize impressions. The CAPE-V, or the Consensus on Auditory Perceptual Evaluation of Voice, is a tool created by voice professionals to do just that.

Patients' perception of their voice disorder and how it impacts their daily life is another factor that is important to discuss. Quantification of patients' feelings and impressions of their voice can be achieved using additional rating tools. The Vocal Handicap Index (VHI) is one such tool that measures how a voice problem impacts a patient's quality of life. Other scales are available for measuring patient perception including the Singing Voice Handicap Index and The Voice-Related Quality of Life Scale (VRQOL) (Table 72-1).

6. **What are the parameters of voice that can be affected?**
The three parameters in which patients have vocal complaints are vocal pitch, loudness, and quality.

7. **What are the respective therapeutic interventions for vocal pitch, loudness, and quality?**
There are many therapeutic techniques that can be applied to improve vocal pitch, loudness, and quality. It may be appropriate to use one or more techniques during a course of voice therapy,

Table 72-1. Voice Handicap Index-10

F1	My voice makes it difficult for people to hear me.	0 1 2 3 4
F2	People have difficulty understanding me in a noisy room.	0 1 2 3 4
F8	My voice difficulties restrict personal and social life.	0 1 2 3 4
F9	I feel left out of conversations because of my voice.	0 1 2 3 4
F10	My voice problem causes me to lose income.	0 1 2 3 4
P5	I feel as though I have to strain to produce voice.	0 1 2 3 4
P6	The clarity of my voice is unpredictable.	0 1 2 3 4
E4	My voice problem upsets me.	0 1 2 3 4
E6	My voice makes me feel handicapped.	0 1 2 3 4
P3	People ask, "What's wrong with your voice?"	0 1 2 3 4

based on patient need and therapeutic response. Patient-centered techniques that focus on increasing self-awareness, the practice of good vocal hygiene, counseling, negative vocal practice, redirection of phonation (coughing, throat clearing, laughing, trilling) are used to improve patient understanding of vocal parameters. Additional respiratory training, relaxation, yawn-sigh, laryngeal massage, and digit manipulation are helpful techniques for improvement of all parameters of voice secondary to hyperfunction. Last, changes in loudness, chant talking, chewing, resonance, confidential voice, and head positioning are valuable techniques to elicit optimal voicing.

8. **Describe common stretches and massage techniques used to decrease laryngeal musculoskeletal tension.**
   If laryngeal tension is a primary or secondary cause of dysphonia, then release of tension provides a means of regaining optimal voicing. Stretches of the neck, shoulders, torso, jaw, and tongue as well as laryngeal massage provide release of extrinsic muscle tension (Table 72-2). Stretches and massage should be completed at least once daily.

9. **What are optimal reflux precautions?**
   The presence of gastroesophageal reflux disease (GERD) and laryngopharyngeal reflux (LPR) are commonly present in those patients who present with laryngologic complaints. While treatment via behavioral, pharmacologic, and surgical means can have benefit toward improving vocal quality, a speech-language pathologist (SLP) can incorporate education of behavioral strategies into the session. Behavioral strategies include but are not limited to: elevating the head of the bed, avoiding overeating, remaining upright for at least 60 minutes after eating, not exercising after eating, decreasing consumption of caffeine, alcohol, and carbonated drinks, avoiding foods that can trigger acid, weight reduction, avoiding tight clothing, taking medication appropriately, and avoiding drinking excessive quantities of water right before bed.

10. **What is vocal hygiene?**
   Vocal hygiene is a term that refers to the ongoing maintenance of a patient's vocal health. The vocal health of patients with voice disorders is a high priority for voice therapists and often a continuing focus of voice therapy. The core issues that surround vocal health include adequate hydration, discussion and elimination of excessive caffeine and alcohol intake, optimal nutrition, elimination and behavioral management of laryngeal irritants such as postnasal drainage and allergies, laryngopharyngeal reflux, and identification and elimination of phonotraumatic behaviors including

Table 72-2. Head and Neck Stretches

AREA	DESCRIPTION
Neck	Head side to side Head forward and backward (chin up and chin down positions) Looking over each shoulder Yawn-sigh
Shoulders	Shoulder shrugs Shoulder rolls: forward and backward
Torso	Reach up to ceiling, lean to the sides Clasp hands in front of the body and stretch Clasp hands behind body and stretch
Jaw	Massage at masseter muscle and at the TMJ Grab jaw and gently pull it down, release tongue
Tongue	Stretch tongue out as far as possible Tenderize: gently bite forward and backward on your tongue
Laryngeal Massage	Place fingers on thyroid notch Feel the top edge of the thyroid cartilage with your thumb and middle finger. Press fingers inward to feel the thyrohyoid space, feeling the lower border of the hyoid bone. Gently massage and pull down to unlock tension of the extrinsic musculature.

chronic cough and throat clearing. Poor vocal hygiene contributes to vocal pathology and speech-language pathologists aim to educate patients about the benefits of optimal vocal health. Adherence to optimal vocal health behaviors contributes greatly to success of voice therapy.

11. **What are common voice therapy goals for a patient with muscle tension dysphonia?**
When a patient is referred for behavioral management of muscle tension dysphonia (MTD), goals are created to reduce hyperfunctional or hypofunctional vocal production that contributes to laryngeal muscle tension. As patients with MTD often demonstrate visible signs of increased muscle activity in the head and neck, commons goals for a patient include implementation of passive and active laryngeal, head, and neck stretches. Additionally, management techniques can include biofeedback, improved airflow with speech at the word, phrase, sentence, and conversational levels, achievement of easy vocal onset, use of resonant voice therapy techniques or circumlaryngeal massage. Additionally, behaviors that contribute to phonotrauma such as yelling or chronic throat clearing are discussed and eliminated. The role of stress and its impact on voice is often an important component to examine and discuss for patients with MTD. In some cases, referral for psychosocial management of voice disorder is indicated.

12. **What is resonant voice therapy and when is it indicated?**
Resonant voice therapy techniques aim to achieve optimal vocal resonance in speech with balanced respiratory effort and articulatory control. Dr. Verdolini Abbott developed a formal, programmatic approach to resonant voice therapy she termed "Lessac-Madsen Resonant Voice Therapy" or LMRVT, as a nod to the contributions of Dr. Arthur Lessac and Dr. Mark Madsen to the voice community. The basic goals of LMRVT include achieving a target laryngeal configuration involving vocal production that results in the strongest voice with the least amount of respiratory effort and stress impact on the vocal folds. Thirty- to 45-minute sessions occur once to twice weekly and patients work through a hierarchy of resonant voice tasks with an emphasis on sensory processing and variable practice. These include discussion of vocal hygiene and provision of stretches, along with resonant voice exercises that include speech tasks incorporating resonant production in a variety of functional settings such as in background noise, while discussing emotional topics, or over the telephone.

13. **What is the best therapeutic option for voices affected by Parkinson's disease?**
Common vocal traits of those diagnosed with Parkinson's disease (PD) include monopitch, a weak or breathy voice, vocal tremor, and decreased speech intelligibility. The Lee Silverman Voice Therapy (LSVT) Loud has provided Level 1 efficacy data outcomes for the improvement in vocal quality, intensity, and speech intelligibility in patients with idiopathic PD. Intensive therapy is completed 4 days a week over 4 consecutive weeks with daily homework focusing on 5 integral concepts: (1) think loud; (2) high effort across the speech system; (3) intensive treatment; (4) recalibrating sensory deficits; (5) quantifying improvements.

14. **Discuss treatment for paradoxical vocal fold motion (PVFM)/vocal cord dysfunction (VCD).**
Initial treatment for PVFM/VCD includes making of speech sounds, "s breathing," and "f breathing," which directs emphasis away from the respiratory system therefore relaxing the larynx and dissipating the attack. Additional maneuvers such as panting (rapid shallow breathing) and/or yawning to open up the oropharynx have also been implemented with some success. While these maneuvers may be effective for some patients, others find them ineffective. Pursed lip breathing has also been documented as a successful maneuver to dissipate episodes of PVFM/VCD. The patient is first instructed to relax upper body tension and use diaphragmatic breathing. The patient should take a gentle but short sniff (1 second) via the nose/mouth and then gently exhale via pursed lips (2 to 3 seconds). Using pursed lip breathing allows the building of back pressure to open and relax the airway, reversing the episode of PVFM/VCD. The application of PLB is tailored to the individual and may be used for retraining, pretreating, and the moments of attacks.

15. **What is a speech-language pathologist's role with patients with laryngeal cancer?**
A speech-language pathologist can provide patients who are postsurgical and postradiotherapy with vocal techniques to improve voicing, as well as promotion of vocal hygiene. Therapeutic outcomes are also impacted by the degree to which the mucosal wave has been preserved.

A speech-language pathologist should also be contacted prior to treatment of laryngeal cancers for education and counseling of dysphagia. Patients typically benefit from ongoing therapy during and after surgical and radiologic treatment.

If a patient is to undergo a laryngectomy, a speech-language pathologist is an essential part of the medical team because laryngectomy alters respiration, swallowing, and speech. The SLP can also provide education, recommendations, and training/therapy of postlaryngectomy communication options including esophageal speech, electrolarynx, and tracheoesophageal voice restoration.

16. **What are hypernasality, hyponasality, and assimilative nasality?**
Hypernasality is an excessive and inappropriate amount of perceived nasal cavity resonance during phonation. Velopharyngeal dysfunction (VPD) or velopharyngeal insufficiency (VPI) are terms used to describe this phenomenon whether due to impaired motion of the VP mechanism, tissue insufficiency or both. Characteristics of this include inappropriate nasal emissions, decreased intraoral pressure, and increased nasal resonance during speaking tasks.

Hyponasality is reduced nasal resonance for /m/, /n/ and "ing" sounds. This is typically as a result of an anatomic obstruction, including but not limited to large adenoids/tonsils, deviated septum, choanal atresia, nasal cavity turbinate swelling, or allergic rhinitis. Articulation substitutions of /b/, /d/, and /g/ are typically seen.

Assimilative nasality appears when the speaker's vowels or voiced consonants present as nasal when adjacent to nasal consonants. This occurs because the velopharyngeal port opens too soon and remains open inappropriately. This may be due to faulty speech patterns or an exaggerated regional dialect.

17. **What should be completed for a clinical evaluation of nasal resonance disorders?**
Patients with resonance disorders are evaluated in a similar manner to patients with other voice disorders. Clinicians should listen carefully to voice during spontaneous conversation, vowels in isolation, and sentences loaded with only oral phonemes and sentences loaded with nasal phonemes. Speech samples loaded with oral phonemes or nasal phonemes help the listener distinguish between hyponasality, hypernasality, and assimilative nasality. Another informal screening tool involves having the patient say these two sentences while pinching the nares shut: "My name means money" and "Mary made lemon jam." If the sentence produced sounds "plugged" with both open and occluded nares, the patient has a hyponasal voice quality. If there is a significant difference between the two sentences, hypernasality may be suspected. Stimulability testing, articulation testing, and oral examination are also included in a patient with a resonance disorder.

18. **What additional laboratory diagnostics should be completed for a thorough nasal resonance disorders evaluation?**
Various aspects of nasal resonance are measured. Aerodynamic instrumentation includes pressure transducers and pneumotachometers that measure relative air pressures and airflows emitted simultaneously from the nasal and oral cavities during speech. Acoustic measures may include use of a Nasometer, a noninvasive microcomputer-based system that measures the relative amount of oral to nasal acoustic energy in an individual's speech. The ratio of oral intensity to nasal intensity is described as nasalance. Spectrography may also be used as part of acoustic analysis. Radiographic instruments and visual probing via endoscopy are other available instruments that can be used to describe the appearance and function of speech mechanisms, such as the velopharyngeal mechanism during speech.

19. **What are treatment options for hypernasality?**
Treatment approaches for a person with hypernasal voice depends on organic or functional causes of the underlying hypernasality. If functional causes exist, voice therapy will be initiated with focus on altering tongue position during speech, change of loudness, auditory feedback, establishing optimal pitch, counseling, opening of mouth, and respiration training. When a physical inadequacy of the velopharyngeal port is suspected, the patient may be referred to an otolaryngologist for surgical options or a prosthodontist to determine the necessity of a palatal lift, obturator, or prosthesis. The speech-language pathologist shares the results of the patient evaluation and can make recommendations related to optimal surgical approach or to suggest which dental appliances may work best for the patient.

20. **What are treatment options for hyponasality?**
Appropriate medical therapy should precede voice therapy for hyponasality to rule out and manage organic causes such as severe nasopharyngeal obstruction or infection. When indicated, voice therapy for increasing nasal resonance may include auditory feedback, counseling, nasal-glide stimulation, and focus of directing tone into a facial mask with speech.

BIBLIOGRAPHY

American Speech-Language-Hearing Association: *The roles of otolaryngologists and speech-language pathologists in the performance and interpretation of strobovideolaryngoscopy [Relevant Paper]*. Available from www.asha.org/policy, 1998.

Boone DR, McFarlane SC, Von Berg SL: *The Voice and Voice Therapy*, ed 7, Boston, 2005, Pearson.

Hicks M, Brugman SM, Katial R: Vocal cord dysfunction/paradoxical vocal fold motion, *Prim Care* 35:81, 2008.

Hodges H: Speech therapy for the treatment of functional respiratory disorders. In Anbar RD, editor: *Functional Respiratory Disorders When Respiratory Symptoms Do Not Respond to Pulmonary Treatment*, New York, 2012, Humana Press, p 251.

Huber J, Stathopoulos E, Ramig L, et al: Respiratory function and variability in individuals with Parkinson disease: pre and post Lee Silverman Voice Treatment (LSVT®), *J Medical Speech-Lang Pathol* 11:185, 2003.

Rosen CA, Lee AS, Osborne J, et al: Development and validation of the Voice Handicap Index-10, *Laryngoscope* 114(9):1549–1556, 2004.

Sapienza C, Hoffman Ruddy B: *Voice Disorders*, ed 2, San Diego, 2013, Plural, pp 59–61, 75–84, 87–93, 95–97, 103–105, 217–220, 224.

Stemple JC, Glaze LE, Gerdeman Klaben B: *Clinical Voice Pathology Theory and Management*, ed 3, San Diego, 2000, Singular.

St. Louis KO, Rusello D: *Oral Speech Mechanism Screening Examination*, ed 3, Austin, 2000, PRO-ED.

Verdolini Abbott K: *Lessac-Madsen Resonant Voice Therapy Clinician Manual*, San Diego, 2008, Plural.

COUGH

Ronald Balkissoon, MD

CHAPTER 73

KEY POINT

1. The American College of Chest Physicians (ACCP) current guidelines define acute and chronic cough, and outline treatment recommendations for these disorders.

Pearl

1. The nucleus tractus solitarius is a key area for modifying cough through both long-term and short-term neuroplasticity.

QUESTIONS

Definitions

1. **How does the definition of chronic cough differ from acute cough and subacute cough?**
   The American College of Chest Physicians (ACCP) current guidelines define acute cough as symptoms lasting less than 3 weeks, subacute cough as symptoms lasting 3 to 8 weeks, and chronic cough as symptoms lasting longer than 8 weeks.

2. **What is meant by the terms "unexplained cough" and "neuropathic cough"?**
   "Unexplained cough" describes a cough that persists despite a comprehensive diagnostic evaluation, exclusion of common causes, and appropriate therapeutic trials for common causes of cough. The term unexplained cough was chosen over idiopathic cough because it implies that there may be as yet unidentified causes for the cough or that it may be multifactorial. *Cough hypersensitivity syndrome* has been applied to individuals that appear to have common causes for cough and despite appropriate therapy have a persistent cough response. The underlying pathophysiology for this remains undefined but has been proposed to follow mechanisms similar to those for chronic pain (lower threshold for stimulation of afferent pain receptors). This has also led to the term neuropathic cough being applied to this group of patients.

3. **What is the burden of illness related to chronic cough?**
   It has been estimated that annually in the United States approximately 40% of the 30 million outpatient pulmonary clinic visits are for chronic cough. Approximately 3.6 billion dollars are spent annually on over-the-counter (OTC) medications for chronic cough in the United States.

Pathophysiology of Chronic Cough

4. **What are the different types of afferent cough receptors?**
   Chemoreceptors react to things such as water, ammonia, carbon dioxide, sulfur dioxide, cigarette smoke, milk, gastric contents, and capsaicin. Mechanoreceptors respond to pressure (touch), flow, proprioception, and laryngeal muscle contraction. Laryngeal irritant receptors include nociceptive C fibers and G-protein coupled receptors (GPCR) plus the ion channel receptors Transient receptor potential vanilloid (TRPV-1) and Transient receptor potential ankyrin 1 (TRPA-1). These latter two are actually ion channels in the membrane (Figure 73-1).

5. **Where are these cough receptors distributed?**
   There is a network of afferent sensory receptors found in the subepithelial layer throughout the respiratory tract as well as the GI tract and cardiovascular system that are all capable of triggering

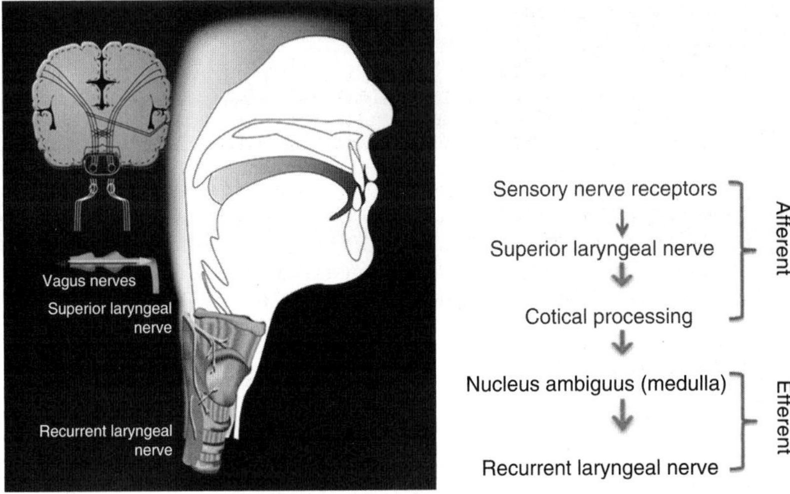

Figure 73-1. Cough reflex neuronal connections.

cough with appropriate and sufficient stimulus. The larynx, trachea, and lower airways have a rich network of cough reflex afferent nerves that are capable of inducing cough. The main inputs are from the cough receptors themselves, slowly adapting pulmonary stretch receptors (SAR), rapidly adapting pulmonary stretch receptors (RAR), bronchial and pulmonary fibers (C-fibers), and Aδ fibers.

6. Describe the physiology of the cough reflex.
When an intense stimulus depolarizes the afferent receptor nerve terminal over the threshold, voltage gated sodium and potassium channels (Kv) are opened and trigger action potentials. Activation of C-fibers can cause mast cell degranulation and release of histamine and bradykinin leading to airway edema and activation of mechanoreceptors and neuropeptides with resultant neurogenic inflammation. The afferent input is relayed to the brainstem where the information can be centrally processed and modulated further before the efferent output leads to the elicitation of a cough. The increased sensitivity of the cough reflex seems to be driven by a complex interaction between C-fiber receptors, rapidly adapting receptors, and the peripheral and central nervous system that remains poorly understood. The nucleus tractus solitarius seems to be a central area for modifying cough through both long-term and short-term neuroplasticity (see Figure 73-1).

7. What role does the nose play in the pathophysiology of chronic cough?
Allergies, infections, and irritants are capable of inducing inflammation in the nose that can lead to symptoms of sneezing, nasal itching, rhinorrhea, and nasal blockage. These responses are likely mediated by trigeminal sensory nerves. Interestingly, it has been shown that intranasal administration of histamine or capsaicin does not cause coughing, but does increase the sensitivity to various tussigenic aerosols.

8. What are the neurologic connections between the gastrointestinal tract and the respiratory tract that contribute to the cough reflex?
Vagal afferents from the esophagus and respiratory tract converge in the brainstem. Esophageal afferents may be triggered simply by significant acid secretion into the esophagus, thus triggering a cough response. Previous studies have demonstrated that acid infusion into the esophagus induces bronchoconstriction, presumably through a vagally mediated esophageal-tracheobronchial reflex, and dual channel pH monitoring correlated with cough both in terms of proximal and distal acid reflux. Further, acid infused into the distal esophagus of patients with chronic cough increased the frequency of coughing and cough reflex sensitivity, a phenomenon that can be blocked with topical lidocaine.

Etiology of Chronic Cough

9. **What are the common causes of chronic cough?**
   Upper airway cough syndrome (previously referred to as postnasal drip), lower airway conditions including bronchial asthma, cough variant asthma, eosinophilic bronchitis, and atopic cough and gastroesophageal reflux disease (GERD) are the most common causes (Box 73-1). Atopic cough is defined as a cough that manifests in atopic individuals without bronchial hyper-responsiveness that responds well to antihistamines alone without inhaled steroids, whereas the other lower airway conditions typically require inhaled steroids. These conditions often coexist in various combinations and failure to address and treat all concurrently may be one of the major impediments to successful amelioration of chronic cough.

10. **What are less common causes of chronic cough?**
   Less common causes include chronic bronchitis, chronic infection, interstitial lung disease, angiotensin converting enzyme inhibitors, cardiac diseases including congestive heart failure and mitral valve disorders, and stimulation of hairs in the external auditory canal (Arnold's nerve reflex). There have been several occupational and environmental exposures also associated with chronic cough (Box 73-2).

11. **What distinguishes upper airway cough syndrome from postnasal drip?**
   What previously was referred to as chronic postnasal drip has more recently been labeled as upper airway cough syndrome (UACS) in recognition of the fact that posterior nasal drainage may result from several conditions of the sinuses and nasal passages (Box 73-3). Inflammatory signaling and possible neurogenic mechanisms originating in the upper airway may contribute to development of cough in addition to the physical and possible chemical irritation of posterior nasal drainage. While allergic rhinitis is often a culprit, other common causes include chronic rhinosinusitis, nasal polyposis, chronic bacterial overgrowth, fungal disease, anatomic anomalies, and postsurgical changes.

   Secondly, the "unified airway" hypothesis proposes that processes that cause upper airway congestion and postnasal drainage induce inflammation in the lower airways. Such changes may lead to increased sensitivity of the cough receptors in the lower airways independent of direct stimulation by the postnasal drainage itself. Further, there is evidence that intense irritant exposures

Box 73-1. Most Common Causes of Chronic Cough

- Upper Airway Cough Syndrome
- Asthma/Eosinophilic bronchitis/Atopic cough
- Gastroesophageal Reflux Disease

Box 73-2. Causes of Upper Airway Cough Syndrome

- Allergic rhinitis
- Perennial nonallergic rhinitis
- Vasomotor rhinitis
- Nonallergic rhinitis with eosinophilia (NARES)
- Postinfectious rhinitis
- Following upper respiratory tract infection
- Bacterial sinusitis
- Allergic fungal sinusitis
- Rhinitis due to anatomic abnormalities
- Rhinitis due to physical or chemical irritants
- Occupational rhinitis
- Rhinitis medicamentosa
- Rhinitis of pregnancy

Box 73-3. Occupational and Environmental Exposures Associated with Chronic Cough

- Occupational Exposures:
  - Coal and hard rock mining
  - Tunnel workers
  - Concrete manufacturing
- Environmental Exposures:
  - Secondhand smoke
  - Particulate matter
  - Irritant gases and fumes
  - Mold
  - Perfumes
  - Mixed pollutants

to the nose may cause the release of cytokines and various other mediators into the systemic circulation that induce changes in the lower respiratory tract that may enhance lower airway cough reflex sensitivity.

Findings such as these form the basis for the adoption of the term upper airway cough syndrome in place of postnasal drip, to reinforce that cough may be triggered by immune/inflammatory signaling and neuroplastic changes increasing cough receptor sensitivity rather than simply being the result of mechanical and/or irritant receptor triggering by postnasal secretions collecting in the larynx and or lower respiratory tract.

12. What is cough variant asthma?

Cough variant asthma is diagnosed in individuals without wheezing, shortness of breath, or chest tightness who report coughing as their sole symptom when exposed to strong odors, exercise, or other triggers and who have a positive methacholine challenge. Spirometry testing is commonly normal and there may be no bronchodilator response.

13. What is nonasthmatic eosinophilic bronchitis?

Individuals with eosinophilic bronchitis report symptoms very similar to asthma and are often initially diagnosed with asthma but exhibit a negative methacholine challenge. Studies of sputum reveal that they have eosinophils and typically respond well to inhaled corticosteroids.

14. What are the mechanisms by which reflux from the gastrointestinal tract contributes to chronic cough?

There are several different mechanisms by which gastrointestinal reflux may contribute to chronic cough. This is supported by the observation that PPI therapy alone rarely resolves GERD-related cough. First there is a convergence of vagal afferents from the esophagus and respiratory tract in the brainstem as outlined earlier (see Questions 5 and 6). Esophageal dysmotility may lead to esophageal reflux to the larynx that may be aspirated into the lungs or simply irritate the laryngeal mucosa.

Aspiration of gastric contents may or may not be associated with typical symptoms of GERD such as heartburn, regurgitation, water-brash, sour taste, chest pain, globus sensation or pharyngeal symptoms such as dysphonia, hoarseness, and sore throat depending on whether it is predominantly acid or nonacid reflux. Individuals with nonacid reflux often report no significant reflux symptoms but demonstrate signs of aspiration on bronchoscopic lavage with increased lymphocytes or neutrophils and possibly endobronchial signs of squamous metaplasia.

15. What is the prevalence of cough related to ACE inhibitors?

Cough induced by ACE inhibitors is estimated to occur in 5% to 35% of users and is reported to be more common in women and nonsmokers. It has also been noted to be more common in patients on ACE inhibitors for congestive heart failure compared to those taking it for other cardiovascular diseases such as hypertension. It may cause cough with the first dose or after months of use.

16. Is there any difference in incidence of chronic cough with ACE inhibitors and angiotensin receptor blockers?

Studies suggest that the incidence of cough with ARBs is less than that with ACE inhibitors and there is no contraindication to trying ARBs if a patient develops a cough related to ACE inhibitor use.

They should be aware of the possibility that the cough may return with ARB use and inform their physician if this occurs.

Clinical Evaluation

17. Discuss an initial diagnostic approach to chronic cough.

The ACCP guidelines recommend that if there are signs and symptoms suggestive of upper airway cough syndrome, asthma, nonasthmatic eosinophilic bronchitis, or GERD (which accounts for 80% of all causes of chronic cough) all disorders suspected should be treated empirically at the same time to see if there is a resolution or significant reduction of the cough. Patients who smoke should be encouraged to stop smoking (Figure 73-2).

If there are any symptoms or physical signs suggestive of cardiopulmonary disease or any suspicion for lung cancer, interstitial lung disease, or bronchiectasis, a chest radiograph should be performed. If there is partial resolution of the cough related to treating any of these entities, the treatment should be continued. It must be emphasized that more than one process may contributing to the chronic cough and all must be treated at the same time.

18. What other tests are useful in evaluation of reflux-associated cough?

- Barium esophogram is useful to assess for hiatal hernia, gastroesophageal reflux, and esophagolaryngeal reflux. It is also useful to evaluate other esophageal anomalies.
- Impedance probe testing allows for evaluation of both acid and nonacid reflux in addition to distal versus proximal events and whether there is any correlation between cough, throat clearing, hoarseness, chest pain, and reflux events. Studies have been varied in showing good correlation between cough events and reflux events. If the cough is being triggered solely by acid events in the lower esophagus then there may very well be a strong correlation between cough events and reflux events. However, if the mechanism is related to laryngopharyngeal reflux with or without aspiration, this may lead to a general increased sensitivity to a variety of irritant exposures.
- Esophagogastroduodenoscopy (EGD) is helpful to look for esophageal changes related to reflux or significant damage indicating Barrett's esophagitis.
- Esophageal manometry can be useful to assess if there are significant motility issues that may be contributing to reflux issues and/or determine whether a patient may be a candidate for a gastric fundoplication.

19. What should be the next step(s) if empiric treatment for the common causes of chronic cough fails?

It is imperative that all causes of cough are treated concurrently and optimally. If the cough continues to be present, depending on the clinical history, a number of further tests may be considered.

A CT scan of the chest can be helpful to rule out cough caused by things that may be missed by plain chest radiograph such as interstitial lung diseases, bronchiectasis, chronic infections such as atypical mycobacterial infections, lung cancer, aspiration, or mitral valve disease.

A CT scan of the sinuses can identify anatomic anomalies, polyps, persistent inflammation, and ostial obstruction.

Skin testing can be used to evaluate for significant environmental allergens that may be contributing to UACS. Identifying pet, dust mite, cockroach, or mold allergies can lead to remediation that may significantly reduce upper airway congestion and inflammation.

20. When should bronchoscopy be considered in evaluation of chronic cough?

The current ACCP guidelines suggest there is not enough evidence for the routine use of bronchoscopy as part of an evaluation of patients with chronic cough. If a thorough pulmonary workup has been performed without identifying a cause, or there is concern for reflux-associated cough or a cough from a chronic low-grade infection such as mycobacteria or mycoplasma, then bronchoscopy may be helpful. BAL may show evidence of high neutrophils and/or lymphocytes which have previously been associated with aspiration and cultures will reveal the presence of noncommensal microbes that may indicate chronic infection/colonization. Biopsies may show changes of squamous metaplasia that are associated with aspiration.

21. What are useful tests to rule out a cardiac cause of chronic cough?

Chest radiographs to look for signs of congestive heart failure and mitral valve calcification are useful but a CT scan of the chest may be more sensitive in this regard. An echocardiogram is helpful to rule out mitral valve disease and cardiac wall motion abnormalities.

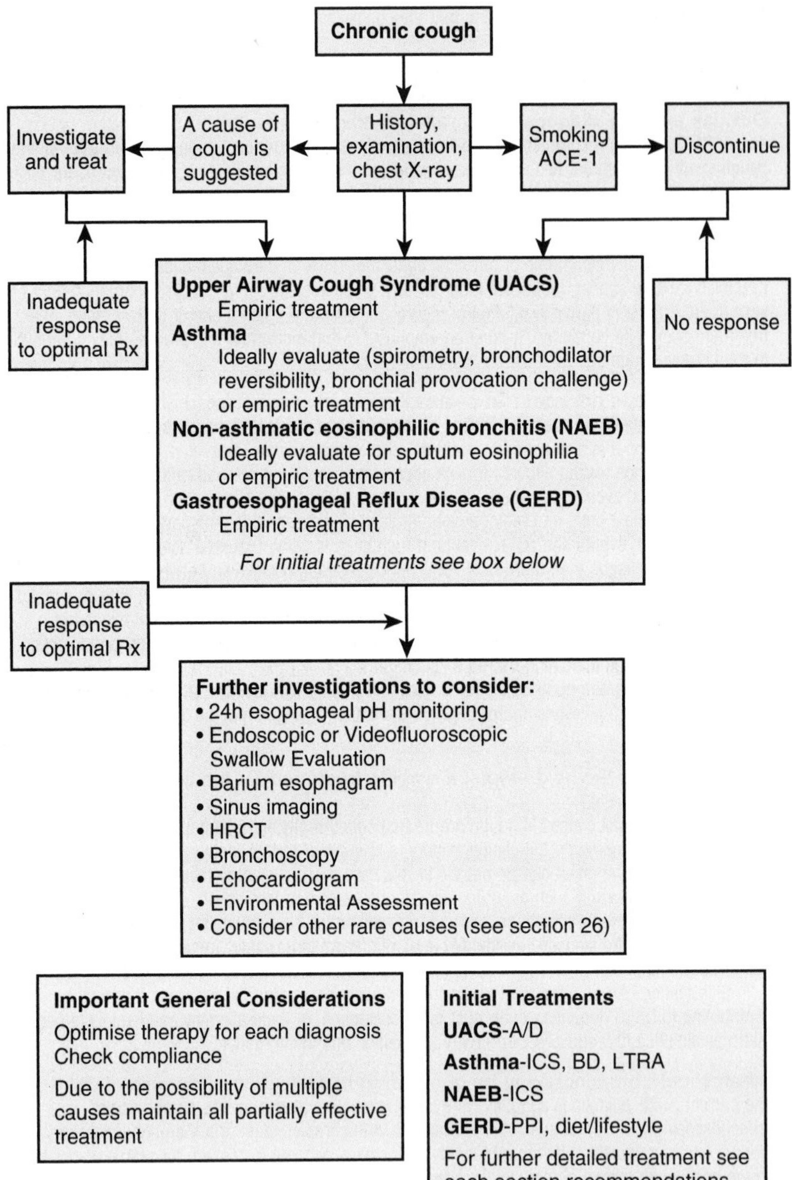

Figure 73-2. ACCP Guidelines Diagnostic Approach to chronic cough. *(Adapted with permission from ACCP Guidelines for Evaluation of Chronic Cough, Irwin et al. Chest, 2006.)*

Therapeutic Approach

22. **What are treatment options for UACS?**
First-generation antihistamines such as bromopheniramine, chlorpheneramine, and promethazine have been shown to have central cough suppressive properties while newer generation nonsedating antihistamines do not have this property. Decongestants can be combined with first-generation antihistamines and are offered in several combinations. Some studies have suggested that for patients with significant nasal and/or sinus congestion saline nasal rinses can be helpful, although evidence is limited.

23. **When should one consider discontinuing ACE inhibitors to see if they are the cause of the cough?**
If there are not signs or symptoms suggestive of more common causes of cough, then discontinuation of ACE inhibitors and appropriate replacement therapy should be attempted right away. A cough caused by ACE inhibitor use will generally subside within 2 to 4 weeks. If there are other factors present that may explain a chronic cough but 4 weeks of an empiric treatment fails to lead to substantial resolution, then discontinuation of an ACE inhibitor is indicated. If the cough persists despite being off the ACE inhibitor for 4 weeks, it is unlikely to be the cause and it can be restarted. If the cough does stop, the ACE inhibitor can be tried again after 2 to 3 months but discontinued permanently if the cough returns.

24. **What if substitution of an ACE inhibitor is not an option?**
Medication commonly used to suppress cough can be tried, including sodium cromoglycate, theophylline, sulindac, indomethacin, amlodipine, ferrous sulfate, and picotamide.

25. **What are medication options for treating unexplained cough?**
Persistent cough may be related to cough habituation and also neuropathic changes (peripheral and central) created by the cough itself. Central cough suppressants such as dextromethorphan or codeine containing products are effective for some but there are concerns about long-term use of narcotics. Benzonatate is reported to reduce stretch receptor sensitivity in the lungs. Some patients respond to baclofen, transdermal lidocaine patches, or nebulized lidocaine. Peripheral afferent cough suppressants are proposed to block sensory receptors peripherally, and have been shown to suppress cough in randomized controlled trials, but these are not available in the United States (e.g., moguisteine and levodropropizine).
Given the theories that chronic cough is somewhat akin to chronic pain syndrome, it is not surprising that there are recommendations for use of such agents as tricyclic antidepressants and gabapentin, but data are limited as far as their efficacy for neuropathic cough.

26. **What is the role of speech therapy in treatment of chronic cough?**
Speech therapy techniques for cough suppression, throat clearing suppression, and throat relaxation play a vital role in breaking the viscious cycle of chronic cough. Techniques used to treat paradoxical vocal fold motion disorder (commonly referred to as vocal cord dysfunction (VCD)) may be helpful in this group as a number of patients exhibit both chronic cough and VCD.

Bibliography

Bascom R, Pipkorn U, Proud D, et al: Major basic protein and eosinophil-derived neurotoxin concentrations in nasal-lavage fluid after antigen challenge: effect of systemic corticosteroids and relationship to eosinophil influx, *J Allergy Clin Immunol* 84(3):338–346, 1989.

Black HR, Bailey J, Zappe D, et al: Valsartan: more than a decade of experience, *Drugs* 69(17):2393–2414, 2009.

Bolser DC: Older-generation antihistamines and cough due to upper airway cough syndrome (UACS): efficacy and mechanism, *Lung* 186(Suppl 1):S74–S77, 2008.

Bolser DC: Pharmacologic management of cough, *Otolaryngol Clin North Am* 43(1):147–155, xi, 2010.

Carr MJ, Undem BJ: Bronchopulmonary afferent nerves, *Respirology* 8(3):291–301, 2003.

Chung KF: Currently available cough suppressants for chronic cough, *Lung* 186(Suppl 1):S82–S87, 2008.

Chung KF, McGarvey L, Mazzone SB: Chronic cough as a neuropathic disorder, *Lancet Respir Med* 1(5):414–422, 2013.

Committee for the Japanese Respiratory Society Guidelines for Management of cough, Kohno S, Ishida T, Uchida Y, et al: The Japanese Respiratory Society guidelines for management of cough, *Respirology* 11(Suppl 4):S135–S186, 2006.

Desai D, Brightling C: Cough due to asthma, cough-variant asthma and non-asthmatic eosinophilic bronchitis, *Otolaryngol Clin North Am* 43(1):123–310, x, 2010.

Dicpinigaitis PV: Angiotensin-converting enzyme inhibitor-induced cough: ACCP evidence-based clinical practice guidelines, *Chest* 129(1 Suppl):169S–173S, 2006.

Dicpinigaitis PV: Cough: an unmet clinical need, *Br J Pharmacol* 163(1):116–124, 2011.

D'Urzo A, Jugovic P: Chronic cough. Three most common causes, *Can Fam Physician* 48:1311–1316, 2002.
Fujimori K, Suzuki E, Arakawa M: [A case of chronic persistent cough caused by gastroesophageal reflux], *Nihon Kyobu Shikkan Gakkai Zasshi* 31(10):1303–1307, 1993.
Gibson PG, Vertigan AE: Speech pathology for chronic cough: a new approach, *Pulm Pharmacol Ther* 22(2):159–162, 2009.
Ing AJ, Ngu MC, Breslin AB: Pathogenesis of chronic persistent cough associated with gastroesophageal reflux, *Am J Respir Crit Care Med* 149(1):160–167, 1994.
Irwin RS, Baumann MH, Bolser DC, et al: Diagnosis and management of cough executive summary: ACCP evidence-based clinical practice guidelines, *Chest* 129(1 Suppl):1S–23S, 2006.
Irwin RS, French CL, Curley FJ, et al: Chronic cough due to gastroesophageal reflux: clinical, diagnostic, and pathogenetic aspects, *Chest* 104(5):1511–1517, 1993.
Jang DW, Lachanas VA, Segel J, et al: Budesonide nasal irrigations in the postoperative management of chronic rhinosinusitis, *Int Forum Allergy Rhinol* 3(9):708–711, 2013.
Javorkova N, Varechova S, Pecova R, et al: Acidification of the oesophagus acutely increases the cough sensitivity in patients with gastro-oesophageal reflux and chronic cough, *Neurogastroenterol Motil* 20(2):119–124, 2008.
Jervis-Bardy J, Boase S, Psaltis A, et al: A randomized trial of mupirocin sinonasal rinses versus saline in surgically recalcitrant staphylococcal chronic rhinosinusitis, *Laryngoscope* 122(10):2148–2153, 2012.
Jervis-Bardy J, Wormald PJ: Microbiological outcomes following mupirocin nasal washes for symptomatic, *Staphylococcus aureus*-positive chronic rhinosinusitis following endoscopic sinus surgery, *Int Forum Allergy Rhinol* 2(2):111–115, 2012.
Kardos P, Berck H, Fuchs KH, et al: Guidelines of the German Respiratory Society for diagnosis and treatment of adults suffering from acute or chronic cough, *Pneumologie* 64(11):701–711, 2010.
Krouse JH, Altman KW: Rhinogenic laryngitis, cough, and the unified airway, *Otolaryngol Clin North Am* 43(1):111–121, ix-x, 2010.
Lai K, Chen R, Lin J, et al: A prospective, multicenter survey on causes of chronic cough in China, *Chest* 143(3): 613–620, 2013.
Magni C, Chellini E, Zanasi A: Cough variant asthma and atopic cough, *Multidiscip Respir Med* 5(2):99–103, 2010.
Malacco E, Santonastaso M, Vari NA, et al: Comparison of valsartan 160 mg with lisinopril 20 mg, given as monotherapy or in combination with a diuretic, for the treatment of hypertension: the Blood Pressure Reduction and Tolerability of Valsartan in Comparison with Lisinopril (PREVAIL) study, *Clin Ther* 26(6):855–865, 2004.
Mazzone SB, Undem BJ: Cough sensors. V. Pharmacological modulation of cough sensors, *Handb Exp Pharmacol* 187:99–127, 2009.
McGarvey LP: Does idiopathic cough exist?, *Lung* 186(Suppl 1):S78–S81, 2008.
Mitchell JE, Campbell AP, New NE, et al: Expression and characterization of the intracellular vanilloid receptor (TRPV1) in bronchi from patients with chronic cough, *Exp Lung Res* 31(3):295–306, 2005.
Morice AH, McGarvey L, Pavord I, et al: Recommendations for the management of cough in adults, *Thorax* 61(Suppl 1):i1–i24, 2006.
Morice AH: Chronic cough hypersensitivity syndrome, *Cough* 9(1):14, 2013.
Pavord ID, Chung KF: Management of chronic cough, *Lancet* 371(9621):1375–1384, 2008.
Prakash UB: Uncommon causes of cough: ACCP evidence-based clinical practice guidelines, *Chest* 129(1 Suppl): 206S–219S, 2006.
Pratter MR: Overview of common causes of chronic cough: ACCP evidence-based clinical practice guidelines, *Chest* 129(1 Suppl):59S–62S, 2006.
Pratter MR: Chronic upper airway cough syndrome secondary to rhinosinus diseases (previously referred to as postnasal drip syndrome): ACCP evidence-based clinical practice guidelines, *Chest* 129(1 Suppl):63S–71S, 2006.
Snidvongs K, Pratt E, Chin D, et al: Corticosteroid nasal irrigations after endoscopic sinus surgery in the management of chronic rhinosinusitis, *Int Forum Allergy Rhinol* 2(5):415–421, 2012.
Ryan NM, Gibson PG: Characterization of laryngeal dysfunction in chronic persistent cough, *Laryngoscope* 119(4): 640–645, 2009.
Tarlo SM: Cough: occupational and environmental considerations: ACCP evidence-based clinical practice guidelines, *Chest* 129(1 Suppl):186S–196S, 2006.
Undem BJ, Carr MJ: Targeting primary afferent nerves for novel antitussive therapy, *Chest* 137(1):177–184, 2010.
van den Berg JW, de Nier LM, Kaper NM, et al: Limited evidence: higher efficacy of nasal saline irrigation over nasal saline spray in chronic rhinosinusitis—an update and reanalysis of the evidence base, *Otolaryngol Head Neck Surg* 150(1):16–21, 2014.
Widdicombe J, Tatar M, Fontana G, et al: Workshop: tuning the "cough center," *Pulm Pharmacol Ther* 24(3):344–352, 2011.

DYSPHAGIA AND ASPIRATION

Lisa Treviso-Jones, MS, CCC-SLP and Kaylee Skidmore, MA, CCC-SLP

CHAPTER 74

KEY POINTS

1. As many as 15 million people will suffer from some level of dysphagia during their lifetime, with 1 million receiving a new diagnosis of dysphagia every year.
2. Over 60,000 Americans die from complications associated with dysphagia, most commonly aspiration pneumonia. Aspiration pneumonia is one of the leading causes of death among the elderly.
3. The cost of managing a patient with a feeding tube is reported to average over $31,000 per patient per year. PEG tubes increase length of stay in the hospital and increase patient expenses.
4. Dysphagia profoundly impacts patients and often leads to depression due to change of lifestyle and overall decreased quality of life.

Pearls

1. Which cranial nerves are involved in swallowing?
   There are 6 cranial nerves that contribute to both swallowing and speech, they include:
   a. CN V: Trigeminal Nerve
   b. CN VII: Facial Nerve
   c. CN IX: Glossopharyngeal Nerve
   d. CN X: Vagus Nerve
   e. CN XI: Spinal Accessory Nerve
   f. CN XII: Hypoglossal Nerve
2. Keeping a cuff inflated on a tracheostomy tube does not mechanically prevent aspiration, as liquids aspirated to the level of the cuff can still leak around it.
3. The less viscous the food material (e.g., liquids), the more likely it is to be aspirated. This is why the 3-oz water test has been successful in indentifying aspiration risk.

QUESTIONS

1. **How do you define normal swallowing?**
   Normal swallowing is divided into phases: (a) the preoral anticipitory phase, (b) the oral preparatory phase, (c) the oral transport phase, (d) the pharyngeal phase, and (e) the esophageal phase.
   - Preoral anticipitory phase: This phase begins with seeing, smelling, and tasting food. When our senses are triggered we produce saliva which is designed to make chewing food easier.
   - Oral preparatory phase: After food enters the oral cavity it is manipulated by the tongue, lips, cheeks, palate, and jaw. The masticated food is formed into a bolus by the tongue in preparation for swallowing.
   - Oral transport phase: The transport phase of a swallow involves propelling the bolus back along the palate until the bolus reaches the anterior tonsillar pillars. At this point, a swallow reflex is initiated and the oral phase of swallow is concluded. A normal oral phase is approximately 1 second, even with differing food consistencies, age, or sex of the individual.
   - Pharyngeal phase: The pharyngeal phase of a swallow is initiated after the swallow reflex occurs. The pharyngeal phase of a swallow involves four main neuromotor components: (a) velopharyngeal closure to prohibit oral contents from entering the nasal cavity, (b) peristaltic contraction with the pharyngeal constrictors moving the bolus through the pharynx, (c) airway protection via laryngeal elevation and laryngeal closure to prevent aspiration, and (d) upper esophageal opening to allow the bolus to pass from the pharynx into the esophagus.
   - Esophageal phase: The esophageal phase of a swallow occurs when the bolus has passed through the upper esophageal sphincter at the base of the pharynx. The bolus is then carried through the esophagus via peristaltic movement of the constrictor muscles of the esophagus.

2. **Define dysphagia.**
   Dysphagia is the symptom of difficulty in swallowing, usually as a result of nerve or muscle injury, that can occur at different phases within the swallowing process as described above.

3. **What are the most common causes of dysphagia?**
   Dysphagia is generally caused by either a neurologic and/or anatomic injury usually occuring from a disease of the cerebral cortex and brainstem, cranial nerves, and/or muscles of swallowing. Cerebral vascular accident (CVA) is the most common neurologic cause of dysphagia. If only a single cerebral hemisphere is affected by CVA, swallowing can be preserved because the brainstem still receives input from the other, noninjured hemisphere.

   Dysphagia can occur in any phase of the swallow. In the oral prepatory phase, swallowing is controlled by both the cortex and the brainstem and is voluntary (i.e. not a reflex). Disorders in the oral phase include decreased lip closure, decreased buccal tension, decreased strength and/or coordination in the musculature needed for adequate mastication, and decreased tongue range of motion and coordination. The pharyngeal phase of swallowing is an involuntary phase that is controlled by the brainstem. Pharyngeal phase impairments can include a delayed swallow reflex; decreased velopharyngeal closure resulting in nasal regurgitation, decreased epiglottic retroflexion, and laryngeal elevation thus increasing risk for airway exposure during the swallow; and damage to the opening and closing of the upper esophageal sphincter, which limits the ability to successfully pass the bolus to the esophagus.

4. **How is dysphagia typically diagnosed?**
   There are three techniques widely used to diagnose dysphagia: (a) bedside swallow evaluation, (b) fluoroscopic examination called a modified barium swallow (MBS), and (c) fiber-optic endoscopic evaluation of swallowing (FEES). Although bedside tests are safe, relatively straightforward, and easily repeated they have variable sensitivity and interrater reliability. They are also poor at detecting silent aspiration. Modified barium swallow studies allow a real time view of both anatomic and physiologic function. Modified barium swallow tests also allow testing of different swallow techniques to decrease the presence of penetration/aspiration. Fiber-optic endoscopy allows swallow assessment and sensory testing but requires specialized equipment.

5. **How do you define penetration and aspiration?**
   Whether a swallow has been triggered or not, the main path of any food or liquid should be directed toward the esophagus. However, when food or liquid is misdirected into the laryngeal vestibule but stays above the level of the true vocal cords, this is referred to as "penetration." If penetration into the laryngeal vestibule occurs during swallowing but clears with no residue once swallowing is complete, it is known as "transient" penetration. Aspiration occurs once material has dropped below the level of the true vocal cords and airway protection has been compromised. "Silent" aspiration indicates that material has dropped below the level of the true vocal cords, without any overt signs and symptoms of aspiration (i.e., coughing, throat clearing, etc.).

6. **What are the steps involved in a bedside swallowing evaluation?**
   A bedside swallow evaluation is a screening process used by speech-language pathologists (SLPs) to assess dysphagia. The purpose is to determine the etiology of dysphagia, assess the patient's ability to adequately protect the airway, assess the possibility of oral feeding, recommend alternative means of nutrition management if needed, assess the need for additional diagnostic tests or referrals, and establish baseline function versus current level of function. SLPs look for signs or symptoms of possible oral or pharyngeal dysphagia when given oral trials. A thorough exam will include a comprehensive chart review, oral motor assessment, assessment of vocal quality, strength of cough, anterior-posterior transport of material, pharyngeal constriction, hypolaryngeal excursion, laryngeal elevation, and assessing overt signs and symptoms of penetration and/or aspiration. When results are inconclusive, an SLP will often perform a more objective measure (MBS or FEES) to further evaluate swallowing function.

   For a patient with a tracheostomy tube, a bedside swallowing evaluation will begin with cuff deflation and finger occlusion to first determine the patient's ability to move air around the tracheostomy tube and the vocal cords and into the oral and nasal cavities. If no difficulty is observed, an SLP will place a Passy Muir valve (PMV) prior to performing PO trials to increase subglottic pressure and allow for increased airway protection. Food and liquid are often dyed blue to check for aspiration (see Question 8).

7. **What do signs and symptoms of penetration/aspiration look like at the bedside?**
Clinicians utilize a variety of symptoms and signs as indicators of oral-pharyngeal dysphagia and subsequently penetration/aspiration. These include coughing, wheezing, recurrent pneumonia, gagging, choking, chest congestion, tachypnea, bradycardia, oxygen desaturations, noisy or wet breathing, delayed swallows, and vocal changes. Additionally, signs such as gurgly respiration or wet vocal quality can be associated with hypopharyngeal or laryngeal pooling of secretions or pharyngeal residue of food materials.

8. **What is a blue dye test and what is the purpose of its use?**
The modified Evan's blue dye test (MEBDT) is a simple and inexpensive way of assessing aspiration in the tracheotomized patient. Blue dye is placed in food and liquids provided to the patient during a bedside assessment. The patient is deep suctioned to see if any blue material has entered the airway. If nothing is recovered during procedure and assessment, the SLP will wait 24 hours for evidence of delayed aspiration before allowing oral intake and notify both nursing and respiratory therapy that a MEBDT has been provided. Sensitivity of the MEBDT in predicting aspiration among individuals in one specific study was 82%; however, this test can provide a false negative result, therefore the absence of of blue dye does not automatically guarentee a patient is not aspirating.

9. **What portion from an "oral mechanism exam" provides the most insight into a person's risk for aspiration?**
The goal of an oral mechanism examiniation is to provide information regarding structures, structural relationships, movement function of the tongue and lips, and to identify sensory function within the immediate extra- and intraoral structures. Studies have shown that incomplete lingual range of motion will make a person more likely to aspirate than those with complete lingual range of motion, regardless of complete labial closure and intact facial symmetry. Identifying oral motor weaknesses will raise a heightened awareness during the bedside swallowing assessment.

10. **How do tracheostomy tubes and one-way speaking valves impact a patient's risk for aspiration?**
In tracheostomy patients, there is a high incidence (50% to 87%) of aspiration and pneumonia. Many studies have looked at the incidence of aspiration with open and closed tracheostomy tubes, and found that with the use of finger occlusion or an obturator the incidence of aspiration was significantly reduced in comparison to those with an open tracheostomy tube. Similarly, the use of one-way valves to occlude the tracheostomy tube has been found to significantly reduce the incidence and severity of aspiration of thin liquids. One reason for the reduction in aspiration is that the one-way valve increases subglottic air pressure and activation of mechanoreceptors, which are lost when the tracheostomy tube is open. Additionally, improved sensation may also increase the patient's ability to expel material through the throat by coughing and/or throat clearing.

11. **FEES vs. MBS—which test is "better"?**
Both evaluations provide visualization of the swallow mechanism including the pharynx and larynx. A FEES is portable to the bedside for patients who are difficult to position/transport due to size. Additionally, you are able to test real food items and for full meal duration. With an MBS, you have a view of oral, pharyngeal, and esophageal phases of a swallow. You are limited to small amounts of food mixed with barium in different consistencies. You are unable to view the soft tissues or the pharynx/larynx. It is an assessment that is of very short duration and is not sensitive to the effect of fatigue on the swallowing mechanism. Additionally, it is dependent on radiology scheduling which limits the flexibility of the procedure.

12. **What is the Penetration Aspiration Scale and why is it so widely used during MBS?**
The Penetration Aspiration Scale (PAS) is an 8-point scale that was developed to provide an objective and consistent way to evaluate a persons penetration and/or aspiration during a MBS. It is widely used due to its favorable intra- and interrater reliability and the ability to easily track outcomes according to changes made on the PAS (Table 74-1).

13. **What is the 3-oz water test and is it effective in determining risk for aspiration?**
The 3-oz water swallow test is a screening tool that is used to identify patients who are at risk for clinically significant aspiration and who will require a more objective swallow evaluation. Individuals are required to drink 3 ounces of water without interruption. If they cough, choke, or show a wet-hoarse vocal quality during the test or for one minute afterward, they are considered to have

Table 74-1. Penetration Aspiration Scale

SCORE	DESCRIPTION
1	Material does not enter the airway
2	Material enters the airway, remains above the vocal cords, and is ejected from the airway
3	Material enters the airway, remains above the vocal cords, and is not ejected from the airway
4	Material enters the airway, contacts the vocal cords, and is ejected from the airway
5	Material enters the airway, contacts the vocal cords, and is not ejected from the airway
6	Material enters the airway, passes below the vocal cords, and is ejected into the larynx or out of the airway
7	Material enters the airway, passes below the vocal cords, and is not ejected from the trachea despite effort
8	Material enters the airway, passes below the vocal cords, and no effort is made to eject

failed. This test relies on overt signs and symptoms of aspiration, but most specifically the cough reflex to determine a patient's risk for aspiration; therefore it is weak in its ability to detect silent aspiration. In recent studies, the 3-oz water swallow test was able to identify 80% of patients aspirating compared to a subsequent videofluoroscopic modified barium swallow examination. It more easily identifies patients with severe dysphagia aspirating larger amounts or thicker consistencies of test material.

14. **What is the incidence of dysphagia following intubation?**
Literature has shown that pharyngeal muscle atrophy begins after 24 hours of intubation. However, literature regarding dysphagia frequency following endotracheal intubation is variable, ranging from 3% to 62%. In a recent study, the highest incidence of dysphagia was seen in patients experiencing intubation longer than 24 hours. Age greater than 55 years, medical comorbidities, and a prior history of dysphagia were also found to increase a person's risk for aspiration following intubation.

15. **Why are infiltrates seen in the RLL more indicative of an aspiration pneumonia?**
Aspirated material is drawn to gravity-dependent portions of the respiratory system, especially since most patients are sitting in an upright position when eating and drinking. The right main stem bronchus is more vertically positioned in most adults than the left, hence the attribution of right lower (or middle) lobe pneumonias to aspiration and dysphagia.

16. **How do speech-language pathologists (SLPs) treat dysphagia?**
Depending on the patient's diagnosis, the treatment plan will differ and focus on either oral, pharyngeal, or esophageal phases of swallowing or a combination thereof. Below is an outline of the area of dysfunction and corresponding treatment methods that can be utilized to assist in improving dysphagia.
   - Oral preparatory phase:
     - Labial weakness results in anterior spillage of material from the oral cavity. Modifications focus on reducing anterior spillage such as using a pincer grasp to assist in closing the weaker labial side and labial strengthening exercises. Neuromuscular electrical stimulation (NMES) can provide assistance in increasing symmetry and improving labial strength.
     - Lingual weakness results in poor bolus formation and presents with difficulty in anterior-posterior movement of a food bolus and "pocketing of food." Isometric tongue exercises can be used to assist in improving strength. External aids such as mirrors can provide visual feedback for pocketed material and anterior spillage. A syringe or modified spoon is used to assist with anterior-posterior transport, as well as education regarding use of finger sweep or lingual sweep of cheek sulcus to remove any pocketed material. Thermal stimulation techniques can also be used to assist in increasing sensation to the oral cavity and head tilt positions to assist in moving material to the stonger side of the oral cavity.

- Pharyngeal phase:
  - Delayed pharyngeal initiation of swallow can be treated with thermal stimulation, sour bolus trials, verbal cueing, and NMES.
  - Dysfunction of intrinsic/extrinsic pharyngeal musculature results in poor pharyngeal constriction and inability to effectively move material through the pharynx. The Mendelson manuever can be used to provide an isometric hold of the pharynx during contraction to build strength and prolong hyolaryngeal elevation, keeping the cricopharyngeus (upper esophageal sphincter) open longer. NMES can provide a consistent pharyngeal contraction with use of electrical stimulation in combination with bolus trials and initiation of swallowing. Head turning to the weaker side will initiate use of the stronger side to adequately move material through the pharynx.
  - Decreased tongue base retraction will also result in poor transit of material through the pharynx by decreasing epiglottic tilt and increasing pooling in the vallecular space. Swallowing manuevers such as the supraglottic swallow will adduct the vocal cords and increase the patients' abilty to protect their airway. The Masako manuever assists in providing an isolated exercise to the tongue base to increase strength.
  - Poor laryngeal elevation/excursion will reduce a person's ability to anteriorly displace their trachea to adequately protect the airway. Several therapies exist to help laryngeal motion including the Shaker exercise, Mendelson manuever, biofeedback, and effortful swallow. Postural changes will also help to increase a patient's ability to protect the airway such as chin tuck and head turn positions.

17. **What is neuromuscular electrical stimuation (NMES), more specifically Vital Stim®?**
Vital Stim® is a noninvasive, external electrical stimulation that has been approved by the FDA for treatment of dysphagia. It is seen to be most effective in conjunction with traditional swallowing therapies. Different electrode placements target specific areas of muscle dysfunction. Depending on signs and symptoms seen during MBS, appropriate placements are determined to improve functional swallowing outcomes. See controversies for more information regarding NMES.

18. **Why is it easier for persons with oral-pharyngeal dysphagia to swallow liquids with thicker viscosity?**
One of the most common causes of dysphagia is delayed initiation of pharyngeal swallow. A common treatment measure for patients with this is to thicken their liquids. This compensatory measure allows slower oral-pharyngeal transit time, while creating a more cohesive bolus that is easier to transport through both the oral and pharyngeal cavities. The more viscous the liquid, the slower the transit, allowing patients with delayed pharygneal swallowing enough time to safely move material through their pharynx and into their esophagus.

19. **What is the Frazier water protocol and who is appropriate for this?**
The Frazier water protocol (FWP) allows people with dysphagia and aspiration free access to water. Unlike soda or coffee, water has a neutral pH level. Therefore, it is well tolerated by the lungs and is quickly absorbed into the bloodstream. The key to this protocol is good oral hygiene to reduce the bacterial load of the mouth and thus reduce the risk of bacterial exposure to the lungs. Patients who are NPO for aspiration or on a modified diet may try the FWP. Its benefits include reducing the risk of dehydration and improving patient compliance with swallowing precautions. It also improves quality of life.

20. **Are there medications that are more likely to cause dysphagia?**
Medication-induced dysphagia is far more common than reports in medical literature suggest. When dysphagia occurs as a side effect of a medication it is usually caused by decreasing muscle function, coordination, and/or sensation needed for swallowing. Additionally, medications that cause dry mouth (xerostomia) can interfere with swallowing by impairing the ability to transport food in the mouth. A list of such medications is provided in Table 74-2.
The therapeutic effects of medications can also contribute to dysphagia. When used over a long period of time and in high doses, some medications can cause muscle deterioration resulting in dysphagia. A list of such medications is in Table 74-3.

21. **How does breathing pattern impact swallowing function?**
There are four patterns of breathing that take place during the initation and completion of the swallow: EX/EX (expiration/expiration), EX/IN (expiration/inspiration), IN/EX (inspiration/expiration), IN/IN (inspiration/inspiration). EX/EX appears to be the most common respiratory pattern in normal

Table 74-2. Medication-Induced Dysphagia

Anticholinergic or Antimuscarinic	Atropine (Atropar) Oxybutynin (Ditropan) Tolterodine (Detrol)
Neuromuscular Blocking Agents	Atracurium (Tracrium) Cisatracurium (Nimbex) Tubocurarine (Tubarine)
Medications that cause xerostomia	Trycyclic antidepressants Antihistamines Diuretics
Local Anesthetics	Benzocaine (Americaine, Dermoplast) Lidocaine (Xylocaine)
Antipsychotic/Neuroleptic Medications	Haloperidol (Haldol) Chlorpromzine (Thorazine) Loxapine (Loxitane)

(From Balzer KM: Drug-induced dysphagia, Int J MS Care 2(1):40–50, 2000.)

Table 74-3. Medical Treatments That Can Cause Dysphagia

Antineoplastics and Immunosuppressants	Azathioprine (Imuran) Carmustine Cyclosporine Daunorubicin
High-Dose Corticosteroids	Dexamethasone (Decadron) Prednisolone (Delta Cortef) Prednisone (Deltasone)
Antiepileptic, Benzodiazepines, Narcotics, Skeletal muscle relaxants	Gabapentin (Neurontin) Phenytoin (Dilantin) Carbamazepine (Tegretol) Alprazolam (Xanax) Clonazepam (Klonopin) Diazepam (Valium) Baclofen (Lioresal) Cyclobenzaprine (Flexeril)

(From Balzer KM: Drug-induced dysphagia, Int J MS Care 2(1):40–50, 2000.)

swallowing adults. However, in adults over the age of 65 and in chronic diseases such as COPD, this respiratory pattern appears to change and can increase the risk for aspiration. The IN/IN (inspiration/inspiration) breathing pattern is the least frequent respiratory pattern. Interestingly, it has been found to be the dominant respiratory pattern in those recieving head and neck cancer treatments, placing them at significantly higher risk for aspiration.

22. **What effect does chemoradiation to the head and neck have on swallowing function?**
Swallow dysfunction is prevalent in patients following intensive chemoradiotherapy (CRT) for head and neck cancer. Some patients will receive a PEG tube prior to CRT that may result in complete cessation of oral intake during treatment. This inactivity has been known to cause atrophy of the swallowing muscles. Following radiation, patients have reduced epiglottic retroflexion, delayed initiation of a swallow, and uncoordinated timing of the swallow and respiration, all of which

promote aspiration. Additionally, the base of tongue does not retract to meet the posterior pharyngeal wall, which often leads to decreased cricopharyngeal opening ultimately causing pooling in both the piriform sinuses and vallecula, which can contribute to aspiration post swallow. Post-swallow aspirations are typically "silent," where the aspiration does not elicit a cough reflex, or the cough is delayed and noneffective in clearing residue. This has been reported in 22% to 42% of patients receiving head and neck CRT. Aspiration pneumonia is an important complication of CRT for patients suffering head and neck cancer.

23. **What treatment methods have been shown to be beneficial in restoring swallowing function after chemoradiation?**
Continued muscle activation throughout treatment and posttreatment periods to prevent or limit the necessity of tube feeding and maintain swallowing function should be encouraged whenever possible. Education by an SLP is an imperative piece in preserving muscle function for swallowing during CRT and cannot be encouraged enough. Some exercises have been seen to provide some improvement on severely atrophied and even radiated musculature.

CONTROVERSIES

24. **Is NMES an appropriate treatment method for dysphagia?**
With NMES being a relatively newer treatment option for dysphagia (it was approved by the FDA in 2002 for dysphagia), some will argue that there is not enough research to support its use. In support of NMES, one of the largest trials performed (Xia et al., 2011) reported 120 patients with dysphagia who were post-stroke and randomly assigned to one of three groups: traditional swallowing treatment alone, e-stim alone, or e-stim plus traditional swallowing treatment. The experimental group that added e-stim to traditional treatment made significantly greater improvements in all four outcome measures than the traditional treatment alone group or the e-stim alone group. The authors thus concluded that the addition of e-stim to traditional treatment resulted in better patient outcomes than traditional treatment alone.
Those against e-stim argue that there is not enough research to support this modality and that concurrent stimulation with swallowing reduces hyolaryngeal mobility, a movement important to successful swallowing.

25. **Do tracheostomy tubes contribute to dysphagia?**
While some studies assert that a tracheostomy tube will not alter the elevation and anterior rotation of the hyoid bone and larynx, others indicate that tracheostomy tubes have been known to cause altered sensory and motor functions that may decrease swallowing efficiency and cause an anchoring effect limiting laryngeal elevation. It is more likely that the need for a tracheotomy indicates comorbidities (e.g., respiratory failure, trauma, stroke, advanced age, reduced functional reserve, and medications used to treat the critically ill) that by themselves predispose patients for dysphagia and aspiration rather than the tracheostomy tube itself.

BIBLIOGRAPHY

Balzer KM: Drug-induced dysphagia, *Int J MS Care* 2(1):40–50, 2000.

Blonsky E, Logemann J, Boshes B, et al: Comparison of speech and swallowing function in patients with tremor disorders and in normal geriatric patients: a cinefluorographic study, *J Gerontol* 30:299–303, 1975.

Buchholz D: Neurologic causes of dysphagia, *Dysphagia* 1:152–156, 1987.

Carter J, Humbert IA: E-stim for dysphagia: yes or no. Asha Leader, April 24, 2012.

DePippo KL, Holas MA, Reding MJ: Validation of the 3 oz water test for aspiration following stroke, *Arch Neurol* 49:1259–1261, 1992.

Gross RD, Mahlmann J, Grayhack J: Physiologic effects of open and closed tracheostomy tube on pharyngeal swallowing, *Ann Otol Rhinol Laryngol* 112:2, 2003.

Leder SB, Suiter DM, Murray J, et al: Can an oral mechanism exam contribute to the assessment of odds of aspiration?, *Dysphagia* 28:370–374, 2013.

Mandelstam P, Lieber A: Cineradiographic evaluation of the esophagus in normal adults, *Gastroenterology* 58:32–38, 1970.

Martin-Harris B, Brodsky MB, Michel Y, et al: Breathing and swallowing dynamics across the adult lifespan, *Arch Otolaryngol Head Neck Surg* 131(9):762–770, 2005.

Pauloski BR: Rehabilitation of dysphagia following head and neck cancer, *Phys Med Rehabil Clin N Am* 19:889–928, 2008.

Xia W, Zheng C, Lei Q, et al: Treatment of post-stroke dysphagia by vital stim therapy coupled with conventional swallowing training, *J Huazhong Univ Sci Technolog Med Sci* 31(1):73–76, 2011.

CHAPTER 75

BENIGN VOCAL FOLD LESIONS AND MICROSURGERY

Sean X. Wang, MD, Mark S. Courey, MD and Matthew S. Clary, MD

KEY POINTS

1. Phonomicrosurgery is usually reserved for patients who have attempted and failed nonsurgical management except in the cases of very large vocal fold lesions.
2. Videolaryngostroboscopy should be performed during the evaluation of a vocal fold lesion to assess mucosal vibratory property and glottic closure.
3. Many vocal fold lesions caused by excessive phonotrauma will inevitably recur if the underlying vocal behavior is not corrected.

Pearls

1. The primary management of vocal fold nodules is voice therapy.
2. To have the best voice outcome after phonomicrosurgery, the depth of dissection should be limited to the superficial lamina propria.

QUESTIONS

1. **What's the definition of phonomicrosurgery?**
   One of the founding fathers of modern day laryngology, Hans von Leden, originally introduced the term "phonosurgery" in 1963 to describe procedures that alter vocal quality and pitch. As technology and the understanding of the delicate vocal fold anatomy advanced, the term "phonomicrosurgery" became popularized. It is usually performed using very fine micro instruments aided by a high-powered microscope to remove the vocal fold lesion and maximize preservation of normal anatomy.

2. **What are the indications for phonomicrosurgery?**
   The most common indication for phonomicrosurgery is for the removal of benign lesions to restore the normal prephonatory glottic configuration of the larynx. It may also be used to resect precancers and early cancers of the glottis.

3. **How is phonomicrosurgery different from the traditional vocal fold stripping with regard to the management of vocal fold lesions?**
   Vocal fold stripping is usually performed by grabbing the lesion with a cup forceps and "tearing" it off the vocal fold. There is no fine control of the depth of injury with vocal fold stripping. Furthermore, the lack of precision may result in excessive removal of normal tissue.

4. **What are the layers of the membranous vocal fold?**
   Stratified squamous epithelium, basement membrane, the superficial lamina propria (SLP), the vocal ligament (the intermediate and deep lamina propria), and the vocalis muscle (Figure 75-1).

5. **What is the histology of the lamina propria?**
   Fibroblasts make up the main cellular component of the lamina propria, while glycosaminoglycans and proteoglycans occupy the interstitial spaces within the extracellular matrix.

6. **Why is the SLP often referred to as Reinke's space?**
   The superficial lamina propria has often been described incorrectly as a potential space. It is about 0.5 mm in thickness and is a distinct anatomic structure. Thus the eponym of Reinke's space is a misnomer.

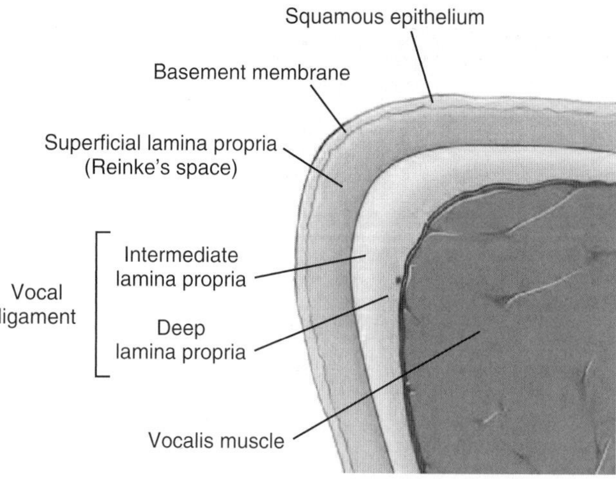

Figure 75-1. The layers of the vocal fold. *(From Rosen CA, Simpson CB: Operative Techniques in Laryngology, New York, 2008, Springer, p. 6.)*

7. **What are the components of the SLP?**
   The SLP is composed mostly of extracellular matrix proteins, water, and loosely arranged fibers of collagen and elastin. The SLP is mostly gelatinous in nature.

8. **What are the components of the vocal ligament?**
   It is composed mostly of elastin and collagen. As the vocal ligament transitions from the intermediate to the deep layer of lamina propria, there is a denser arrangement of collagen.

9. **What is the body-cover model of vocal fold motion?**
   The cover of the vocal fold includes the epithelium and the SLP. The vocal ligament and the vocalis muscle make up the body. Some authors consider the vocal ligament as a transition zone. As air passes between the vocal folds from the lung, the loose mucosa (epithelium and SLP) moves like a wave over the denser vocal ligament and vocalis muscle.

10. **How do laryngeal lesions cause dysphonia?**
    By altering the cover viscosity, interfering with the body-cover relationship, and distorting prephonatory glottic configuration.

11. **What are the principals of phonomicrosurgery?**
    The principals are based on the body-cover model of the vocal fold vibration. Given the importance of the interaction between the cover and the body, phonomicrosurgery for most benign lesions has evolved to limit the dissection to the depth and extent of the lesion and to maximize the preservation of normal microarchitecture. For removal of malignancy, the same principal applies; however, the primary goal is to achieve a negative margin, thus normal tissue may be sacrificed to ensure cancer extirpation.

12. **What is the plane of dissection for most phonomicrosurgery?**
    Dissection is within the SLP. Usually after incising the epithelium of the vocal fold, the SLP can be easily entered using a flap elevator. The vocal ligament is dense and appears to be pearly white (Figure 75-2).

13. **Can you use a laser to achieve the similar control and precision as cold steel instruments?**
    Yes. Modern laser technology such as the carbon dioxide (CO_2) laser with an articulating arm can be attached to an operative microscope. With specific software and hardware modifications, one can achieve precise control of the depth and thickness (Figure 75-3).

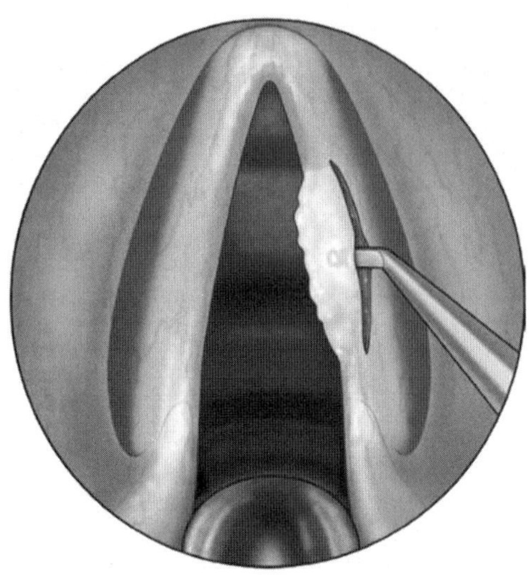

Figure 75-2. Elevating a leukoplakic lesion off the epithelium of the vocal fold using microflap technique. *(From Rosen CA, Simpson CB: Operative Techniques in Laryngology, New York, 2008, Springer, p. 125.)*

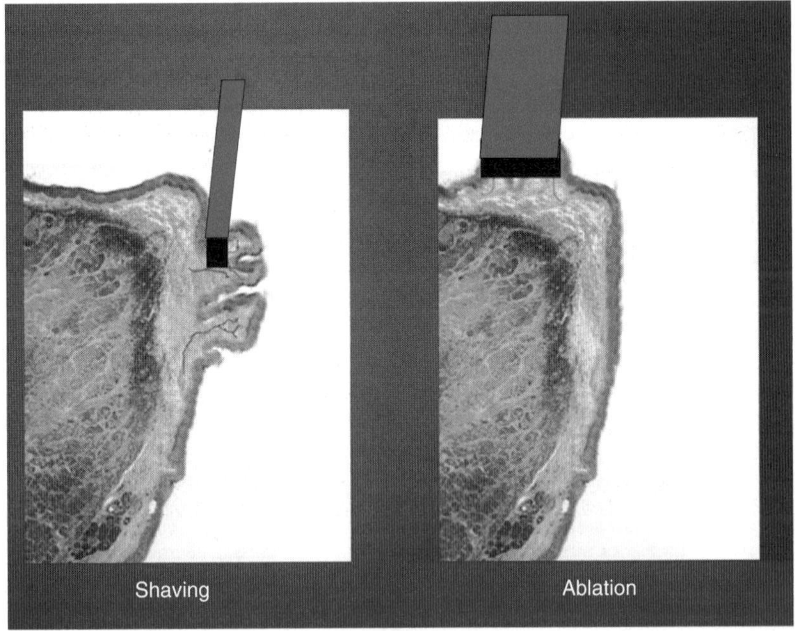

Figure 75-3. Microphonosurgery with a CO_2 laser. Left figure demonstrates shaving of respiratory papilloma off the free edge of the vocal fold. Right figure demonstrates ablating papilloma off the superior surface of the vocal fold. *(Courtesy of Mark S. Courey, MD.)*

14. **Why is laryngostroboscopy a vital part of the preoperative evaluation for phonomicrosurgery?**
Stroboscopy can assess vibratory property and glottic closure pattern of the vocal folds. These findings allow the clinician to predict the type and depth of the lesion. In other words, stroboscopy is the only clinically available tool that allows clinicians to assess the "suppleness" of the vocal folds. High-speed photography is another method to evaluate the vibratory property; however, this is rarely feasible due to the cost and size of the equipment. A detailed discussion of the specific findings on laryngostroboscopy is beyond the scope of this chapter; interested readers are referred to the publication by Kitzing in the reference section.

15. **What are the common benign laryngeal lesions treated with phonomicrosurgery?**
Vocal fold polyps and cysts, polypoid corditis (Reinke's edema), and recurrent respiratory papilloma.

16. **What are vocal fold nodules?**
These are bilateral and symmetric midmembraneous vocal fold lesions that are usually due to inefficient voice use. On laryngostroboscopy, there is minimal alteration in the normal vibratory property of the vocal folds. They tend to resolve with behavioral modification and voice therapy. Vocal fold nodules are rarely managed surgically.

17. **What are vocal fold polyps?**
These lesions are classically exophytic and can be clear or vascularized in appearance. Chronic vocal strain may lead to the formation of clear appearing, gelatinous polyps. Some phonotraumatic polyps may develop aberrant vessels and present as vascularized polyps. The vascularized polyps may hemorrhage into the vocal fold if there is an acute episode of violent cough or phonotrauma. Polyps can present unilaterally or bilaterally and usually do not lead to significant perturbation of the normal vibratory properties when they are small; however, most polyps do not respond completely to voice therapy.

18. **What are vocal fold cysts?**
These lesions can be unilateral or bilateral. There is the subepithelial type which is thought to be the product of an obstructed mucous gland and may cause mild change in the vibratory properties. A deeper intraligamentous (in the vocal ligament) type may cause significant impairment to vocal fold vibration. Vocal fold cysts usually do not respond to voice therapy and eventually require surgery.

19. **What underlying etiologies are shared by some benign lesions such as vocal fold nodules, polyps, and cysts?**
The development of these vocal fold lesions is often related to the patient's inefficient phonatory pattern that leads to excessive vocal fold collision and trauma. Sometimes the traumatic phonatory pattern may be a compensatory behavior due to glottic insufficiency.

20. **What is Reinke's edema (also known as polypoid corditis)?**
Reinke's edema presents as diffuse swelling of one or both vocal folds. As the result of significant increase in vocal fold mass, the patient speaks with a lower-pitched and harsher voice. The degree of reduction in mucosal wave correlates with the size of the lesion. In extreme cases, bilateral Reinke's edema can cause obstruction of the glottic airway. This lesion is usually associated with tobacco abuse. Often patients are asked to quit smoking before surgical excision is attempted.

21. **What are vocal fold scars or sulcus vocalis?**
When there is irreversible loss of viscoelasticity to the superficial lamina propria, a scar or sulcus vocalis forms. These patients normally have a history of voice abuse. If the tissue loss is significant, the patient may also experience glottic insufficiency. Phonomicrosurgery rarely improves the mucosal wave vibration. Augmenting the vocal fold with an injectable or permanent implant may correct the glottic insufficiency and thus provide more vocal projection and volume.

22. **What kinds of precancerous and cancerous lesions can be treated with phonomicrosurgery?**
Dysplasia, squamous cell carcinoma in situ, and early vocal fold squamous cell carcinoma.

23. **What are the different techniques for endoscopic excision of early glottic cancer?**
Squamous cell carcinoma in situ and superficial early stage squamous cell carcinomas can be removed with a microflap technique staying superficial to the vocal ligament. If the lesion extends

into or through the vocal ligament, endoscopic carbon dioxide laser–assisted cordectomy is an excellent treatment modality that rivals radiation therapy in cure rate.

24. **What's the most important predictor of voice outcome following endoscopic vocal fold cordectomy for cancer resection?**
The deeper the excision the more unpredictable the voice outcome becomes.

25. **What common pathologies can lead to glottic insufficiency?**
Vocal fold paralysis or paresis and vocal fold atrophy as related to aging or neurologic disease.

26. **Why is preoperative voice therapy important in the management of many benign laryngeal lesions?**
Voice therapy can ameliorate abusive phonatory patterns, so the patient is less likely to cause further trauma to the vocal folds postoperatively. Furthermore, some patients may be satisfied with their voice after therapy so that they no longer need surgery. Last, for benign laryngeal lesions, phonomicrosurgery is an elective procedure, and one or two sessions of voice therapy can solidify the patient-physician relationship.

27. **What are the potential complications of phonomicrosurgery discussed with the patient preoperatively?**
Since the larynx is part of the airway, there is always a risk for airway obstruction during and after the procedure. Making an incision in the vocal fold may cause scar formation and thus worsen the patient's voice. A rigid laryngoscope provides the surgeon with the exposure of the vocal folds, and the laryngoscope rests on the teeth and tongue; thus dental injury, lip laceration/abrasion, and taste changes can all occur. Lesions that are due to voice abuse may recur if the patient maintains the same vocal behavior.

28. **What equipment is usually needed to perform phonomicrosurgery?**
A specialized laryngoscope is used to expose the larynx. As a general rule, the surgeon should use the largest laryngoscope that the patient can safely tolerate. A suspension system is used to place the laryngoscope in a fixed position. A high-powered operative microscope is used to provide a magnified binocular view of the vocal folds. A 0-degree and/or 70-degree telescope can be used to take operative photos and closely examine the lesion. The main microlaryngeal instruments are small suctions to remove blood and mucus, sickle knife to make incisions, flap elevators to dissect the lesion, forceps to grab and retract the lesion, and scissors to extend the incision. Different lasers can also be used.

29. **What is the typical duration of voice rest after phonomicrosurgery?**
Patients may be placed on complete voice rest for 0 to 14 days and gradually increase their vocal use while working closely with the surgeon and the speech-language pathologist. Some patients may not go back to unrestricted voice use until 30 to 60 days postoperatively, especially professional singers and patients with large lesions. The appropriate amount of prescribed voice rest or conservation is under constant debate. Ultimately, the postoperative care should be individually tailored based on the type and size of the lesion, the degree of tissue deficiency, the patient's current voice use pattern and projected vocal requirement, and the clinical experience.

Bibliography

Goor KM, Peeters AJ, Mahieu HF, et al: Cordectomy by CO_2 laser or radiotherapy for small T1a glottic carcinomas: costs, local control, survival, quality of life, and voice quality, *Head Neck* 29(2):128–136, 2007.

Kitzing P: Stroboscopy—a pertinent laryngological examination, *J Otolaryngol* 14(3):151–157, 1985.

Mitchell JR, Kojima T, Wu H, et al: Biochemical basis of vocal fold mobilization after microflap surgery in a rabbit model, *Laryngoscope* 124(2):487–493, 2014. doi: 10.1002/lary.24263.

Mortuaire G, Francois J, Wiel E, et al: Local recurrence after CO_2 laser cordectomy for early glottic carcinoma, *Laryngoscope* 116(1):101–105, 2006.

Rosen CA: Benign vocal fold lesions and phonomicrosurgery. In Bailey BJ, Johnson JT, editors: *Head and Neck Surgery: Otolaryngology*, ed 4, Philadelphia, 2006, Lippincott Williams and Wilkins, Chapter 60.

Rosen CA, Gartner-Schmidt J, Hathaway B, et al: A nomenclature paradigm for benign midmembranous vocal fold lesions, *Laryngoscope* 122(6):1335–1341, 2012.

Rosen CA, Simpson CB: *Operative Techniques in Laryngology*, New York, 2008, Springer.

Sataloff RT, Hawkshaw MJ, Divi V, et al: Voice surgery, *Otolaryngol Clin North Am* 40(5):1151–1183, ix, 2007.

VOCAL FOLD PARALYSIS

Ameer T. Shah, MD and Thomas L. Carroll, MD

CHAPTER 76

KEY POINTS

1. Understand the embryology and anatomy of the recurrent and superior laryngeal nerves (RLN and SLN). Unilateral or bilateral injury to one or both of these nerves can lead to a range of dysfunction regarding voice, swallowing, and the ability to cough.
2. A comprehensive history focusing on recent surgeries, intubations or viral illnesses is critical in determining the etiology of vocal fold paralysis. A complete head and neck exam to evaluate for other cranial neuropathies or masses is also required. In the setting of unexplained unilateral vocal fold paralysis, a CT scan of the neck from skull base through the aortic arch with contrast is typically obtained to evaluate the entire course of the RLN (Box 76-1).
3. In adults, unilateral vocal fold paralysis typically presents with hoarseness, dysphagia, and dyspnea with speaking, but not dyspnea with exercise. Bilateral vocal fold paralysis typically presents with dyspnea on exertion and inspiratory stridor. Voice and swallowing may be normal in bilateral paralysis. Bilateral RLN paralysis can be life-threatening and may present as an acute airway emergency (Table 76-1).
4. It is rare for a vocal fold paresis to recover after 6 months from the date of insult. Laryngeal electromyography (LEMG) is often helpful in determining prognosis for recovery before 6 months have passed from the date of injury. Temporary vocal fold augmentation is used to bridge the gap before the paralysis is deemed permanent by time or LEMG criteria.
5. Treatment for unilateral vocal fold paralysis is to augment/medialize the immobile vocal fold to allow the mobile, opposite vocal fold to meet it and restore glottic competence. Treatment for bilateral vocal fold paralysis is aimed at enlarging the airway, often at the expense of voice, by removing normal vocal fold tissue or lateralizing one of the paralyzed folds.

Pearls

1. The position of the affected TVF does not correlate with the level or extent of the injury to the vagus nerve or RLN branch. Not all branches of the nerve may recover and the position of the paralyzed or immobile vocal fold may vary over time.
2. Laryngeal EMG is a tool to measure motor unit recruitment. When muscle is denervated, fibrillation potentials and positive waves are seen, whereas polyphasic motor units are seen when reinnervation occurs.
3. Augmenting a unilateral TVF immobility does not eliminate the risk of aspiration when there is also a sensory deficit from an affected SLN. However, improving the patient's ability to cough more effectively may be enough to protect the lungs and tolerate some aspiration.
4. Early augmentation with temporary injection in symptomatic patients with unilateral TVF immobility offers better long-term outcomes and decreased need for permanent augmentation.
5. In bilateral complete vocal fold immobility, tracheostomy may initially be required, but many of these patients can later be decannulated after surgeries to enlarge the glottic airway.

QUESTIONS

1. **Describe the anatomy of the vocal folds as part of the larynx.**
   The larynx is divided into the supraglottis, glottis, and subglottis (Figure 76-2A). The glottis is comprised of the paired true vocal folds (TVF). The supraglottis encompasses all the tissue of the larynx above the TVFs. The laryngeal ventricles extend laterally and superiorly, under the false vocal folds, and end blindly in the laryngeal saccule. The subglottis begins approximately 1 cm below the

Box 76-1. Key Historical Questions in a Patient Presenting with Vocal Fold Paralysis

- Symptom frequency, associations, relieving/exacerbating factors, onset, duration
- Avoiding communication because of the effort required?
- Decreased ability to complete everyday tasks/work?
- Decreased participation in strenuous sports/activities?
- Conversion to a relatively sedentary lifestyle? (more common in bilateral paralysis)
- History of aspiration pneumonia/swallowing difficulty?
- Previous neurologic, head and neck, carotid or cardiothoracic surgery?
- History of alcohol and tobacco use?
- Is it difficult to project the voice?
- History of endotracheal intubation?

Table 76-1. Signs and Symptoms of Vocal Fold Paralysis

Unilateral	• Dysphonia (hoarseness, breathy speech, soft voice) • Dyspnea and fatigue with speaking (but lack of stridor or dyspnea on exertion) • Episodic coughing with thin liquids/dysphagia • Recurrent aspiration pneumonia • Nasopharyngeal regurgitation if high vagal injury • Signs of other cranial nerve involvement, e.g., tongue paralysis or loss of gag • Signs of thoracic malignancy (cough, dyspnea, hemoptysis, etc.)
Bilateral	• Normal voice is possible • Dyspnea on exertion • Stridor with or without activity • Acute airway compromise/stridor post operatively • Worsening of symptoms after upper respiratory infection

rima glottis (the area where the TVFs meet during phonation), extending to the inferior border of the cricoid cartilage. The TVFs are involved in phonation, whereas the false vocal folds are typically not. The false vocal folds are formed of mucosa overlying the superior aspect of the thyroarytenoid muscle and other connective tissue. The TVFs are covered by stratified squamous epithelium, differentiating them from the ciliated pseudostratified columnar epithelium of the remainder of the respiratory tract. Deep to the squamous epithelium of the TVFs is the superficial lamina propria (Reinke's space), which together comprise the vocal cover that affords vibration during phonation. Deeper are the intermediate and deep lamina propria, making the vocal ligament. The vocal ligament sits on top of the vocalis muscle (the medial portion of the thyroarytenoid muscle) and is the superior extent of the conus elasticus, a fibrous tissue condensation extending up from the cricoid cartilage.

2. **Other than phonation, what are the functions of the vocal folds?**
Although phonation is an important function, it is not the primary role of the true and false vocal folds. Protection of the lower airway during swallowing is the most crucial function of the larynx, and the vocal folds are imperative to this. In addition, the TVFs provide the ability to cough and clear the airway and allow increased intra-abdominal pressure to build during a Valsalva maneuver. A Valsalva affords the ability to equalize middle ear pressure, lift weight, and bear down for bowel movements and child birth.

3. **Describe the innervation of the larynx.**
The larynx is innervated by various sensory and motor branches of the vagus nerve (CN X). After the vagus exits the skull base it gives off a branch, the superior laryngeal nerve (SLN). The SLN then divides into internal and external branches. The internal branch carries sensory information from the laryngeal mucosa above the TVFs. The external branch innervates the cricothyroid muscle, which

contracts to bring the thyroid cartilage closer to the cricoid cartilage, thus lengthening the TVFs and allowing pitch elevation of the voice. After giving off the superior laryngeal nerve, the vagus descends into the neck within the carotid sheath, along with the internal carotid artery and internal jugular vein (posterolateral to the internal carotid artery and posteromedial to the internal jugular vein). As the vagus enters into the thoracic cavity, it sends a branch cephalad, which is the recurrent laryngeal nerve (RLN). The right RLN splits from the right vagus nerve at the cervicothoracic junction, passing posterior to the right subclavian artery, and ascending posterior to the common carotid along the tracheoesophageal groove. One percent of right RLNs arise at the level of the thyroid gland and can be more readily injured during thyroidectomy. The left RLN takes off from the vagus nerve at the aortic arch, wrapping posteriorly underneath the ligamentum arteriosum and ascending cephalad in the tracheoesophageal groove. The RLNs enter the larynx near the cricothyroid joint and then split into anterior and posterior branches. The RLN innervates all the intrinsic muscles of the larynx (thyroarytenoid (TA), lateral cricoarytenoid (LCA), interarytenoid (IA) and posterior cricoarytenoid (PCA)), except the cricothyroid muscle. It also supplies sensory innervation to the mucosa of the TVFs and below.

4. **If innervation to the larynx is injured, what can happen?**
It should be understood that the innervation to the larynx is more complex than described above. There are anastamoses of the motor and sensory system as well as between the right and left sides. When the RLN and/or SLN sustains an injury, repair and reinnervation is often incomplete and variable among the smaller, terminal branches. Because the RLN carries adductor (TA, LCA, and IA) and abductor (PCA) fibers, damage to the nerve severe enough to cause Wallerian degeneration results in "cross-wiring" or synkinetic reinnervation and lack of purposeful motion to the affected muscles. Synkinetic TVFs will have good tone and often a normal interference pattern on LEMG whereas completely denervated TVFs will atrophy.

5. **Describe the embryology pertinent to the RLN.**
The larynx develops from the branchial arch system. The supraglottis and superior laryngeal nerve arise from the fourth arch. The cricoid cartilage and recurrent laryngeal nerve arise from the sixth arch. On the right the sixth segmental artery disappears completely, and the fourth arch artery remains as the subclavian artery. This explains why the right recurrent laryngeal nerve passes under only the right subclavian vessels and has a shorter distance to travel back to the larynx. In contrast, on the left side, the sixth arch artery persists as the ductus arteriosus, which later fibroses to become the ligamentum arteriosum. This remnant necessitates a longer course for the left recurrent laryngeal nerve, forcing it to descend into the chest before returning to the larynx. The effect of this embryologic development on the course of the RLN explains why intrathoracic processes can result in unilateral vocal fold paralysis (Table 76-2).

Table 76-2. Causes of Vocal Fold Paralysis/Immobility

Idiopathic (postviral neuropathy)	Tumors of the head and neck
Thyroid or parathyroid surgery	Laryngeal ventricle or piriform sinus mass
Skull base surgery	Intrathoracic, mediastinal neoplasm
Vagal neoplasm	Thoracic/cervical trauma
Anterior cervical fusion surgery	Aortic aneurysm
Carotid surgery	Left atrial dilation ('Ortner syndrome')
Traumatic intubation/extubation	Brainstem infarction (bulbar palsy)-rare
Arytenoid dislocation	Wallenberg syndrome
Cricothyroid joint fixation	Multiple sclerosis
Rheumatoid arthritis	ALS
Osteomyelitis of skull base	Poliomyelitis
Tuberculosis	Lupus
Chronic alcohol abuse	Granulomatous disease (e.g., sarcoidosis)
Fibrosis from radiation to head and neck	Diabetic polyneuropathy
Endotracheal tube cuff injury to RLN	Polyarteritis nodosum
Thoracic surgery	
Surgery of/near aortic arch	

6. **What is the difference between vocal fold immobility, vocal fold paralysis, and vocal fold paresis?**
It is important to use the correct terminology when evaluating vocal folds that do not move, as it refers to the etiology of their dysfunction. *Immobility* is a general term that does not indicate a cause; it refers to the lack of movement of the vocal folds from any cause, neurologic or mechanical. In addition, any nonmobile vocal fold that has yet to be designated as one with permanent motion impairment is called *immobile* rather than paralyzed. In contrast, *paralysis* of the vocal folds specifically refers to lack of movement (or immobility) from a permanent neurologic cause. If a vocal fold has a partial motion abnormality that is yet to be designated as permanent (i.e., a patient who presents with a new onset partial vocal TVF motion abnormality) it is called *hypomobile*; it is only given the diagnosis of a TVF *paresis* when it is 6 months or older with no other mechanical explanation, and is therefore from a permanent neurologic cause.

7. **Describe the findings on laryngoscopy and stroboscopy seen in vocal fold paralysis.**
In a complete unilateral paralysis, the fold will neither abduct nor adduct and will sit in a neutral position somewhere between adducted and abducted. The position of the immobile or paralyzed TVF does not necessarily distinguish between vagus and RLN injury. As reinnervation occurs in RLN injury, not all minor branches of the nerve may recover, and the position of the affected vocal fold often changes over time. The healthy, opposite vocal fold will have full abduction and adduction capability, and will try to cross the midline to meet the paralyzed fold (Figure 76-1). The arytenoid

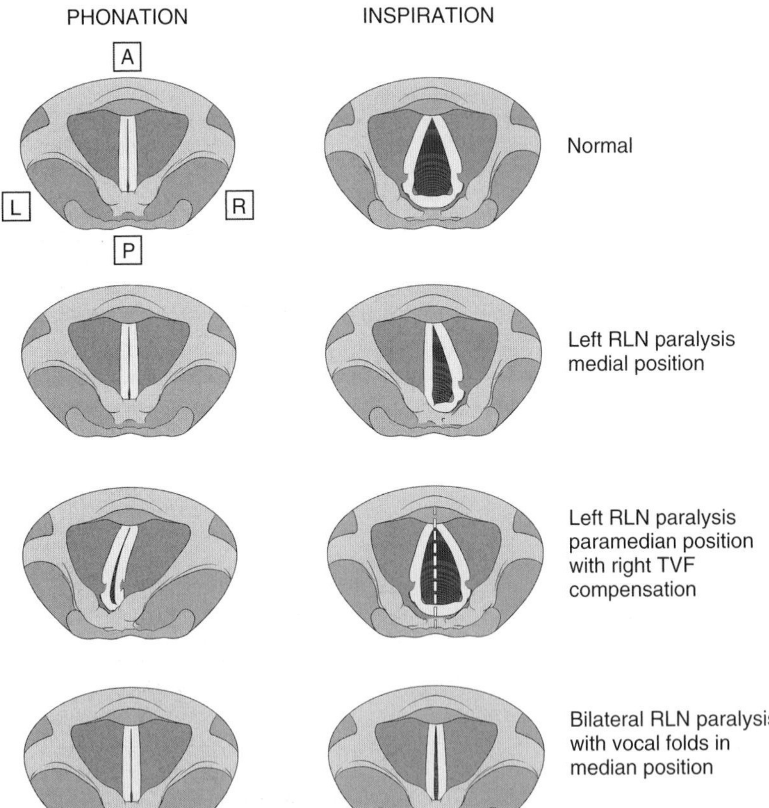

Figure 76-1. Vocal cord paralysis diagrams.

cartilage on the side of denervation most often falls anteriorly into the airway, but the appearance of the arytenoid does not give any definitive information on the neurologic status of the affected RLN. On stroboscopy one may see a transglottic gap without significant vibration or a complete (but dominantly open) closure pattern with asymmetry depending on the position of the immobile TVF. Denervation atrophy after a few weeks or months may lead to greater vibratory amplitude. There is typically supraglottic hyperfunction (secondary muscle tension) due to the compensatory effort by the surrounding intrinsic laryngeal muscles, which may even cause pain/discomfort.

In bilateral vocal fold paralysis, it is important to differentiate between those patients with bilateral midline TVFs and those with TVFs that remain paramedian with a glottic gap. When the folds are immobile in the midline, patients typically experience a normal voice but significant airway compromise and respiratory distress. On the contrary, when the TVFs lie in a paramedian position, the patient will not routinely have airway compromise but the voice will be severely affected with a transglottic gap on stroboscopy.

8. **What is a glottic gap/glottic insufficiency?**
A glottic gap refers to a pathologic space between the true vocal folds during phonation. It is possible to see this grossly in the setting of severe atrophy or vocal fold paralysis/immobility. Often, laryngovideostroboscopy (flexible laryngoscopy modality that uses a strobe light to give better visualization of the movement and closure pattern of the vocal folds) is needed to identify a more subtle glottic gap due to small benign lesions, paresis/hypomobility, early atrophy or scar. Glottic insufficiency is the pathologic and excess loss of air from the vocal folds due to a glottic gap. Glottic insufficiency typically is the cause of secondary muscle tension dysphonia that presents on exam as hyperfunctional behaviors of the supraglottic structures that are attempting to compensate for the glottic insufficiency. In females, a posterior glottic gap is often physiologic and normal.

9. **What is the role of laryngeal electromyography in evaluating vocal fold paralysis?**
Laryngeal electromyography (LEMG) is a test to help characterize the innervation status of an immobile vocal fold. It uses the body's own electricity to demonstrate whether or not the RLN is sending signals to the muscle's motor units or if the muscle is just firing on its own without any input. LEMG can determine if an immobile TVF is from a neurologic cause or a mechanical cause, such as cricoarytenoid joint dislocation, with the latter demonstrating normal LEMG activity. If the muscle is normally innervated, multiple action potentials from many motor units will overlap into a normal *interference pattern* and there is no spontaneous/random electrical activity. Alternatively, if the muscle is denervated, fibrillation potentials and positive waves are spontaneously seen. During the time when reinnervation is occurring or after incomplete reinnervation, polyphasic motor units are present. LEMG may indicate the potential for return of neuromuscular activity months before a clinical exam shows vocal fold motion. Synkinesis or other poor prognostic findings such as persistent positive waves/fibrillation potentials after serial LEMGs a few months apart help the physician recommend early permanent augmentation.

10. **Which other tests should be included in the workup of unexplained unilateral TVF immobility or paralysis?**
In patients with new onset unilateral TVF paralysis that cannot be explained by a recent surgery, intubation, trauma or known pathology, it is important to consider extrinsic causes, specifically masses compressing the recurrent laryngeal nerve anywhere along its course. A CT scan with contrast from the skull base through the aortic arch is the initial test of choice as a chest X-ray is rarely helpful. If the CT is negative and the history and neurologic exam suggests multiple cranial neuropathies, an MRI of the brain and brainstem is indicated. If there is associated stridor that cannot be explained by laryngoscopy, tracheobronchoscopy should be performed.

11. **What are the potential sequelae of unilateral true vocal fold immobility?**
Aspiration pneumonia is a potentially fatal sequela and early injection augmentation is offered preventatively in acute TVF immobility in an effort to improve "pulmonary toilet" (the ability to cough and clear secretions). Augmenting a unilateral TVF immobility by no means guarantees improvement in dysphagia or prevention of aspiration pneumonia, as it may be related to a sensory deficit from SLN dysfunction. However, improving the patient's ability to cough more effectively may be enough to protect the lungs from small aspirations and will also improve voice.

12. **What are the potential sequelae of bilateral true vocal fold paralysis?**
Airway compromise is the primary concern in bilateral TVF paralysis. Most patients do not tolerate the insult if it occurs acutely. Patients who have long-standing bilateral paralysis (or who had a gradual onset) may have stridor at rest or with exercise but function to a satisfactory level when they are otherwise healthy. However, as in the setting of an acute upper respiratory infection, even a small amount of edema in an already narrow glottis can significantly decrease the cross-sectional area of the airway and lead to a life-threatening situation.

13. **What are the treatment options for new onset unilateral vocal fold immobility?**
When underlying causes have been ruled out or are concurrently being treated, the first step to manage a unilateral TVF immobility in a *symptomatic* patient is temporary injection augmentation of the affected TVF. This can be performed in the office, at the bedside or in the operating room with a material that typically lasts 2 to 6 months. Early augmentation has been shown to improve long-term voice outcomes and decrease the need for permanent augmentation (the reason for this phenomenon is incompletely understood). LEMG is performed as early as 3 weeks from the time of injury and can be repeated 2 months later, affording prognostic information. Various factors such as patient age, occupation, comorbid conditions, and preferences all play a role in management. Watchful waiting is satisfactory in many who can swallow and communicate sufficiently.

14. **What are the treatment options for a long-standing unilateral vocal fold paralysis?**
Treatment options include injection laryngoplasty, medialization laryngoplasty with or without arytenoid adduction, and RLN reinnervation. Reinnervation procedures can be performed to re-establish tone to the intrinsic muscles of the larynx but these will not produce motion of the TVF and often require augmentation to improve voice during the period of nerve regrowth. No procedure to treat unilateral TVF paralysis will ever restore actual purposeful motion of the affected TVF.

Injection laryngoplasty, deep into the TA muscle, is accomplished via a percutaneous or peroral route in the office, or via suspension laryngoscopy in the operating room. The materials available for long-term (>6 months) augmentation include: calcium hydroxylapatite, micronized dermis, hyaluronic acid, and autologous fat (fat is considered the only permanent injectable by many and is only performed in the OR because of harvesting). Injection laryngoplasty can be very effective for a small glottic gap when the paralyzed vocal fold is midline or paramedian. For larger glottic gaps, injection is often less than satisfactory and medialization laryngoplasty is a more effective treatment (Figure 76-2A).

Medialization laryngoplasty, or laryngeal framework surgery, involves the placement of a carved silastic block, Gore-Tex® strip, or prefabricated implant within the paraglottic space, pushing the affected TVF medially (see Figure 76-2B). An adjunctive treatment to medialization laryngoplasty includes arytenoid adduction with or without arytenopexy. The arytenoid cartilage is repositioned by anchoring sutures into a more physiologic position for phonation. This is employed when there is a large posterior glottic gap or mismatch of the height of the vocal processes of the arytenoid cartilages (Figure 76-2B).

15. **What are the treatment options for acute bilateral vocal fold immobility?**
Patients with bilateral incomplete paralysis can experience partial or even full recovery, and LEMG is employed in this setting to help with prognosis. Treatment options aim to both preserve and protect the patient's airway, while awaiting one or both sides to recover motion. Suture lateralization of one vocal fold or tracheostomy is typically used to overcome the acute insult. Theoretically, both of these treatments are reversible.

16. **What are the treatment options for permanent bilateral TVF paralysis?**
For cases of permanent bilateral TVF paralysis where the airway is affected and voice is normal, unilateral or bilateral cordotomy with medial or total arytenoidectomies can be performed. This is typically accomplished in a serially, progressively destructive fashion, until a balance between airway and voice loss is acceptable. These destructive procedures will often lead to a breathier voice but afford enough airway improvement to avoid/remove a tracheotomy tube. Alternatively, lateralization procedures of either the vocal fold itself or the arytenoid (arytenoid abduction) can be performed. In bilateral complete vocal fold paralysis, tracheostomy may be initially required, but with surgeries to enlarge the airway at the glottic level many bilateral TVF paralysis patients can

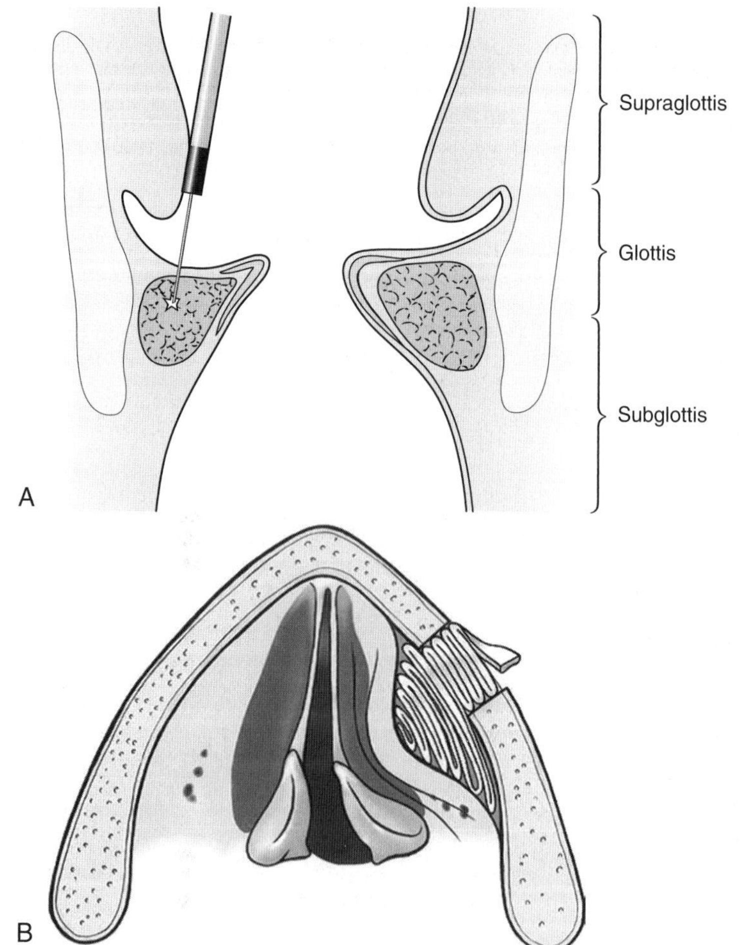

Figure 76-2. A, Coronal section of the larynx, demonstrating depth of needle placement and location deep in the thyroarytenoid muscle for injection laryngoplasty. **B,** Axial section glottis showing Gore-Tex® medialization *(Adapted from Rosen CA, Simpson CB: Operative Techniques in Laryngology, Berlin, 2008, Springer.)*

eventually be decannulated. When the voice is affected by paramedian bilateral paralyzed TVFs, medialization and injection augmentation can be used to close the glottic gap, but tracheotomy is often necessary.

17. **What is the long-term prognosis in patients with vocal fold paralysis?**
In cases of unilateral vocal fold paralysis, the outcomes are generally good. With augmentation procedures, most patients can achieve a functional voice with the exception of certain scenarios like singing or projecting one's voice loudly. As discussed, patients with vocal fold paralysis are at risk for aspiration, as they cannot always protect the airway. This is especially true when the etiology is a high vagal insult that includes a laryngeal sensory deficit. Augmentation of the affected TVF in no way guarantees swallowing improvement, though it often helps. In the setting of a complete, unilateral RLN injury without SLN involvement, many patients swallow effortlessly.

BIBLIOGRAPHY

Arviso LC, Johns MM, Mathison CC, et al: Long-term outcomes of injection laryngoplasty in patients with potentially recoverable vocal fold paralysis, *Laryngoscope* 120:2237–2240, 2010.

Carroll TL, Rosen CA: Trial vocal fold injection, *J Voice* 24(4):494–498, 2010.

Friedman AD, Burns JA, Heaton JT, et al: Early versus late injection medialization for unilateral vocal cord paralysis, *Laryngoscope* 120:2042–2046, 2010.

Lichtenberger G: Reversible lateralization of the paralyzed vocal cord without tracheostomy, *Annals Otol Rhinol Laryngol* 111(1):21–26, 2002.

Morris L, Afifi S: *Tracheostomies: The Complete Guide*, New York, 2010, Springer.

Oertli D, Udelsman R: *Surgery of the Thyroid and Parathyroid Glands*, New York, 2007, Springer, pp 13–20.

Ossoff RH, Shapshay SM, Woodson GE, et al: *The Larynx*, Philadelphia, 2003, Lippincott Williams & Wilkins, pp 3–14, 267–305.

Rosen CA, Simpson CB: *Operative Techniques in Laryngology*, Berlin, 2008, Springer-Verlag, p 105, 240, 248.

Statham MM, Rosen CA, Nandedkar SD, et al: Quantitative laryngeal electromyography: Turns and amplitude analysis, *Laryngoscope* 120:2036–2041, 2010.

Vaccha B, Cunnane MB, Mallur P, et al: Losing your voice: etiology and imaging features of vocal fold paralysis, *J Clin Imaging Sc* 3:15, 2013.

CHAPTER 77

INTUBATION AND TRACHEOTOMY

Justin Casey, MD and Kenneth T. Bellian, MD, MBA

KEY POINTS

1. A general rule for determining airway size in children, is **Age/4 + 3** for a cuffed tube, and **Age/4 + 4** for an uncuffed tube. It is generally safer to choose a smaller ET tube if debating between two tube sizes.
2. Tracheostomy does not prevent chronic aspiration.
3. Inspiratory stridor with muffled voice and usually a lack of cough are concerning symptoms for epiglottitis, a possible emergent airway. If the patient is stable, a lateral neck x-ray may demonstrate a "thumb sign" indicating a swollen epiglottis.
4. Biphasic stridor with barking cough is consistent with subglottitis, or "croup." An AP neck x-ray may demonstrate a "steeple sign" indicating subglottic narrowing.
5. Significant bleeding from a tracheostomy should be taken seriously and investigated to rule out trachea-innominate fistula, a surgical emergency that carries a mortality rate of 73%.

Pearls

1. A vertical incision can be used in newborns to decrease the risk of subglottic stenosis.
2. The trachea is the anatomic location in the head and neck with the highest rate of cocaine absorption.
3. A cuff pressure of 34 cm H_20 will compromise capillary blood flow to tracheal mucosa and cause pressure necrosis.
4. What is the management for an airway fire?
   - Turn off the flow of O_2
   - Douse fire with saline
   - Remove damaged tube
   - Reintubate as atraumatically as possible
   - Administer IV steroids and antibiotics
   - Bronchoscopy before leaving the OR to remove any charred tissue or other debris, and evaluate extent of airway injury
   - Delayed extubation with repeat endoscopic airway examinations

QUESTIONS

1. **What are common airway grading systems to consider prior to intubation?**
Friedman Palate Position (Figure 77-1):

I—Visualization of entire uvula and tonsils/tonsillar pillars
II—Visualization of the uvula, but not tonsils
III—Visualization of the soft palate, but no uvula
IV—Visualization of hard palate only

Similarly, the Mallampati Score (more commonly used in anesthesiology):

Class I—Soft palate, uvula, fauces, pillars visible
Class II—Soft palate, uvula, fauces visible
Class III—Soft palate, base of uvula visible
Class IV—No soft palate visible

The higher the score, the more difficult exposure of the larynx may be during intubation.

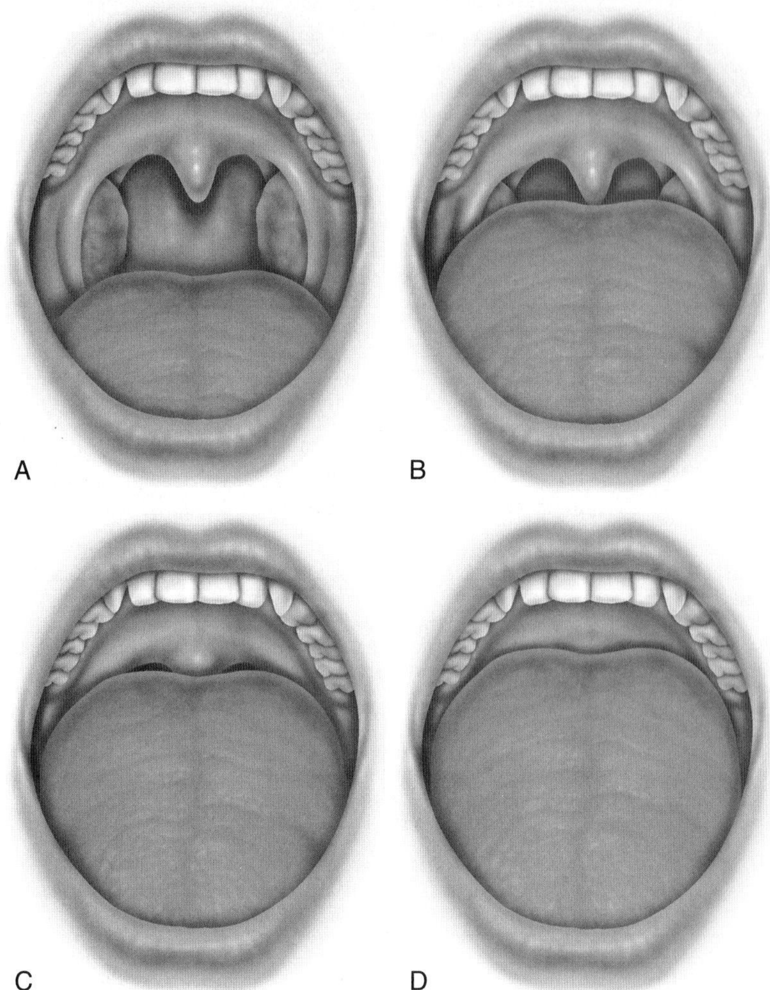

Figure 77-1. Friedman Palate Position. **A,** I—Visualization of entire uvula and tonsils/tonsillar pillars. **B,** II—Visualization of the uvula, but not tonsils. **C,** III—Visualization of the soft palate, but no uvula. **D,** IV—Visualization of hard palate only. *(From Friedman M, Hani I, Bass L: Clinical staging for sleep disordered breathing, Otolaryngol Head Neck Surg 127:13–21, 2002.)*

2. What does the size of the endotracheal tube refer to?
   The number refers to the inner diameter of the endotracheal tube. Thus, a 5.0 ET tube will have an inner diameter of 5 mm, a 5.5 ET tube will have an inner diameter of 5.5 mm, and so on. The outer diameter of the ET tube can vary by material, manufacturer, and type of tube.

3. How can you quickly estimate the properly sized endotracheal (ET) tube for children?
   - Cuffed tube = age/4 + 3
   - Uncuffed tube = age/4+4

     This is generally accurate for children ages 1 through 12.

Table 77-1. Suggested ETT Size for Age

AGE	ENDOTRACHEAL TUBE SIZE
Neonate	2.5–3.0
Infant 1–6 months	3.0–3.5
Infant 6–12 months	3.5–4.0
Toddler	4.0–5.0
Adult Female	6.0–7.0
Adult Male	7.0–8.0

4. **How are ET tube sizes chosen for other patients?**
See Table 77-1.

As a general rule, if between two ET tube sizes it is safer to put in a slightly smaller ET tube rather than one that is too large and difficult to pass. If ventilation is difficult with a small tube, some ventilation can be administered to stabilize the patient, and a tube exchanger can be used to change the ET tube, with very low risk of losing the airway.

5. **What is the common airway classification measured during intubation?**
Cormack-Lehane Classification grades the view of the larynx during direct laryngoscopy:

Grade I—Visualization of entire glottis
Grade II—Partial view of glottis
Grade III—Visualization of the epiglottis only
Grade IV—Not even epiglottis is visible

6. **What are the typical sounds of obstruction at different levels of the airway?**
- Trachea—Usually expiratory, occasionally inspiratory
- Subglottis—biphasic stridor, barking cough, hoarse voice
- Glottis—biphasic or inspiratory stridor, hoarse voice
- Supraglottic—inspiratory stridor, muffled voice, inability to feed, no cough
- Oropharynx/nasopharynx—stertor, muffled or hyponasal voice

7. **What are some conservative interventions for upper airway obstruction?**
Chin lift with jaw thrust, oropharyngeal airway, and *nasopharyngeal airway* are anatomic manipulations that can help alleviate upper airway obstruction. The first two are generally used for unconscious patients. The latter is best used for patients with oral obstruction (i.e., trauma, Ludwig's angina), or in neonates with nasal obstruction who are obligate nasal breathers. *Heliox* can be used to deliver oxygen in cases of airway obstruction. Heliox is a mixture of helium and oxygen and is a lower density gas compared to room air or pure oxygen. This allows a higher flow rate, which reduces turbulent flow past an obstruction delivering more oxygen distally to the lungs. This reduced turbulent flow also decreases the pressure gradient needed to move air across an obstruction, thus reducing airway resistance and work of breathing. Typical concentrations are 21%:79% oxygen to helium. Helium is inert, insoluble in human tissues, and noncombustible. Heliox is used as a temporizing measure while planning to perform a more definitive airway stabilization.

8. **What other noninvasive interventions can improve upper airway obstruction?**
- *Racemic epinephrine*—administered via nebulizer to cause vasoconstriction and reduce mucosal edema. Racemic epinephrine has been shown to help treat croup and postextubation stridor from laryngeal edema. Racemic epinephrine is not as effective for epiglottitis and the practice of trying to administer it can be dangerous because agitation for these patients can cause acute obstruction by the swollen epiglottis.
- *IV steroids*—glucocorticoids, such as dexamethasone, are used to reduce airway inflammation and edema. This is thought to occur through reduced capillary dilation and decreased plasma

extravasation and inflammatory mediator release. They are also indicated for croup and laryngeal edema, and are often used for other causes of upper airway obstruction (i.e., abscess or other infectious edema including epiglottitis, angioedema). IV steroids act gradually, unlike racemic epinephrine, which acts fairly rapidly.

9. **What are the indications for fiber-optic intubation (FOI)?**
   - History of difficult intubation requiring FOI
   - Micrognathia or other craniofacial anomalies
   - Cervical spine issues (fused disks, unstable C-spine)
   - Facial trauma
   - Upper airway obstruction (glottis level or above)
   - Necessity for awake intubation (cannot mask ventilate)
   - Trismus

10. **What are the most common indications for tracheostomy?**
   - Emergent upper airway obstruction or inability to intubate
   - Prolonged intubation/ventilatory support
   - Glottic/supraglottic obstruction (including tumor, infection, trauma, surgical changes)
   - Pulmonary toilet
   - Chronic aspiration (relative indication)
   - Severe sleep apnea not controlled by CPAP or less-invasive surgery

11. **What is the difference between tracheostomy and tracheotomy?**
   A tracheotomy is any procedure that cuts an opening into the trachea. Tracheostomy is technically a term for a more permanent tract that is formed from trachea to skin. In reality, a trache*otomy* is typically performed, which naturally becomes a trache*ostomy* as the tract from skin to airway matures. However, a tracheostomy can be performed at the time of a tracheotomy by suturing skin to the trachea, thus allowing a more stable airway in case of accidental decannulation. These terms are often used interchangeably.

12. **What are the surgical landmarks for tracheotomy?**
   Using a surgical marking pen, the thyroid notch, the cricoid cartilage, and sternal notch should be marked.

13. **On what area on the trachea should the tracheotomy be made?**
   Between the second and third tracheal rings. Above this, the tube may erode or fracture the cricoid cartilage, which can lead to subglottic stenosis. Below this, there is risk to mediastinal structures such as the innominate artery.

14. **What are the basic steps of a tracheotomy?**
   1. The procedure starts with positioning the patient supine with the neck extended. A shoulder roll is very effective in maximizing this extension.
   2. Next, the proper landmarks are marked, and the neck is injected with a mixture of lidocaine and epinephrine.
   3. The tracheostomy tube cuff is tested with inflation of the balloon, completely deflated, and then lubricated for ease of insertion. During insertion, the balloon can tear and the lubricant minimizes the trauma to the balloon.
   4. An incision is made in the skin in either a vertical or horizontal direction depending on surgeon preference and age of patient. This incision is centered over the second to third tracheal rings, which can be approximated by incising two fingerbreadths above the sternal notch. Incision is carried through skin, subcutaneous fat, and platysma. Anterior jugular veins may be encountered during this portion of the dissection.
   5. Strap muscles are encountered next, and are divided vertically along the midline raphe to reveal pretracheal fascia and the thyroid isthmus inferiorly. By staying in the midline with your dissection, you will minimize bleeding and inadvertent injury to other structures.
   6. The thyroid isthmus is either retracted inferiorly or superiorly depending on its mobility. If it lacks mobility then the isthmus is transected to expose the trachea.
   7. At this point, the anesthesia team should be notified. The anterior surface of the trachea is cleared of its fascial and soft tissue attachments, and any bleeding is attended to in order to ensure a clear vision of the trachea prior to incision.

8. Incision into trachea is made between second and third rings. This is done with cold steel to avoid risk of airway fire with electrocautery. Most commonly, either a square section of tracheal cartilage is removed ("tracheal window") or a Björk flap (described later in this chapter) is created.
9. The ETT is slowly removed by anesthesia under direct visualization by surgery team. Once it has moved past the opening in the trachea, the tracheostomy tube is inserted using the obturator. The ETT remains in place until the tracheostomy tube location is confirmed and the tube is fixed in place.

15. **What are the proper steps and precautions after the tracheostomy tube has been placed into the airway?**
One hand should be kept on the tube AT ALL TIMES. The obturator should be removed and the inner cannula is inserted into the tracheostomy tube. The cuff should be inflated. Next, the anesthesia circuit is immediately connected and ventilation should be administered. Several items should immediately be assessed: (1) CO_2 return, (2) chest rise, (3) the connection to the tracheostomy tube is checked for condensation, (4) integrity of the balloon is confirmed, and (5) passage of a flexible suction catheter through the tracheostomy tube confirms patency. The anesthesiologist may listen for equal breath sounds. The tube is then sutured into place, and a trach collar is applied.

16. **What is a cricothyroidotomy?**
In contrast to the tracheotomy procedure described above, a cricothyroidotomy is an emergency procedure to establish an airway during a life-threatening situation. Many believe that this procedure is easier and quicker than a tracheotomy for the vast majority of medical personnel. There are several kits and techniques that can be used for a percutaneous or open cricothyroidotomy, but it typically begins with proper positioning and palpation of the cricothyroid membrane between the inferior border of the thyroid cartilage and superior border of the cricoid. The membrane is approximately 1 cm in height, depending on neck positioning. Next, a vertical incision is made through the overlying skin. The cricothyroid membrane is then palpated again, visualized, and a horizontal incision is made into the airway. Following the visualization of air bubbling from the wound, the wound is retracted open (using a tracheal hook, Trousseau dilator, or curved hemostat, etc.), and the tube can be placed with direct visualization of the airway. Some kits involve placing a needle percutaneously, followed by guide wire passage and dilation through a Seldinger technique.

17. **Tracheotomy versus cricothyroidotomy?**
For a planned procedure, a tracheotomy is preferred because it is a long-term and stable airway. A cricothyroidotomy should be converted to a tracheotomy as soon as possible to prevent erosion of the cricoid cartilage or tracheal stenosis.

In emergent procedures, there is some debate. Some ENT surgeons feel they are used to tracheotomies, so they should do this in an emergent situation as well. Others feel that a cricothyrotomy is quicker, with less blood loss, and generally a more reliable landmark in patients with anatomic differences (i.e., short and/or obese necks).

Infants and young children do not have a cricothyroid membrane, thus a tracheotomy is required in these populations.

18. **What are the most important intraoperative complications of tracheotomy?**
Complications can be avoided with appropriate communication with your anesthesiologist and operating room staff. For example, an airway fire is one of the more devastating complications. This can result from the use of electrocautery during tracheotomy if the FiO_2 concentration is too high. It is imperative to inform your anesthesiologist to turn down the FiO_2 several minutes before there is any chance of inadvertently cutting into the trachea with electrocautery. Prior to this point, a high FiO_2 may be needed to properly preoxygenate the patient for extubation and placement of the tracheostomy tube. The ETT should be slowly removed under direct visualization by the surgeon through the tracheotomy incision. If possible, the anesthesiologist may also watch over the surgical drape barrier. There should be constant communication between surgeon and anesthesiologist during this period.

Additional perioperative complications include subcutaneous emphysema, pneumothorax, and/or pneumomediastinum. Subcutaneous emphysema is thought to occur when air is forced through the incision into tissue planes of the neck. The mechanisms of pneumothorax or pneumomediastinum are less well understood. Pneumomediastinum is thought to occur when subcutaneous emphysema is forced further into the chest, through negative intrathoracic pressure or a cough that forces air into deep tissue planes of the neck and mediastinum. One theory for formation of a pneumothorax is through direct injury to the pleural apices when operating low in the neck. Another is progressive pneumomediastinum causing pleural injury followed by air tracking into the thoracic cavity.

19. **What is the first intervention for subcutaneous emphysema in a postoperative tracheotomy patient?**
Cutting sutures and inflating the cuff (if it is not already) is the first step. This is followed by a stat chest x-ray and further investigation into the cause.

20. **What are other life-threatening postoperative complications of tracheotomy?**
- Bleeding and/or tracheo-innominate fistula
- Mucus plugging
- Accidental decannulation
- False passage during placement of tracheotomy tube

21. **What is a tracheo-innominate (TI) fistula?**
A TI fistula occurs from erosion of the tracheotomy tube through the tracheal wall into the innominate (brachiocephalic) artery. This is an emergency requiring immediate intervention. The fistula typically comes from pressure necrosis from the inflated cuff or distal tip of the tracheostomy tube. Contributing factors include an overinflated cuff, poor wound healing, and a poorly fitting tube. Fistula formation usually occurs at about 2 weeks post-op, but has been described as early as 2 days. Mortality rate is approximately 73%. Classically, a "sentinel bleed" is described hours or even days prior, wherein there is a brief and intense period of bleeding that spontaneously resolves. This is important to identify, and a CTA may be used to evaluate a stable patient.

22. **How do you handle an urgent bleed in a patient with a tracheotomy?**
If there is a large amount of bleeding from in or around the stoma, the first step is to inflate or overinflate the cuff. If the tube is cuffless, or the patient is coughing up blood through the tube despite overinflation, it should be replaced with a cuffed 6.0 ET tube. The cuff should be placed distal to the site of bleeding and inflated. Finally, if TI fistula is suspected, an index finger should be placed through the tracheotomy in an attempt to apply pressure anteriorly against the innominate artery such that it is compressed against the sternum. The patient should then be taken emergently to the OR.

23. **What is a Björk flap?**
A Björk flap is created by utilizing the section of tracheal cartilage that is normally removed during tracheotomy. Superior and lateral cuts are made into the cartilage, but the inferior portion of the cartilage is left intact, leaving an inferiorly based cartilage flap. This flap is then sutured to muscle/fascial layers and skin of the stoma, such that it serves as the "floor" of the stomal tract. This assists in maintaining a patent stoma in the case of accidental decannulation. The Björk flap creates a tracheostomy that is less likely to spontaneously close upon decannulation (a tracheocutaneous fistula), therefore it is generally used in patients who will have the tracheostomy long term (Figure 77-2).

24. **What is the basic postoperative care for a tracheotomy?**
Some practitioners prefer to obtain a postoperative chest x-ray to ensure there is no pneumothorax. However, recent literature has demonstrated that this is generally low-yield in patients without signs or symptoms of a complication such as pneumothorax. Patients are typically admitted to the surgical ICU for airway monitoring.

A standard protocol for tracheotomy care is necessary to avoid a number of the frequent postoperative issues. The suctioning should be very frequent early on and it can even be necessary every 15 minutes for the first few hours. As the secretions change and lessen, it will be needed less frequently. The nurse and respiratory staff should instill saline lavage with suctioning to avoid any mucus plugging, and humidified air is administered to avoid crusting and plugging issues as the innate humidification system of the upper airway has been bypassed due to the tracheotomy.

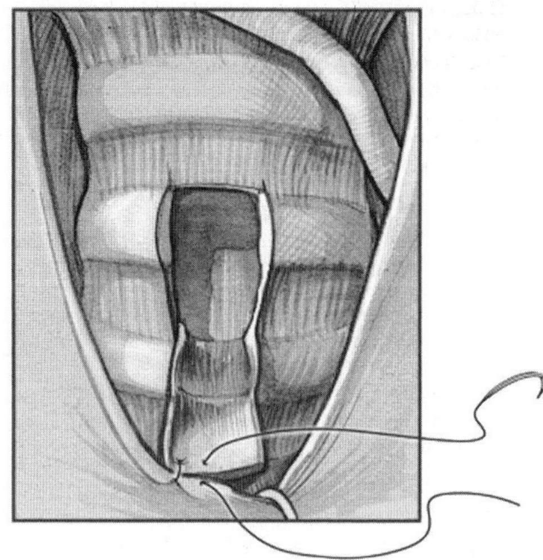

Figure 77-2. Björk flap. *(From Scurry Jr WC, McGinn JD: Operative tracheotomy. Operative Techniques Otolaryngol-Head Neck Surg 18(2):85–89, 2007.)*

CONTROVERSIES

25. **When is a cuffed tracheotomy tube indicated? Do they help prevent aspiration?**
A cuffed tube is used when positive airway pressure is needed for ventilation. This includes complete ventilatory support, as well as BiPAP/CPAP. Cuffed tubes can also help *slow* aspiration in patients not controlling their secretions. Otherwise, cuffs should always be left deflated. This will allow phonation and reduce the risk of pressure-induced injury to the tracheal mucosa.

Tracheotomy is generally not indicated for aspiration. Cuffed tracheotomy tubes may be helpful in dealing with pulmonary toilet/suctioning of the aspirating patient, or decreasing secretions from entering the lungs in patients with sensory or muscle problems of the upper airway. However, cuffed tubes do not prevent chronic aspiration. In fact, tracheotomies can increase the risk of aspiration, by preventing proper hyolaryngeal elevation during swallowing.

26. **What are advantages of an open versus percutaneous tracheotomy?**
Open tracheotomy is a surgical procedure that takes place in the OR. It involves an open wound, with the advantage of better visualization of the trachea prior to entering into the airway. It also allows for the identification and control of structures such as small and large blood vessels or the thyroid gland, which theoretically may allow for fewer minor and major complications during the procedure, as well as less postoperative bleeding. However, there have been several large-scale studies looking at the safety of bedside percutaneous tracheotomy in an ICU setting, usually through a dilatational/Seldinger method. The vast majority of these studies have suggested that they are as safe as OR procedures and with similar long-term complications, even in obese patients. Proponents argue that these procedures are faster and far more cost efficient than open tracheotomies. Critics, however, argue that there is a lack of prospective data, and that potentially complicated airways require open procedures. Some critics feel that a potentially catastrophic complication such as transecting a high-riding innominate artery during a percutaneous tracheotomy is enough risk to avoid such procedures. Additionally, in forcing somewhat blunt objects through the skin and trachea, tracheal rings can be crushed, causing long-term tracheal stenosis and/or tracheomalacia.

Bibliography

Ball JAS, Rhodes A, Grounds RM: A review of the use of helium in the treatment of acute respiratory failure, *Clinical Intensive Care* 12:105–113, 2001.

Benjamin BR: Prolonged intubation injuries of the larynx: endoscopic diagnosis, classification, and treatment, *Ann Otol Rhinol Laryngol Supple* 160:1–15, 1993.

Dennis BM, Eckert MJ, Gunter OL, et al: Safety of bedside percutaneous tracheostomy in the critically ill: evaluation of more than 3,000 procedures, *J Am Coll Surg* 216(4):858–865, 2013.

Depuydt S, Nauwynck M, Bourgeois M, et al: Acute epiglottitis in children: a review following an atypical case, *Acta Anaesth Belg* 54:237–241, 2003.

Durbin CG Jr: Tracheostomy: why, when, and how?, *Respir Care* 55(8):1056–1068, 2010.

Fernandez R, Tizon AI, Gonzalez J, et al: Intensive care unit discharge to the ward with a tracheostomy cannula as a risk factor for mortality: a prospective, multicenter propensity analysis, *Crit Care Med* 39(10):2240–2245, 2011.

Friedman M, Hani I, Bass L: Clinical staging for sleep disordered breathing, *Otolaryngol Head Neck Surg* 127:13–21, 2002.

Goldenberg D, Gov EG, Golz A, et al: Tracheotomy complications: a retrospective study of 1130 cases, *Otolaryngol Head Neck Surg* 123:495–500, 2000.

Kairys SW, Olmstead EM, O'Conner GT: Steroid treatment of laryngotracheitis: a meta-analysis of the evidence from randomized trials, *Pediatrics* 83:683–693, 1989.

Lalwani AK: *Current Diagnosis & Treatment in Otolaryngology: Head & Neck Surgery*, New York, 2008, McGraw-Hill Medical. Print.

CHAPTER 78

LARYNGEAL TRAUMA

Brook K. McConnell, MD and Jeremy D. Prager, MD

KEY POINTS

1. Laryngeal fractures are uncommon injuries that may be associated with life-threatening airway compromise.
2. The first and most important step in the management of laryngeal trauma is to secure a safe airway.
3. Esophagoscopy should be performed in any patient going to the operating room to rule out concomitant injury.
4. The most common cause of internal laryngeal trauma is endotracheal intubation, especially in the setting of prolonged intubation.
5. Arytenoid dislocations are rare and may present similarly to unilateral vocal cord paralysis.

Pearls

1. An experienced physician should manage the airway, and endotracheal intubation should only be performed under adequate visualization and when the larynx and trachea are in known continuity.
2. Intubating a patient blindly can convert a stable airway to an unstable airway.
3. Avoiding prolonged intubation is the most effective way to prevent internal laryngeal trauma.
4. Choosing the smallest endotracheal tube that will provide adequate ventilation will help minimize mucosal trauma.
5. Laryngeal trauma should be included in the differential diagnosis when evaluating a patient with vocal cord paralysis.

QUESTIONS

External Laryngeal Trauma

1. What is the incidence of external laryngeal trauma?
External laryngeal trauma is rare and occurs with an estimated incidence of 1 in 137,000 inpatient admissions and 1 in 30,000 emergency room visits. Laryngeal injuries in the pediatric patient are even more uncommon and account for $<0.5\%$ of trauma admission compared to 1% of adult trauma admissions. The occurrence of blunt trauma injuries has decreased in the past several decades due to improved automobile safety. However, the incidence of penetrating trauma has increased with a rise in violent crimes.

2. What anatomic features are protective against laryngeal trauma?
   - **Surrounding structures:** Multiple surrounding structures shield the larynx and provide protection from external trauma. These structures include the mandible superiorly, the sternum and clavicles inferiorly, the sternocleidomastoid muscles laterally, and the vertebrae posteriorly. Anterior soft tissue including strap muscles provides minimal protection from anteriorly directed force. In pediatric patients, the larynx is located higher in the neck in relation with the mandible and is thus further protected.
   - **Laryngeal mobility:** The larynx is mobile in multiple directions, most prominently in the lateral plane, but also in the anterior/posterior and superior/inferior planes. This mobility allows it to be pushed out of the way by external forces.
   - **Tissue pliability:** In adults, ossification of the larynx increases the chances of fracture in the setting of blunt trauma. In children, laryngeal cartilages remain pliable and are consequently more resistant to fracture.

3. **Discuss the etiology of external laryngeal trauma.**

Blunt trauma occurs as the result of an anterior force compressing the larynx against the fixed vertebral column. These injuries classically result from motor vehicle accidents and occur when the hyperextended neck is thrust onto the dashboard or steering wheel during rapid deceleration. Another subset of these injuries are "clothesline" injuries in which a thin horizontal structure (e.g., barbed wire fence) is struck.

The severity of trauma is variable and depends on multiple factors. The speed at which the patient is traveling is key because injury severity is generally proportional to velocity. The size and configuration of the surface against which the neck makes contact is also important to consider because a larger force distributed over a smaller surface area is more likely to result in penetrating trauma rather than blunt trauma.

Penetrating trauma more commonly occurs as a result of violent crime and military conflict. The energy of the penetrating object is an important factor in determining the potential for airway injury. Any additional information regarding the penetrating object is helpful as it can help predict the extent of collateral damage.

4. **What are the main symptoms and signs of blunt laryngeal trauma?**

Physical exam may range from the asymptomatic to the critically ill and symptoms alone may not denote severity. Dysphonia, dysphagia, pain, and difficulty breathing are the most common initial symptoms. Patients may present with mild symptoms and progress to airway compromise over minutes to hours due to progressive edema, hematoma or instability of the laryngotracheal framework. Observation is recommended if history and physical are at all concerning. A disrupted airway may present with cervical crepitus, particularly in the patient who has been managed with positive pressure ventilation. In these critically ill patients, look for/anticipate pneumomediastinum, pneumothorax, and worsening respiratory status. Note that these patients are often at risk for cervical spine and vascular trauma as well. Loss of anatomic landmarks on neck palpitation may indicate hyoid or laryngeal fracture, or hematoma. Hemoptysis is indicative of mucosal disruption at the least.

5. **Discuss the management of acute airway compromise following laryngeal trauma.**

The first step in airway management is to determine whether the patient displays signs and symptoms of impending airway compromise such as stridor, dyspnea, respiratory distress, or aphonia. If a patient exhibits signs of airway compromise, a secure airway must be obtained as soon as possible. There are several methods that are appropriate to secure the airway in the setting of laryngeal trauma including intubation, tracheostomy, and cricothyroidotomy.

Several factors must be taken into consideration when choosing which method will be used to secure the airway, including patient stability and injury severity. Control of the airway should occur in the emergency room or, when possible, the operating room to allow for optimal direct and endoscopic evaluation. For endotracheal intubation to proceed, the larynx and trachea must be clearly intact and in continuity to prevent mucosal disruption, laryngotracheal separation, false passage of the endotracheal tube surrounding soft tissue, and further respiratory compromise. It is important to note that intubation should be performed by an experienced physician to help prevent intubation-related trauma (Figure 78-1).

Cricothyroidotomy is reserved for those patients with a rapidly deteriorating airway, those who do not meet the optimal conditions for intubation, or those patients in whom tracheostomy is not possible due to patient factors or availability of physicians experienced in the surgical airway. Cricothyroidotomy is dependent on continuity of the cricoid and trachea. Cricothyroidotomy should subsequently be converted to a tracheostomy to prevent the development of subglottic stenosis. Following emergent management of the airway, these patients should undergo endoscopic evaluation of the aerodigestive tract in the operating room.

6. **Discuss important aspects of the evaluation and management of a stable patient with external laryngeal trauma.**

A. History:
   1. Mechanism of injury: Be suspicious in the setting of high velocity impact directed anteriorly to the neck.
   2. Temporal evolution: Determine if symptoms are getting worse.

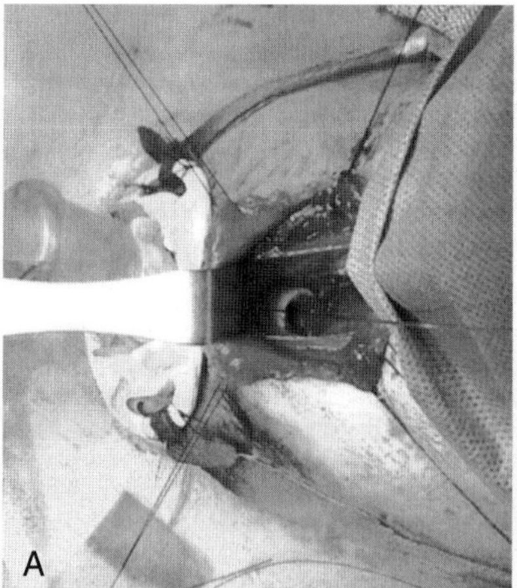

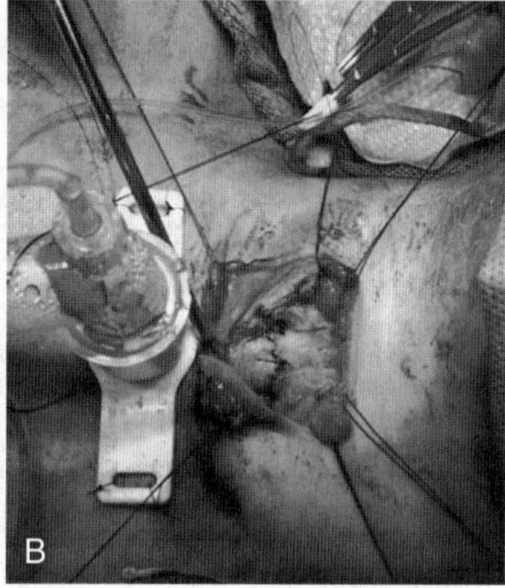

Figure 78-1. Clothesline injury followed by intubation in the field resulting in complete separation of the larynx and trachea. **A,** Patient was managed by low tracheostomy followed by neck exploration. The airway was separated between the cricoid and the first tracheal ring, which was crushed and fractured. **B,** The second tracheal ring and cricoid were anastomosed.

B. Physical exam:
   1. Head and neck exam: Bony and soft tissue trauma, voice quality, respiratory effort, loss of landmarks, crepitus
   2. Associated injuries: Neurological, vascular, or spinal injuries

C. Flexible laryngoscopy: Damage to mucosa of supraglottis, damage to vocal folds (mucosal tears, hematoma, exposed muscle or cartilage), vocal fold mobility

D. Definitive management:
   1. Nonsurgical management
      a. Appropriate for "reversible injuries" due to blunt trauma: endolaryngeal edema, hematoma, contusion, abrasion, non-displaced fractures and small lacerations. These patients commonly have dysphonia, neck pain and tenderness to palpation.
      b. Observe for 12–24 hours following injury. +/- Steroids; +/- Proton Pump Inhibitor; +/- Cool mist.
      c. Controversy regarding plating/repairing all laryngeal framework fractures. Some authors prefer plating even non-displaced fractures due to concerns of displacement over time.
   2. Surgical management: Goal is preservation of airway patency and function. Earlier intervention is associated with better outcomes. Surgical approach may require some or all of the following:
      a. Midline thyrotomy
      b. Repair of mucosal lacerations, muscle disruption, cartilage repair
      c. Stenting may or may not be used. Surgeon experience/preference will determine this.
      d. Repair laryngeal skeletal fractures with wires, sutures, plating. Plating may be difficult in the more cartilaginous pediatric larynx.

7. **What is the preferred imaging modality for the assessment of laryngeal trauma?**
In the patient with a stable airway, CT scan is the preferred imaging modality due to its fast acquisition and adequate imaging of the larynx and surrounding structures. It is important to note that airway management should not be delayed for imaging. Imaging is particularly helpful in patients with blunt injury in whom it is difficult to ascertain severity of injury and/or when the continuity of the endolarynx/trachea is unknown.

8. **What associated injuries should be ruled out in laryngeal trauma patients?**
A. Cervical spine injury: Based on the National Emergency X-Radiography Utilization Study (NEXUS) criteria, laryngeal trauma qualifies as a "distracting injury" and cervical radiography is indicated

to evaluate for the presence of cervical spine injuries. Since a CT scan may be obtained to evaluate the larynx, a cervical spine protocol may be added.

B. Pharyngeal/Esophageal Injuries:
- Infrequent in penetrating and blunt laryngeal injuries (4% to 6%) but potentially catastrophic
- Rigid esophagoscopy recommended in all patients undergoing surgical treatment of external airway injuries
- Barium esophagram may also be useful in nonsurgical patients.

9. **Propose an algorithm for evaluation and management of external laryngeal trauma.**
See Figure 78-2.

10. **What anatomic factors affect laryngeal trauma in the pediatric patient?**
There are several differences between the pediatric larynx and adult larynx that affect laryngeal trauma in the pediatric population. Some of these factors are protective, but some also convey increased risk. First, the larynx lies at the level of C3 in young children and descends gradually until the age of three when it takes on a more adult location at the level of C6. The relatively high location of the pediatric larynx provides some additional protection afforded by the overhanging mandible. Another protective feature of the pediatric larynx is its pliability. Compared to an adult larynx, which is relatively rigid due to ossification, the pediatric larynx remains pliable. The flexibility allows for compression without fracture in the setting of external blunt trauma.

Conversely, the child's larynx is relatively smaller than the adult airway, which translates to greater potential compromise from edema. Furthermore, the submucosal tissue in a pediatric patient is loosely adherent to the underlying perichondrium when compared to the adult, resulting in the potential for greater soft tissue injury, edema, and hematoma formation. This combination of factors translates to greater risk of airway compromise in these patients despite the protective factors discussed above.

Internal Laryngeal Trauma

11. **Discuss the etiology of internal laryngeal trauma.**
The predominant cause of internal laryngeal trauma is iatrogenic injury related to endotracheal intubation. The injury can result from the act of intubation or the presence of an endotracheal tube: risk factors include prolonged intubation, excessive endotracheal tube (ET) size, intubation in the emergency setting, and intubation without neuromuscular blockade. Acute complications include mucosal lacerations, arytenoid dislocation, and tracheal rupture, among others. Trauma related to prolonged intubation is the result of long-standing excessive pressure from the ET or the cuff, leading to tissue necrosis, inflammation, and subglottic stenosis from scar formation. Longer duration correlates with greater histologic damage.

There are several locations that are at risk for injury from prolonged intubation, including the narrowest portions of both the adult and pediatric airway—the glottis and subglottis, respectively. In children, intubation injury in the subglottis can result in subglottic stenosis. In adult patients, damage at the level of the glottis generally occurs posteriorly and can result in posterior glottic stenosis and even bilateral vocal cord immobility (Figure 78-3).

12. **What is the incidence of subglottic stenosis following endotracheal intubation?**
The incidence in pediatric patients (those most at risk) ranges from approximately 1% to 8%. More recent reports indicate an incidence between 0% and 2%. Of patients with acquired subglottic stenosis, approximately 90% of cases are due to endotracheal intubation.

13. **What are other causes of internal laryngeal trauma?**
Caustic injections and inhalational burns are two other causes of internal laryngeal injury. The larynx is involved in 40% of caustic ingestions. Thermal injury of the larynx occurs in 30% of burn patients. These injuries tend to produce more severe stenosis compared to postintubation trauma.

14. **What is arytenoid dislocation?**
Arytenoid dislocation is a rare injury that can occur as the result of external laryngeal trauma with disruption of the laryngeal framework or more commonly as a result of upper aerodigestive tract instrumentation (intubation). Dislocation occurs either anteriorly or posteriorly. Anterior dislocation

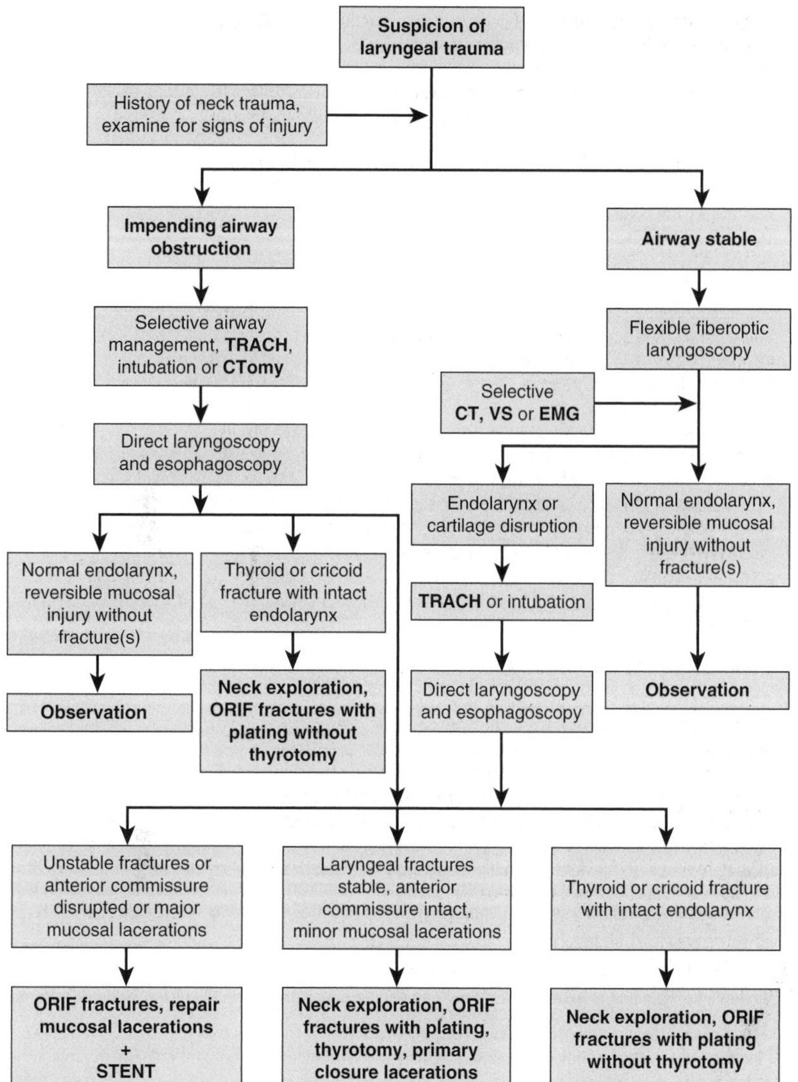

Figure 78-2. Algorithm for early treatment of acute external laryngeal trauma. CT = computed tomography; Ctomy = Cricothyroidotomy; EMG = electromyography of the larynx; ORIF = open reduction and internal fixation of laryngeal skeletal fractures; STENT = endolaryngeal stent or lumen keeper; TRACH = tracheotomy; VS = videostroboscopy of larynx. *(Used with permission Schaefer SD. Management of acute blunt and penetrating external laryngeal trauma, Laryngoscope 124(1):233–244, 2014.)*

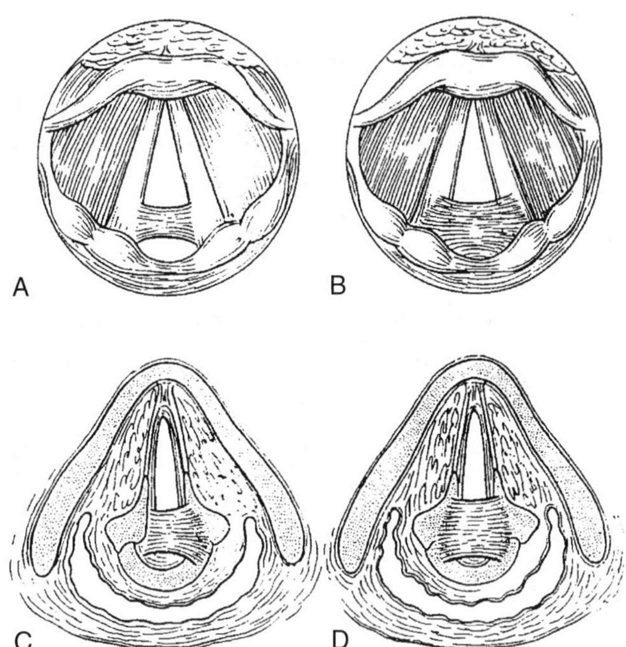

Figure 78-3. Posterior subglottic stenosis. **A,** Interarytenoid adhesion with a mucosally lined tract posteriorly. **B,** Posterior commissure and interarytenoid scar without a mucosally lined tract posteriorly. **C,** Posterior commissure scar extending into the right cricoarytenoid joint. **D,** Posterior commissure scar extending into both cricoarytenoid joints. *(From Zalzal GH, Cotton RT: Glottic and subglottic stenosis. In Flint PW, Haughey BH, Lund VJ, et al, editors: Cummings Otolaryngology: Head and Neck Surgery, ed 5, Philadelphia, 2010, Mosby, Elsevier, p 2916.)*

results from anterior displacement of the cartilage during laryngoscope or ET insertion, whereas posterior cartilage displacement can result from forces applied by the ET as it passes through the glottis. Another possibility includes extubation with an inflated cuff, which translates posteriorly directed forces on the cartilage.

15. **How common is arytenoid dislocation?**
Arytenoid dislocation is extremely rare with an estimate incidence of 0.1% of tracheal intubations.

16. **How does an arytenoid dislocation present?**
Common presenting symptoms include dysphonia, vocal fatigue, cough, and inability to project the voice due to reduced vocal cord mobility. Some patients may also experience swallow dysfunction. In the acute phase after laryngeal trauma, the patient may also note sore throat or pain with swallowing.

Flexible fiber-optic laryngoscopy and/or videostroboscopy demonstrates diminished ispilateral vocal cord movement with abnormal position of the arytenoid cartilage as well as a height discrepancy between the vocal cords (CT scans may also reveal incorrect position of the arytenoid cartilage). Laryngeal electromyography can distinguish vocal cord paralysis from arytenoid dislocation as paralysis will be associated with the absence of electrical activity and arytenoid dislocation should be associated with normal electrical activity.

17. **Describe treatment for arytenoid dislocation.**
Early intervention is recommended to prevent joint ankylosis. Microlaryngoscopy with arytenoid repositioning is effective in the majority of patients who undergo this treatment. Voice therapy as adjunctive treatment is also helpful.

BIBLIOGRAPHY

Bent JP 3rd, Silver JR, Porubsky ES: Acute laryngeal trauma: a review of 77 patients, *Otolaryngol Head Neck Surg* 109(3 Pt 1):441–449, 1993.

Esteller-More E, Ibanez J, Matino E, et al: Prognostic factors in laryngotracheal injury following intubation and/or tracheostomy in ICU patients, *Eur Arch Otorhinolaryngol* 262:880, 2005.

Flint PW, Haughey BH, Lund VJ, et al, editors: *Cummings Otolaryngology: Head and Neck Surgery*, Philadelphia, PA, 2015, Saunders Elsevier.

Hoffman JR, Mower WR, Wolfson AB, et al: Validity of a set of clinical criteria to rule out injury to the cervical spine in patients with blunt trauma, *N Engl J Med* 343:94, 2000.

Jewett BS, Shockley WW, Rutledge R: External laryngeal trauma analysis of 392 patients, *Arch Otolaryngol Head Neck Surg* 125(8):877–880, 1999.

Nahum AM: Immediate care of blunt laryngeal trauma, *J Trauma* 9(2):112–125, 1969.

Norris BK, Schweinfurth JM: Arytenoid dislocation: an analysis of contemporary literature, *Laryngoscope* 121:142, 2011.

Schaefer SD: Management of acute blunt and penetrating external laryngeal trauma, *Laryngoscope* 124(1):233–244, 2014. doi: 10.1002/lary.24068. [Epub 2013 Jun 26].

Schaefer SD: The acute management of external laryngeal trauma. A 27-year experience, *Arch Otolaryngol Head Neck Surg* 118(6):598–604, 1992.

Schaefer SD: The treatment of acute external laryngeal injuries. "State of the art," *Arch Otolaryngol Head Neck Surg* 117(1):35–39, 1991.

Schaefer SD: Management of acute blunt and penetrating external laryngeal trauma, *Laryngoscope* 124:233, 2014.

Walner DL, Loewen MS, Kimura RE: Neonatal subglottic stenosis—incidence and trends, *Laryngoscope* 111(1):48–51, 2001.

Zalzal GH, Cotton RT: Glottic and subglottic stenosis. In Flint PW, Haughey BH, Lund VJ, et al, editors: *Cummings Otolaryngology: Head and Neck Surgery*, ed 5, Philadelphia, 2010, Mosby, Elsevier, p 2916.

INDEX

Page numbers followed by "*f*" indicate figures, "*t*" indicate tables, and "*b*" indicate boxes.

I

J

K

P

S